Slee's

Health Care Terms

Slee's
Health Care Terms

Fifth Edition

Debora A. Slee, JD
Vergil N. Slee, MD
H. Joachim Schmidt, JD

JONES AND BARTLETT PUBLISHERS

Sudbury, Massachusetts

BOSTON   TORONTO   LONDON   SINGAPORE

World Headquarters

Jones and Bartlett Publishers	Jones and Bartlett Publishers	Jones and Bartlett Publishers
40 Tall Pine Drive	Canada	International
Sudbury, MA 01776	6339 Ormindale Way	Barb House, Barb Mews
978-443-5000	Mississauga, Ontario L5V 1J2	London W6 7PA
info@jbpub.com	Canada	United Kingdom
www.jbpub.com		

Jones and Bartlett's books and products are available through most bookstores and online booksellers. To contact Jones and Bartlett Publishers directly, call 800-832-0034, fax 978-443-8000, or visit our website, www.jbpub.com.

Substantial discounts on bulk quantities of Jones and Bartlett's publications are available to corporations, professional associations, and other qualified organizations. For details and specific discount information, contact the special sales department at Jones and Bartlett via the above contact information or send an email to specialsales@jbpub.com.

This publication is designed to provide accurate and authoritative information in regard to the subject matter covered. It is sold with the understanding that the publisher is not engaged in rendering legal, accounting, or other professional service. If legal advice or other expert assistance is required, the service of a competent professional person should be sought.

Production Credits
Publisher: Michael Brown
Associate Editor: Katey Birtcher
Senior Production Editor: Julie Champagne Bolduc
Production Assistant: Jessica Steele Newfell
Marketing Manager: Sophie Fleck
Composition: Shawn Girsberger
Cover Design: Kristin E. Ohlin
Cover Image: © Brueghel, Pieter the Elder, Tower of Babel; Kunsthistorisches Museum,
    Vienna, Austria/The Bridgeman Art Library
Printing and Binding: Malloy, Inc.
Cover Printing: Malloy, Inc.

Library of Congress Cataloging-in-Publication Data
Slee, Debora A.
  Slee's health care terms / Debora A. Slee, Vergil N. Slee, H. Joachim Schmidt. -- 5th ed.
    p. ; cm.
  Vergil Slee's name appears first on the previous edition.
  Includes bibliographical references.
  ISBN-13: 978-0-7637-4615-5 (alk. paper)
  1. Medical care--Dictionaries. 2. Public health--Dictionaries. 3. Medical laws and legislation--Dictionaries. 4. Medicine--Dictionaries. I. Slee, Vergil N., 1917- II. Schmidt, H. Joachim (Herbert Joachim), 1948- III. Title. IV. Title: Health care terms.
  [DNLM: 1. Delivery of Health Care--Terminology--English. 2. Health Planning--Terminology--English. 3. Health Services Administration--Terminology--English. W 15 S632h 2007]
  RA423.S55 2007
  362.103--dc22
                       2007011155

6048

Printed in the United States of America
11 10 09 08 07   10 9 8 7 6 5 4 3 2 1

This book is dedicated to the memory of
Beth Ellen Stoke Slee (1915–2007). ❧

Contents

Preface

History of Slee's Health Care Terms

Healthcare consumers demanded this book. To be sure, in 1985, when the first edition was put together, they weren't called "consumers." They were called physicians, trustees, hospital administrators, and the spouses of all of these professionals, It was at a conference of Estes Park Institute where critical mass was reached in the cumulative frustration of those charged with providing, understanding, and making decisions about health care—for themselves and for their communities.

Estes Park Institute (EPI) has held the Hospital Medical Staff and Trustee Conference since the 1960s for physicians in leadership positions, hospital and other healthcare administrators, and trustees of healthcare institutions. EPI's mission is "to educate teams of physicians, board members, and health care managers so that they can better serve their patients and all people in their local communities and can exercise leadership in the field."

During the conference sessions, a concurrent Healthcare Seminar for Spouses was presented by EPI faculty, highlighting important changes in the healthcare industry, particularly issues of concern to patients and community members.

Early on, the spouses let it be known that one of the greatest barriers to their understanding the current healthcare scene and its problems was the language used. Different terms were often applied to the same thing, and many terms had multiple meanings (a "sanction," for example, could be either a punishment or a support). In addition, new terms were appearing daily in healthcare circles, some dealing with technology, some with forms of organization, and some with legal and financing developments.

Many terms were part of the jargon and slang that are the natural means of communication among insiders. Among the most irritating impediments to the "outsiders" (the spouses) were the abbreviations and acronyms. The faculty spouses began a movement, spearheaded by Beth Slee and Mary Ya Deau, to obtain relief.

A glossary was clearly needed. Finding nothing that covered the breadth of the field with which the healthcare professionals were dealing, EPI faculty member Vergil Slee drafted (on an Otrona Attache, a "pre-PC" portable computer) about a dozen pages of essential terms: medical staff, credentials, Hill-Burton, Darling case, HCFA. Copies were made to hand out to the spouses and set out on a table. By the end of the day, all copies were gone, but the spouses were complaining. The glossary had been snatched up by the doctors, trustees, and administrators!

The truth was out: although each professional was proficient in the language of her or his own discipline, no one could keep up with the proliferation of jargon. Each group had been suffering in silence while the others used terms that "everybody understood." In fact, many terms used within one group (physicians or administrators, for example) are not familiar to members of another group; and, in the case of new terminology, often no one really knows what it means.

The most pressing need appeared to be in the areas of healthcare regulation, administration, organization, financing, and the law. But it was soon found that other areas had to be included. For example, some clinical terms, particularly those dealing with new technology (lithotripsy, for instance), couldn't be looked up handily by trustees and concerned citizens. Nor could many terms dealing with medical and other professional education—on which trustees had to increasingly focus because of problems of financing education under prospective payment, and because of changing governmental attitudes—easily be found. Organizational development and human resources development have languages all their own. And on and on.

So *Slee's Health Care Terms*, the book, was first published in 1986 (with Vergil Slee as the senior author), and is now in its fifth edition. It has greatly expanded from the 150 pages of the first edition and now includes almost 8,000 terms (over 1,200 more than the fourth edition!). Its audience has expanded to all healthcare consumers—students, policymakers, health professionals, patients, journalists—who need access to this information.

PURPOSE

Health Care Terms serves to enable communication among those involved in health care, so that understanding is enhanced and better decisions can be made. Language is a critical tool.

Those in control of the language retain to a large extent control of the discussion. It is important that we—all who have a stake in our country's health care—share this control.

Most new terms coming into play, or old terms taking on new usage, do so innocently: a new thing can't carry the same label as something else, and it is the nature of language for meanings to change over time. But in health care, as in other fields, some of the changes are mischievous.

A disturbing trend is the "trademarking" of new terms, to restrict their expression and use. This seems to be the antithesis of cooperation, and a direct attempt to stifle the expansion of human knowledge and advancement by placing private gain, control, or prestige above the common welfare.

J.M. Juran, one of our major quality gurus, knew the importance of clarity of expression. He observed that some changes in terminology are the products of "deliberate efforts of human beings to create and use terminology to secure benefits for their organizations and for themselves."

> The prime need is to discover the realities under the labels, i.e., the deeds, activities, or things which the other fellow is talking about. Once these are understood, accurate communication can take place whether the labels are agreed upon or not. In contrast, if communication is purely through labels, it is easy to be deluded into believing there is an understanding despite the fact that each of the parties literally does not know what the other fellow is talking about.[1]

This book is intended to help us understand what the other person is talking about.

USER NOTES

Each definition is intended to present a concept and show how that concept relates to the healthcare field, and at the same time serve as a quick reference (reminder) for those already familiar with the concept. The emphasis of the work is on breadth, not depth. In certain instances, however, some depth is necessary to explain the term (coding, for example); in others, such as with the highly technical (and changing) computations used in the Medicare payment system, no attempt has been made to give detail. Technical terms, such as those from the fields of law, medicine, and accounting, are defined simply; they are not intended to be authoritative or to take the place of professional advice.

Alphabetization is strictly letter-by-letter, disregarding spaces and hyphens.

Cross-references are indicated by **bold italics**.

One word or two? The world hasn't decided: it's both "health care" and "healthcare." This book (mostly) uses "healthcare" when the term is used as an adjective ("healthcare financing"), and "health care" when the main term is "care" ("higher quality health care"). The exception is a proper name or title—such as *Health Care Terms*.

---

1 Juran, J.M. "A Wistful Postscript on Terminology" from *Quality Control Handbook*. McGraw-Hill, 1974.

The word "hospital" is often used in a context that would clearly apply to other types of healthcare institutions as well. The purpose is to keep the definitions, as much as possible, simple and clear. Thus, hospital is used to represent all healthcare institutions in these instances. Similarly, "physician" or "nurse" might be used to denote healthcare professionals generally.

When geographic and governmental terms—national, federal, state, and so forth—are used without modifiers, they refer to the United States. We have included a significant number of international references, but we make no claim to cover the "world" of health care outside the United States. Although our focus is local, we are mindful of the many significant healthcare developments occurring globally. Whenever one of these developments may have a likely effect on the United States, we make an effort to include it.

A note regarding comprehensiveness. The number of terms used in health care is very large, and growing constantly. The authors have attempted thoroughness in this volume, but are aware that not all terms have been included. Therefore, the exclusion of a specialty, professional, institution, or any other term should not be taken as a diminution of the importance of that term. Rather, it should be taken as either an editorial decision (excluding very commonly understood terms, for example) or an oversight by the authors. Readers are urged to bring to the authors' attention any terms that the reader believes should be included in future editions, as well as comments regarding the definitions.

ACKNOWLEDGMENTS

One of the continuing pleasures of working on this book is the help and support received from many people.

We are especially grateful to Kristin Alline, MD, MPH; Richard Ament; Samuel P. Asper, MD; Richard Bates, MD; Robert Bednarek; Robert Cress; Elaine Deppe, RN; Linda Haddad, JD; John S. Hoff; William Hogan, MD, LLB; John Horty, LLB; Kathy Jamerson; Charlotte S. Jefferies, JD; Leland Kaiser, PhD; Hon. John Kitzhaber, MD; U. Beate Krinke, PhD, MPH, RD; Jack Lewin, MD; Jack McConnell, MD; Betsy Moore; Dan Mulholland, JD; Charles F. Petet; Richard G. Rockefeller, MD; Bobbi Ryan; Margaret VanAmringe, MHS; Fay Coker Walker, MSW; Barbara Wilcox, RN; Kenneth J. Williams, MD; and Richard Ya Deau, MD.

List of Figures and Tables

A

AA See *anesthesiologist assistant*.

AAA See *animal-assisted activities* and *area agency on aging*.

AAAHC See *Accreditation Association of Ambulatory Healthcare*.

AA-C See *Certified Anesthesiologist Assistant* under *anesthesiologist assistant*.

AACN See *American Association of Colleges of Nursing* and *American Association of Critical-Care Nurses*.

AACRN See *Advanced AIDS Certified Registered Nurse* under *HIV/AIDS nursing*.

AAFP See *American Academy of Family Physicians*.

AAHA See *American Association of Homes for the Aging*.

AAHC See *American Association of Healthcare Consultants*.

AAHP See *American Association of Health Plans*.

AAHSA See *American Association of Homes and Services for the Aging*.

AAIHDS See *American Association of Integrated Healthcare Delivery Systems*.

AAMC See *Association of American Medical Colleges*.

AAMD See *American Academy of Medical Directors*.

AAMSI See *American Association for Medical Systems and Informatics*.

AAN See *American Academy of Nursing*.

AANP See *American Academy of Nurse Practitioners*.

AAP See *Association of American Physicians*.

AAPA See *American Academy of Physician Assistants*.

AAPC See *American Academy of Professional Coders*.

AAPCC See *average adjusted per capita cost*.

AAPS See *American Association of Physician Specialists* and *Association of American Physicians and Surgeons*.

AARP A national membership organization of people age 50 and older. It is a leading advocate on issues affecting older Americans, including health and long-term care, and provides a wide range of services and publications. The organization's acronym comes from its former name, American Association of Retired Persons. **www.aarp.org**

AAT See *animal-assisted therapy*.

AATA See *American Art Therapy Association*.

ABA See *American Board of Anesthesiology*.

ABAI See *American Board of Allergy and Immunology*.

abandonment A *tort* in which the wrongdoing consists of leaving a patient without treatment when there is still a doctor-patient relationship requiring the physician to continue treatment.

ABBM See *American Board of Bariatric Medicine*.

ABC codes A national coding system designed for complementary and alternative medicine (CAM), nursing, and other integrative healthcare providers. The initials ABC stand for "advanced billing concept." The five-character (plus two alphanumeric characters as modifiers) codes are designed to be compatible with current healthcare information systems, and can be used in a similar fashion to other coding systems such as CPT and HCPCS codes (such as with the form UB-92). The main part of the ABC code has a very hierarchical structure, with the first letter representing a major section, such as "A" for clinical practice charges, "E" for supplies, and "N" for nursing. Interestingly there is an entire section ("G") dedicated to "Herbs and natural substances." The next four letters "drill down" to ever greater detail for what the code represents. The ABC modifier currently describes 13 types of licensed healthcare practitioners, and allows the addition of 1,283 more if needed.

ABC codes began to be developed in 1996 by a private company called Alternative Link (now ABC Coding Solutions), which in 1999 handed over code development and updating to the Foundation for Integrative Healthcare (FIHC), a nonprofit 501(c)(3) organization, and its practitioner association members. ABC codes are developed in a manner similar to the method used by the Uniform Code Council in the retail industry, with the intention that every "product" in the healthcare "store" would have the equivalent of a Universal Product Code (UPC). Early in 2003 the Department of Health and Human Services approved ABC codes as an optional, but not mandatory, code set for alternative medicine, nursing, and other integrative healthcare practices. **www.abccodes.com**

ABCP See *American Board of Clinical Pharmacology*.

ABCRS See *American Board of Colon and Rectal Surgery*.

ABD See *American Board of Dermatology*.

ABEM See *American Board of Emergency Medicine*.

ABFM See *American Board of Family Medicine*.

ABFPRS See *American Board of Facial Plastic and Reconstructive Surgery*.

ABGC See American Board of Genetic Counseling and *Certified Genetic Counselor* under *genetic counselor*.

ABHPM See *American Board of Hospice and Palliative Medicine*.

ABIM See *American Board of Internal Medicine*.

ABMG See *American Board of Medical Genetics*.

ABMM See *American Board of Medical Management*.

ABMS See *American Board of Medical Specialties*.

ABN See *advance beneficiary notice*.

ABNM See *American Board of Nuclear Medicine*.

ABNS See *American Board of Neurological Surgery*.

ABO See *American Board of Ophthalmology*.

ABOC See *Board Certified Dispensing Optician* under *dispensing optician*.

ABOC-AC See *Board Certified Dispensing Optician—Advanced Certification* under *dispensing optician*.

ABODM See *American Board of Disaster Medicine*.

ABOG See *American Board of Obstetrics and Gynecology*.

ABOM See *Master in Ophthalmic Optics* under *dispensing optician*.

ABOS See *American Board of Orthopaedic Surgery*.

ABOto See *American Board of Otolaryngology*.

ABP See *American Board of Pathology* and *American Board of Pediatrics*.

ABPM See *American Board of Pain Medicine* and *American Board of Preventive Medicine*.

ABPMR See *American Board of Physical Medicine and Rehabilitation*.

ABPN See *American Board of Psychiatry and Neurology*.

ABPS See *American Board of Plastic Surgery*.

ABR See *American Board of Radiology*.

ABS See *American Board of Surgery*.

abstract A summary of data or information. Also a verb; see *abstracting*.

case abstract See *discharge abstract*.

discharge abstract A coded summary of selected data in the patient's hospital medical record, prepared after discharge. It contains a standardized set of items in a form ready for computer processing in order to provide statistics, medical record indexes, submission of bills, patient care quality review, and healthcare research. The core content is usually the Uniform Hospital Discharge Data Set (UHDDS) prescribed by the federal government. Synonym: case abstract.

abstracter See *medical record abstracter*.

abstracting The process of extracting information from a document in order to create a summary, called an abstract, of that document. The process of abstracting should not introduce the abstracter's judgment; that is, the resulting abstract must carry exactly the same information as in the original document for those items that have been extracted.

ABT See *Asian bodywork therapy* under *bodywork therapy*.

ABTS See *American Board of Thoracic Surgery*.

ABU See *American Board of Urology*.

abuse (generally) Misuse, mistreatment, or improper treatment. In some cases, may be used to mean failure to do things that ought to be done, such as provide adequate food, clothing, and medical treatment when necessary.

abuse (healthcare) The improper or excessive use of healthcare products and services. Abuse may result from excessive (unnecessary) use of diagnostic tests, unnecessary surgical and other procedures, and so forth. Abuse may be either intentional or unintentional, and may or may not be illegal. The laws governing Medicare, for example, make certain referral arrangements illegal because they create opportunity for abuse, even though there may be no actual abuse or intent to abuse. See *fraud and abuse*.

abuse of process A *tort* where the wrongdoing consists of using the legal system for an improper purpose. For example, initiating involuntary commitment proceedings to hospitalize a person to stop him from doing something (such as leaving town), rather than because he legitimately needs treatment, is abuse of process. Unlike a lawsuit for malicious prosecution, a plaintiff alleging abuse of process does not need to win the improper suit, nor prove a lack of probable cause for that suit.

AC Affiliated contractor; see *Comprehensive Error Rate Testing*.

Academy for Health Services Research and Health Policy (AHSRHP) See *AcademyHealth*.

AcademyHealth An organization formed in 2000 by the merger of the Alpha Center and the Association for Health Services Research. A "think tank" and "professional home and technical assistance resource for researchers and policy professionals." Its mission is to improve health and health care by "generating new knowledge and moving knowledge into action." Its "tagline" is "Advancing Research, Policy and Practice." Also home to the *Coalition for Health Services Research*. Formerly called Academy for Health Services Research and Health Policy (AHSRHP). **www.academyhealth.org**

ACC See *American College of Cardiology*.

A-CCC See *Continuity of Care Certification, Advanced*, under *case manager*.

accelerated compensation event (ACE) See *health court*.

accelerated death benefit An amount paid to an individual, under a life insurance contract, when that individual has been diagnosed with a specific medical condition (generally a terminal illness). Thus it can be used to pay for the immediate needs of the individual. After that person's death, the balance is paid to the beneficiary just like any other life insurance. See also *viatical benefits*.

acceptable daily intake (ADI) A measure of the amount of a substance in food that can be ingested daily in the diet over a lifetime without appreciable risk, based on all facts known at the time. "Without appreciable risk" refers to the practical certainty that injury will not result, even after a lifetime of experience. There is a built-in safety margin, so excess levels are not necessarily toxic. The concept, developed principally by the World Health Organization (WHO) and the Food and Agriculture Organization (FAO), is applied to chemicals such as food additives, pesticide residues, and veterinary drugs.

access (physical) The ability to get to doctors, facilities, and information. Hospitals, clinics, and other resources must be located where they can be reached, and designed without barriers. Information systems, as well, need to be accessible to all regardless of ability. Adaptations such as extra-large type size, high-contrast colors, talking computers, and so forth are available. See also *Americans with Disabilities Act (ADA)*.

access (to health care) The ability to obtain health care. Access includes available physicians and facilities, transportation, acceptance by the facility, means of communication (no language barriers), and means of payment. "Access" is often used specifically to mean eligibility for (access to) insurance benefits, because lack of insurance can be a formidable barrier to receiving health care. Individuals who are above a given state's definition of the poverty level for qualification for Medicaid but are unable to afford health insurance are said to be denied access. In 2005, for example, when the federal poverty threshold was $19,350 for a family of four, access was very different in a state that had its Medicaid threshold at $5,000 (family income above this amount disqualifies the family for Medicaid) than in a state where the threshold was $19,350. Thus an unemployed (or employed low income) person who cannot be insured through an employer might not qualify for public assistance, either.

Access Agency See *Health Resources and Services Administration*.

access control The ability and responsibility of a healthcare organization to control and account for access to medical records and other protected health information (PHI). With the shift towards the electronic health record (EHR) and having access to it over computer networks, access control has become increasingly important. This is reflected in such legislation as HIPAA. Access control is implemented using *authentication* methods. As technology becomes more sophisticated, it will become increasingly possible to restrict what health information is seen by whom, likely leading to efforts taking advantage of greater access control.

ACCME See *Accreditation Council for Continuing Medical Education*.

account An arrangement between a buyer and a seller in which goods or services are exchanged and payment is to be made at a later time.

closed account An account upon which full payment has been made; the account is thus "closed."

open account An account upon which not all payments have been made.

accountability (data) See *data accountability*.

accountability (governance) The duty to provide, to all concerned, the evidence needed to: (1) establish confidence that the task or duty for which one is responsible is being or has been performed; and (2) describe the manner in which that task is being or has been carried out. When accountability has been fulfilled, the authority that delegated the responsibility can be satisfied by evidence (rather than simply assertion) that the duties or tasks that have been delegated are being or have been adequately performed.

Accountability must be defined in conjunction with responsibility. An individual or organization has responsibility (that is to say, a duty) because some individual or body with authority has granted or delegated that responsibility. Failure to carry out the duty carries with it liability. A responsible party is entitled to delegate duties, that is, to get help in carrying out the duty, but not to delegate the duty itself. The responsible party, therefore, must have reasonable ground on which he or she can render account (be accountable) for the duties that have been delegated. So the delegation of duties, as a matter of law, carries with it the requirement of "accountability" to the source of the delegation of the duties.

A hospital, for example, is delegated certain duties by "society," by government. For this purpose, the hospital's responsibility is accepted and held by its governing body. The governing body must render account for its performance (it holds accountability) to society, through specific reporting mechanisms, voluntary efforts to provide society evidence of its performance, and defending itself against liability suits. In turn, the governing body delegates tasks to the chief executive officer (CEO) and demands accounting from that individual; the CEO, in turn, delegates tasks to departmental heads and demands accountability from them.

Similarly, the governing body gives the medical staff duties, for example, with respect to the credentialing of applicants for medical staff membership. The medical staff incurs, along with the duty, the obligation of accountability—it must provide the evidence needed to establish the governing body's confidence that it, the medical staff, has indeed performed the task, and the evidence must be presented in enough detail to permit the governing body to assess the quality of performance of the duty. See also *duty (legal)*, *governing body*, *liability (legal)*, and *transparent*.

accountable health partnership (AHP) See *accountable health plan*.

accountable health plan (AHP) A form of health plan proposed in legislation in the early 1990s as a feature of the "managed competition" approach to healthcare reform. The AHP would be accountable for meeting federal requirements for providing certain standardized health services. Synonyms: accountable health partnership (AHP), approved health plan (AHP). See also *community care plan*.

accountant An individual who specializes in examining, interpreting, or managing financial records.

> **public accountant (PA)** An individual who performs a variety of functions, such as audit of an organization's financial statements and design of financial systems. Use of the term and the designation as "PA" require state licensure, and the PA is under state regulation. Most healthcare organizations employ a certified public accountant (CPA) for these functions.

> **Certified Public Accountant (CPA)** An individual who has met the requirements of the American Institute of Certified Public Accountants (AICPA). www.aicpa.org

accounting of disclosures (AOD) A right given to patients as a result of HIPAA, allowing persons who have received healthcare services to request from their providers an accounting of disclosures (AOD) made of their *protected health information (PHI)*. The person making the request is entitled to information including the date of the disclosure, the name of the entity that received the PHI, the purpose of the disclosure, and a brief description of what was actually disclosed. The patient's rights typically do not extend to being able to prevent the disclosure—the "prior authorization" requirements were removed from the rule before it was enacted. If an entity is obliged under HIPAA to provide an AOD, it must do so under a single point of access, freeing requestors from having to contact different departments of the same provider. It must also keep this information available for a period of six years after the disclosure. The provision is in HIPAA Sec. 164.528.

accounting period The time, usually a month, a quarter, or a year, covered by a financial statement.

accounts payable (AP) Amounts on open account (see *account*) owed to creditors for goods and services.

accounts receivable (AR) Amounts owed by others on open account for goods or services.

accreditation A process of: (1) evaluation of an institution or education program to determine whether it meets the standards set up by an accrediting body, and (2) if the institution or program meets the standards, granting recognition of the fact. Accreditation is a process performed by a nongovernmental agency at the request of the institution or education program. Although governmental agencies carry out evaluation and recognition processes on a mandatory basis for licensure purposes, these processes are not accreditation.

Healthcare institutions are accredited by the Joint Commission on Accreditation of Healthcare Organizations (JCAHO) in the United States and by the Canadian Council on Health Facilities Accreditation (CCHFA) in Canada. Healthcare education programs are accredited by other bodies. See also *compliance*.

Accreditation Association of Ambulatory Healthcare (AAAHC) A national association that offers voluntary accreditation for ambulatory care organizations, including ambulatory healthcare clinics, birthing centers, diagnostic imaging centers, multispecialty group practices, occupational health centers, and many other types of facilities. Compare to the *Joint Commission on Accreditation of Healthcare Organizations (JCAHO)*, which also provides accreditation for ambulatory care. www.aaahc.org

Accreditation Council for Continuing Medical Education (ACCME) A nonprofit organization that provides a method for accreditation of continuing medical education (CME) programs. See *medical education* under *education*. www.accme.org

Accreditation Council for Graduate Medical Education (ACGME) A nonprofit organization that provides accreditation for post-MD clinical training programs (medical residencies). See *medical education* (under *education*) and residency. **www.acgme.org**

accreditation decision grid A numerical summary of an institution's survey scores and findings, which the institution may obtain from the Joint Commission on Accreditation of Healthcare Organizations (JCAHO) on request. Its purpose is to provide an overview of the institution's performance.

accreditation manual A book setting out the criteria for accreditation. For example, the Joint Commission on Accreditation of Healthcare Organizations (JCAHO) annually publishes manuals delineating current JCAHO standards in several areas. In 2007 the major publications were:

Comprehensive Accreditation Manual for Ambulatory Care (CAMAC)
Comprehensive Accreditation Manual for Behavioral Health Care (CAMBHC)
Comprehensive Accreditation Manual for Critical Access Hospitals (CAMCAH)
Comprehensive Accreditation Manual for Home Care (CAMHC)
Comprehensive Accreditation Manual for Hospitals: The Official Handbook (CAMH)
Comprehensive Accreditation Manual for Laboratory and Point-of-Care Testing (CAMLAB)
Comprehensive Accreditation Manual for Long Term Care (CAMLTC)
Comprehensive Accreditation Manual for Office-Based Surgery Practice (CAMOBS)
Joint Commission International Accreditation Standards for Ambulatory Care
Joint Commission International Accreditation Standards for the Care Continuum
Joint Commission International Accreditation Standards for Clinical Laboratories
Joint Commission International Accreditation Standards for Disease- or Condition-Specific Care
Joint Commission International Accreditation Standards for Hospitals, Second Edition (first published in 2001)
Joint Commission International Accreditation Standards for Medical Transport Organizations

accredited Formally recognized by an accrediting body as meeting its standards for accreditation.

Accredited Record Technician (ART) See *Registered Health Information Technician* under *health information technician*.

Accredited Standards Committee (ASC) See *ASC (organization)*.

ACE Accelerated compensation event; see *health court*. See also *angiotensin-converting enzyme*.

ACE-CPT See *ACE Certified Personal Trainer* under *personal trainer*.

ACEP See *American College of Emergency Physicians*.

ACF See *Administration for Children & Families*.

ACGME See *Accreditation Council for Graduate Medical Education*.

ACHA See *American College of Hospital Administrators*.

ACHCA See *American College of Health Care Administrators*.

ACHE See *American College of Healthcare Executives*.

ACHPN See *Advanced Practice Certified Hospice and Palliative Nurse* under *hospice and palliative nursing*.

ACLS See *Advanced Cardiovascular Life Support* under *life support*.

ACMG See *American College of Medical Genetics*.

ACMQ See *American College of Medical Quality*.

ACNHA See *American College of Nursing Home Administrators*.

ACNM See *American College of Nurse Midwives*.

ACNP See *Acute Care Nurse Practitioner* under *acute care nursing*.

ACOG See *American College of Obstetricians and Gynecologists*.

ACP See *American College of Physicians*.

ACPE See *American College of Physician Executives*.

acquired immunodeficiency syndrome (AIDS) See *AIDS*.

ACR See *adjusted community rate* or *adjusted community rating* (under *rating*). Also, *American College of Radiology*.

ACRN See *AIDS Certified Registered Nurse* under *HIV/AIDS nursing*.

ACR-NEMA American College of Radiology and the National Electronic Manufacturers Association. An effort underway since 1985 to develop standards for the transmission of medical images and other medical information; see *DICOM*.

ACS See *American Cancer Society* and *American College of Surgeons*. Also approved clinical supervisor; see *counselor*.

ACSH See *American Council on Science and Health*.

ACSM Certified Personal Trainer See under *personal trainer*.

Action Learning Lab (ALL) An intensive training program that brings diverse agencies and programs together to tackle priority issues in maternal and child health. The Association of Maternal and Child Health Programs (AMCHP) designed the labs to promote collaboration at the state level and improve family health programs. **www.amchp.org/allguide**

activities director The individual responsible for providing activities to patients in a long-term care facility (LTCF) in order to promote continuing involvement in activities of daily living (ADL) and to retard or prevent disabilities.

activities of daily living (ADL) Functions that are ordinarily done for oneself, such as combing hair, brushing teeth, eating, dressing, and taking care of bodily functions. In the case of bedfast and paralyzed persons, the definition is restricted to activities that do not require mobility, such as combing hair and brushing teeth. See also *Instrumental Activities of Daily Living (IADL) scale*.

activities therapist See *therapeutic recreation specialist*.

actuarial analysis A forecast developed by specialized actuarial methods, giving the probability of future events for a given population, such as life expectancy, frequency of hospitalization, or probability of loss from fire. A common use of such forecasts is the calculation of insurance premiums and, for the insurer, the necessary reserves.

actuary A mathematician who specializes in estimating risks, rates, premiums, and other factors for insurance companies.

acuity Acuteness, as of an illness. The term is used a great deal in reference to nursing needs and demands for other healthcare resources: the greater the acuity, the more nursing care or other services are needed.

acupressure The therapeutic use of pressure applied to specific "acupoints" in the body; similar to acupuncture.

acupuncture An alternative or complementary therapy of Asian origin in which fine needles are inserted in the body along "meridians" of the body, carefully rotated, and then removed. Acupuncture is used for various purposes, such as treatment of various conditions, control of pain, and surgical anesthesia. Under some circumstances, the needles, when gold, are purposely broken off and left in the body permanently.

   medical acupuncture The medical discipline involving the integration of acupuncture into current biomedical practice.

acupuncturist A person who uses acupuncture to help or treat people. Most states have laws governing the practice of acupuncture.

   Diplomate in Acupuncture (Dipl. Ac.) An acupuncturist who has met the requirements for eligibility and passed an examination of the National Certification Commission for Acupuncture and Oriental Medicine (NCCAOM). **www.nccaom.org**

   Diplomate of the American Board of Medical Acupuncture (DABMA) A licensed physician who has completed additional training in acupuncture in an approved program and passed an examination of the American Board of Medical Acupuncture (ABMA). **www.medicalacupuncture.org**

ACURP See *American College of Utilization Review Physicians*.

acute With respect to an illness, having a short course, which often is relatively severe. The term is also used for the portion or portions of an illness, ordinarily in its early stages, in which symptoms are most severe and the patient may be at greatest risk. The period following acute is referred to as "postacute." Distinguished from *chronic*.

acute care Care for short-term patients; see *acute*.

acute care nursing Nursing care for people with injuries or acute illness.

    Acute and Critical Care Clinical Nurse Specialist (CCNS) See under *critical care nursing*.

    Acute Care Nurse Practitioner (ACNP) A nurse practitioner who specializes in acute care. Formerly, ACNP was a credential offered by the American Nurses Credentialing Center (ANCC) (**nursingworld.org/ancc**) in conjunction with the AACN Certification Corporation (**www.certcorp.org**). Now, registered nurses with a graduate degree who pass the credentialing examination for acute care nurse practitioners and otherwise qualify receive the credential APRN, BC (Advanced Practice Registered Nurse, Board Certified).

AD See *associate degree*.

ADA See *American Dental Association*, *American Dietetic Association*, and *Americans with Disabilities Act*.

ADAMHA See *Alcohol, Drug Abuse, and Mental Health Administration*.

ad damnum clause The part of a legal complaint (the document that initiates a lawsuit) that states the amount of money (damages) the plaintiff demands. Some states prohibit a plaintiff from demanding any specific dollar amount other than that required for the court's jurisdiction (for example, "a sum greater than $10,000"). This requirement helps avoid tabloid headlines such as, "Patient Sues Physician for $10 Billion Over Hangnail."

added qualification See *certificate of added qualification*.

addiction See *substance dependence*.

addiction counselor A counselor with special training in substance dependence.

    Master Addiction Counselor (MAC) An addiction counselor with at least a master's degree who has been certified by NAADAC, the Association for Addiction Professionals (formerly the National Association of Alcohol and Drug Abuse Counselors, **naadac.org**).

    National Certified Addiction Counselor (NCAC) An addiction counselor who has been certified by NAADAC, the Association for Addiction Professionals (formerly the National Association of Alcohol and Drug Abuse Counselors, **naadac.org**). There are two levels of certification, Level I and Level II. (Level II requires a bachelor's degree.)

addictionist See *addictionologist*.

addiction medicine The medical specialty focusing on alcoholism and other addictions. Credentials in this specialty are offered by the American Society of Addiction Medicine (ASAM, **www.asam.org**) and the American Board of Psychiatry and Neurology (ABPN, **www.abpn.com**). Sometimes called addictionology.

addictionologist An individual, usually a physician, who specializes in *addiction medicine*. Also called addictionist.

addictionology See *addiction medicine*.

addictions nursing The nursing specialty concerning the prevention, intervention, treatment, and management of addictive disorders, including alcohol, nicotine, and other drug dependencies; eating disorders; and process addictions such as gambling.

    Certified Addictions Registered Nurse (CARN) A specialist in addictions nursing who has met the requirements of the Addictions Nursing Certification Board (ANCB). **www.intnsa.org**

    Certified Addictions Registered Nurse—Advanced Practice (CARN-AP) A Certified Addictions Registered Nurse who has met advanced requirements of the Addictions Nursing Certification Board (ANCB). **www.intnsa.org**

ADE See *adverse drug event*.

adenine (A) See *DNA*.

ADFS See *alternative delivery and financing system*.

ADI See *acceptable daily intake*.

adjusted community rate (ACR) A term used by CMS in its Medicare risk contracts with HMO/CMPs to mean the premium the HMO would charge for providing exactly the same Medicare-covered benefits to a community rated group, adjusted to allow for the greater intensity and frequency of utilization by Medicare recipients. See *community rating* and *adjusted community rating*, both under *rating*.

adjustment (bookkeeping) A bookkeeping entry made to correct errors, adjust balance-sheet balances to their true balance, and so forth.

administrative adjustment A bookkeeping entry to a patient's bill to account for services rendered but not billed to the patient's account for some reason, such as in settlement of a disagreement between hospital and patient.

contractual adjustment See *contractuals*.

adjustment (statistics) A statistical term referring to a procedure for correcting for differences in the composition of two or more populations. The correction is made, for example, so that valid comparisons can be made between populations. The factors most commonly adjusted for are age and sex. Such adjustments are essential if the rates of occurrence of a disease, for example, are to be compared without distortion (see *rate (ratio)*). Adjustments are used in a specific procedure called *standardization*.

adjuvant A drug that, when given in conjunction with another ("main") drug (usually by incorporating the adjuvant into the formulation), changes the action of the main drug in a predictable manner.

ADL See *activities of daily living*.

ADM See *Advanced Diabetes Management Certification* under *diabetes management*. AdM is sometimes used for *addiction medicine*.

administration (government) A division of the federal government; a subdivision within a department. For example, the Food and Drug Administration is an agency within the Department of Health and Human Services (HHS).

administration (management) The direction and management of an organization.

functional administration (FA) The traditional type of administration of an organization. In a hospital, FA focuses on the organization's functional components, such as nursing and pathology.

healthcare administration The profession dealing with the management of healthcare organizations.

market administration (MA) A type of administration of an organization in which the focus is on the institution's markets. In a hospital, MA focuses on the hospital's markets, such as women, the elderly, or specific payers.

product administration (PA) A type of administration of an organization in which the focus is on products. In a hospital, PA would focus on such "products" as surgery and internal medicine.

Administration for Children and Families (ACF) The agency within the Department of Health and Human Services (HHS) responsible for federal programs that "promote the economic and social well-being of families, children, individuals, and communities." Its programs include the Administration for Native Americans; Administration on Children, Youth and Families (ACYF); Administration on Developmental Disabilities; Child Support Enforcement; Head Start Bureau (HSB); Healthy Marriage Initiative; Office of Refugee Resettlement (ORR); and more. **www.acf.dhhs.gov**

Administration on Aging (AoA) The federal agency within the Department of Health and Human Services (HHS) charged by the Older Americans Act (OAA) with serving the senior citizens in the United States. Among the programs within the agency are the National Family Caregiver Support Program (NFCSP), the Older Americans Act Nutrition Program (OAANP), and the Long-Term Care Ombudsman Program (LTCOP). Web resources include an "Alzheimer's Resource Room" (**www.aoa.gov/alz**) and an "Eldercare Locater" (**www.eldercare.gov**). **www.aoa.dhhs.gov**

administrative adjustment See under *adjustment (bookkeeping)*.

administrative agency See *agency (administrative)*.

administrative engineer A hospital engineer who has administrative (planning or management) responsibility. Typically there is one person with this title, the highest rank among the engineers of the institution. Synonyms: director of buildings and grounds, chief engineer, plant engineer.

administrative law The body of law that governs administrative rules and regulations, the powers of administrative agencies, the process of agency decision making, and the procedures by which a party can challenge an adverse decision of an agency. See also *Code of Federal Regulations*.

administrative process The process by which an administrative agency (see *agency (administrative)*) makes a decision. In the context of hospitals, an example would be the procedure for obtaining a certificate of need (CON). This would include a petition for the certificate, setting of a hearing date and notice to all interested parties, the hearing itself (which is normally less formal than a court hearing), and a decision by the agency. The decision may be appealed within the administrative agency. After the complete administrative process is "exhausted," meaning that all avenues have been tried, a party dissatisfied with the result can go to the courts to challenge the decision.

administrative residency See *residency*.

Administrative Simplification Compliance Act (ASCA) A federal law passed in 2001 that extended the time for hospitals to comply with the electronic transactions standards issued under the administrative simplification provisions of HIPAA. Pub. L. No. 107-105, 115 Stat. 1003 (2001).

administrative simplification provisions (ASP) A portion of *HIPAA* (42 U.S.C. §§ 1320d–1320d-8 (2004)) that calls for the Secretary of the Department of Health and Human Services (HHS) to standardize certain administrative and financial transactions in order to improve efficiency and effectiveness within the healthcare system. It is also this section's goal to protect the security and privacy of health information. HHS has issued rules in the following areas:

- Transactions (see *electronic transactions standards*)
- Data (see *data standards*)
- Privacy (see *Privacy Rule*)

HHS maintains a web site for this topic at **aspe.os.dhhs.gov/admnsimp**.

administrator The individual responsible for carrying out policies established by the organization or agency for which he or she is employed. An administrator is a line official, that is, an employee with authority over others. When the authority is over the entire hospital, the individual is *the* administrator, and current usage is to call this person the *chief executive officer (CEO)*. When a person is referred to as "the administrator," it usually means the CEO.

admissible A legal term referring to whether evidence (such as a witness's testimony, medical record entry, or blood test result) will be allowed to be presented to the judge or jury to prove a legal case. There are specific rules of evidence governing admissibility. For example, even though a plaintiff obtains a medical record during discovery, portions of the record may not be admissible in court because they are irrelevant to the plaintiff's case, protected by law (see *privileged communication*), not properly authenticated, or for other reasons.

admission (hospital) Formal acceptance of a patient by a hospital or other healthcare institution in order to provide care. See also *readmission*.

   elective admission An admission that can be scheduled in advance because the illness or injury is not life-threatening.

   emergency admission An admission that must take place immediately, or else death or serious disability is likely to result.

   emergency department admission Admission of a patient, who needs prompt attention, to an emergency department, a department or facility that gives care for a single encounter.

By definition, patients may not become continuing patients of an emergency department; the entire episode of emergency care is one visit. Also called an emergency outpatient admission.

inpatient admission Admission to an institution that provides lodging and continuous nursing services.

> **newborn inpatient admission** See *newborn admission.*

newborn admission Admission by virtue of being born in a hospital. Only a baby born in a given hospital can be a newborn admission to that hospital. A newborn delivered elsewhere (even on the way to the hospital or in its emergency department [ED]) is a pediatric admission or a transfer. Synonym: newborn inpatient admission.

outpatient admission (OP admission) Admission to a facility of the hospital that gives care but does not provide lodging. An outpatient facility is ready to furnish a series of services to the same patient over a period of time (as contrasted with the emergency department, which can give a patient service only once for one episode).

> **clinic outpatient admission** Admission of a patient to a hospital outpatient clinic. This is a specific kind of outpatient admission.

> **emergency outpatient admission** See emergency department admission.

> **referred outpatient admission** A special kind of outpatient admission in which the patient is to receive only the diagnostic procedures or treatments specified by the referring physician or institution.

pediatric admission Admission of a child, with the upper age defined by the hospital (perhaps 15 to 20 years of age, depending on the clinical problem), except for infants born in the hospital (who are newborn admissions).

transfer admission Admission of a patient by transfer: (1) from another institution where the individual was also a patient; or (2) from another division of the hospital, as when a newborn remains after discharge of the mother and becomes a "transfer admission" from the newborn service to the pediatric service of the hospital.

urgent admission An admission of a patient whose condition is less critical than emergency (less life- or serious-disability threatening), but more critical than elective. An "urgent admission" stands between these two in priority.

admission (law) A statement made by a party to a lawsuit, which affirms or denies a material fact concerning the lawsuit. A "material fact" is one that is essential to the plaintiff's or defendant's case. Admissions are used to streamline the legal process, so that time is not wasted in court proving facts about which the parties do not disagree, such as the parties' names and addresses, whether the plaintiff was in fact a patient at the hospital, and so forth. If a party denies such a fact in bad faith, and the other party has to prove it at trial, the party acting in bad faith is penalized.

admitting department The hospital department that carries out the administrative tasks connected with admission, discharge, and transfer of patients.

admitting manager See *admitting officer.*

admitting officer A hospital official, usually not a physician, who is responsible for the processes of admission (hospital) and discharge of patients, and who is in charge of the admitting department. Synonyms: admitting manager, registrar.

admitting privileges See *privileges.*

ADN Associate Degree in Nursing.

ADP See *advanced dependent practitioner* under *allied health professional.*

ADR Adverse drug reaction (see *adverse drug event*) and *alternative dispute resolution.*

ADS See *alternative delivery system.*

ADTR See *Academy of Dance Therapists Registered* under *dance therapist.*

adult day care See under *day care.*

adult day health services Medical and other healthcare services provided to patients whose condition permits them to return home or to another facility at night. When such care is regularly scheduled, it may be termed partial hospitalization. Synonym: day healthcare services.

adult foster home See *family care home*.

adult health nursing See *adult nursing*.

adult nursing The nursing specialty concerning the needs of adult patients. Sometimes called adult health nursing.

Adult Nurse Practitioner (ANP) A nurse practitioner specializing in adult nursing. Formerly, ANP was a credential offered by the American Nurses Credentialing Center (ANCC, **nursingworld.org/ancc**). Now, registered nurses with a graduate degree who pass the ANCC credentialing examination for adult nurse practitioners and otherwise qualify receive the credential APRN, BC (Advanced Practice Registered Nurse, Board Certified).

Clinical Specialist in Adult Health Nursing A clinical nurse specialist in adult nursing, which the American Nurses Credentialing Center (ANCC) defines as providing medical-surgical nursing "care for individuals who have a known or predicted physiological alteration." A registered nurse with a graduate degree who otherwise qualifies may take the ANCC examination in this area and receive the credential APRN, BC (Advanced Practice Registered Nurse, Board Certified). **nursingworld.org/ancc**

advance beneficiary notice (ABN) A written form notifying a Medicare beneficiary that Medicare may deny payment for a specific procedure or treatment, and that the beneficiary will be personally responsible for full payment if Medicare denies payment. A hospital or physician must provide this to the beneficiary before the procedure or treatment in order to bill the patient for any uncovered services. The ABN form requires (1) identification of the test, service, or procedure; (2) documentation of the reason Medicare is unlikely to pay; and (3) an estimate of what the out-of-pocket cost will be to the beneficiary. An ABN form is not required for services that Medicare never covers, such as routine physicals, screening tests, and personal comfort items.

advanced billing concept codes See under *ABC codes*.

advanced dependent practitioner (ADP) See under *allied health professional*.

advanced emergency medical procedure See under *procedure*.

advance directive A statement executed by a person while of sound mind as to that person's wishes about the use of medical interventions for him- or herself in case of the loss of his or her own decision-making capacity. A number of forms of advance directives have been proposed and are used; some are described below. See also *Patient Self-Determination Act* and *value inventory*.

durable power of attorney A power of attorney that remains (or becomes) effective when the principal becomes incompetent to act for herself. It should be noted that in most states, even an agent with a durable power of attorney cannot make medical treatment decisions for an incompetent patient, unless state law provides that she can or a court has given her specific authority.

healthcare proxy A document that authorizes a designated person (who is called a "proxy") to make healthcare decisions in the event that the signer is incapable of making those decisions. State law governs whether such a document is valid, how it must be created, and to what extent the proxy is authorized to make healthcare decisions. For example, a proxy may not be able to consent to electroconvulsive therapy or sterilization.

instructional advance directive (IAD) An advance directive in which an attempt is made to allow the person executing the directive to record quite specifically those interventions that are not to be attempted in case of the loss of the person's own decision-making capacity.

living will A will concerning the life of the individual executing the will, in contrast with the usual "last will and testament" in which the subject matter is the disposition of property (this could be thought of as a "property will") and custody of minor children. In many states, individuals may execute "living wills" concerning the circumstances under which they wish to refuse, or discontinue the use of, life-support measures administered to themselves should they become incompetent. Living will statutes (also known as right to die laws or natural death acts) govern the execution and enforcement procedures for living wills. At least one state (New Hampshire) calls the living will a "terminal care document." Some call it a "will to live."

The "life-sustaining procedures act," proposed by the National Conference of Commissioners on Uniform State Laws, suggests the following language for a living will: "If I should have an incurable or irreversible condition that will cause my death within a relatively short time, and if I am unable to make decisions regarding my medical treatment, I direct my attending physician to withhold or withdraw procedures that merely prolong the dying process and are not necessary to my comfort or to alleviate pain."

The Medical Directive An instructional advance directive document published in the New England Journal of Medicine (NEJM) in 1989 that has been made available to the lay public. The Medical Directive describes four clinical scenarios, each of which affects the patient's own decision-making capacity, and then lists a series of medical diagnostic or therapeutic interventions. The person who completes the document checks off whether she or he would choose the interventions in the case of each of the scenarios. The completed document is interpreted as an advance directive for the person who completes it.

values history A guide to family and medical care providers in making medical decisions for people no longer competent to decide for themselves. The values history is not a legal document such as the advance directive or the durable power of attorney. The values history could be in one of two formats: (1) a questionnaire completed by the patient, or (2) the product of a discussion between the physician and the patient much like the traditional family history and medical history. Currently, taking a values history is not part of the physician's responsibility, but the need for a values history is justified in three ways: (1) it breaks the silent relationship between the physician and patient; (2) it is a strong way for patients to exercise their autonomy in medical decision making; and (3) the values history provides clear evidence of the patient's views toward heroic and life-saving measures. If the patient has a values history in his or her chart, the physician does not need to rely so heavily on statements the patient might have made to family members. The National Values History Project was launched in 1988 to develop the values history idea and form. A values history form might include, for example, questions about the patient's need for independence or control, their religious background, who their closest relations are with, and what their overall attitude toward life is. Ultimately, the values history stimulates conversation between physician and patient, which protects the autonomy of the patient.

advanced life support (ALS) See *life support*.

advanced practice nurse (APN) A nurse with advanced skills, education, and training in a *nursing specialty*. Each specialty has specific requirements for eligibility, education, training, and certification and/or licensure of its practitioners. State laws govern the scope of practice. See also *clinical nurse specialist* and *nurse practitioner*.

Advanced Practice Registered Nurse, Board Certified (APRN,BC) A credential given to advanced practice nurses (nurse practitioners and clinical nurse specialists) with graduate degrees who have qualified in their areas of expertise. Offered by the American Nurses Credentialing Center (ANCC). **nursingworld.org/ancc**

Advanced Practice Sonographer (APS) See *diagnostic medical sonographer*.

advanced qualifications The term sometimes used for a credential given a health professional who has passed an examination and met other requirements in a specialized field. The next step after certification. See also *certificate of added qualification*.

Advanced Research Projects Agency (ARPA) See *Defense Advanced Research Projects Agency*.

Advanced Research Projects Agency Network (ARPANET) See *Defense Advanced Research Projects Agency*.

Advanced Technology Institute (ATI) A consulting firm dedicated to advancing technology through collaboration. Its healthcare efforts include enabling organizations to effectively share health information (see **Healthcare Information Technology Standards Panel**) and providing technology to improve care in rural and underserved communities. **www.aticorp.org**

adverse drug event (ADE) One of a series of terms frequently appearing in the healthcare literature dealing with the prevention of harm (illness or injury) to humans as a consequence of drug usage. The following list of terms is so closely intertwined, it is more meaningful to discuss them together:

    medication error ("med error")
    adverse drug event (ADE)
      potential adverse drug event (PADE)
    adverse drug reaction (ADR)
      expected ADR
      unexpected ADR
      preventable ADR
    serious ADE or serious ADR

It should be noted that the harm need not be directly caused by the drug itself to fall into the ADE category. (For the purposes of this discussion, "medication" and "drug" are treated as synonymous.) Several keys are useful to understanding these terms:

- Not all errors lead to harm—some mistakes turn out to be harmless. This is just as true for drug use as it is for the rest of life.
- It is just as possible for harm to flow from drugs that are *not* given to a person as from those that are. Failing to give the proper heart medication in a timely manner to a patient with a severe heart condition will just as likely harm the patient as giving the patient an overdose or the wrong medication.
- Harm from a drug may be expected or unexpected. This may seem nonsensical—why would you give a patient a drug where you "expected" harm? The answer is that almost all drugs have known side effects, with varying degrees of harm. The "expected" harm of mild nausea or drowsiness, for example, is often accepted as a worthwhile compromise for significantly reduced pain.

A **medication error** is a failure of some kind in the process of drug administration. The medication process begins when the physician (or other practitioner) in the hospital writes a medication order (distinguished from drug prescription). It is often transcribed (perhaps by a clerk or secretary), then communicated to the hospital pharmacy, where the order is filled and the medication sent back to the patient care unit (PCU). A nurse (or other qualified professional) gives the medication to the patient, observing the 5 R's of medication administration: (1) right medication, (2) right dosage, (3) right patient, (4) right time, and (5) right route of administration (for example, oral, intravenous [IV], or intramuscular [IM]). Mistakes can happen at any one or more points along way. For example, the pharmacy may dispense the wrong drug, or the nurse may give it to the wrong patient. Any of these is a medication error, although the term is sometimes used more narrowly to refer to a nursing error.

A medication error may be harmless or have serious consequences, and there may be disagreement as to what in fact constitutes an error (for example, a ten-minute delay might constitute serious error in one instance, but be totally insignificant in another, depending upon the drug and the patient's condition). A written medication error report is usually completed for each error as part of the hospital's quality management process. Only through careful analysis of medication errors can it be determined whether errors are due to lack of skill, lack of education, or problems with the process itself. (The term "medication error" does not refer to inappropriate *usage* of drugs; drug usage in general is reviewed by the medical staff. See **drug utilization review** and **pharmacy and therapeutics**.) When a medication error results in harm it becomes an "adverse drug event" (ADE).

An **adverse drug event (ADE)** is broadly defined as any injury related to the use of a drug. The harm may be trivial or fatal. It may be expected or unexpected, caused by the drug or by an allergic reaction (or unknown cause), due to error (by a health professional or the patient), or unpreventable. Sometimes the term **adverse event (AE)** is used as a synonym for ADE. A worldwide surveillance system for ADEs is being developed; see *Adverse Event Reporting System*. The term **potential adverse drug event (PADE)** is sometimes used for a medication error that has the capacity to cause harm but fails to do so, whether by chance or because it was intercepted before it reached the patient.

An **adverse drug reaction (ADR)** is defined by the World Health Organization (WHO) as an adverse event that is "noxious and unintended and occurs at doses used in man for prophylaxis, diagnosis, therapy, or modification of physiologic functions." This includes the "bad side effects" of many drugs. If the side effect is known and anticipated, it leads to an "expected ADR." If the side effect was not previously known, it is called an "unexpected ADR." If the ADR is caused by an error, it is said to be a "preventable ADR."

ADRs in a hospital may be detected not only by specific ADR reports, but also by other events which suggest that a patient may have had a reaction: discontinuation of the medication, decrease in dosage, ordering of certain laboratory tests, specific test abnormalities, and low white blood cell counts. A questionnaire called a Naranjo algorithm can also be used to assess whether a change in clinical status was due to an ADR. Increasingly, computer software used in the healthcare setting is being programmed to "flag" the existence of ADRs (and ADEs more generally) in an effort to reduce their occurrence.

An ADE or an ADR, regardless of its cause, may be classified as "serious" or not. The WHO defines a **serious adverse drug reaction** as an event that, at any dose:

- Results in death,
- Requires inpatient hospitalization or prolongation of existing hospitalization,
- Results in persistent or significant disability/incapacity, or
- Is life-threatening.

In this context, the WHO distinguishes the term "severe" because it is relative; a headache may be severe, but not serious.

Finally, harm may result from intentional drug abuse by an individual, including such circumstances as committing suicide via drug overdose. Most studies and reports in the healthcare field treat cases falling into this category differently from other ADE occurrences, possibly because it is more of a mental health issue than a medication issue.

adverse drug reaction (ADR) Not synonymous with, but defined and discussed under, *adverse drug event*.

adverse event (AE) See *adverse drug event* and *adverse patient occurrence*.

Adverse Event Reporting System (AERS) A postmarketing safety surveillance system of the Center for Drug Evaluation and Research of the FDA for all approved drug and therapeutic biologic products. Reports of *adverse drug events (ADEs)* are sent to the system by drug manufacturers (required by federal regulations) and by health professionals and consumers (voluntarily via the *MedWatch* program). **www.fda.gov/cder/aers**

adverse occurrence See *adverse patient occurrence*.

adverse patient occurrence (APO) An instance of substandard (or possibly substandard) patient care. Some examples are: (1) a patient is injured, whether or not the hospital may be liable; (2) the admission was the result of an adverse result of outpatient care; (3) the patient was readmitted because of complications or incomplete care in the previous admission; (4) there were deficiencies in documentation, such as in informed consent procedures or in the medical record; (5) unplanned surgery was done; (6) procedures were employed that did not meet the hospital's criteria for appropriateness; (7) a problem occurred with use of blood or blood components; (8) a nosocomial (hospital-acquired) infection occurred; (9) drug usage was inappropriate; (10) cardiac or respiratory arrest or death occurred; (11) there was an incident (such as a patient fall); (12) abnormal laboratory or x-ray findings were not followed up; (13) the stay was unusually short or long for the condition; (14) there were problems in obtaining services; or (15) there was patient or family dissatisfaction. These criteria are paraphrased from the Medical Management Analysis (MMA) system for review of care, which depends heavily on screening for and reporting of APOs.

Sometimes an APO is called an incident, but these terms are not necessarily synonymous. "Incident" is sometimes more narrowly used to refer only to accidents (such as falls) or behavioral problems. If an APO involves medications or drugs, it may be an **adverse drug event (ADE)**. See also **medical harm**, **sentinel event**, and **unanticipated outcome** (under **outcome**). Synonyms: adverse event, adverse occurrence.

adverse reaction Not synonymous with, but defined and discussed under, **adverse drug event**.

adverse selection A situation in which patients with greater than average need for medical and hospital care enroll in a prepaid health plan in greater numbers than they occur in a cross-section of the population. A plan that somehow encouraged or allowed people to sign up when they were already ill would suffer from adverse selection.

advocacy Attempting to persuade others of the rightness of a cause, or of a point of view on an issue. Such educational efforts—for example, health education—are increasingly undertaken by hospitals and other nonprofit organizations, but if they are addressed at passing or defeating legislation, they may be classified as lobbying and therefore endanger the organization's tax-exempt status.

AE Adverse event; see **adverse drug event**.

AED See **automated external defibrillator** under **defibrillator**.

aerospace medicine The branch of preventive medicine that deals with the special problems of flying, both within and outside the atmosphere.

AERS See **Adverse Event Reporting System**.

AFCR See **American Federation for Clinical Research**.

affiliated contractor (AC) See **Comprehensive Error Rate Testing**.

affiliation Any one of a number of arrangements among providers outlining their relationships and their individual responsibilities. The relationships are contained in documents that range from broad letters of intent to detailed contracts. In the past, such arrangements were often called "alliances," but this term was preempted in the healthcare reform movement by proposals for specific organizations labeled "healthcare alliances," which were often referred to merely as "alliances."

AFS See **alternative financing system**.

after care Care during the period of convalescence following hospitalization.

against medical advice (AMA) See **discharge against medical advice** under **discharge**.

age- and sex-specific capitation See **capitation**.

Age Discrimination in Employment Act (ADEA) Federal legislation prohibiting discrimination based on age in employment practices. This law applies to everyone, regardless of whether they receive federal funding or not. Physician recruitment program criteria based on age or years out of medical school may violate the ADEA. 29 U.S.C. § 621 (2005).

agency (administrative) A part of state or federal government, created by the legislature, that has specific administrative duties and functions, often including *regulation* of a profession or industry. A state board of medical examiners, for example, is an administrative agency. There is a body of law (administrative law) that governs the powers of administrative agencies, the process of agency decision making, and the procedures by which a party dissatisfied with a decision of an agency can challenge it. Ordinarily, any person who wishes to contest an administrative agency decision must go through all of the channels of appeal within the agency before challenging the decision in the courts.

agency (legal) A legal relationship in which one person acts on behalf of another. A written agency agreement is called a power of attorney.

agency (organization) An organization set up to carry out services such as home health care, "meals on wheels," or registration of tumor patients. In this usage, the agency may be part of either the public sector or the private sector. If the agency is private, it may be either nonprofit or for-profit.

Agency for Health Care Policy and Research (AHCPR) Former name of the *Agency for Healthcare Research and Quality.*

Agency for Healthcare Research and Quality (AHRQ) The lead federal agency for research to improve the quality of health care, reduce its cost, and broaden access to essential services. A component of the Department of Health and Human Services (HHS). See also *Office of Health Technology Assessment*. Formerly the Agency for Health Care Policy and Research (AHCPR), renamed by reauthorizing legislation in 1999. www.ahrq.gov

Agency for Toxic Substances and Disease Registry (ATSDR) See *National Center for Environmental Health/Agency for Toxic Substances and Disease Registry* under *Centers for Disease Control and Prevention*.

agent (facilitator) An instrument or means by which something is done. Often used to describe a person working within an organization.

change agent A person whose efforts, by design or not, facilitate change in an organization. Such a person may not even be aware of causing change.

energy agent A term that more accurately describes the role of an individual who provides leadership, from within the organization or outside it, to enhance the productivity and satisfaction of individuals. For many years the emphasis has been on change agents; however, at least as much effort must be employed for entropy prevention as for change. The term "energy agent" covers both of these tasks of management (as well as individuals who are effective in creating and maintaining an organization's enthusiasm and productivity).

agent (representative) A person who acts for another person, who is called the principal. An agent can legally bind the principal. An agent may or may not be an employee, but an employee is always an agent of the employer.

actual agent A person who has been authorized by another (the principal) to act for that other person. The term "actual" is used to describe the fact that the principal has, in fact, authorized the agent. Usually the nature and limits of the agent's authority are specific. In some circumstances, the law will impose liability on a principal even though the agent was not actually authorized; see *apparent agent*.

apparent agent A person who has not been authorized to act on behalf of another (the principal), but who appears, to other people, to have such authority. In cases where the principal is responsible (or partly responsible) for this appearance, the principal may be held legally responsible for the acts of the apparent agent. See also *actual agent*.

agent (substance) A chemical substance or biological substance or an organism capable of producing an effect.

infectious agent A microorganism (a germ, virus, or other living microscopic organism) that can cause a disease by invading the tissues and multiplying within the body. It is contrasted with other agents, such as chemicals, which can cause disease, but are not live and therefore are not capable of multiplying within the body.

noxious agent An agent that causes harm.

therapeutic agent An agent that heals or aids healing.

aging in place Growing older without having to move from one's residence. This requires that necessary healthcare and other needed services be available. Recently, the term is being used to describe facilities that can provide the full range of services and levels of care required during aging, so that residents do not have to relocate when their needs change. However, one must first move to the facility before the aging "in place" can happen. See also *continuing care retirement community* and *naturally occurring retirement community*.

agroterrorism The threat of or the deliberate introduction of an animal or plant disease that would affect a population's food system. See also *bioterrorism* and *terrorism*.

AHA See *American Heart Association* and *American Hospital Association*.

AHA Guide to the Health Care Field An annual directory of hospitals, multihospital systems, healthcare networks, health-related organizations, and American Hospital Association (AHA) members, published by the AHA. Often called simply the *AHA Guide*. Contains a great amount of information, including chief executive officers, addresses, phone numbers, facilities and services, number of beds, census, expenses, and so forth. Also includes national organizations (for example, Emergency Nurses Association, Society of Critical Care Medicine); resources (Indoor Air Quality Information Clearinghouse, Grief Recovery Helpline, Tourette Syndrome Association); Blue Cross and Blue Shield plans; hospital associations; licensing agencies; state health planning and development agencies; state and provincial government agencies; health maintenance organizations (HMOs); freestanding ambulatory surgery centers, hospices, and accredited long-term care; psychiatric facilities; substance abuse programs; and much more. See also *Hospital Statistics*.

AHCPR See *Agency for Health Care Policy and Research*.

AHFS DI See *American Hospital Formulary Service Drug Information*.

AHIC See *American Health Information Community*.

AHIMA See *American Health Information Management Association*. Formerly the American Medical Records Association (AMRA).

AHIP See *America's Health Insurance Plans*.

AHLTA The U.S. military's *electronic health record (EHR)* for Uniformed Services members, retirees, and their families. Developed by the Department of Defense (DoD), AHLTA will be interoperable, globally accessible, protected, and always available. It is planned to be fully implemented by 2011.

AHME See *Association for Hospital Medical Education*.

AHN-BC See *Advanced Holistic Nurse—Board Certified* under *holistic nursing*.

AHP See *allied health professional*. Also accountable health partnership, accountable health plan, approved health plan; see *accountable health plan* and *association health plan*.

AHQA See *American Health Quality Association*.

AHR See *Alliance for Health Reform*.

AHRC See *allied health review committee*.

AHRQ See *Agency for Healthcare Research and Quality*.

AHRQ Quality Indicators (QIs) See under *quality indicator*, under *indicator*.

AHSRHP Academy for Health Services Research and Health Policy. See *AcademyHealth*.

AI See *artificial intelligence*.

A/I A specialist in allergy and immunology. See *medical specialty*.

AI/AN American Indians and Alaska Natives, the populations served by the Indian Health Service.

aide A person who assists a patient, a patient's family, or another care provider.

    home care aide A person who provides housekeeping services for ill, elderly, or disabled persons in their homes. Services may include cleaning, cooking, meal planning, grocery shopping, changing linens, and so on. The National Association for Home Care & Hospice (NAHC) has a national certification program for home care aides.
    www.nahc.org/community_education.html

    home health aide A person who helps ill, elderly, or disabled persons in their homes. Health services provided may include administering oral medications; checking pulse, temperature, and respiration; assisting with exercises; changing dressings; and helping with braces and artificial limbs. A home health aide may also provide housekeeping and personal care services.

    nursing aide A person who, under the supervision of an authorized member of the nursing staff, carries out nonspecialized duties and personal care activities. See also *nursing assistant*.

personal care aide A person who helps ill, elderly, or disabled persons with basic personal care such as bathing, dressing, and eating. Personal care aides often also perform tasks of the home health and care aides.

AIDS (acquired immunodeficiency syndrome) The disease caused by HIV (human immunodeficiency virus). The official definition of AIDS, a disease that was first described in 1981, has been changed repeatedly as the disease has become better understood. The first official definition took effect in 1985. The second, in 1987, required that the patient also have any one of several dozen specified *opportunistic infections* (see under *infection*) associated with HIV. The 1992 definition stated that any person with a blood count revealing fewer than 200 CD4 lymphocytes (also known as helper T cells) per cubic millimeter (mm^3) was considered to have full-blown AIDS.

At the same time, the 1992 definition removed the requirement that there must be accompanying opportunistic infections. This change was stimulated by two things. First, the treatments for the opportunistic infections became increasingly effective. Newer drug therapy either eliminated or delayed the development of the opportunistic infections in HIV-infected individuals. Furthermore, the natural history of AIDS was better known, and other studies confirmed that the lowered CD4 cell count is a change that can be attributed to AIDS during a latent period between infection of the patient and the development of other symptoms and effects. Secondly, although HIV infections were still increasing in numbers, applying the 1987 definition in the face of fewer or later opportunistic infections made the incidence of AIDS appear to be slowing down or decreasing.

Thus the changes in definition affected morbidity statistics (dealing with the incidence and prevalence of the disease in the population) but not the mortality statistics: The 1985 definition resulted in an increase in the reported incidence of AIDS of 3% to 4% over the period when there was no official definition. The 1987 definition, by adding a number of diagnoses to the list of those diagnoses that, coupled with evidence of the HIV infection, labeled the patient as having AIDS, increased the reported incidence by 19% to 24%. The 1992 definition increased the reported incidence by nearly another 50%, despite its removal of the requirement that there be the designated accompanying infections.

One should also be aware that labeling of the individual patient as having or not having AIDS has serious social, employment, and financial consequences, so the definition is important to that patient.

AIDS nursing See *HIV/AIDS nursing*.

AIHQ Fellow See *Fellow of the American Institute for Healthcare Quality* under *quality management professional*.

air and surface transport nursing See *flight nursing*.

Alcohol, Drug Abuse, and Mental Health Administration (ADAMHA) A former administration within the Department of Health and Human Services (HHS) of the executive branch of the federal government. See *Substance Abuse and Mental Health Services Administration (SAMHSA)*.

alcoholism Dependence on the use of alcohol, which leads to interference with health and to social and economic problems. Withdrawal of alcohol from a person with alcoholism leads to psychological and physical symptoms.

alcoholism counselor A counselor specializing in the needs of individuals suffering from alcoholism.

Aldrete score A post-anesthesia recovery score developed by J. Antonio Aldrete, MD, published first in 1970 and revised in 1995. Its use is encouraged by the Joint Commission on Accreditation of Healthcare Organizations (JCAHO), especially to evaluate the condition of patients who have undergone conscious sedation. Numerical values are given for the patient's condition with regard to (1) activity, (2) respiration, (3) circulation, and (4) consciousness; possible scores range from 1 to 10. A sufficiently high total score must be attained before the patient is considered adequately recovered from the anesthesia.

alert See *clinical alert*.

alert practitioner A phrase sometimes used to describe a clinician who is exceptionally observant, especially at detecting patterns among patients. Important discoveries have been made by alert practitioners. For example, some major causes of birth defects, including thalidomide and rubella, were first identified by individuals who noticed an increase in birth defects and hypothesized a cause. The hypotheses led to controlled studies, which established the link. Similarly, the connection between heart valve deformities and a combination of two weight loss drugs, fenfluramine and phentermine ("fen-phen") was discovered by an observant and persistent echocardiogram sonographer in Fargo, North Dakota (see *fen-phen*).

algorithm A set of rules for carrying out a process, such as the care of a patient with a given set of problems, or the calculation of a statistic. The rules are such that a specific set of steps is required in sequence, with each step dependent on the preceding step.

Naranjo algorithm A questionnaire that can be used to assess whether a change in clinical status of a patient was due to an adverse drug reaction (ADR).

alien FMG See *foreign medical graduate (FMG)*.

ALL See *Action Learning Lab*.

allele Any one of a series of two or more different genes that may occupy the same locus on a specific chromosome. Autosomal (nonsex) chromosomes are paired, so each autosomal gene is represented twice in normal somatic cells. If the same allele occupies both units of the locus, the individual or cell is homozygous for this allele. If the alleles are different, the individual or cell is heterozygous for both alleles.

Dominant traits or conditions (such as brown eyes) are caused by inheritance of a single allele from either parent; **recessive** ones (blue eyes) by inheritance of a relevant allele from each parent. With the advent of DNA technology, the allele has become the focus of intense scrutiny, as molecular biologists attempt to track down genes responsible for physical and behavioral traits, and for the 3,500 human diseases that have been identified as chromosomally linked. Paired with radioisotopes or fluorescent dyes, alleles may serve as probes that allow for the identification of such genes.

allergist A physician specializing in the diagnosis and treatment of patients with disorders due to allergy. This is a branch of internal medicine.

allergy An acquired condition of the body causing it to react abnormally to a chemical substance or physical agent, such as cold.

allergy and immunology The study of diseases due to allergy and disorders of the immune system.

alliance In common usage, any one of a variety of collaborative arrangements among individuals or institutions. In the past, hospitals have formed alliances or affiliations, for example, among those furnishing primary, secondary, and tertiary care.

Alliance for Health Reform (AHR) A nonpartisan, nonprofit organization formed in 1991 to provide unbiased information on U.S. health care and its problems to opinion leaders such as elected officials and their staffs, journalists, policy analysts, and advocates. **www.allhealth.org**

Alliance for Nursing Informatics (ANI) A collaboration of organizations involved in nursing informatics. ANI represents more than 3,000 nurses and brings together 20 distinct nursing informatics groups in the United States that function separately at local, regional, national, and international levels. ANI's purpose is to "advance the efforts of nursing informatics professionals in improving the delivery of patient care." It is sponsored by the American Medical Informatics Association (AMIA) and the Healthcare Information and Management Systems Society (HIMSS). **www.allianceni.org**

allied health professional (AHP) A term loosely used to refer to health professionals who are not physicians or nurses; see *health science discipline*. However, it has a more precise meaning to describe nonphysician health professionals who have clinical contact with patients within the hospital, but are not necessarily hospital employees. The hospital is responsible for *credentialing* these professionals and specifying what they are permitted to do. There are three categories:

licensed independent practitioner (LIP) A health professional who, by license and hospital policy, is permitted to practice independently in the hospital without supervision or direction of a physician. LIPs include, for example, audiologists, clinical psychologists, social workers, optometrists, and in some states podiatrists and dentists. They may operate independently or be employed by the hospital. LIPs are granted *clinical privileges* (see under *privileges*) and may or may not be *medical staff members*, depending on hospital policy.

advanced dependent practitioner (ADP) A health professional who is licensed or certified and works under the supervision or direction of a physician. ADPs include advanced practice registered nurses (APRNs) and physician assistants (PAs). They are granted *clinical privileges* (see under *privileges*) that restrict their practice to working with a physician *medical staff member*. An ADP may be employed by the physician or contracted or employed by the hospital. The Joint Commission on Accreditation of Healthcare Organizations (JCAHO) requires ADPs to be credentialed through the medical staff credentialing process or an equivalent process; however, the Centers for Medicare and Medicaid Services (CMS) requires that the medical staff process be used. This credentialing is necessary even if the ADP is employed by the hospital.

dependent practitioner (DP) A health professional who may or may not be licensed or certified, who practices under the supervision or direction of a physician. A DP may be employed by the physician or be contracted or employed by the hospital. Examples are first assistants, therapists, technicians, and nurses who accompany an attending physician. CMS requires that any DP who provides a "medical level" of care must be credentialed through the medical staff credentialing process. The Joint Commission on Accreditation of Healthcare Organizations (JCAHO) requires that before a DP may practice within the hospital, the DP's qualifications and competence must be "assessed by the hospital and be determined to be commensurate with the qualifications and competence required if the individual were to be employed by the hospital to perform the same or similar services." The DP must also be reevaluated by the hospital with the same frequency as an equivalent employee. The assessments may or may not go through the medical staff process, depending on hospital policy.

allied health review committee (AHRC) A hospital committee charged with reviewing the credentials and performance of *allied health professionals (AHPs)* and making recommendations as to clinical privileges to be granted or modified. See also *credentialing*, *credentials committee*, and *privileges*.

allograft An organ or tissue transplanted (grafted) from one individual to another, both of the same species. Most organ transplants today are allografts. Synonym: homograft.

allopathy See *medicine (system)*.

all-payer system A system in which prices for healthcare services and payment methods are the same for all, regardless of payer. All those financing health care—government, individual, insurance company, health plan, self-insured employer—pay the same rates. Healthcare providers may not shift costs from one payer to another, as is often the case in the United States. Maryland hospitals presently operate under this system.

ALOS Average length of stay. See *length of stay*.

Alpha Center A nonprofit, private research organization, focusing on healthcare financing and organizational issues, which merged into *AcademyHealth*.

alphanumeric A string of characters containing both letters of the alphabet and numerals. The term is usually applied to codes, which are typically either alphabetic (letters only), numeric (numerals only), or alphanumeric (both).

alpha testing See under *testing*.

ALS See *advanced life support* (under *life support*) and *amyotrophic lateral sclerosis*.

alternative billing concept codes Now called "advanced billing concept codes." See under *ABC codes*.

alternative delivery and financing system (ADFS) A general term that covers any kind of alternative organizational arrangement for the delivery of health care, such as a health maintenance organization (HMO), in which payment for physician services is other than fee-for-service (FFS). Thus, an ADFS is a combination of an alternative delivery system (ADS) and an alternative financing system (AFS).

alternative delivery system (ADS) (care) An alternative to traditional inpatient care, such as substitution of ambulatory care, home health care, hospice, or ambulatory surgery (same-day surgery). Synonym: alternative delivery mode.

alternative delivery system (ADS) (organization) An alternative to the traditional arrangements of healthcare providers into solo practice or group practice. Examples include the independent/integrated physician association (IPA), preferred provider organization (PPO), health maintenance organization (HMO), and healthcare organization (HCO). The method of purchase of service or payment of physicians (fee-for-service [FFS] or capitation, for example) does not govern the term in this usage.

alternative dispute resolution (ADR) Methods of settling claims and disagreements other than by the "traditional" method in the United States—a lawsuit. See also *early offer* and *health court*.

arbitration A form of alternative dispute resolution in which providers and patients would agree in advance to have any disputes resolved without resorting to litigation. A single arbitrator or panel of arbitrators is chosen by the parties to hear the case, and the parties agree to be bound by the arbitrator's decision. The arbitrator's decision is usually final; a court will not overrule it unless there was fraud or partiality involved.

mediation A method of settling disputes by bringing the parties together to agree on a solution, rather than having a third party (such as an arbitrator, judge, or jury) make the decision for them. Mediation, usually done with the assistance of a mediator (someone trained in dispute resolution), may be private or may be connected to the court system. Some states have laws requiring or encouraging mediation as an alternative or supplement to costly, time-consuming lawsuits or trials.

alternative financing system (AFS) An alternative to the fee-for-service (FFS) payment system, such as a healthcare organization (HCO), health maintenance organization (HMO), or competitive medical plan (CMP) in which some other mechanism, usually capitation, is the method of payment to the organization and sometimes to the physician.

Alternative Link See *ABC codes*.

alternative medicine See *complementary and alternative medicine*.

AMA Against medical advice. See *discharge against medical advice* under *discharge*. See also *American Medical Association*.

AMA Physician Masterfile A database created and maintained by the American Medical Association (AMA), the nation's largest association representing doctors. The AMA assigns each new medical student a *medical education number* when he or she begins training, and uses that number to track that person from then on. Each Masterfile record includes the physician's name, medical school and year of graduation, gender, birthplace, and birth date. Additional data (residency training, state licensure, board certification, geographical location and address, type of practice, present employment, and practice specialty) are added from primary data sources or from surveying the physicians directly as the physicians' training and career develop. Physicians are never removed from the database, even after death.

Although only about 40% of U.S. doctors are dues-paying members of the AMA, the Masterfile has detailed information, including the DEA number, on all doctors licensed in the United States. The DEA number can be used to cross-reference specific physicians with other databases that contain information about them. The AMA has maintained the Masterfile for nearly 100 years, and has licensed it to other companies for more than 50. For example, marketing firms in the pharmaceutical industry consider the Masterfile the "gold standard" for reference information about doctors. Coupled with the records of pharmacy sales, which these firms also have access to, the Masterfile helps create profiles of individual doctors. The AMA states that there are some restrictions on licensing the Masterfile, including that it cannot be sold to tobacco companies, and it cannot be used to deceive physicians or the public. Any doctor may ask the AMA to exclude his or her name from lists that are sold to third parties (though doctors who are not AMA members may not be aware of the Masterfile).

ambulatory A term that specifically means "able to walk," but which in health care refers to a person who is not bedridden. Thus a person who requires a wheelchair is ambulatory, and can come in for treatment and return home.

ambulatory care Care provided to a patient without hospitalization.

ambulatory care center A facility that provides health and allied services to patients who do not require overnight lodging in an inpatient facility. To be designated an ambulatory care center, the facility is expected to have an organized professional staff (see *staff (group)*).

Ambulatory care centers are either freestanding or hospital-based. Those that are freestanding seem to be classified into several levels, whereas hospital-based centers are not. Freestanding ambulatory care centers of the highest level are stated to be able to provide emergency care; those of a lower level, urgent care; and those at the lowest level, primary care. Hospital-based ambulatory care centers, on the other hand, do not seem to be divided into these categories. No doubt the usage will be clarified with time.

ambulatory care nursing The nursing specialty concerned with the health needs of individuals and families in a variety of settings other than inpatient.

Certified Ambulatory Care Nurse A registered nurse with an associate degree or diploma, or a Bachelor of Science in Nursing or higher degree, who is qualified in ambulatory care nursing and has passed an examination of the American Nurses Credentialing Center (ANCC, **nursingworld.org/ancc**). The credential is RN,C (Registered Nurse, Certified).

Ambulatory Care Quality Alliance (ACQA) Original name of the *AQA*.

ambulatory care system Although people use this phrase, such as in "the U.S. ambulatory care system," it has no specific meaning.

ambulatory medical record (AMR) An electronic medical record (EMR) system in use in an outpatient setting, such as a physician's office.

Ambulatory Patient Category (APC) A grouping method used in the Ambulatory Patient Group (APG) classification system for outpatients. The term was easily confused with the Ambulatory Payment Classification because both have the same initialism—APC.

Ambulatory Patient Group (APG) The precursor to the *Ambulatory Payment Classification*.

Ambulatory Payment Classification (APC) The basis for payment for care in the outpatient prospective payment system (OPPS) (see under *prospective payment system*). APCs evolved from Ambulatory Patient Groups (APGs), which were developed in the early 1990s and initially put into use in the Iowa Medicaid program. The APC is used in a fashion similar to the way DRGs (Diagnosis Related Groups) are used for payment for inpatients. Both APCs and DRGs are intended to represent groups of patients that are similar clinically and that also have roughly the same resource consumption. But there is a significant difference between them: APCs depend on the *procedures* performed whereas DRGs depend on the *diagnoses* treated. The primary reference in determining the APC assignment of a case is the HCPCS, which uses CPT plus other codes supplied by CMS.

Unlike inpatients, where each case is assigned to a single DRG, outpatients may receive a number of separate services during a single episode, and so a case (claim) can have multiple APCs, each of which has a fixed prospective price. DRGs apply to the entire hospital admission, whereas APCs relate to individual encounters. A complex set of rules governs the final price for the case, depending on the prices for each of its APCs and a number of other factors. In general, the highest-priced APC payment amount is allowed, while other APCs for the case are discounted through a formula that is found in the *Outpatient Code Editor*. Adjustments to the payment rate are made for geographic variations in labor rates and for certain facility types.

ambulatory perianesthesia nursing See *Certified Ambulatory Perianesthesia Nurse* under *perianesthesia nursing*.

Ambulatory Quality Alliance See *AQA*.

ambulatory surgical center (ASC) A facility that specializes in *ambulatory surgery* (see under *surgery (treatment)*). May be part of another institution, such as a hospital, or free standing.

ambulatory visit group (AVG) A counterpart of the DRG classification (scheme), but designed for use for ambulatory care rather than hospital care. Patients, as in DRGs, undergo classification (process) into diagnosis groups (in this case, AVGs rather than DRGs) for which a predetermined or prenegotiated fee can be established.

AMCRA American Managed Care and Review Association. See *American Association of Health Plans*.

American Academy of Family Physicians (AAFP) A national association of specialists in family medicine, with more than 94,000 members. **www.aafp.org**

American Academy of Medical Directors (AAMD) The previous name of the *American College of Physician Executives (ACPE)*.

American Academy of Nurse Practitioners (AANP) A national membership organization based in Washington, DC, which provides advocacy and information concerning legislative, regulatory, and clinical practice issues affecting nurse practitioners. **www.aanp.org**

American Academy of Nursing (AAN) An organization whose goal is to transform health-care policy and practice through nursing knowledge. AAN members are authorized to use the credential "Fellow of the American Academy of Nursing" (FAAN). **www.aannet.org**

American Academy of Physician Assistants (AAPA) A national professional society representing physician assistants (PAs) in all areas of medicine. The society was founded in 1968 and has chapters in all fifty states. **www.aapa.org**

American Academy of Professional Coders (AAPC) A national membership organization of physician practice and outpatient coding specialists. **www.aapcnatl.org**

American Accreditation HealthCare Commission See *URAC*.

American Art Therapy Association (AATA) A nonprofit organization representing art therapy professionals. **www.arttherapy.org**

American Association for Medical Systems and Informatics (AAMSI) A national organization interested in the application of computers to medical problems. It was formed by the merger of the Society for Computer Medicine (SCM) and the Society for Advanced Medical Systems (SAMS) in August 1981. In 1990, the AAMSI was one of three organizations that merged to become the *American Medical Informatics Association*.

American Association of Colleges of Nursing (AACN) An organization of institutions offering baccalaureate and higher degree programs in nursing. The purpose of the AACN is to provide its members with a framework through which to advance the quality of baccalaureate and graduate programs, promote research, and develop academic leaders. **www.aacn.nche.edu**

American Association of Critical-Care Nurses (AACN) A professional organization of nurses specializing in critical care nursing. It was established in 1969 to help educate nurses working in newly developed intensive care units. The AACN is now the largest specialty nursing organization in the world, representing the interests of more than 400,000 nurses. **www.aacn.org**

American Association of Healthcare Consultants (AAHC) A national organization of professional consultants in health care. AAHC grants credentials to qualified individuals; see *healthcare consultant*. **www.aahc.net**

American Association of Health Plans (AAHP) An association of more than 1,000 health maintenance organizations (*HMO*s), preferred provider organizations (*PPO*s), and other network-based health plans, that was dedicated to a "Philosophy of Care" that put the patient first, and encouraged active partnerships between patients and their physicians. AAHP was created in 1996 by the merger of the Group Health Association of America (GHAA) and the American Managed Care and Review Association (AMCRA). AAHP has merged into *America's Health Insurance Plans.*

American Association of Homes and Services for the Aging (AAHSA) A national organization that represents over 5,600 nonprofit nursing homes, continuing care retirement communities, assisted living residences, senior housing facilities, and community service organizations for the elderly. A major focus is development of an integrated continuum of chronic or long-term care services that includes supportive housing. Programs include the Certified Aging Services Professional (CASP) program (formerly the Certification Program for Retirement Housing Professionals [RHP Program]), with the University of North Texas (UNT), and AAHSA conferences and educational programs. **www.aahsa.org**

American Association of Homes for the Aging (AAHA) The original name for the *American Association of Homes and Services for the Aging.*

American Association of Integrated Healthcare Delivery Systems (AAIHDS) A nonprofit organization dedicated to the educational advancement of provider-based managed care professionals involved in integrated healthcare delivery, such as through managed care organizations, health systems, physician-hospital organizations, and independent practice associations. **aaihds.org**

American Association of Physician Specialists (AAPS) A national membership organization of allopathic and osteopathic physicians with twelve affiliated Academies of Medicine offering continuing medical education for a number of medical specialties. **www.aapsga.org**

American Board of Allergy and Immunology (ABAI) A medical specialty board that grants a general certificate in allergy and immunology and a subspecialty certificate in clinical and laboratory immunology. It is a conjoint board of the American Board of Internal Medicine and the American Board of Pediatrics. Member of the American Board of Medical Specialties (ABMS). **www.abai.org**

American Board of Anesthesiology (ABA) A medical specialty board that grants a general certificate in anesthesiology and subspecialty certificates in critical care medicine and pain medicine. Member of the American Board of Medical Specialties (ABMS). **www.abanes.org**

American Board of Bariatric Medicine (ABBM) A medical specialty board that grants certification in bariatric medicine. **www.abbmcertification.org**

American Board of Clinical Pharmacology (ABCP) A medical specialty board that grants certification in clinical pharmacology. **www.abcp.net**

American Board of Colon and Rectal Surgery (ABCRS) A medical specialty board that grants a general certificate in colon and rectal surgery. Member of the American Board of Medical Specialties (ABMS). **www.abcrs.org**

American Board of Dermatology (ABD) A medical specialty board that grants a general certificate in dermatology and subspecialty certificates in clinical and laboratory dermatological immunology and dermatopathology. Member of the American Board of Medical Specialties (ABMS). **www.abderm.org**

American Board of Disaster Medicine (ABODM) A medical specialty board that grants a certificate in disaster medicine. An affiliate of the American Board of Physician Specialties (ABPS). **www.abpsga.org**

American Board of Emergency Medicine (ABEM) A medical specialty board that grants a general certificate in emergency medicine and subspecialty certificates in medical toxicology, pediatric emergency medicine, sports medicine, and undersea and hyperbaric medicine. Member of the American Board of Medical Specialties (ABMS). **www.abem.org**

American Board of Facial Plastic and Reconstructive Surgery (ABFPRS) A medical specialty board that grants a certificate in facial plastic and reconstructive surgery. Applicants must have earned prior certification from the American Board of Otolaryngology, the American Board of Plastic Surgery, or the Royal College of Physicians and Surgeons of Canada in otolaryngology-head and neck surgery or plastic surgery. **www.abfprs.org**

American Board of Family Medicine (ABFM) A medical specialty board that grants a general certificate in family medicine and, in conjunction with the American Board of Internal Medicine (ABIM), a certificate of added qualifications (CAQ) in geriatric medicine. A CAQ in adolescent medicine is offered in conjunction with the American Board of Pediatrics (ABP) and the ABIM. The ABFM also offers a CAQ in sports medicine jointly with the ABIM, the ABP, and the American Board of Emergency Medicine (ABEM). Member of the American Board of Medical Specialties (ABMS). **www.theabfm.org**

American Board of Genetic Counseling (ABGC) An organization that certifies genetic counselors and accredits genetic counseling training programs. **www.abgc.net**

American Board of Hospice and Palliative Medicine (ABHPM) A medical specialty board that grants certification to physicians specializing in hospice and palliative medicine. **www.abhpm.org**

American Board of Internal Medicine (ABIM) A medical specialty board that grants a general certificate in internal medicine and subspecialty certificates in cardiovascular disease, endocrinology, diabetes, metabolism, gastroenterology, hematology, infectious disease, medical oncology, nephrology, pulmonary disease, and rheumatology. Certificates of added qualifications are granted in adolescent medicine, clinical cardiac electrophysiology, critical care medicine, geriatric medicine, interventional cardiology, sleep medicine, sports medicine, and transplant hepatology. Member of the American Board of Medical Specialties (ABMS). **www.abim.org**

American Board of Medical Genetics (ABMG) A medical specialty board that grants several general certificates in medical genetics: clinical genetics (MD), clinical biochemical genetics, clinical cytogenetics, clinical molecular genetics, and PhD medical genetics. The ABMG also offers a subspecialty certificate in molecular genetic pathology, jointly with the American Board of Pathology (ABP). Member of the American Board of Medical Specialties (ABMS). **www.abmg.org**

American Board of Medical Management (ABMM) The former specialty board for physicians specializing in medical management. This board will no longer exist after 2007, when all certificates it has granted expire. The new certifying body is the Certifying Commission in Medical Management (CCMM).

American Board of Medical Specialties (ABMS) The umbrella organization for twenty-four of the boards certifying medical specialties in the United States. These boards are titled "American Board of (Specialty)." Associate members of ABMS include the Accreditation Council for Graduate Medical Education, Accreditation Council for Continuing Medical Education, American Hospital Association, American Medical Association, Association of American Medical Colleges, Council of Medical Specialty Societies, Educational Commission for Foreign Medical Graduates, Federation of State Medical Boards, and National Board of Medical Examiners. **www.abms.org**

American Board of Neurological Surgery (ABNS) A medical specialty board that grants a general certificate in neurological surgery. Member of the American Board of Medical Specialties (ABMS). **www.abns.org**

American Board of Nuclear Medicine (ABNM) A medical specialty board that grants a general certificate in nuclear medicine. Member of the American Board of Medical Specialties (ABMS). **abnm.snm.org**

American Board of Obstetrics and Gynecology (ABOG) A medical specialty board that grants a general certificate in obstetrics and gynecology and subspecialty certificates in maternal-fetal medicine, reproductive endocrinology and infertility, and gynecologic oncology. Member of the American Board of Medical Specialties (ABMS). **www.abog.org**

American Board of Ophthalmology (ABO) A medical specialty board that grants a general certificate in ophthalmology. Member of the American Board of Medical Specialties (ABMS). **www.abop.org**

American Board of Orthopaedic Surgery (ABOS) A medical specialty board that grants a general certificate in orthopaedic surgery, a subspecialty certificate in orthopaedic sports medicine, and a certificate of added qualifications (CAQ) in surgery of the hand. Member of the American Board of Medical Specialties (ABMS). **www.abos.org**

American Board of Otolaryngology (ABOto) A medical specialty board that grants a general certificate in otolaryngology-head and neck surgery. ABOto offers subspecialty certificates in pediatric otolaryngology, neurotology, and plastic surgery within the head and neck. Member of the American Board of Medical Specialties (ABMS). **www.aboto.org**

American Board of Pain Medicine (ABPM) A medical specialty board that grants a specialty certificate in pain medicine. **www.abpm.org**

American Board of Pathology (ABP) A medical specialty board that grants general certificates in anatomic pathology and clinical pathology, anatomic pathology, and clinical pathology. Subspecialty certificates are offered in blood banking/transfusion medicine, chemical pathology, cytopathology, dermatopathology, forensic pathology, hematology, medical microbiology, molecular genetic pathology, neuropathology, and pediatric pathology. Member of the American Board of Medical Specialties (ABMS). **www.abpath.org**

American Board of Pediatrics (ABP) A medical specialty board that grants a general certificate in pediatrics and certificates in the following pediatric subspecialties: adolescent medicine, cardiology, clinical and laboratory immunology, critical care medicine, developmental-behavioral pediatrics, emergency medicine, endocrinology, gastroenterology, hematology-oncology, infectious diseases, neonatal-perinatal medicine, nephrology, pulmonology, and rheumatology. A certificate of added qualifications (CAQ) is offered for medical toxicology, neurodevelopmental disabilities, pediatric transplant hepatology, and sports medicine. Member of the American Board of Medical Specialties (ABMS). **www.abp.org**

American Board of Physical Medicine and Rehabilitation (ABPMR) A medical specialty board that grants a general certificate in physical medicine and rehabilitation and subspecialty certificates in pain medicine, pediatric rehabilitation medicine, and spinal cord injury medicine. Member of the American Board of Medical Specialties (ABMS). **www.abpmr.org**

American Board of Physician Specialties (ABPS) The umbrella organization for nine of the boards certifying medical specialties in the United States. These boards are titled "Board of Certification (BOC) in (Specialty)," with the exception of the American Board of Disaster Medicine (ABODM). **www.abpsga.org**

American Board of Plastic Surgery (ABPS) A medical specialty board that grants a general certificate in plastic surgery and a subspecialty certificate in surgery of the hand. Member of the American Board of Medical Specialties (ABMS). **www.abplsurg.org**

American Board of Preventive Medicine (ABPM) A medical specialty board that grants general certificates in aerospace medicine, occupational medicine, and public health/general preventive medicine, and subspecialty certificates in medical toxicology and undersea and hyperbaric medicine. Member of the American Board of Medical Specialties (ABMS). **www.abprevmed.org**

American Board of Psychiatry and Neurology (ABPN) A medical specialty board that grants general certificates in psychiatry, neurology, and neurology with special qualifications in child neurology, and subspecialty certificates in addiction psychiatry, child and adolescent psychiatry, clinical neurophysiology, forensic psychiatry, geriatric psychiatry, neurodevelopmental disabilities, neuromuscular medicine, pain medicine, psychosomatic medicine, sleep medicine, and vascular neurology. Member of the American Board of Medical Specialties (ABMS). **www.abpn.com**

American Board of Radiology (ABR) A medical specialty board that grants general certificates in diagnostic radiology, radiation oncology, and radiologic physics, and subspecialty certificates in neuroradiology, nuclear radiology, pediatric radiology, and vascular and interventional radiology. Member of the American Board of Medical Specialties (ABMS). **www.theabr.org**

American Board of Surgery (ABS) A medical specialty board that grants a general certificate in general surgery, and subspecialty certificates in pediatric surgery, surgical critical care, surgery of the hand, and vascular surgery. Member of the American Board of Medical Specialties (ABMS). **www.absurgery.org**

American Board of Thoracic Surgery (ABTS) A medical specialty board that grants a general certificate in thoracic surgery. Member of the American Board of Medical Specialties (ABMS). **www.abts.org**

American Board of Urology (ABU) A medical specialty board that grants a general certificate in urology, which includes pediatric urology. There are no subspecialty certificates. Member of the American Board of Medical Specialties (ABMS). **www.abu.org**

American Cancer Society (ACS) A national organization dedicated to eliminating cancer by prevention, saving lives, and diminishing suffering from cancer, through research, education, advocacy, and service. ACS is the largest source of private, nonprofit cancer research funds in the United States. **www.cancer.org**

American College of Cardiology (ACC) A national organization of physicians specializing in cardiology. **www.acc.org**

American College of Emergency Physicians (ACEP) A national organization of physicians specializing in emergency medicine. **www.acep.org**

American College of Health Care Administrators (ACHCA) A nonprofit association of administrators of long-term care (LTC) facilities, formerly called the American College of Nursing Home Administrators (ACNHA), founded in 1962. **www.achca.org**

American College of Healthcare Executives (ACHE) A professional society of more than 30,000 healthcare executives who lead hospitals, healthcare systems, and other healthcare organizations. ACHE has educational and credentialing programs for its members. **www.ache.org**

American College of Hospital Administrators (ACHA) The former name (until 1985) of the *American College of Healthcare Executives*.

American College of Medical Genetics (ACMG) An association of biochemical, clinical, cytogenetic, medical, and molecular geneticists, genetic counselors, and other health professionals committed to the practice of medical genetics. **www.acmg.net**

American College of Medical Quality (ACMQ) An organization to provide leadership and education in healthcare quality management. Founded in 1973 as the American College of Utilization Review Physicians. Its affiliated American Board of Medical Quality offers the Certified in Medical Quality (CMQ) credential to those with an MD, DO, DDS, DPM, or DMD who qualify and pass a certification examination. **www.acmq.org**

American College of Nurse-Midwives (ACNM) An organization dedicated to development and support of the profession of midwifery as practiced by Certified Nurse-Midwives and Certified Midwives (see *midwifery*). With roots dating to 1929, ACNM is the oldest women's healthcare organization in the United States. **www.acnm.org**

American College of Nursing Home Administrators (ACNHA) Former name of the *American College of Health Care Administrators*.

American College of Obstetricians and Gynecologists (ACOG) A national organization of physicians specializing in obstetrics and gynecology. **www.acog.org**

American College of Physician Executives (ACPE) The national professional association that serves, recognizes, and certifies physician executives. Individuals who are certified by the ACPE (see *Certified Physician Executive* under *physician executive*) may be granted fellowship in the ACPE and may then use the designation FACPE (Fellow of the American College of Physician Executives). Formerly, ACPE was known as the American Academy of Medical Directors (AAMD). **www.acpe.org**

American College of Physicians (ACP) A national organization of physicians that is the nation's largest medical specialty society. Members are physicians in general internal medicine and related subspecialties, including cardiology, gastroenterology, nephrology, endocrinology, hematology, rheumatology, neurology, pulmonary disease, oncology, infectious diseases, allergy and immunology, and geriatrics. Qualified members may achieve Fellowship status and may use the credential, "Fellow of the American College of Physicians" (FACP). This status is also available to those who have not been members previously who are elected as Fellows, and to those selected by the College as Honorary Fellows (FACP (Hon)).

ACP was created by the merger of two former organizations, the American College of Physicians (ACP), founded in 1915, and the American Society of Internal Medicine (ASIM), founded in 1956. In 1998, they merged to become the American College of Physicians—American Society of Internal Medicine (ACP-ASIM). Finally the name was changed again to simply the American College of Physicians (ACP). **www.acponline.org**

American College of Radiology (ACR) A national organization of physician specialists in radiology. Its 30,000 members include radiologists, radiation oncologists, medical physicists, interventional radiologists, and nuclear medicine physicians. **www.acr.org**

American College of Surgeons (ACS) A national scientific and education association of surgeons founded in 1913 to improve the quality of surgical care. Its members are called "Fellows" and use the credential "Fellow of the American College of Surgeons" (FACS). There are also "Associate Fellow" members. It is the largest surgeons' organization in the world, with over 70,000 members. **www.facs.org**

American College of Utilization Review Physicians (ACURP) Former name of the *American College of Medical Quality*.

American Council on Science and Health (ACSH) An independent, nonprofit consumer education consortium established to help Americans distinguish between real and hypothetical health risks. ACSH has a board of 350 experts in a wide variety of fields. Areas of focus include Activists/Hype, Chemicals/Environment, Children/Infants, Diseases, Food Safety, Nutrition/Lifestyle, Pharmaceuticals, Terrorism, and Tobacco. **www.acsh.org**

American Dental Association (ADA) The national professional association of dentists in the United States. It was founded in 1859 by twenty-six dentists in Niagara Falls, New York. ADA now has over 153,000 members. **www.ada.org**

American Dietetic Association (ADA) The primary professional association for dietitians and nutritionists in the United States, with nearly 65,000 members. It was founded in 1917 by a group of women dedicated to helping the government conserve food and improve the public's health and nutrition during World War I. **www.eatright.org**

American Federation for Clinical Research (AFCR) Former name of the *American Federation for Medical Research*.

American Federation for Medical Research (AFMR) A multi-disciplinary, international organization of scientists engaged in all areas of biomedical investigation. Members are located at government facilities, medical centers, research institutions, and private industry in all fifty states and throughout the world. Founded in 1940 as the American Federation for Clinical Research (AFCR). **www.afmr.org**

American Health Information Community (AHIC) A federally chartered public-private group of stakeholders charged with providing input to the Department of Health and Human Services (HHS) on how to make health records digital and interoperable, and assure that the privacy and security of those records are protected. The goal of the collaboration is to develop and adopt an architecture, standards, a certification process, and a method of governance for ongoing implementation of health information technology (HIT). AHIC was chartered in 2005 for two years with the option to renew for no more than five years, after which it would be replaced with a private-sector **health information community initiative (HICI)** that would set additional needed standards, certify new health information technology, and provide long-term governance for HIT.

American Health Information Management Association (AHIMA) The national association of health information management professionals. AHIMA operates a publishing business; offers professional practice, library, and professional certification services; and develops standards for the accreditation of health information management degree-granting programs (see *Commission on Accreditation for Health Informatics and Information Management Education*). AHIMA also approves certificate-level coding education programs. Formerly the American Medical Record Association (AMRA), it was founded in 1928 to improve the quality of medical records. **www.ahima.org**

American Health Quality Association (AHQA) An educational, nonprofit association of the nation's quality improvement organizations (QIOs). AHQA is dedicated to improving healthcare quality and patient safety through educational programs; community-based, independent quality evaluation and improvement programs; and other quality and safety initiatives. **www.ahqa.org**

American Heart Association (AHA) A nonprofit organization whose mission is to reduce disability and death from cardiovascular diseases and stroke. These include heart attack, stroke, and related disorders. Its efforts include research and education. AHA was founded in 1924 in New York City by six cardiologists. See also *life support*. **www.americanheart.org**

American Hospital Association (AHA) The national association of hospitals in the United States. Nonhospital healthcare organizations and individuals may also hold membership. In addition to membership activities, it maintains a major reference library of hospital literature, and publishes a number of titles, including the magazine *Hospitals and Health Networks* and two standard annual reference volumes, *Hospital Statistics* and *AHA Guide to the Health Care Field*. See also *Personal Membership Group*. **www.aha.org**

American Hospital Formulary Service Drug Information (AHFS DI) A standard reference on drugs, published annually by the American Society of Health-System Pharmacists (ASHP). **www.ashp.org/ahfs**

American Hospital System Although this term is often used, there really is no such thing as the "American Hospital System," except that the nation's hospitals and other healthcare facilities, along with health professionals and allied health professionals, do make up an informal network across the country through which care is provided. The "American Hospital System" simply means what actually exists—community hospitals, university hospitals, nonprofit hospitals, investor-owned hospitals, government hospitals, and the like.

American Managed Care and Review Association (AMCRA) See *American Association of Health Plans*.

American Medical Association (AMA) The major national association of physicians in the United States, whose mission is to promote the art and science of medicine and the improvement of public health. AMA was founded in 1847 at the Academy of Natural Sciences in Philadelphia. It is now the largest physician organization in the United States. **www.ama-assn.org**

American Medical Informatics Association (AMIA) A national organization whose members are committed to the promotion of medical informatics, as well as education and training related to this interest. AMIA's mission is to advance health care through information technology. The AMIA Annual Symposium (formerly SCAMC) is the largest conference for medical informatics professionals in the United States, and usually takes place in Washington, DC, in the fall. See also *medical informatics* under *informatics*. **www.amia.org**

American Medical Record Association (AMRA) The former name of the national association for professionals in medical record science, now called the *American Health Information Management Association (AHIMA)*.

American Medical Society on Alcoholism and Other Drug Dependencies (AMSAODD) The former name of the *American Society of Addiction Medicine (ASAM)*.

American National Standards Standards officially approved by *ANSI*.

American National Standards Institute (ANSI) See *ANSI.*

American Nurses Association (ANA) The professional association for registered nurses in the United States, made up of fifty-four constituent member associations (CMAs) in the states, the District of Columbia, Guam, and the Virgin Islands, plus the Federal Nurses Association (FedNA). The ANA works for better health standards and nursing services, high standards of nursing, and the professional development and economic and general welfare of nurses. It is concerned with nursing ethics and serves as spokesperson for nursing, nationally and internationally. The ANA was founded in New York City in 1896. It now has approximately 150,000 members. **www.nursingworld.org**

American Nurses Credentialing Center (ANCC) An independent organization (originally established by the American Nurses Association) that provides recognition of the professional achievement of nurses. Since 1991, ANCC has certified over 150,000 nurses in 40 specialty and advanced practice areas of nursing (see *nursing specialty*). ANCC also provides accreditation of education providers and approvers, recognition of excellence in nursing services, and education of the public in the value of professional nursing credentialing. **nursingworld.org/ancc**

American Organization of Nurse Executives (AONE) A national organization of over 5,000 nurse executives. AONE is a subsidiary of the American Hospital Association (AHA). **www.aone.org**

American Osteopathic Association (AOA) The major national association of osteopathic physicians (DOs) in the United States. The AOA was founded in 1897, and now has more than 56,000 members. The AOA serves as the primary certifying body for DOs, and is the accrediting agency for all osteopathic medical colleges and healthcare facilities. **www.osteopathic.org**

American Osteopathic Board of Anesthesiology (AOBA) An osteopathic specialty board that grants a general certificate in anesthesiology and added qualifications in pain management. Member of the Bureau of Osteopathic Specialists (BOS).

American Osteopathic Board of Dermatology (AOBD) An osteopathic specialty board that grants a general certificate in dermatology and added qualifications in dermatopathology and Mohs-micrographic surgery. Member of the Bureau of Osteopathic Specialists (BOS). **www.aocd.org/qualify/board_certification.html**

American Osteopathic Board of Emergency Medicine (AOBEM) An osteopathic specialty board that grants a general certificate in emergency medicine and certificates of added qualifications in emergency medical services, medical toxicology, and sports medicine. Member of the Bureau of Osteopathic Specialists (BOS). **www.aobem.org**

American Osteopathic Board of Family Physicians (AOBFP) An osteopathic specialty board that grants a general certificate in family practice and added qualifications in geriatric medicine and sports medicine. Member of the Bureau of Osteopathic Specialists (BOS). **www.aobfp.org**

American Osteopathic Board of Internal Medicine (AOBIM) An osteopathic specialty board that grants a general certificate in internal medicine; special qualifications in allergy/immunology, cardiology, endocrinology, gastroenterology, hematology, infectious disease, pulmonary diseases, nephrology, oncology, and rheumatology; and added qualifications in addiction medicine, clinical cardiac electrophysiology, critical care medicine, geriatric medicine, interventional cardiology, and sports medicine. Member of the Bureau of Osteopathic Specialists (BOS). **www.acoi.org/CertGen.html**

American Osteopathic Board of Neurology and Psychiatry (AOBNP) An osteopathic specialty board that grants general certificates in neurology and psychiatry, special qualifications in child neurology and child/adolescent psychiatry, and added qualifications in neurophysiology and geropsychiatry. Member of the Bureau of Osteopathic Specialists (BOS).

American Osteopathic Board of Neuromusculoskeletal Medicine (AOBNMM) An osteopathic specialty board that grants a general certificate in neuromusculoskeletal medicine and osteopathic manipulative medicine. Member of the Bureau of Osteopathic Specialists (BOS). www.academyofosteopathy.org/certification_neuro.cfm

American Osteopathic Board of Nuclear Medicine (AOBNM) An osteopathic specialty board that grants a general certificate in nuclear medicine and added qualifications in nuclear cardiology, nuclear imaging and therapy, and in vivo and in vitro nuclear medicine. Member of the Bureau of Osteopathic Specialists (BOS).

American Osteopathic Board of Obstetrics and Gynecology (AOBOG) An osteopathic specialty board that grants a general certificate in obstetrics and gynecology and special qualifications in gynecologic oncology, maternal and fetal medicine, and reproductive endocrinology. Member of the Bureau of Osteopathic Specialists (BOS). www.aobog.org

American Osteopathic Board of Ophthalmology and Otolaryngology—Head and Neck Surgery (AOBOO-HNS) An osteopathic specialty board that grants general certificates in ophthalmology, otolaryngology, and otolaryngology/facial plastic surgery, and a certificate of added qualifications in otolaryngic allergy. Member of the Bureau of Osteopathic Specialists (BOS). www.aoboo.org

American Osteopathic Board of Orthopedic Surgery (AOBOS) An osteopathic specialty board that grants a general certificate in orthopaedic surgery, and a certificate of added qualifications in hand surgery. Member of the Bureau of Osteopathic Specialists (BOS). www.aobos.org

American Osteopathic Board of Pathology (AOBP) An osteopathic specialty board that grants general certificates in laboratory medicine, anatomic pathology, and anatomic pathology and laboratory medicine; special qualifications in forensic pathology; and added qualifications in blood banking/transfusion medicine, chemical pathology, cytopathology, dermatopathology, hematology, immunopathology, medical microbiology, and neuropathology. Member of the Bureau of Osteopathic Specialists (BOS).

American Osteopathic Board of Pediatrics (AOBP) An osteopathic specialty board that grants a general certificate in pediatrics and special qualifications in neonatology, pediatric allergy/immunology, pediatric endocrinology, and pediatric pulmonology. Member of the Bureau of Osteopathic Specialists (BOS). www.aobp.org

American Osteopathic Board of Physical Medicine and Rehabilitation (AOBPMR) An osteopathic specialty board that grants a general certificate in physical medicine and rehabilitation. Member of the Bureau of Osteopathic Specialists (BOS). www.aobpmr.org

American Osteopathic Board of Preventive Medicine (AOBPM) An osteopathic specialty board that grants general certificates in preventive medicine/aerospace medicine, preventive medicine/occupational-environmental medicine, and preventive medicine/public health-community medicine, and a certificate of added qualification in occupational medicine. Member of the Bureau of Osteopathic Specialists (BOS). www.aobpm.org

American Osteopathic Board of Proctology (AOBP) An osteopathic specialty board that grants a general certificate in proctology. Member of the Bureau of Osteopathic Specialists (BOS).

American Osteopathic Board of Radiology (AOBR) An osteopathic specialty board that grants general certificates in diagnostic radiology and radiation oncology, and subspecialty certificates in body imaging, neuroradiology, nuclear radiology, pediatric radiology, and vascular and interventional radiology. Member of the Bureau of Osteopathic Specialists (BOS). www.aocr.org/certification

American Osteopathic Board of Rehabilitation Medicine (AOBRM) The former name of the American Osteopathic Board of Physical Medicine and Rehabilitation (AOBPMR).

American Osteopathic Board of Surgery (AOBS) An osteopathic specialty board that grants general certificates in general surgery, neurological surgery, plastic and reconstructive surgery, thoracic cardiovascular surgery, urological surgery, and vascular surgery, and added qualifications in surgical critical care. Member of the Bureau of Osteopathic Specialists (BOS). www.aobs.org

American Psychiatric Association (APA) The major national organization of psychiatrists in the United States. **www.psych.org**

American Psychological Association (APA) A national scientific and professional organization representing the interests of psychologists and the field of psychology. **www.apa.org**

American Public Health Association (APHA) The national association that embraces all public health professionals. Founded in 1872, it now has more than 50,000 members from over fifty occupations of public health. It is concerned with a broad range of issues affecting personal, public, and environmental health. **www.apha.org**

American Red Cross (ARC) A humanitarian organization, led by volunteers, committed to providing relief to victims of disasters and helping people prevent, prepare for, and respond to emergencies. The collection and distribution of blood are its major activities. Another important service, mandated by Congress, is to assist families in communicating with members of the armed services in times of emergency; this is handled by the Armed Forces Emergency Services (AFES) section of the ARC.

The American Red Cross, established in 1881, is modeled after the International Red Cross, created in 1863 in Geneva, Switzerland, to provide nonpartisan care to the wounded and sick in times of war. The Red Cross emblem was adopted at this first International Conference as a symbol of neutrality. There are now about 181 national Red Cross societies. Clara Barton was instrumental in establishing the American Red Cross, which extended its services from battlefield assistance to disaster relief. **www.redcross.org**

American Registry of Radiologic Technologists (ARRT) An organization that provides certification and registration to *radiologic technologist*s. **www.arrt.org**

American Roentgen Ray Society (ARRS) The first and oldest radiology society in the United States, founded in 1900. Dedicated to advancing medicine through the science of radiology and its allied sciences. **www.arrs.org**

American Society for Bariatric Surgery (ASBS) The national society for surgeons specializing in surgery for the treatment of obesity. **www.asbs.org**

American Society for Quality (ASQ) A national organization dedicated to quality, with over 100,000 individual and organizational members. ASQ offers technologies, concepts, tools, and training to quality professionals, quality practitioners, and consumers. Areas of focus include education, government, health care, manufacturing, and service. See also *Baldrige National Quality Program*. **www.asq.org**

American Society for Testing and Materials (ASTM) See *ASTM*.

American Society of Addiction Medicine (ASAM) A national medical specialty organization dedicated to educating physicians and improving the treatment of individuals suffering from alcoholism and other addictions. ASAM provides certification for physicians who pass an examination. See also *medical review officer*. **www.asam.org**

American Society of Anesthesiologists Physical Status Classification See ASA *Physical Status Classification*.

American Society of Clinical Investigation (ASCI) A medical "honor society" of physician-scientists from all medical specialties. Members, who must be under age 45 at time of admission, are elected because of their outstanding records of scholarly achievement in biomedical research. Founded in 1908, it now has about 2,800 members. **www.asci-jci.org**

American Society of Health-System Pharmacists (ASHP) A national membership organization of 30,000 pharmacists who practice in hospitals, health maintenance organizations, and other components of healthcare systems. It works to prevent medication errors and to help people make the best use of medicines. ASHP publishes *American Hospital Formulary Service Drug Information* (AHFS DI) and the *American Journal of Health-System Pharmacy* (AJHP). **www.ashp.org**

American Society of Internal Medicine (ASIM) See *American College of Physicians*.

Americans with Disabilities Act (ADA) A federal law enacted in 1990 that ushered in a new era of social policy pertaining to people with disabilities (see *disability*). In effect, the act extended the *Rehabilitation Act* of 1973 to the private sector. The substantive provisions of the act are divided into five titles:

- Title I requires that employers provide reasonable accommodations on the job unless it would be unduly hard to do so.
- Title II provides that no qualified individual with a disability shall be excluded from a program or benefit sponsored by state or local government.
- Title III holds that no individual shall be discriminated against on the basis of a disability in the full and equal enjoyment of goods, services, facilities, privileges, or advantages of public accommodation by anyone who runs, owns, or leases such accommodation. Churches are exempt from this requirement.
- Title IV provides that the Federal Communications Commission (FCC) shall ensure that interstate and intrastate telecommunications services are available to the disabled.
- Title V consists of other miscellaneous provisions.

Pub. L. No. 101-336, 104 Stat. 327 (1990), codified at 42 U.S.C. § 12101 et seq.

America's Health Insurance Plans (AHIP) A national association representing nearly 1,300 health insurance plans, which collectively provide health benefits to over 200 million Americans. AHIP's principal purpose is to represent the interests of its members on legislative and regulatory issues at the federal and state levels, and with the media, consumers, and employers. **www.ahip.org**

AMI Acute *myocardial infarction*; see under *infarction*.

AMIA See *American Medical Informatics Association*.

amino acid A molecule that is the building block of a protein.

AMR See *ambulatory medical record*. Sometimes used to mean automated medical record.

AMRA See *American Medical Record Association*.

AMSAODD American Medical Society on Alcoholism and Other Drug Dependencies. The former name of the *American Society of Addiction Medicine*.

amyotrophic lateral sclerosis (ALS) A serious neurological disease that attacks the nerve cells that control voluntary muscles. It may begin with muscle twitching or weakness in an arm or leg, or with slurring of speech. Eventually, ALS affects the ability to control the muscles needed to move, speak, eat, and breathe. As of 2007, neither a cause nor a cure has been found; treatment focuses on relieving symptoms. In the United States, people diagnosed with ALS are automatically enrolled in Medicare Part A. ALS is commonly called Lou Gehrig's disease, after Hall of Fame baseball player Lou Gehrig of the New York Yankees, who died of the disease in 1941.

ANA See *American Nurses Association*.

anatomy The structure of organs and tissues, rather than their activities (see *physiology*). The study of anatomy includes gross anatomy and histology; see below.

gross anatomy The study of the body to the degree of detail visible to the naked eye.

histology The study of body tissues as visible under the microscope. Synonym: microscopic anatomy.

microscopic anatomy See *histology* (above).

ANCC See *American Nurses Credentialing Center*.

ancillary personnel Personnel other than physicians and nurses.

ancillary services Hospital services other than room and board. In a hospital, nursing services are included as part of "room and board"; because normal nursing services are not billed for separately, they are not ancillary services.

The Oregon Health Plan defines ancillary services as those services that are considered to be integral to successful treatment of a condition. Examples given are hospital services, laboratory services, radiation therapy, prescription drugs, medical transportation, rehabilitation, and maternity case management, and hospice services.

andrologist A physician specializing in diseases of the male sex.

anencephaly A severe birth defect where infants are born without portions of the brain and skull including the cerebral cortex and hemispheres. The infants usually have the brain stem, which regulates the lungs and heart, but are never conscious. The infant rarely lives beyond a few days. A difficult issue arises when the infant has transplantable organs. Technically, the anencephalic infant is not dead under the Uniform Determination of Death Act, but to wait for the actual brain death would cause the viable organs to no longer be suitable for transplanting. Some states allow a parent to terminate life support for the infant, others do not. Some argue for an extension of the Uniform Determination of Death Act to include these infants, others are wary of extending the definition of death to meet various societal needs.

anesthesia The condition of having lost feeling or sensation. This condition may arise because of the administration of a drug, the use of another agent or method (cold, for example) that depresses sensation, or neurological (nervous system) impairment. Words such as "ether" and "spinal" are commonly used to modify "anesthesia"; they refer to the anesthetic used, the route of administration, the area involved in the anesthesia, and the like.

anesthesiologist A physician specializing in anesthesiology, which, in modern hospitals, includes consultation in cardiopulmonary resuscitation (CPR), respiratory therapy (RT), and special problems in the relief of pain. Note that a physician may be called an "anesthetist," but only a physician may be called an "anesthesiologist."

anesthesiologist assistant (AA) A health professional who develops and implements anesthesia care plans under the direction of an anesthesiologist. May also be called an anesthetist, but an anesthetist is not necessarily an AA.

Certified Anesthesiologist Assistant (AA-C) An AA with a master's degree who has met the requirements of the National Commission for the Certification of Anesthesiologist Assistants (NCCAA). **aa-nccaa.org**

anesthesiology The study of anesthesia, including its pharmacology and physiology, and related fields, such as respiratory therapy, resuscitation, and the relief of chronic pain.

anesthetic A drug or other agent that depresses feeling or the sensation of pain.

inhalation anesthetic An anesthetic agent administered as a gas, by breathing.

anesthetist A person who administers anesthesia. An anesthetist may be a nurse, dentist, physician, or other individual. If a nurse administers the anesthesia, it is considered the practice of nursing; administration of anesthesia by an anesthesiologist is considered the practice of medicine. See also *anesthesiologist* and *anesthesiologist assistant*.

Certified Registered Nurse Anesthetist (CRNA) An advanced practice nurse who has met the requirements of the American Association of Nurse Anesthetists (AANA) (**www.aana.com**). CRNAs were the first clinical nursing specialists, beginning in the late 1800s. They are the sole anesthesia providers in nearly 50% of all hospitals and more than 65% of rural hospitals in the United States.

anesthetizing location The area of a building designated to be used for administering inhalation anesthetics.

angiotensin-converting enzyme (ACE) A class of blood pressure–reducing drugs. ACEs are thought to act by suppressing the renin-angiotensin-aldosterone system, but they are also effective at times in patients with low-renin hypertension. Synonym: kininase.

ANH See *artificial nutrition and hydration*.

ANI See *Alliance for Nursing Informatics*.

animal See *animal-assisted activities*, *animal-assisted therapy*, and *service animal*.

animal-assisted activities (AAA) The provision of a variety of benefits through the interaction of animals and humans. AAA seeks to enhance quality of life in a variety of settings, such as schools and nursing homes, by "meet and greet" activities introducing animals to people. It should be distinguished from *animal-assisted therapy*, which is tailored to a particular person or medical condition. Services are provided by professionals or volunteers who have received special training. The animals also must meet specific criteria to ensure their health and dispositions. Examples of animals used are dogs, cats, guinea pigs, rabbits, horses (see *hippotherapy*), goats, llamas, donkeys, potbellied pigs, cockatoos, African gray parrots, and chickens. See also *Delta Society*.

animal-assisted therapy (AAT) The use of animals to improve human physical, social, emotional, and/or cognitive functioning. AAT is directed by a health professional and provided by an individual with special training in this area. The therapy is tailored to the needs of the individual patient; there are specific goals for the treatment, and progress is measured. The animal used may be called a "therapy animal" (see also *service animal*). AAT is sometimes called "pet-facilitated therapy" or "animal-facilitated therapy." Specialists in this area reject the term "pet therapy" as inaccurate and misleading. See also *animal-assisted activities*, *Delta Society*, and *hippotherapy*.

animal rights movement The name adopted by the current movement to stop experimentation on animals in the course of medical and veterinary research. The movement threatens essential progress in a number of areas of medicine, particularly senile dementia, stroke, and cancer, in which other techniques, such as computer modeling, are not applicable and/or sufficient. Synonym: antivivisectionism.

anonymization See *de-identification*.

ANP See *Adult Nurse Practitioner* under *adult nursing*.

ANSI American National Standards Institute. A nonprofit, privately funded *standards development organization (SDO)* whose mission is the development of U.S. national standards on a voluntary basis. Standards are developed in a variety of fields, including health care, occupational safety, medical devices, and medical informatics, and are referred to as "American National Standards." Because members who agree on these standards are typically the major players in the area involving the standards (the "stakeholders"), being officially approved by ANSI gives any standard the virtual effect of law.

ANSI also represents the United States to nontreaty international standards organizations, such as the *ISO (International Organization for Standardization)*, for which it was a charter member. Founded in 1918, ANSI has a diverse membership consisting of private companies; professional, labor, and consumer organizations; and government agencies. ANSI also audits and provides accreditation for other SDOs. See also *CEN (organization)* and *Healthcare Information Technology Standards Panel*. www.ansi.org

ANSI ASC X12N ANSI Accredited Standards Committee Electronic Data Interchange Insurance Subcommittee. Develops the most widely implemented *electronic data interchange* (EDI) standards that interact with a multitude of e-commerce technologies and serves as the premier source for integrating electronic applications. EDI standards relating to health care include claims, payment and remittance advice, health plan eligibility, enrollment/disenrollment, premium payments, first report of injury, claim status, referral authorization, and certification. More at the *Data Interchange Standards Association* (DISA) web site. www.disa.org

ANSI HISB See *Healthcare Informatics Standards Board*.

ANSI HISPP See *Healthcare Information Standards Planning Panel*.

ANSI HITSP See *Healthcare Information Technology Standards Panel*.

ANSI IISP See *Information Infrastructure Standards Panel*.

anthrax A disease caused by a spore-forming bacterium (*Bacillus anthracis*) that lives in the soil. It generally infects hoofed animals, such as cattle, sheep, and camels. It can be transmitted to humans via the skin (through a cut or abrasion), by inhalation of the spores, or by eating undercooked meat from infected animals. Cases have occurred sporadically in the United States, most frequently as an industrial hazard among persons handling animal hides, hair (especially goat hair), bone and bone products, and wool (one synonym for anthrax is "woolsorters disease"). Veterinarians and agriculture and wildlife workers are also occasionally infected.

Inhalation anthrax is rare in the United States (only eighteen cases, all incurred occupationally, were reported in the 20th century), and is far more serious than the skin infection, which is more responsive to antibiotics. It is much harder to become infected by inhaling the spores, however, because a high concentration of spores is required, and they are difficult to disperse in the air.

Research on anthrax as a biological weapon was reported in the 1920s, but it was suspended or terminated by most nations after the Biological Weapons Convention (BWC) in the early 1970s. Beginning in late 2001 anthrax spores were transmitted through the U.S. mail as a form of terrorism, infecting a number of people (eleven cases of inhalation anthrax with five deaths and eleven cases of cutaneous anthrax with no deaths as of May 2002). The Centers for Disease Control and Prevention (CDC) has a web site for information on anthrax: **www.bt.cdc.gov/agent/anthrax**

anthropometric assessment See under *nutrition assessment*.

anthropometry See *anthropometric assessment* under *nutrition assessment*.

antibiotic Originally a class of natural compounds that inhibit the growth of or kill microorganisms. Compounds of the same class have subsequently been synthesized (i.e., created in the laboratory). Sometimes the term "antibiotic" is used in the context of affecting bacteria, while the term "**antimicrobial**" is used in the context of affecting all microorganisms.

antibiotic resistance The development by a microorganism of the ability to resist the effect of an antibiotic. Antibiotic resistance is generally specific to an individual antibiotic, so that often another antibiotic may be used effectively against that microorganism. However, an increasing number of microorganisms have become resistant to a number of antibiotics, and there is a constant race between antibiotic developers and microorganisms.

antibody A substance in the body that reacts with another substance called an antigen. An antibody may be created by the body in response to stimulation of the body by the antigen, or it may be present without this stimulation. Vaccination against a disease is a method that uses a disease antigen to stimulate the body to produce an antibody to that antigen (and thus the disease that produces the antigen).

anticodon See under *DNA*.

Anti-Dumping Act See *Emergency Medical Treatment and Labor Act*.

antigen A substance, such as a bacterium, virus, or protein, that, when coming into contact with an appropriate tissue in an animal body, stimulates that tissue to produce a state of resistance or sensitivity to infection by the organism (bacterium or virus) or to a toxic substance (such as dust). The adjective is "antigenic."

Antikickback Statute Federal legislation that makes it a felony for a person to receive or offer any bribe or kickback in exchange for a referral from another person in Medicare, Medicaid, or any federally financed state healthcare programs. The law is aimed at providers who receive compensation for referring patients to other providers, perhaps needlessly, which ultimately drives up the cost of Medicare and Medicaid. Because this legislation is written in very broad language, it is not always clear what kind of conduct is allowed and what is prohibited. The Office of Inspector General (OIG) has created safe harbors for providers; see *safe harbor regulations*. See also *fraud and abuse*. 42 U.S.C. § 1320a-7b (2004).

antimicrobial See *antibiotic*.

antitrust That branch of law which seeks to prevent monopolies and unfair competition. A "trust" was originally a combination of several corporations (each maintaining its separate identity) to eliminate competition, control prices, and the like. The term "antitrust" now broadly covers any activity (or conspiracy) to eliminate competition and control the marketplace. It includes actions that unreasonably restrain trade. Such activities are illegal, and severe penalties are imposed by antitrust laws. For example, the trust may be broken up, and anyone who suffers injury to his or her business or property as a result of the combination or conspiracy may collect treble damages. Federal antitrust laws (principally the Sherman Act of 1890, the Clayton Act of 1914, and the Federal Trade Commission Act of 1914) apply to companies doing business in interstate commerce. Many states also have antitrust laws.

Antitrust problems may arise for hospitals when they place limitations on medical staff membership, for example, or when several hospitals seek to combine services. Careful legal guidance is required in any area in which a hospital's actions may affect competition or regulate prices.

Antitrust issues are of concern in healthcare reform because of the fear that innovative approaches to healthcare organization and delivery of service may be deemed to be in violation of the antitrust regulations. Serious consideration is being given to amending the laws or providing for exceptions in order to stimulate and facilitate experimentation, and avoid unnecessary duplication of services.

Also, antitrust law is becoming more of an issue in the healthcare industry as providers are becoming more responsive to consumer preferences, which is fueling competition. However, applying antitrust law is problematic in the healthcare industry because the market lacks many competitive characteristics of other markets and the pervasive regulation questions whether the market is ever truly private. Some states have enacted statutes that exempt HMOs, hospital mergers, and joint ventures from their state antitrust laws. Issues of antitrust in the healthcare setting revolve around credentialing, staff privileges, price fixing, fee schedules and boycotts, and situations where physicians contract with third-party payers to enhance their market power (by forming ventures to provide goods and services related to their professional practice).

Problems have arisen trying to determine what is anticompetitive collusion versus cooperation among healthcare providers that results in enhanced efficiency. This is a hot topic as healthcare financing changes. The Department of Justice has scrutinized physician-hospital organizations (PHOs), for example, requiring some to agree to consent decrees that forbid more than 30% of the doctors in the PHO's market to have an ownership interest in the PHO. Mergers and acquisitions (M & A) between hospitals have withstood antitrust scrutiny if they have not resulted in producing one dominant hospital or excessive concentration in a market, much like mergers in other industries. See also *McCarran-Ferguson Act* and the *Health Care Quality Improvement Act*.

antiviral A class of drugs designed to attack virus infections.

antivivisectionism Against *vivisection*. See also *animal rights movement*.

any willing provider A law in some states that requires a managed care organization, such as an HMO, to grant participation to any provider who is legally qualified as a practitioner and who is willing to become a member of the organization. Such laws are enacted to protect the patient's freedom of choice. However, they often interfere seriously with the efforts of the managed care organization to achieve high quality and efficiency by limiting its provider network to caregivers with the best performance records, to hospitals in convenient geographic locations, and to selected pharmacies.

AOA See *Administration on Aging* and *American Osteopathic Association*.

AOBA See *American Osteopathic Board of Anesthesiology*.

AOBD See *American Osteopathic Board of Dermatology*.

AOBEM See *American Osteopathic Board of Emergency Medicine*.

AOBFP See *American Osteopathic Board of Family Physicians*.

AOBIM See *American Osteopathic Board of Internal Medicine*.

AOBNM See *American Osteopathic Board of Nuclear Medicine*.

AOBNMM See *American Osteopathic Board of Neuromusculoskeletal Medicine*.

AOBNP See *American Osteopathic Board of Neurology and Psychiatry*.

AOBOG See *American Osteopathic Board of Obstetrics and Gynecology*.

AOBOO See *American Osteopathic Board of Ophthalmology and Otolaryngology*.

AOBOS See *American Osteopathic Board of Orthopedic Surgery*.

AOBP See *American Osteopathic Board of Pathology*, *American Osteopathic Board of Pediatrics*, and *American Osteopathic Board of Proctology*.

AOBPM See *American Osteopathic Board of Preventive Medicine*.

AOBPMR See *American Osteopathic Board of Physical Medicine and Rehabilitation*.

AOBR See *American Osteopathic Board of Radiology*.

AOBRM American Osteopathic Board of Rehabilitation Medicine. Now the *American Osteopathic Board of Physical Medicine and Rehabilitation*.

AOBS See *American Osteopathic Board of Surgery*.

AOCN See *Advanced Oncology Certified Nurse* under *oncology nursing*.

AOCNP See *Advanced Oncology Certified Nurse Practitioner* under *oncology nursing*.

AOCNS See *Advanced Oncology Certified Clinical Nurse Specialist* under *oncology nursing*.

AOD See *accounting of disclosures*.

AONE See *American Organization of Nurse Executives*.

AORN Association of perioperative registered nurses. **www.aorn.org**

AOT See *assisted outpatient treatment*.

AP See *accounts payable*.

APA See *American Psychiatric Association* and *American Psychological Association*.

APACHE III A system designed to predict an individual's risk of dying in a hospital, generally used to measure the severity of illness of intensive care unit (ICU) patients. Twenty-seven objective facts—such as vital signs, results of certain blood tests, and age—are provided to the computer system, which then compares the patient's profile to nearly 18,000 cases in the database and makes a prognosis that, on the average, is 95% accurate. The APACHE III result can be useful in deciding whether treatment is effective, as well as whether "heroic measures" (see *extraordinary treatment* under *treatment*) should be used to keep a patient alive. APACHE is an acronym for Acute Physiology and Chronic Health Evaluation.

APAMI See *Asia Pacific Association for Medical Informatics* .

APC See *Ambulatory Patient Category* and *Ambulatory Payment Classification*. Also means "aspirin, phenacetin, and caffeine."

AP-DRG See *All Patient DRG* under *DRG*.

APG See *Ambulatory Patient Group*.

Apgar score A method devised by Virginia Apgar, an American anesthesiologist, for giving a numeric score to the physical condition of a newborn infant. Points are given for the infant's color, heart rate, respiratory effort, muscle tone, and response to stimulation. Ten is the highest score possible.

APHA See *American Public Health Association*.

apheresis The process of withdrawing blood, selectively removing one or more components (plasma, platelets, or red blood cells), and then returning the remainder of the blood to the donor. Also called hemapheresis.

APM See *admission pattern monitoring* under *monitoring*.

APN See *advanced practice nurse*.

APNG See *Advanced Practice Nurse in Genetics* under *genetic nursing*.

APO See *adverse patient occurrence*.

appliance A device that is used to provide function to a part of the body or for treatment. The term is used most commonly in orthodontics.

applied health science See *health science discipline*.

appointment The process of admitting a physician or other qualified health professional to the medical staff, and granting, along with the membership, specific privileges.

appropriateness The degree to which care (which may include tests, medication, procedures, hospitalization, education, and other services) is clearly indicated, adequate, not excessive, and provided in the setting best suited to the patient's needs.

approved health plan (AHP) See *accountable health plan*.

APR-DRG See *All Patient Refined DRG* under *DRG*.

APRN Advanced Practice Registered Nurse; see *advanced practice nurse*.

APRN,BC See *Advanced Practice Registered Nurse, Board Certified* under *advanced practice nurse*.

APRN,BC-ADM Advanced Practice Registered Nurse, Board Certified—Advanced Diabetes Management. See *Advanced Diabetes Management Certification* under *diabetes management*.

APS See *Advanced Practice Sonographer* under *diagnostic medical sonographer*.

APS-DRG See *All-Payer Severity-adjusted DRG* under *DRG*.

AQA A coalition developing standardized clinical *performance measures* for physicians (individuals and groups). Its goal is to build a strategy to measure, report on, and improve physician performance. The group was formed in 2004 by the American Academy of Family Physicians (AAFP), American College of Physicians (ACP), America's Health Insurance Plans (AHIP), and the Agency for Healthcare Research and Quality (AHRQ), and includes over 150 member organizations (physician specialty organizations, consumer groups, employers, government agencies, health insurance plans, and accrediting and quality organizations). AQA is working in three areas: performance measures, data aggregation, and data reporting.

AQA recommended that performance measures be selected that:
- are reliable, doable, evidence-based, and easy to implement;
- represent consensus;
- are endorsed by the National Quality Foundation (NQF);
- evaluate cost-of-care in relationship to quality;
- reflect a continuum of care; and
- are developed through a transparent process.

The first set of 26 **physician performance measures** approved by AQA focused on primary care and shared many of the measures in the Health Plan Employer Data and Information Set (HEDIS). These include screenings for breast cancer, colorectal cancer, and cervical cancer; tobacco use; vaccinations for influenza and pneumonia; use of beta blockers after a heart attack; pharmacologic therapy for asthma; and antidepressant use. By 2007, eighty measures had been adopted for practitioners in twenty-five surgical and medical specialties.

AQA also established principles to guide data sharing and aggregation. These include transparency with respect to framework, process and rules, reporting of data that are useful to physicians and consumers, standardized and uniform rules associated with measurement and data collection, collection of both public and private sector data so that performance can be assessed as comprehensively as possible, accountability for the accuracy and completeness of data, compliance with privacy and confidentiality rules, and minimal cost and burden. Guidelines were also set for reporting to the public, and reporting to hospitals and physicians.

Originally called the Ambulatory Care Quality Alliance, AQA changed its name when its mission broadened to incorporate all areas of physician practice. Sometimes called the AQA Alliance or the Ambulatory Quality Alliance. See also *pay-for-performance*, *Physician Consortium for Performance Improvement*, *Quality Alliance Steering Committee*, and *transparency initiative*. www.aqaalliance.org

AQA-HQA Steering Committee See *Quality Alliance Steering Committee*.

AR See *accounts receivable*.

arbitration See under *alternative dispute resolution (ADR)*.

arbitrator A person, not serving in the capacity of a court officer, chosen by the parties to a dispute to make a final, binding decision concerning the dispute. See *arbitration* under *alternative dispute resolution (ADR)*.

ARC See *American Red Cross*.

Arden Syntax A standardized language (similar to a computer language) used to write very detailed clinical decision rules called Medical Logic Modules (MLMs). These MLMs are designed to be used by healthcare providers in their clinical decision support systems to respond to certain events ("triggers") that cause the programmed logic (rule) in the MLM to execute. Each MLM is written so it contains sufficient logic to make a single clinical decision. For example, an MLM might automatically remind (alert) a physician to switch a patient from non-oral (NPO) to oral (PO) medication when there is a change in the patient's diet. The MLM may do this by continuously monitoring the patient's electronic medical record (EMR) to see if "diet order = intravenous (IV)," and when it changes, to automatically print out a new diet order suggesting the use of more cost-effective oral medications. In order for the Arden Syntax MLMs to be effective, however, the healthcare provider must already have some kind of information system in place that is capable of providing the properly structured and coded data to "trigger" the MLMs.

Obvious applications for MLMs include safety measures (prevent medication errors) as well as providing more cost-effective health care. Arden Syntax derives its name from the place where its development began: Columbia University's Arden Homestead Conference Center, where medical researchers met in 1989 to discuss how electronic medical knowledge-bases might be shared.

area agency on aging (AAA) An agency established in a community under the federal Older Americans Act (OAA) of 1973 to respond to the needs of those age sixty and over. The OAA also helps fund Native American programs, known as Title VI, for older American Indians, Aleuts, Eskimos, and Hawaiians. The primary purpose of the AAAs and Title VI programs is to provide services that make it possible for older individuals to remain in their homes, preserving their independence and dignity. The agencies coordinate and support a wide range of home- and community-based services, including information and referral, home-delivered and congregate meals, transportation, employment services, senior centers, adult day care, and a long-term care ombudsman program.

In 2007, there were 655 AAAs and over 230 Title VI programs in the United States. To find an agency or program, call the toll-free Eldercare Locator at 1-800-677-1116 or go to **www.n4a.org/locator**. See also *National Association of Area Agencies on Aging*.

Area Health Education Center (AHEC) A collaborative effort between a health science center (such as a university hospital or medical school) and the local community to foster health professions education. These centers arose from concerns about the supply, distribution, retention, and quality of health professionals. A major focus for AHECs is the shortage of primary care physicians in rural (underserved) areas. The name arose from a 1970 report by the Carnegie Commission that recommended the development of a nationwide system of "Area Health Education Centers." Since the early 1970s, federal and state support has made the implementation of AHEC programs possible in many states. Each center is unique.

One of the oldest AHECs is the Mountain Area Health Education Center (MAHEC) in Asheville, North Carolina. Its home facility, housed in its own buildings between two hospitals' adjoining campuses, contains a library, classrooms, administrative offices, and an audio-visual service. MAHEC also operates a health museum at a downtown site. It has a family medicine residency program and an obstetrics-gynecology residency program as satellites from the University of North Carolina. It also has a dental health center and general practice dental residency program. It provides area hospitals with such services as helping design the hospitals' education programs and being their intermediary in obtaining continuing education credit for those programs, preparing audio-visual materials such as lantern slides, and conducting Internet and library searches for their physicians and other health professionals. MAHEC's library contains, in addition to a good selection of books and periodicals, several thousand health education videotapes that are available to healthcare organizations, schools, and so forth. **www.mahec.net**

area wage adjustment A component of the payment formula under the prospective payment system (PPS) to allow for differences in wage scales in different parts of the country.
arithmetic mean See *mean*.

arm's-length transaction A transaction conducted "at arm's length"—a legal term meaning that it is beyond the reach of personal influence or control. A transaction not conducted at arm's length isn't necessarily unfair or unreasonable, but it is often subjected to closer scrutiny than one that is.

ARPA See *Defense Advanced Research Projects Agency*.

ARPANET Advanced Research Project Agency Network. See *Defense Advanced Research Projects Agency*.

ARRS See *American Roentgen Ray Society*.

ARRT See *American Registry of Radiologic Technologists*.

ART Accredited Record Technician. See *Registered Health Information Technician* under *health information technician*.

artificial intelligence (AI) A term used to describe a type of system in which the computer appears to be "thinking," and thus exhibits intelligence. Although the system appears to think, it really does not; rather, it has been given a number of "rules" to follow. A simple example would be a billing system that follows the rule: If there has been no payment within thirty days, send letter "A"; if there has been no payment within sixty days, send letter "B." Another example would be a program that looks up "unfamiliar" words (those not in its memory): If the word is a synonym for or similar to a word to which the system should respond and take action, it will either go ahead with the action or ask a human to confirm its "decision." There is some tendency for computer salespeople to overuse the term "artificial intelligence" to gain a sales advantage; this leads the customer to believe that AI systems are invariably better for every task than other systems.

artificial neural network See *neural network*.

artificial nutrition and hydration (ANH) Provision of nourishment and fluids by means of a tube inserted into the stomach (either by mouth or through a percutaneous endoscopic gastrostomy (PEG), a relatively simple operation that places a tube between the stomach and outside abdomen), or by intravenous means. It is a form of life-sustaining treatment; some people may indicate in their advance directives that they wish "no ANH."

art therapist A health professional qualified to practice art therapy.

Board Certified Registered Art Therapist (ATR-BC) A *Registered Art Therapist* who has passed a written examination of the Art Therapy Credentials Board (ATCB). **www.atcb.org**

Registered Art Therapist (ATR) An art therapist with at least a master's degree and/or ten years of art therapy experience, who has met all requirements for registration of the Art Therapy Credentials Board (ATCB). **www.atcb.org**

art therapy (AT) The use of art media, images, and the creative art process and responses to help people reconcile conflicts, develop social skills, manage behavior, reduce anxiety, increase self-esteem, and solve problems.

ASAM See *American Society of Addiction Medicine*.

ASA Physical Status Classification A way to describe the preoperative condition of a patient, used by anesthesiologists. It was originally devised by the American Society of Anesthetists (predecessor of the American Society of Anesthesiologists) to permit collection and tabulation of statistical data in anesthesia. It has now become a routine, international "shorthand" for anesthesiologists to use in assessing a patient prior to surgery. There are six classes: (P1) a normal healthy patient; (P2) a patient with mild systemic disease; (P3) a patient with severe systemic disease; (P4) a patient with severe systemic disease that is a constant threat to life; (P5) a moribund patient who is not expected to survive without the operation; (P6) a declared brain-dead patient whose organs are being removed for donor purposes. Also called PS score, PS classification.

ASBS See *American Society for Bariatric Surgery*.

ASC (facility) See *ambulatory surgical center*.

ASC (organization) Accredited Standards Committee. A committee chartered by ANSI to work on standards in a particular area of commerce, such as the insurance industry. See *ANSI ASC X12N*.

ASCA See *Administrative Simplification Compliance Act*.

ASCI See *American Society of Clinical Investigation*.

ASCP American Society for Clinical Pathology. Its Board of Registry is one credentialing body for *clinical laboratory technicians*, *clinical laboratory technologists*, and *clinical laboratory specialists*.

ASC X12N See *ANSI ASC X12N*.

aseptic See *sterile (aseptic)*.

ASH See *Assistant Secretary for Health*.

ASHP See *American Society of Health-System Pharmacists*.

ASHRHP See *Academy for Health Services Research and Health Policy*.

Asia Pacific Association for Medical Informatics (APAMI) A regional group of the International Medical Informatics Association. Formed in 1993, APAMI's mission is to promote regional cooperation, information dissemination, research and development, and standards in medical informatics among Asia Pacific countries. Member countries include Australia, China, Hong Kong, Indonesia, Japan, Korea, Malaysia, New Zealand, Philippines, Singapore, Taiwan, Thailand, and Vietnam. **www.apami.org**

ASIM American Society of Internal Medicine. See *American College of Physicians*.

ASO Administrative services only. Used in connection with health plans where a third party is contracted to provided only administrative services, such as claims processing and billing.

ASP See *administrative simplification provisions*.

ASQ See *American Society for Quality*.

AS-SCORE index One of the methods devised for classifying patients as to severity of illness. It uses five factors: age, stage of disease, physiological systems involved, complications, and response to therapy.

assessment procedure A term used by the Joint Commission on Accreditation of Healthcare Organizations (JCAHO) to describe the process used by a hospital to obtain information about each individual seeking care at a healthcare facility, so that the individual's needs may be matched with appropriate care.

asset An object (property or money, for example), a right (to royalties, for example), or a claim (a title to a debt, for example) that its owners consider to be of benefit to them. Assets in hospitals include property and equipment (which may have less value than their original cost because of depreciation), investments, accounts receivable (claims to money owed to the institution), and the other items that are listed as "assets" on the balance sheet of the institution.

capital asset An asset with a life of more than one year that is not bought and sold in the ordinary course of business.

current asset An asset with a life of less than one year, such as inventory.

fixed asset Long-term assets that are not bought or sold in the normal course of business. Typically, fixed assets are land, equipment, and buildings.

intangible asset An asset that is not physical. Examples include goodwill and patents.

noncurrent asset An asset with a life of more than one year.

tangible asset An asset that is physical, such as a building and equipment.

asset reduction Selling or giving away one's assets (house, stocks, etc.) in order to be eligible for public assistance, such as Medicaid.

assignment of benefits A voluntary decision by the beneficiary to have insurance benefits paid directly to the provider rather than to the beneficiary him- or herself. The act requires the signing of a form for the purpose. The provider is not obligated to accept an assignment of benefits; it may refuse and instead require the beneficiary to handle the collection procedure.

Conversely, the provider may insist on assignment in order to protect its revenue; if the provider accepts the assignment, it ordinarily assumes responsibility for the collection paperwork.

Assistant Secretary for Health (ASH) The senior advisor on health and science to the Secretary of the Department of Health and Human Services (HHS), and head of the *Office of Public Health and Science (OPHS)* and the U.S. *Public Health Service (PHS)*. www.hhs.gov/ash

assisted living The provision of services, including housing, health care, and support services, to those who need help with the *activities of daily living*. The idea is to allow people to remain as independent as possible.

assisted outpatient treatment (AOT) Treatment (usually for mental illness) ordered by a court as a condition of remaining in the community (rather than being institutionalized) for individuals who have a history of *noncompliance* with medication. Also called "outpatient commitment." See *Kendra's Law*.

assisted suicide See under *suicide*.

Assize of Bread Generally considered to be the first English language law regulating food safety and quality. In 1202, King John of England proclaimed this law, which prohibited adulteration of bread with such ingredients as ground peas or beans. Although regulation of food in the United States dates from early colonial times, the best known original federal food and drug law was the *Federal Food and Drugs Act of 1906 (the "Wiley Act")*.

associate degree (AD) A degree given by a two-year community college upon successful completion of a program in a given field.

Association for Health Services Research (AHSR) A national, nonprofit organization formed to promote the field of health services research. See *AcademyHealth*.

Association for Hospital Medical Education (AHME) A national, nonprofit professional organization concerned with all phases of medical education—undergraduate, graduate, and continuing medical education. AHME's more than 600 members represent hundreds of teaching hospitals, academic medical centers, and consortia nationwide. Founded in 1956 as the Association for Hospital Directors of Medical Education (AHDME). www.ahme.org

Association for Pharmacoeconomics and Outcomes Research (APOR) Former name (until 1997) of the *International Society for Pharmacoeconomics and Outcomes Research*.

association health plan (AHP) A concept by which small businesses band together to gain an advantage in purchasing health insurance for their employees. Such plans have not been legal in all states, although federal legislation was introduced in 2001 (the "Small Business Health Fairness Act") to permit the formation and regulation of AHPs. See also *multiple employer welfare arrangement*.

Association of American Medical Colleges (AAMC) An organization committed to improving the health of the public by enhancing the effectiveness of academic medicine. Its members include the 125 accredited U.S. medical schools, the 17 accredited Canadian medical schools, nearly 400 major teaching hospitals and health systems, 96 academic and professional societies representing nearly 109,000 faculty members, and the nation's medical students and residents. Among its many activities, AAMC administers the *Medical College Admission Test (MCAT)* and is a sponsor of the *National Resident Matching Program (NRMP)* and *Summer Medical and Dental Education Program (SMDEP)*. www.aamc.org

Association of American Physicians (AAP) An association of physician scholars established in 1885 by seven physicians, including Dr. William Osler, for "the advancement of scientific and practical medicine." AAP now has about 1,000 active members and 550 emeritus and honorary members from the United States, Canada, and other countries. Membership in the AAP is by invitation. www.aap-online.org

Association of American Physicians and Surgeons (AAPS) A national organization of physicians in all types of practices and specialties, devoted to preserving freedom in the one-on-one patient-physician relationship and the practice of private medicine. Established in 1943. www.aapsonline.org

Association of State and Territorial Health Officials (ASTHO) A nonprofit public health organization representing the state and territorial public health agencies of the United States, the U.S. Territories, and the District of Columbia. ASTHO's members, the chief health officials of these jurisdictions, are dedicated to formulating and influencing sound public health policy, and to assuring excellence in state-based public health practice. Areas of current activity include access to care, environmental health, infectious disease, prevention, public health information infrastructure, and public health preparedness. **www.astho.org**

assuming company See *reinsurance* under *insurance*.

assumption of risk A legal defense to a lawsuit when the lawsuit is based on negligence. If a person knowingly and voluntarily exposes him- or herself to a risk of harm, he or she is said to "assume the risk," meaning that he or she has agreed to accept it. This may release the defendant from liability. This defense is not usually successful in malpractice suits, because courts do not consider that the patient has "consented" to malpractice, even though he or she may have consented to the treatment (surgery, for example).

ASTHO See *Association of State and Territorial Health Officials*.

Astler-Coller system A method of staging tumors. See *staging (tumors)*.

ASTM American Society for Testing and Materials. A scientific and technical organization, founded in 1898, for the development of standards on characteristics and performance of materials, products, systems, and services, and the promotion of related knowledge. It is the world's largest source of voluntary consensus standards. It originally concerned itself with industrial materials, but its scope has broadened to include, for example, medical devices and services, standardized investigation of sexual assault, ambulance driving standards, civilian search and rescue operations, and the electronic health record (EHR). See *ASTM E31 Committee on Health Informatics*. **www.astm.org**

ASTM E31 Committee on Health Informatics The technical committee of ASTM that develops standards related to the architecture, content, storage, security, confidentiality, functionality, and communication of information used within health care and healthcare decision making, including patient-specific information and knowledge. Established in 1970, by 2007 E31 had approximately 300 members, including clinicians, provider institutions, administrators, patient advocates, vendors, and others from throughout the healthcare industry Approved standards are published annually in the *Annual Book of ASTM Standards*, Volume 14.01.

asymmetry of information See *knowledge asymmetry*.

asynchronous At different times; the opposite of simultaneously.

ATC Alcoholism treatment center. Also, ATC designates a *Certified Athletic Trainer*; see under *athletic trainer*.

ATGC See *genetic code*.

athletic trainer A health professional who specializes in the prevention, treatment, and rehabilitation of athletic injuries and illness. See also *personal trainer*.

Certified Athletic Trainer (ATC) An athletic trainer who has met the requirements of the Board of Certification (BOC) (formerly associated with the National Athletic Trainers' Association (NATA)). **www.bocatc.org**

ATI See *Advanced Technology Institute*.

ATLS See *advanced trauma life support* under *life support*.

atmosphere absolute (ATA) See *hyperbaric*.

atom The smallest particle of an element that can enter into a chemical combination. The term "atom" was used in this sense before it was known that an atom consisted of a nucleus and electrons, and before it was known that for most elements the atoms did not all have the same mass (weight).

A simplified picture describes an atom as a nucleus containing a number of protons (Z) and neutrons (N), surrounded by the number of electrons (E) equal to the number of protons. Protons are particles that have mass *and* electrical charge; neutrons have mass but *no* electrical charge. The symbol Z indicates the number of protons in the nucleus, and the symbol N indicates the number of neutrons. Thus, $N + Z = A$, the mass number of the atom. Z also represents the atomic number of the element.

For example, carbon (C) has atomic number 6, meaning that it has six protons in its nucleus, that is, $Z = 6$. If a given atom of carbon also has six neutrons, its mass number is 12 (6 + 6), and modern notation would label it as

$$^{12}_{6}C$$

The small mass differences among atoms occur when their nuclei have different numbers of neutrons. For example, another carbon atom could have eight neutrons, and thus would have an atomic mass of 14 (6 + 8) and would be shown as $^{14}_{6}C$. This atom is sometimes referred to as carbon-14. These two carbon atoms are called isotopes of carbon because they have the same number of protons (thus both are carbon) and differ only in the numbers of neutrons and mass numbers. The chemical properties of these carbon atoms are the same; the small mass differences among them do not affect the way they enter into chemical combination.

In nuclear science, the important particle is the nucleus; thus a new word, "nuclide," was coined to indicate a nucleus with a specific mass. This term allows one to describe the different atoms of carbon that have different atomic masses. See *nuclide* for more information.

atomic notation See *nuclide*.

atomic number See under *nuclide*.

ATR See *Registered Art Therapist* under *art therapist*.

ATR-BC See *Board Certified Registered Art Therapist* under *art therapist*.

ATSDR See *National Center for Environmental Health/Agency for Toxic Substances and Disease Registry (NCEH-ATSDR)* under *Centers for Disease Control and Prevention*.

audiologist A professional who examines, evaluates, and provides treatment for persons with hearing loss. Some states require licensure.

Certificate of Clinical Competence in Audiology (CCC-A) A credential granted to audiologists who meet the requirements of the American Speech-Language-Hearing Association (ASHA). **www.asha.org**

audiology The science of hearing. The practice of audiology involves examination, diagnosis, evaluation, and therapy for persons with hearing defects.

audiometrician A person who administers hearing tests.

audit A systematic review. When used alone, the term usually means a fiscal audit, in which the organization's financial statement, and the degree to which the statement reflects the actual affairs of the organization, is examined. An audit also includes a review of the procedures used to keep records, prevent losses of funds and equipment, and the like. An audit may be an internal audit or an external audit. When the term is used without a modifier, "audit" refers to an external audit by a public accountant (PA).

An audit may also be made of the organization's compliance with its own policies and with grant and contract duties, of its management efficiency, or of its quality management.

clinical audit (patient care) The term used in Great Britain for the *patient care audit*. It is aimed at improving care and outcomes. It is used by the National Health Service (NHS).

clinical audit (reimbursement) A review of the patient's medical record to see that all Medicare, HIPAA, and other requirements for reimbursement are met. Includes evaluation of medical necessity, admission, length of stay, procedures, readmission, transfers, DRG verification, eligibility, payment coverage, coding, billing, etc., according to relevant rules and regulations. Also called clinical chart audit. See also *clinical auditor*.

clinical chart audit See *clinical audit (reimbursement)*.

external audit An audit carried out by an independent auditor. "Independent" means that the auditor is not an employee of the audited organization, and does not have certain other forbidden connections with the organization.

fiscal audit An audit of the financial (fiscal) affairs of the institution. The fiscal audit has been developed over many years by the accounting profession, and standards for its conduct are well established.

internal audit An administrative process carried out in organizations, by the organization's own employees, in an effort to determine the extent to which the organization's internal operations conform with its own intended procedures and practices. When a similar review is done by an outside group, it is called an external audit.

patient care audit (PCA) The preferred term for the process also called "medical audit" or "medical care evaluation study." A patient care audit is a retrospective review of the quality of care of a group of patients, ordinarily a group with the same diagnosis or therapy. The review is based on medical records, and matches the care against standards of care. "Patient care audit" is the preferred term because it indicates that the focus of the study is the care received by the group of patients, rather than the performance of physicians, nurses, or other caregivers.

quality management audit An audit of the quality management of an institution, similar in intent and conduct to a fiscal audit, but addressed at the quality function rather than the fiscal function.

audit log In the context of the electronic health record, a list of individuals (users) who have accessed the record, and also typically the date and time of the access. Increasingly there is a demand for accountability in the handling of healthcare information, especially when it is *protected health information (PHI).*

audit trail A means of accessing original data in order to verify statistics or other information. In an acceptable data system, the audit trail is an integral part of the data flow, providing a step-by-step record by which aggregated data can be verified by a straightforward process. The trail must be sufficiently detailed so that one can go back to the original data and reconstruct any figure in a financial statement or statistical tabulation, for example.

The audit trail principle, although well recognized, is not presently part of our national health information system. We lack an audit trail for medical diagnoses, which are aggregated directly into categories (using a process known as category coding). A proper audit trail would require retention of the individual diagnoses that go into the categories; instead they are, at best, kept only in narrative form in the original medical records. The effort necessary to get back to the detail in these circumstances is prohibitive, and the audit trail principle is violated. Thus our statistics on incidence of disease, and other statistics, cannot be verified or broken down by exact diagnosis.

In addition, the *Privacy Rule* now requires that there be an "audit trail" by which every step in the "movement" of a medical record is imprinted with an identifier of each person who handled the record and stating for what purpose. This usage is somewhat similar to the legal "chain of custody" demanded for identification of documents or other items to be introduced as evidence in a trial. This can readily be accomplished with electronic health record (EHR) systems, which should be designed so that every time the record is accessed there is a date and time stamp that carries the identity of the individual making or seeking access. The system could also require a statement of the purpose before access is permitted. See also *audit log.*

authentication Providing evidence that can be used to prove (in the legal sense) the source, authorship, or ownership of a written or electronic record. Forms of authentication include, for example, a written signature, initials, a symbol, and an electronic signature. The Joint Commission on Accreditation of Healthcare Organizations (JCAHO) permits authentication of a medical record entry by the use of a rubber-stamp signature if certain requirements are met as to possession and use of the stamp. As the medical record moves increasingly into the electronic world, specific legislation such as HIPAA also addresses authentication issues.

Authentication also means providing evidence to prove that you are who you say you are. In this context, forms of authentication include picture IDs, fingerprints, digital certificates, passwords, voiceprints, and retinal scans.

auto-authentication A method for permitting a physician to "sign" a document (usually dictation) after it has been prepared by computer by recording his approval on a list of the documents. Presumably this method is acceptable if the physician has the opportunity and ability to verify the accuracy of the documents.

patient authentication See *National Patient Identifier*.

autograft An organ or tissue transplanted (grafted) from one location to another in the same individual.

autologous Related to the self. The term is found most frequently in autologous blood transfusion, a transfusion using the person's own blood, which was stored in advance for that purpose. Often such blood is stored in the frozen state in an autologous frozen blood program.

autologous blood transfusion A transfusion of an individual using his or her own blood, which was drawn previously and stored for later use, typically in elective surgery. This procedure, although used for many years primarily to avoid transfusion reactions (an individual does not react against his or her own blood), is gaining adherents because of the threat of AIDS and other diseases that may be transmitted by transfusion.

autologous frozen blood program A program in which an individual may deposit one or more units of his or her own blood to be kept in the frozen state in a special blood bank under close supervision for his or her later use in case of elective surgery or emergency. Autologous frozen blood programs are gaining adherents because of the threat of transmission of AIDS, as well as other diseases, by transfusion.

automated external defibrillator (AED) See under *defibrillator*.

autonomy A principle of *ethics (moral)* which states that the individual has the right to self-determination; in health care, this means that he or she is free to make decisions concerning his or her life and health. See also *informed consent*.

autopsy A postmortem (after death) examination of a body. An autopsy is usually performed by an anatomical pathologist, a physician trained in this specialty. Although hospital or other policy may require that an anatomical pathologist perform autopsies, the law does not impose such a requirement; another physician or even a nonphysician may perform the examination, and it will still be called an autopsy.

Usually the consent of the deceased person's next of kin or legal representative is required for an autopsy. However, under certain circumstances prescribed by state law, an autopsy must be performed. These circumstances may include death by homicide (murder), death in an automobile accident, death under suspicious circumstances, unexpected death of a younger person, or a suspected sudden infant death syndrome (SIDS) death. Synonyms: necropsy, postmortem, PM.

epidemiologic autopsy The use of data from autopsies for epidemiologic studies. A method has been described for carrying out such studies by using only "surprise" findings, that is, evidence of disease other than that for which the patient was treated, and which the physician did not know the patient had. Suitable statistical adjustments are made so that the findings are deemed applicable to the general or a specific population.

hospital autopsy An autopsy performed on the body of a patient who dies in the hospital, or who has been a patient of the hospital. There seems to be no requirement as to how recent the hospitalization must have been in order for an autopsy to be called a "hospital autopsy." Hospitals compute autopsy rates using hospital autopsies as here defined as the numerator and "hospital deaths" (deaths in the hospital) as the denominator.

autosomal disease A genetic disease caused by a mutation on any chromosome other than a sex chromosome (X and Y). Either parent can pass it along.

autosome See under *chromosome*.

auxiliary Providing help. As a noun, it means an organization that provides help.

hospital auxiliary An organization whose membership is from the community, and whose purpose is to assist the hospital. Often called simply the auxiliary.

average A mathematical term that, unless otherwise stated, means the arithmetic mean. The average is the result of adding together two or more quantities, and then dividing the sum of the quantities by the number (count) of the quantities. For example, the average length of stay (ALOS) for four people, who stay in the hospital for periods of 1, 4, 5, and 8 days, is 4.5 days (1 + 4 + 5 + 8 = 18 divided by 4).

An average may be "weighted" or not. If it is not weighted (or, logically, weighted by the value of one), it is a "mean." If it is weighted by a factor other than one, it is referred to as a "weighted average." For example, one healthcare provider in a locale charges $25 for a brief office visit, while another provider in the same locale charges $30 for the same service. The simple, unweighted average (mean) of the fees is $27.50, calculated as follows: ($25 + $30) ÷ 2. Assuming, however, that the provider who charged $25 was much larger, and had five clinics where $25 was charged as opposed to the two clinics of the other provider, the "weighted average" would be only $26.43 ($25 × 5) + ($30 × 2) ÷ 7. The $25 fee is said to be weighted by a factor of five to reflect its greater significance, while the other is weighted by a factor of two. If a relatively equal number of patients visited each of the seven clinics in this locale, the average fee of $26.43 would more accurately reflect the amount being paid by residents of this locale for brief office visits.

See also *median*. Synonym: mean.

average adjusted per capita cost (AAPCC) A dollar amount arrived at by actuarial projection, which is meant to represent the average annual cost for a Medicare beneficiary in a particular geographic area. Prior to 1997, the AAPCC was the basis of the government's payment to health maintenance organizations (HMOs) and other risk-based providers for Medicare beneficiaries. CMS paid the HMO 95% of the AAPCC. If the Medicare beneficiaries were relatively healthy in a particular region, the 95% capitated payment resulted in the government paying more than if the same beneficiaries were enrolled in a fee-for-service plan. This payment method therefore had a built-in incentive for HMOs to attempt to enroll only the healthier Medicare beneficiaries (see *cherry picking*).

average daily census (ADC) See under *census*.

average length of stay (ALOS) A standard hospital statistic. A **length of stay (LOS)** is the number of days between a single patient's admission and discharge. The day of admission is counted as a day, while the day of discharge is not.

To determine the average length of stay (ALOS) for a group of patients, their total lengths of stay are added together, and that total is divided by the number of patients in the group. A hospital uses the ALOS statistic to evaluate care within the hospital, and for comparison with other hospitals.

The ALOS may be calculated not only for the entire hospital, but also for specific age groups or DRGs, for example. It may also be calculated in a more refined ("normalized") manner by making an adjustment for the case mix of the hospital. An ALOS that adjusts for the age distribution of the patients, for example, makes for fairer comparisons between hospitals than one without such an adjustment; adjusting for additional factors, such as the distribution of patients among DRGs, further improves the statistic for interhospital comparison purposes.

AVG See *ambulatory visit group*.

axis In classifications, an axis is a conceptual framework consisting of one of the universes of objects for which categories or pigeonholes are provided. A telephone book typically has two classifications, each with a different axis: in the white pages, the single axis is the name of the subscriber; in the yellow pages, the primary axis is the type of product or service provided, and the secondary axis is the name of the vendor. In a classification of medicine, there are a number of universes, such as body "systems," causes of the disorder, physiological disturbances, and anatomic sites. All parts of the body would "be found along" the *anatomic* axis; all causes of disease would be arranged in an *etiologic* axis.

One classification of diseases could have a single axis, such as the diseases themselves. Another classification of diseases could have a different single axis, such as the parts of the body affected. Another might have primary and secondary (or more) axes. For example, the primary axis could be anatomical and the secondary could be etiologic, in which case for each body site, the causes would be categorized. The *International Classification of Diseases* (see **ICD (classification)**) is described as a "variable multiaxial classification," because in its various parts, different axes are used; for example, infectious diseases are classified according to the organism that causes them, whereas injuries are classified by both the site of the injury and its nature, such as fracture or laceration.

ayurvedic medicine See under *medicine (system)*.

B

BAA See *business associate agreement*.

baby boomers Those born in the United States from 1946–1964, inclusive, during the post-World War II "baby boom."

Baby Doe case A legal case involving an infant born with Down's syndrome and with esophageal atresia, a condition that prevented him from eating normally but that was surgically correctable. His parents decided not to consent to the corrective surgery or to intravenous feeding. The hospital administration sought a court order to override the parents' decision. The court ruled that the parents had the right to withhold consent. Before an attempted appeal could be processed, the baby died. The case raised the public consciousness about the issues surrounding the withholding of treatment from seriously ill newborns, and legislatures acted to protect newborns from *medical neglect* (see under *neglect*). Among the resulting laws were the federal *Baby Doe regulations* and *Child Abuse Amendments*, and numerous state laws making medical neglect one form of child abuse and neglect. *Indiana ex rel. Infant Doe v. Monroe Cir. Ct.*, No. 482S140 (Ind. Sup. Ct. Apr. 16, 1982).

Baby Doe Law See *Child Abuse Amendments*.

Baby Doe regulations Regulations promulgated by the federal government in 1985 aimed at preventing the withholding of medically indicated treatment from a seriously ill infant ("Baby Doe") with a life-threatening condition, except under certain specific circumstances where treatment would be futile. These regulations were ruled invalid, but the federal *Child Abuse Amendments* of 1984 (also passed in response to Baby Doe) made such withholding of treatment a form of child neglect, and thus provided an avenue of legal recourse for health professionals or other interested persons who believe that medical decisions concerning seriously ill newborns are not being made appropriately.

baccalaureate program in nursing A nursing education program offered by a college or university that leads to a baccalaureate degree with a major in nursing. This degree provides eligibility for licensure as a registered nurse (RN).

Bachelor of Science in Nursing (BSN) The degree awarded by a college or university with a baccalaureate program in nursing.

bacteria One-celled microscopic organisms of a particular class (Schizomycetes). Some bacteria (pathogenic bacteria) are able to cause disease in animals. The singular is "bacterium."
  resistant bacteria Bacteria that are not susceptible to available antibacterial drugs. Some bacteria of this nature exist because no drugs or other antibacterial agents have yet been found to which they are susceptible. Others, which are causing a great deal of concern, are those that have developed resistance to drugs to which they were formerly susceptible. This is an increasing problem in the care of patients with infectious diseases, and some of the bacterial agents are **multiply resistant** (i.e., resistant to more than one drug). Tuberculosis is one disease that is reappearing in numbers because of this problem.

bactericide A class of antibiotics or chemicals that kills bacteria, in contrast with a bacteriostat, which only prevents the growth of bacteria.

bacteriologist A person who is specially trained in the study of bacteria.

bacteriology The study of bacteria.

bacteriostat A class of antibiotics or chemicals that prevents the growth of bacteria, in contrast with a bacteriocide, which kills bacteria.

balance billing See *balance billing* under *billing*.

Balanced Budget Act of 1997 (BBA) A 1997 federal law that made many changes to federal and state health programs. Some claim these changes constitute the most significant in health reform in over 30 years. Included was the creation of the $48 billion *State Children's Health*

Insurance Program (SCHIP), as well as reforms aimed at extending the life of the Medicare Trust Fund. This act also created the *Medicare+Choice* program and the provider-sponsored organization (PSO), as well as establishing the National Bipartisan Commission on the Future of Medicare.

Unfortunately the BBA reportedly cut some $30-plus billion more than the intended $72.7 billion cut in hospital spending. Political pressure from healthcare providers and others to increase benefits for Medicare beneficiaries in the years following this law's enactment resulted in the *Balanced Budget Refinement Act of 1999 (BBRA)* and the *Medicare, Medicaid and SCHIP Benefits Improvement and Protection Act of 2000 (BIPA)*. Pub. L. No. 105-33, 111 Stat. 251 (1997).

Balanced Budget Refinement Act of 1999 (BBRA) Effectively an extension of the *Balanced Budget Act of 1997 (BBA)*. Its formal title is "The Medicare, Medicaid, and SCHIP Balanced Budget Refinement Act of 1999, as Incorporated into P.L. 106-113." Before the BBRA, Medicare beneficiaries were required to pay 20% of the entire amount they were charged for an outpatient hospital service, with no limit. After the BBRA, and made effective as if included in the BBA, beneficiaries have to pay no more than the inpatient hospital deductible amount, or $776 in 1999. Other Medicare-related benefits were improved as well.

The Medicare benefits affected under this legislation were significantly increased by the Medicare, Medicaid and SCHIP Benefits Improvement and Protection Act of 2000 (BIPA) enacted the following year.

balance sheet One of the two standard components of a financial statement, on which are shown the assets (what is owned) and the liabilities (what is owed) by the organization (see *liability (financial)*). An organization is most unlikely to find the assets and the liabilities exactly equal, so a third category of entry makes the sheet "balance": a line entitled "profit" or "loss." When assets exceed liabilities, the line shows a profit; when liabilities exceed assets, the line shows a loss. Because most hospitals are nonprofit, a line called "profit" would be inappropriate (although even a hospital could not survive if, over time, it owed more than it owned). Thus, most nonprofit organizations long ago abandoned the term "profit" and in its place adopted a euphemism such as "fund balance." A profit, then, would be called a "positive fund balance"; a loss would be called a "negative fund balance."

The other standard component of a financial statement is the *income and expense statement*.

Baldrige National Quality Program A federal program established in 1987 to recognize U.S. organizations for their achievements in quality and performance and to raise awareness about the importance of quality and performance excellence as a competitive edge. Each year, the **Malcolm Baldrige National Quality Award** may be given in each of these categories: manufacturing, service, small business, education, and health care. Recipients must be judged to be outstanding in seven areas: leadership; strategic planning; customer and market focus; measurement, analysis, and knowledge management; human resource focus; process management; and results.

The award was named for Malcolm Baldrige, a key proponent of quality management, who served as Secretary of Commerce from 1981 until his death in a rodeo accident in July 1987. It is administered by the National Institute of Standards and Technology (NIST), assisted by the American Society for Quality (ASQ). **www.quality.nist.gov**

Balint group A group of physicians who gather to study cases to learn more about the psychology of the doctor-patient relationship. A leader who has been trained in this method facilitates the group. The technique grew out of the work of Michael and Enid Balint, British psychoanalysts. Michael published a book in 1957 entitled *The Doctor, His Patient and the Illness*. The Balint Society (**www.balint.co.uk**) was founded in Great Britain in 1969 to continue this work. There is an active society in the United States as well, the American Balint Society (ABS). **familymed.musc.edu/balint**

bandwidth A term coined in the 1930s to describe a range within a band of wavelengths (measured in Hertz, or simply Hz) of the radio frequency type. Its common usage today refers to the raw carrying capacity of a transmission medium, such as copper wires, fiber-optic cable, or satellite links. The greater the bandwidth, the more information can be transmitted per unit of time. Telephones that also transmit the live picture of the persons speaking require much greater bandwidth than those transmitting the voice alone.

The implication for health care is the limitation on what kinds of information may be shared remotely. Transmitting a detailed x-ray picture to a distant site likely requires significantly greater bandwidth than all the *text* in a patient's medical record, for instance. (See *cybercadaver* for an example of this concept.) The solution, of course, is to increase the transmission medium's bandwidth. A single fiber-optic cable, for example, can carry the same number of telephone conversations as 3,200 copper wires. Increasing bandwidth is usually more of a political and economic issue than a technical one, because implementation of the already existing technology lags behind its development.

bank See *health record bank*.

bar code A machine-readable coding system that uses a pattern of bars and empty spaces to convey a specific meaning. The system is commonly encountered in grocery stores and other retail establishments, where the bar code is read with a scanning device. The system usually calculates the bill, corrects the inventory of the item, and carries out other management and accounting functions.

Bar codes are being increasingly used in the hospital industry for such purposes as recording the receipt of materials and supplies purchased by the hospital, maintaining their inventory, and making charges for them. Other hospital applications include recording services (such as in the laboratory or emergency department), posting the charges to the patient bills and to the appropriate revenue and expense accounts, and inventory control. An example of bar coding can be found on the back cover of nearly any book, on which the book's ISBN number is displayed in both human-readable and machine-readable bar code formats.

The method with which data are encoded into the bars and spaces of the actual bar code is called its "symbology." There are many symbologies in use in different industries, each typically having at least one standard. Most people are familiar with the Universal Product Code (UPC) standard of the retail industry, because nearly every item sold these days is identified by this code. Also, nearly every item of mail now has a POSTNET bar code on it to help speed up delivery. Other standards include Code 39, Code 128, Interleaved 2 of 5, and EAN/5. See also *Health Industry Bar Code (HIBC)* and *identifier*.

Bar Code Medication Administration (BCMA) A system that electronically validates and documents medications for inpatients. Each patient has a wrist ID band with a bar code. Nurses use handheld scanners to check the patient's ID, then use notebook computers at the patient's bedside to access the BCMA system to validate that the medication about to be administered is the correct one, is the exact dose ordered, and is being given at the right time. The system also alerts clinicians to potential adverse drug interactions and allergic reactions. BCMA was developed by the Department of Veterans Affairs (VA). See *VistA*.

BARDA See *Biomedical Advanced Research and Development Authority*.

bare-bones health plan A no-frills health plan or healthcare insurance policy with limited coverage, large deductibles and copayments, and low policy limits. Designed to be affordable to small businesses.

bariatrics The branch of medicine dealing with obesity and related diseases.

barium enema An x-ray examination in which a radiopaque substance, namely a barium compound, is introduced into the bowel by enema, and in which a physician examines the bowel "in action" through a fluoroscope and also makes permanent records by taking x-ray films at appropriate times.

baromedical nursing A nurse specializing in the area of *hyperbaric medicine*.

Certified Hyperbaric Registered Nurse (CHRN) A registered nurse specializing in baromedical nursing who has met the certification requirements of the Baromedical Nurses Association Certification Board (BNACB). **hyperbaricnurses.org**

base (genetics) See *DNA*.

base (measure) A reference quantity or reference time, often a given year. For example, the data used in calculating a consumer price index (CPI) include base prices, which are prices found in the year chosen as the base.

base (rate) A statistical term referring to the "per" number in a given rate. A ratio or proportion is often expressed as a percentage (per 100), but it may also be expressed per 1,000, per 10,000, per 100,000, or even per million. These "per" numbers are called the "base." Thus a percentage is said to have 100 as the base. The base chosen is usually large enough to ensure that the rate will be expressed in whole numbers; the more rare the event, the larger the base used. For example, a death rate of 7 per 10,000 simply is easier to understand than a rate of 0.07%, although both actually give the same information.

base pair See under *DNA*.

base unit A procedure or service used in developing a *relative value scale (RVS)*.

base year Medicare costs A hospital's costs for the base year from which computations are made in the Medicare payment formula. The base year is, by definition, always several years behind the present, and its costs are those as determined according to the federal regulations for cost allocations.

basic nursing care See *intermediate care* under *nursing care*.

BASIS-32 A brief patient self-report survey used to assess psychiatric and behavioral health outcomes, widely used in both inpatient and outpatient settings. Developed in 1985 by Susan V. Eisen, PhD, at McLean Hospital, Belmont, Massachusetts. **www.basissurvey.org**

bassinet See *newborn bed* under *bed*.

bassinet count See *newborn bed count* under *bed count*.

battery A *tort* in which the wrongdoing is the physical touching of another person without that person's consent. The threat of such touching is called an assault. There does not have to be any physical harm for a battery to result in legal liability. Treating or performing surgery upon a patient without the patient's *informed consent*, or going beyond the scope of the patient's consent, is a battery.

Baumol's Disease A "law" of economics identified by William Baumol which states that because productivity in the labor-intensive service sector tends to lag behind manufacturing, costs in service-related businesses end up increasing over time. Health care, a "service industry," is controlled by this law. In manufacturing, productivity can be improved by technological advances and improved efficiency with resulting decreases in costs. Such productivity improvements are not possible in connection with services. There is a finite limit to how little time a physician can spend with a patient, perhaps 5 minutes—a maximum of 12 patients per hour. If payment for services is to keep up with payment in manufacturing, the pay per hour must inevitably increase. Many similar services, such as education, sanitation, and policing, have become too expensive for the private sector and have been taken over by the government.

Bayesian analysis A statistical method based on Bayes's theorem (a theorem in probability theory named for Thomas Bayes) used in clinical decision analysis and in the evaluation of diagnostic tests, disease progression, case control studies, and certain types of clinical trials. Also called Bayesian statistics.

Bayh-Dole Act See *technology transfer*.

BB See *Blood Banking Technologist* under *clinical laboratory technologist*.

BBA See *Balanced Budget Act of 1997*.

BBRA See *Balanced Budget Refinement Act of 1999*.

BC Blue Cross; see *Blue Cross (BC) and Blue Shield (BS)*.

BCA See *Board of Certification in Anesthesiology*.

BC/BS See *Blue Cross (BC) and Blue Shield (BS)*.

BCBSA See *Blue Cross and Blue Shield Association*.

BCC See *Board Certified Chaplain* under *chaplain*.

BCEM See *Board of Certification in Emergency Medicine*.

BCFP See *Board of Certification in Family Practice*.

BCGM See *Board of Certification in Geriatric Medicine*.

BCIM See *Board of Certification in Internal Medicine*.

BCMA See *Bar Code Medication Administration*.

BCNP See *Board Certified Nuclear Pharmacist* under *nuclear pharmacist*, under *pharmacist*.

BCNSP See *Board Certified Nutrition Support Pharmacist* under *nutrition support pharmacist*, under *pharmacist*.

BCO See *Board Certified Ocularist* under *ocularist*.

BCOP See *Board Certified Oncology Pharmacist* under *oncology pharmacist*, under *pharmacist*.

BCOS See *Board of Certification in Orthopedic Surgery*.

BCPP See *Board Certified Psychiatric Pharmacist* under *psychiatric pharmacist*, under *pharmacist*.

BCPS See *Board Certified Pharmacotherapy Specialist* under *pharmacotherapy specialist*, under *pharmacist*.

BCR See *Board of Certification in Radiology*.

BCS See *Board of Certification in Surgery*.

BCT See *Board Certified Trainer* under *drama therapist*.

BEC See *behavioral emergency committee*.

bed A bed for an inpatient in a hospital or other healthcare facility.

> **adult bed** A bed maintained for an adult patient (not for a child or a newborn). Sometimes a hospital's adult beds are subdivided into two categories:
>
> > **adult inpatient bed** A bed maintained for an adult patient who needs round-the-clock inpatient care.
> >
> > **adult outpatient bed** A bed maintained for an adult patient who does not require round-the-clock inpatient care.
>
> **bassinet** See *newborn bed*, below.
>
> **day bed** A bed maintained for use by partial hospitalization patients who need a bed during daytime periods. A bed used similarly during the night is called a night bed.
>
> **hospital bed** When used by itself—that is, without other modifiers—this term implies not only the bed itself, but also the routine accommodations for inpatients: board, lodging, and nursing and certain medical services.
>
> **incubator bed** A special bed (an incubator) maintained by a hospital for an infant who needs control of its environment: temperature, humidity, and breathing (such as supplementary oxygen). Such a bed also provides isolation for the infant. Incubators are used for premature infants and other infants with special problems, whether born in the hospital or elsewhere. Thus incubator beds are not part of the hospital's newborn bed (bassinet) count.
>
> **inpatient bed** A bed maintained by the hospital for inpatient use (see *patient*). When used alone, the term "inpatient bed" could mean a newborn, pediatric, or adult inpatient bed.
>
> **isolation bed** A bed maintained for a patient who requires isolation. For an infant, such isolation may be provided in an incubator bed. Isolation may be provided in a variety of regular beds by "setting up isolation" for beds when needed by the particular patients; techniques include using private rooms, instituting special nursing routines, using separate waste cans, and following other procedures appropriate to the case.
>
> **newborn bed** A bed (bassinet) maintained by a hospital for a child born in the hospital (a newborn admission). A newborn admission to a hospital, by definition, must have been born in that hospital; any other newborn infant is a pediatric patient, and occupies a pediatric bed.

night bed A bed maintained for use by partial hospitalization patients during the night. The counterpart, for day use, is a day bed.

observation bed A bed for patients with a length of stay (LOS) of less than 24 hours.

occupied bed A bed that has a patient assigned to it.

partial hospitalization bed A day bed or a night bed, used in partial hospitalization.

pediatric inpatient bed A bed maintained for a child, other than a newborn admission. (A newborn born in that hospital occupies a newborn bed.)

resident bed A bed for a resident, that is, for a patient who does not require nursing and other hospital care, but who does need custodial and personal care.

specialty bed Generally, a bed maintained by the hospital for patients receiving care within a specific medical or surgical specialty. For example, an "orthopaedic bed" would be a specialty bed normally held ready for patients requiring orthopaedic care.

swing bed A bed that the hospital may, according to changing needs, assign to different kinds of patients. For example, beds may swing between obstetrics and gynecology, or between general surgery and gynecological surgery. More commonly today, the term refers to beds that swing between acute care and long-term care. Often the swinging of beds must be approved by a regulatory agency, such as the state's hospital licensing authority.

temporary bed A bed set up for emergency use, that is, for use when the number of patients temporarily exceeds the number for which beds are regularly maintained.

bed capacity The number of patients a hospital can hold. A hospital may have different bed capacity figures depending on whether one refers to its constructed beds, its licensed beds, or its regularly maintained beds. Thus, a statement of capacity should always tell which is intended. It is possible, though, that bed capacity figures may all be the same for a given hospital at a given moment.

constructed beds The number of beds the hospital was built to accommodate.

licensed beds The number of beds the state licensing agency authorizes the hospital to operate on a regular basis.

regularly maintained beds The number of beds a hospital has set up for daily operation (in units of the hospital in use and staffed) on a regular basis. This number may change from time to time. It would ordinarily be a number smaller than the number of licensed beds or the number of constructed beds. The count is usually expressed in three segments: for adult inpatients, pediatric patients, and newborns. See *bed count*.

bed conversion The reassignment of beds by the hospital from one use to another, for example, the reassignment of beds from acute care to long-term care use. When such a conversion is done in both directions (when it is, depending on changing circumstances, reversible) the beds are usually called swing beds. In some states, certain types of conversion must be permanent and can be made only with permission of the state licensing authority.

bed count The number of beds a hospital maintains regularly for the use of inpatients.

adult inpatient bed count The number of adult inpatient beds (beds exclusive of newborn beds and pediatric inpatient beds) that a hospital maintains in regular use, or that are available for use at the time of the count.

bassinet count See *newborn bed count*, below; a bassinet is a bed for a newborn.

child inpatient bed count See *pediatric bed count*, below.

newborn bed count The number of newborn beds a hospital maintains regularly in use, or that are available at the time of the count. Synonym: bassinet count.

pediatric bed count The number of pediatric inpatient beds a hospital maintains regularly in use. Synonym: child inpatient bed count.

bed day A way to measure the utilization of hospital inpatient facilities.

available bed days The number of bed days that the hospital is set up to provide in a given time period. It is computed by multiplying the number of regularly maintained beds (see *bed capacity*) by the number of days in the time period. Available bed days are ordinarily expressed in three segments: available adult inpatient service days, available newborn bed days, and available pediatric (child) inpatient bed days. See also *bed* and *bed count*.

occupied bed day The period of time between the taking of the hospital census on two successive days (the census is taken at the same hour each day). In counting the length of stay (LOS) of a patient, "the day of admission is an occupied bed day, the day of discharge is not." Application of this rule gives one day of stay to a patient who is admitted and discharged during a single occupied bed day.

bed pan mutual A slang term for a physician-owned professional liability insurance company.

bed turnover rate See under *rate (ratio)*.

behavioral emergency committee (BEC) A hospital committee concerned with incidents involving patients' violent or assaultive behavior toward other patients, employees, visitors, or property.

behavioral genetics See under *genetics*.

behavioral health An umbrella term that includes mental health and substance abuse, and frequently is used to distinguish from "physical" health. Healthcare services provided for depression or alcoholism would be considered behavioral health care, whereas setting a broken leg would be physical health care. See also *parity*.

Behavioral Risk Factor Surveillance System (BRFSS) A state-based system of health surveys that generate information about health risk behaviors, clinical preventive practices, and healthcare access and use primarily related to chronic diseases and injury. It is administered by the Centers for Disease Control and Prevention (CDC), which makes available a standardized questionnaire. States use this to conduct monthly telephone surveys to determine the distribution of risk behaviors and health practices among noninstitutionalized adults. (States may also add their own questions.) The states forward the responses to the CDC, where the monthly data are aggregated for each state. The data are returned to the states, then published on the BRFSS web site. **www.cdc.gov/brfss**

Examples of questions (2007): Do you have any kind of healthcare coverage, including health insurance, prepaid plans such as HMOs, or government plans such as Medicare? Do you now smoke cigarettes every day, some days, or not at all? How often do you use seat belts when you drive or ride in a car? During the past month, other than your regular job, did you participate in any physical activities or exercises such as running, calisthenics, golf, gardening, or walking for exercise? During the past 30 days, how many times have you driven when you've had perhaps too much to drink?

behavior offset An overall percentage decrease in physician fees to be paid by Medicare during the period of transition to the resource-based relative value scale (RBRVS). The assumption was made by HCFA (now CMS) that physicians would attempt to adjust to the RBRVS (which will reduce physician fees for certain services) by increasing their volume of services (i.e., by changing their behavior). Thus the fee reduction to counter this and keep the total Medicare spending for physician services from increasing was termed by HCFA a "behavior offset." The process of adopting the RBRVS also had a "volume adjustment" aimed at the same goal, and a great deal of opposition developed in Congress as well as among physicians against the additional behavior offset.

behavior therapy A therapy designed to influence behavior by focusing on objective behavior rather than on psychological or other causes. The theory is that behavior and certain types of thinking are learned, and can thus be unlearned. Techniques include reinforcement, aversion therapy, conditioning, and biofeedback. Also called behavior modification, behavior management.

BEM therapy See *bioelectromagnetic therapy*.

benchmark Originally, a mark on a permanent object (such as a rock or wall) indicating elevation, such as the points of high and low tide. Benchmark now also means a location, such as a spot from which to measure (surveyor's benchmark). In computer usage, a benchmark is a standard set of processes carried out in order to obtain performance data for comparison among computers or software. These are all precise definitions—"terms of art."

An important use of the term today is in connection with **quality indicators** (see under **indicator**). "Benchmark" is used to label the reference point for each thing being monitored. This can be any of a number of kinds of references—a median, mean, maximum rate, consensus, past experience, and so forth. For example, one suggested clinical quality indicator is "in-hospital mortality following common elective procedures." The benchmark for this indicator is "state, regional, and peer group average."

In the quality indicator context, many use the term "benchmark" as if it were synonymous with "goal," but it is *not*. Obviously, achieving an average mortality rate would not be something to strive for. Rather, the hospital would want to be as far below the average as possible. (Besides, to achieve an average, every superoptimal performance would have to be offset by a suboptimal performance!)

The "goal"—more precisely, *target*—is a value judgment, something decided upon after the benchmark is chosen. Whoever is assessing performance must decide what result is expected or desired. For example, an indicator for obstetrics is the cesarean section rate, which has a benchmark of 15%, based on expert opinion, meaning that there is consensus among obstetricians that not more than 15% of deliveries should require cesarean section. The target is to keep the rate under 15%; if the rate is exceeded, this will trigger investigation into the cause.

benchmarking Comparing the performance of an institution or a physician with regard to a particular **indicator** against that of some other source of data representing "**best practice**." See **benchmark**.

bench-to-bedside See **translational research**.

beneficence A principle of **ethics (moral)** that requires people to act in the best interests of others. In health care, this means that the health professional must strive to do what's best for the patient, and avoid doing any harm. This principle sometimes is at odds with other ethical principles, such as that of **autonomy**, which empowers the patient to decide what is best for him- or herself. See also **patient empowerment** and **informed consent**.

beneficiary The person entitled to benefits from insurance or some other healthcare financing program, such as Medicare—the person "insured" as contrasted with the owner of the policy, for example.

benefit package The array or set of benefits (services covered) included in or provided by a given insurance "policy." The term is widely heard in the healthcare reform discussions; one does not hear it used in connection with automobile insurance, for example.

    basic benefit package A standard benefit package that contains the services that must be the *least* that can be provided to any insured individual. Such a package would be the "floor" under the health benefits given to any individual. States, insurance companies, employers, or others could offer or provide additional benefits at their discretion. Healthcare reform discussions assume the existence of such a package. Also called "core benefit package" or "benchmark benefit package."

    benchmark benefit package See **basic benefit package**, above.

    core benefit package See **basic benefit package**, above.

    defined benefit package See **standard benefit package**, below.

    Medicare benefit package The federal government defines a basic benefit package for Medicare beneficiaries at the federal level for those for whom it provides coverage; Medicare benefits are thus uniform throughout the country. Medicaid benefit packages, on the other hand, are determined by each state.

    standard benefit package A uniform (usually mandated) package of health insurance or health plan benefits. The purposes of standard benefit packages are to permit purchasers to compare among plans as to price and to prevent risk selection by the plans. For true plan comparison, there must also be standard definitions of benefits.

supplemental benefit package Any array or set of benefits to be added to the basic benefit package. Definition or standardization of the contents of the package is not implied in the term, except in the case of Medigap.

uniform benefit package See *standard benefit package*, above.

benefits The money, care, or other services to which an individual is entitled by virtue of insurance. In healthcare insurance, there are two basic kinds of benefits:

indemnity benefits Insurance benefits provided in cash to the beneficiary rather than in services. Indemnity benefits are usual with commercial insurance. Payment may go directly to the provider, or to reimburse the beneficiary.

service benefits Insurance benefits that are the healthcare services themselves, rather than money. Service benefits are traditional with Blue Cross and Blue Shield and Medicare. In fact, the unique nature of service benefits led to special legislation for the Blue Cross and Blue Shield plans when they were established, and the granting of their original nonprofit charters.

Benefit Security Card (BSC) See *Electronic Benefits Transfer*.

benign See *malignant*.

bereavement care Care that assists with the physical, emotional, spiritual, psychological, social, financial, and legal needs of the survivors of a person who has died.

best practice A popular term used to describe a ***benchmark*** against which to compare outcomes or performance. Someone or some body must decide what constitutes "best practice." The source is usually either clinical evidence from the literature or actual performance as observed under similar conditions. There also appears to be increasing usage of "best practice" as meaning "what is OK to do, and what is not OK" when healthcare providers are seeking guidance for compliance with legislative and administrative requirements. See also ***indicator***.

beta testing See under ***testing***.

BHIE Bi-directional Health Information Exchange. See ***Federal Health Information Exchange***.

BHPr See ***Bureau of Health Professions***.

bias A factor or factors that systematically influence the judgments of individuals or the results of investigations so that the judgment is not impartial or so that one outcome of the investigation is unfairly preferred over another.

b.i.d. Latin abbreviation for "bis in die," meaning "twice a day," as used in the prescription of medicines.

Bi-directional Health Information Exchange (BHIE) See ***Federal Health Information Exchange***.

bilateral modifier See ***modifier***.

bill A statement from the provider of the charges for services, drugs, appliances, use of facilities, and other items for a given patient's care, for example, for an emergency department admission or an inpatient episode of care.

billing Notifying patients or their third-party payers of the charges for services rendered, along with the amount due.

balance billing The practice of physicians to charge a patient the balance of charges when the patient's insurance (or other third-party payer) will not pay the entire charge. For example, when Medicare will pay the physician only 80% of her or his usual fee for a given service, the physician sometimes "balance bills" the patient, who then has to pay the balance. A provider who has agreed to accept assignment as payment in full cannot balance bill the patient. See also ***assignment of benefits*** and ***mandatory assignment***.

Federal legislation (OBRA) in 1989 limited the amount a physician could balance bill to 115% of Medicare's approved rates for nonparticipating physicians. About 90% of physicians are participating, and thus must accept the amount Medicare pays them, and Medicare pays them faster, and 5% more, than it pays nonparticipating physicians. Since October 1994, CMS has been required to monitor "excess billing" by nonparticipating physicians, and can now recover refunds or credits from physicians who bill excessive amounts.

combined billing A billing in which the hospital and physician services and their charges are not separately identified. Certain payers, such as Medicare, will not accept such billing.

separate billing Billing that clearly identifies hospital and physician services and charges (and thus permits their separation). This may be accomplished on a properly designed single bill, or through the use of two bills, one for the hospital and one for the physician.

BIM See *Board of Insurance Medicine*.

biobank A collection of specimens of biological material, such as tissue, and their associated data.

biochemical Relating to chemical elements or compounds (biochemicals) involved in living organisms.

biochemical assessment See under *nutrition assessment*.

biochemical genetics See under *genetics*.

biochemist A person expert in the study of the class of chemicals known as biochemicals (chemicals involved in living organisms). Synonyms: physiological chemist, clinical chemist.

biochemistry The chemistry of living organisms; see *chemistry*.

bioelectromagnetic therapy (BEM therapy) Treatment using electromagnetic fields. The theory is that electrical currents in the body produce magnetic fields outside the body, which can be influenced by external magnets, which may in turn produce physical responses.

bioengineer An engineer who specializes in biological applications of engineering principles.

bioethics The field of *ethics (moral)* applied to medicine and the health sciences.

biohazard A biological or chemical agent, an article, or a condition that may be harmful to humans or other living things. Biohazardous waste, for example, includes used hypodermic needles, bloody bandages, and other contaminated materials that may harbor infectious or other dangerous elements. Special precautions are required to make sure the biohazard cannot cause harm.

bioinformatics The National Institutes of Health (NIH) defines bioinformatics as "research, development, or application of computational tools and approaches for expanding the use of biological, medical, behavioral or health data, including those to acquire, store, organize, archive, analyze, or visualize such data." See also *computational biology*.

biological Pertaining to life and to living matter.

biologicals Medicine made from biological substances. These medicines include serums, vaccines, antigens, and antitoxins.

biological substance A substance produced by a living organism, as distinguished from a chemical substance, which is produced by chemistry. Both chemical and biological substances are used in diagnostic procedures and the treatment of disease.

biological therapy The therapeutic use of biological products. Examples include treatment of cancer with laetrile and shark cartilage, and treatment of autoimmune disorders with bee pollen.

biological waste See *hazardous waste*.

biology The science that studies life and living organisms.

Biomedical Advanced Research and Development Authority (BARDA) An agency within the Department of Health and Human Services (HHS) responsible for coordinating and promoting the development of *medical countermeasures (MCMs)*, as required by *Project Bioshield*. Some pharmaceutical companies are reluctant to develop MCMs (which may never be used) due to the high cost of their development (see *valley of death*) and possible liability for their use. BARDA provides a number of encouragements, including paying researchers and manufacturers for reaching certain milestones in the drug development process, such as getting the product to clinical trials. BARDA was created by the Pandemic and All-Hazards Preparedness Act (PAHPA) of 2006.

biomedical concept See the diagram at *natural language*.

biomedical engineer An engineer trained in biological applications of engineering, and who specializes in medical problems. See also *clinical engineer*.

biomedical engineering department The hospital department responsible for medical instruments and equipment. The responsibility may involve testing of equipment being considered, recommendations regarding purchase, maintenance of equipment, training in its use, and, on occasion, the design and construction of equipment. The hospital's biomedical engineering staff is found in this department. Also called clinical engineering department.

biomedical instrumentation technologist (BMIT) A health professional who tests, maintains, and repairs medical equipment. Sometimes called biomedical equipment technician or biomedical engineering technician (BMET). See also *clinical engineer*.

    Certified Biomedical Equipment Technician (CBET) A BMIT who has passed a certification examination and met other requirements of the International Certification Commission for Clinical Engineering and Biomedical Technology (ICC). **www.aami.org**

    Certified Laboratory Equipment Specialist (CLES) A BMIT who has met the requirements of the International Certification Commission for Clinical Engineering and Biomedical Technology (ICC) (**www.aami.org**) for specialization in clinical laboratory equipment.

    Certified Radiology Equipment Specialist (CRES) A BMIT who has met the requirements of the International Certification Commission for Clinical Engineering and Biomedical Technology (ICC) (**www.aami.org**) for specialization in radiology equipment.

biometrics The application of mathematics and statistics to the study of life sciences. Also now used when discussing identifiable biological characteristics of an individual, such as fingerprints, face prints, voice patterns, and other features, in identification technology to provide security in computer systems.

bioprocess A process in which living cells or their components are used to produce a desired end product.

biopsy The surgical removal of a sample of body tissue for clinical analysis, typically to determine if the tissue is malignant or benign. See also *anatomic pathology* under *pathology*.

bioremediation The use of bacteria in the soil to consume contamination.

biosafety Measures taken to ensure that biological agents—for example, dangerous viruses or bacteria—do not cause harm to humans or other living things. This term is used in the context of the clinical laboratory, where specific standards and procedures have been developed to assure safety for those working in the lab, and to contain any biohazards from leaving the lab. The term is also used in relation to weapons of mass destruction and biological warfare.

Bioshield See *Project Bioshield*.

biosurgery The use of biological or biotechnological products or methods in surgery. The most notable example is the use of fly larvae (maggots) to debride wounds: they eat only dead or dying tissue (leaving healthy tissue intact), kill bacteria, and speed healing. Some say biosurgery is a euphemism for "maggot therapy" (MT) or "maggot debridement therapy" (MDT) (also larva therapy, biodebridement), but there are other types of biosurgery. For example, "leech therapy," also known as "hirudotherapy," involves the use of leeches to remove blood from blood-congested limbs.

biotechnology Development of products by a biological process. The process may use intact organisms, such as bacteria and yeasts, or use natural substances from organisms. The manipulations are generally at the molecular genetic level.

biotechnology product A class of therapeutic agents (see *agent (substance)*) produced by using *biotechnology*.

bioterrorism The deliberate release of viruses, bacteria, or other biological agents to cause illness or death in people, animals, or plants. These agents are typically found in nature, but it is possible that they could be altered to increase their ability to cause disease or spread into the environment, or to make them resistant to current medicines. See *agroterrorism* and *terrorism*, and also *zoonosis*, *vector (epidemiology)*, and *enteric disease*.

Bioterrorism Act (BTA) A federal law enacted in 2002 to help protect the United States from bioterrorism attacks. In addition to a number of provisions to enhance preparedness and responsiveness, the BTA imposed specific requirements to protect the food supply: All foreign and domestic food facilities that manufacture, process, pack, or hold food products must register with the Food and Drug Administration (FDA), and the FDA must be given prior notice for most food shipments entering or transiting the United States. The BTA also includes provisions to increase the safety of the drinking water supply and to enhance controls on certain dangerous biological agents and toxins. It also created the **Emergency System for Advance Registration of Volunteer Health Professionals (ESAR-VHP)**. The full name of the act is Public Health Security and Bioterrorism Preparedness and Response Act of 2002. Also called Public Health Security Act.

BIPA See *Medicare, Medicaid and SCHIP Benefits Improvement and Protection Act of 2000*.

Bipartisan Patient Protection Act of 2001 (BPPA) See *Patient's Bill of Rights*.

birth certificate The official record of a person's birth, signed by the attending physician (if the delivery was assisted by a physician) or other authorized person. A record form designated by the state, which specifies the items of information to be included, must be used. The birth certificate is filed with the registrar (vital records) for the local unit of government, who in turn files a copy with the state office of vital statistics.

birthing center See *childbirth center*.

birthing room A "homelike" hospital room that is both a labor room and delivery room. Usually the father is permitted to be present for the delivery. Synonym: birth room.

black box Something that cannot be examined inside to see how it works. It can only be observed from the outside—its behavior, or what happens when something goes into it and something comes out. Certain assumptions can be made or conclusions drawn about the character of the black box, even though reasons or causes remain unknown.

black box epidemiology See under *epidemiology*.

black box warning A warning in *PDR* (*Physicians' Desk Reference*) indicating that a drug has been found to have one or more serious adverse drug reactions (ADRs) (see **adverse drug event**). The warning gets its name because of its typographic presentation within a distinctive, black bordered box.

blacklisting Refusal by insurers to insure high-risk industries, professions, or individuals (especially those who might inherit diseases). If the blacklisting applies to high risks in a given geographical area, it is called "redlining" (this has been a civil rights issue). Refusal to insure a high-risk industry is also called "industry screening."

blended medicine See *complementary and alternative medicine*.

blind Unable to see. This term may be used to distinguish someone with no vision from someone with partial vision. However, to be "legally blind" means having visual acuity of less than 20/200 in the better eye with the best possible correction (perfect vision is 20/20) or having side vision narrowed to 20 degrees or less. Thus, someone who is legally blind may actually have partial vision, but being legally blind will entitle her or him to certain government benefits and services. See also **low vision** and **visually impaired**.

blindness and visual impairment professions See *low vision therapist*, *orientation and mobility specialist*, and *vision rehabilitation therapist*.

blind PPO See *silent PPO*.

blood bank A facility for provision of whole blood and its components for transfusion. Its functions include recruitment of donors for procurement of blood, drawing blood, processing (grouping and typing and testing for safety), storage, and distribution. A pathologist or other physician, or another qualified scientist, is ordinarily in charge of a blood bank. Blood banks may be characterized as of several types, depending on their auspices:

commercial blood bank A blood bank operated as a money-making enterprise. Donors are paid for blood and the blood is sold to hospitals. The profit goes to the owners of the blood bank. Sometimes called a proprietary blood bank.

community blood bank A nonprofit blood bank serving more than one hospital. Fees are charged to cover the costs of operation.

hospital blood bank A blood bank operated by a hospital for the benefit of its own patients. Fees are charged to cover the operating costs.

blood banking The entire process of obtaining, drawing, processing, storing, and distributing blood and its components. See also *blood processing*.

Blood Banking Technologist (BB) See under *clinical laboratory technologist*.

blood components The components ("ingredients") of human blood, for example, red cells, white cells, plasma, and the antihemophilic fraction. Blood components can be separated out by a process called "fractionation." When whole blood is not needed, each blood component can be administered by itself, with greater benefit and safety to the patient than whole blood. Furthermore, each unit of whole blood "goes farther" (can be used to treat more patients) when it is distributed as blood components. See also *leukoreduction*.

blood distribution The issuance, sale, or exchange of blood (both whole blood and blood components) by a blood bank.

bloodless medicine and surgery An increasing number of medical and surgical proce-dures in which techniques are being developed to decrease or eliminate the use of blood transfusions. Technology used to assist in this process includes the use of certain drugs, laser surgery, detailed surgical technique, autotransfusion, hyperbaric chambers, use of blood expanders, and recirculation of the patient's own blood. A major stimulus for developing the techniques is the religious doctrine of Jehovah's Witnesses, which prohibits transfusion, even from a blood relative, and even when death without transfusion is deemed inevitable.

blood processing The testing steps taken to determine the group and type of blood available for transfusion, and its safety, and to prepare it for distribution and use, both as whole blood and as blood components. See also *leukoreduction*.

blood replacement deposit A charge levied against the recipient of blood. It is called a deposit because the intent is to encourage the replenishment of the blood supply of the blood bank rather than to obtain money. If the blood is replaced, the deposit is returned.

blood repository A facility that carries out the storage and distribution functions for a blood bank.

BLS See *basic life support* under *life support*.

Blue Cross (BC) and Blue Shield (BS) The original prepayment health plans, first established in 1929. Blue Cross (BC) was developed and sponsored by hospitals, and was originally restricted to furnishing hospital care (to Texas teachers). Blue Shield (BS) was developed by and sponsored by physicians, and was originally restricted to furnishing physician care (to lumber and mine workers in the Pacific Northwest). In 2007, there were 38 independent companies (most have combined Blue Cross and Blue Shield) in the United States, which collectively covered one in three Americans. Although the plans are similar in principle, each one is autonomous; there are differences in policies, benefit structure, and administration from plan to plan. Sometimes called the "Blue Plans" or "Blue System," or simply the "Blues." Most plans have combined the names and omitted any "and" or slash—for example, Blue-Cross BlueShield of Minnesota.

Blue Cross and Blue Shield Association (BCBSA) The national association of Blue Cross and Blue Shield plans. The original stimulus for the national association was to facilitate the plans entering into "national" contracts—for example, with large corporations having plants or offices in the territories of several independent BC and BS plans. **www.bcbs.com**

Blue Shield (BS) See *Blue Cross (BC) and Blue Shield (BS)*.

Bluetooth The codename for a world-wide technology specification (standard) for small form factor, low-cost, short-range radio (wireless) links between mobile PCs, mobile phones, and other portable devices. The Bluetooth Special Interest Group (SIG) (**www.bluetooth.com**) consists of leaders in the telecommunications and computing industries that are cooperating in a voluntary effort to encourage development of this technology, which helps to overcome the dependence of networked computers and other devices on being connected by wires (cables). It also makes it easier for caregivers in a clinical setting to access current information about their patients, especially in the context of the electronic health record (EHR). Security measures, in the form of encryption (see *cryptography*) and authentication, are designed into the specification.

BMD Bone mineral density.

BMI See *body mass index*.

BMIT See *biomedical instrumentation technologist*.

BNDD Bureau of Narcotics and Dangerous Drugs. See *Drug Enforcement Administration*.

BNDD number Bureau of Narcotics and Dangerous Drugs number. See *DEA number*.

board (credentialing) A licensing or other qualifying or credential awarding body. See also *boards*.

    specialty board A nongovernmental, voluntary body that certifies a health professional as a specialist when that person has met the specialty board's requirements (see *certification (credential)*). Examples of specialty boards in medicine are the American Board of Internal Medicine (ABIM) and the American Board of Surgery (ABS). When the term "specialty boards" (plural) is used, it refers to the examinations. See also *specialty*.

    state medical board The agency in a state that is authorized by that state's legislature to license physicians to practice within the state, and to oversee the practice of medicine by those physicians. In particular, the state medical board reviews the credentials of physicians applying for licensure to practice within the state, administers examinations if required, investigates the background of applicants, and approves or denies licensure.

    When the term "state (medical) boards" (plural) is used, it refers to the examinations given by the agency. See *state boards* under *boards*. Synonyms: state licensing board, state board, state board of medical examiners.

board (governing) A common term for the hospital's governing body, the body that is legally responsible for the hospital's policies, organization, management, and quality of care. "Board" is short for "board of trustees," "board of directors," or "board of governors." It is discussed further under *governing body*.

board admissible See *board eligible*.

board certified The credential granted to a physician, nurse, or other health professional who has passed an examination by a specialty board (see *board (credentialing)*) and has been certified by that board as a specialist in the subject of expertise of the board. See *specialty*.

board eligible The term applied to a physician (or other health professional) who has met or can meet the requirements of a specialty board (see *board (credentialing)*) for eligibility to take the examination required to become board certified. Due to abuse of this term in the past, most specialty boards now use the terms "board admissible" or "board qualified" in place of board eligible.

boarder A person, other than a patient, physician, or employee, who is temporarily residing in a hospital or other healthcare facility. A patient's parent or spouse staying in the hospital would be a boarder.

board in residence A term used to indicate the role of the executive committee and the chief executive officer (CEO) of an organization. When the full board (governing body) is not in session, but its executive committee is, the executive committee is "in residence" and has the authority of the full board in most matters. When the executive committee is not in session, the CEO has the authority of the full board in most matters (unless forbidden by specific board action), especially in response to emergencies.

Board of Certification in Anesthesiology (BCA) A medical specialty board that grants a certificate in anesthesiology. An affiliate of the American Board of Physician Specialties (ABPS).

Board of Certification in Emergency Medicine (BCEM) A medical specialty board that grants a certificate in emergency medicine. An affiliate of the American Board of Physician Specialties (ABPS).

Board of Certification in Family Practice (BCFP) A medical specialty board that grants a certificate in family practice. An affiliate of the American Board of Physician Specialties (ABPS).

Board of Certification in Geriatric Medicine (BCGM) A medical specialty board that grants a certificate in geriatrics. An affiliate of the American Board of Physician Specialties (ABPS).

Board of Certification in Internal Medicine (BCIM) A medical specialty board that grants certificates in internal medicine, dermatology, and psychiatry. An affiliate of the American Board of Physician Specialties (ABPS).

Board of Certification in Orthopedic Surgery (BCOS) A medical specialty board that grants a certificate in orthopedic surgery. An affiliate of the American Board of Physician Specialties (ABPS).

Board of Certification in Radiology (BCR) A medical specialty board that grants certificates in diagnostic radiology and radiation oncology. An affiliate of the American Board of Physician Specialties (ABPS).

Board of Certification in Surgery (BCS) A medical specialty board that grants certificates in surgery, obstetrics and gynecology, ophthalmology, and plastic and reconstructive surgery. An affiliate of the American Board of Physician Specialties (ABPS).

board of directors See *governing body*.

Board of Insurance Medicine (BIM) A medical specialty board that grants certification in insurance medicine. **www.aaimedicine.org**

board of medical examiners See *state medical board* under *board (credentialing)*.

board of trustees See *governing body*.

board qualified See *board eligible*.

boards A term commonly used to describe examinations given by a board (credentialing) to a physician (or medical student) or other health professional.

   national boards Examinations given by the National Board of Medical Examiners (NBME). These are similar to state board examinations in scope and provide "portable" evidence (evidence acceptable in various states), which some states accept in lieu of their own state boards for awarding medical licensure. Part of the National Board examination can be taken by undergraduate medical students.

   specialty boards A short term for "specialty board examinations," examinations given by a voluntary specialty board to eligible health professionals who wish to become board certified. The term "specialty board" (singular) refers to the certifying body.

   state boards Examinations given by a state medical board (of medicine or nursing, for example) to applicants who wish to be licensed to practice a profession or occupation. State boards must be passed by a graduate physician in order for that physician to become licensed to practice medicine in the examining state unless that state (1) accepts national boards in lieu of state boards or (2) grants licensing by reciprocity with another state in which the applicant is already licensed. Similarly, state boards are involved in the licensing of dentists, nurses, and those wishing to practice certain other professions and occupations.

Boards of Certification (BOCs) See *American Board of Physician Specialties*.

BOCO See *Orthotist, BOC-Certified* under *orthotist*.

BOCP See *Prosthetist, BOC-Certified* under *prosthetist*.

body mass index (BMI) A mathematical calculation of a person's weight in kilograms divided by his or her height in meters squared (kg/m^2). Although BMI does not measure body fat directly, it is considered a reliable indicator of body fat. According to the Centers for Disease Control and Prevention (CDC), a healthy BMI is in the range of 18.5 to 24.9. A value from 25 to 29.9 is considered overweight, while 30 and above is considered obese. The quickest way to find out your BMI is to use the online calculator at the National Heart, Lung and Blood Institute (NHLBI) (**www.nhlbisupport.com/bmi**). Or, use the following formula:

   1. Square your height in inches. For example, if you are 6'2" (74 inches):
      $74 \times 74 = 5,476$

2. Divide your weight in pounds by the answer from step 1. For example, if you weigh 170 pounds:
$$170 \div 5{,}476 = 0.031$$
3. Multiply the answer from step 2 by a conversion factor of 703:
$$0.031 \times 703 = 21.8$$

bodywork therapy Any of a number of therapeutic or relaxing techniques that involve physical or energetic manipulation of the human body to enhance the structure and function of the body, stimulate circulation, promote relaxation, reduce pain, and/or promote healing. See also *massage therapy*.

Asian bodywork therapy (ABT) Treatment of the body, mind, and spirit (including the electromagnetic or energetic field surrounding the body) by pressure and/or manipulation. There are a number of forms, including various types of shiatsu, acupressure, and massage therapy.

Diplomate in Asian Bodywork Therapy (Dipl. A.B.T.) A practitioner of Asian bodywork therapy who has met the requirements for eligibility and passed an examination of the National Certification Commission for Acupuncture and Oriental Medicine (NCCAOM). **www.nccaom.org**

boilerplate Standard language in a contract, often in small print. Boilerplate may be distinguished from language that has been written specifically for a certain contract, and that reflects the specific intentions of the unique parties involved. Boilerplate may not always be enforced, especially if it conflicts with the specific, expressed intentions of the parties.

The term "boilerplate" comes from the printing industry, and refers to a piece of metal, resembling a plate from a boiler, upon which text to be printed was cast or stamped. Some items, such as advertisements or syndicated columns, were supplied to newspapers already fixed on a plate, so that they could not be modified by the newspaper. Hence "boilerplate" referring to standard, rather than custom, language.

bond A certificate sold by a corporation or government entity to raise funds. It is basically a form of "IOU" upon which the corporation or government entity will pay interest to the bondholder for a given period of time, and pay the bondholder the amount borrowed (the principal amount) at the end of that time. Some bonds qualify as "tax-exempt," meaning that the bondholder does not have to pay taxes on the interest earned.

performance bond A bond that guarantees correct and timely performance (for example, construction of a facility) and that will pay money if the performance is not completed.

rapid amortization bond A bond with special provisions that permit the principal to be paid off without penalty (i.e., the bond may be retired) prior to its maturity date.

revenue bond A bond payable solely from the revenue generated from the operation of the project being financed, for which the bond was sold. In the case of hospital revenue bond financing, the bonds are typically payable from the gross receipts of the hospital. Such bonds may only be sold by municipalities (or by quasi-municipal organizations, such as hospitals, under special legislation).

tax-exempt bond A bond, the holder of which does not have to pay taxes on the interest she or he receives. Municipalities and, in some instances, nonprofit hospitals, are authorized to sell "tax-exempt" bonds.

bond indenture The contract between a bondholder and the institution (for example, a hospital) issuing the bond.

bone densitometrist This could refer to a physician who specializes in bone density and related diseases, or to any health professional trained in performing and reading the tests that measure bone density.

Registered Technologist—Bone Densitometry (RT(BD)) A *Registered Technologist (RT)* (see under *radiologic technologist*) with an added qualification in bone densitometry from the American Registry of Radiologic Technologists (ARRT). **www.arrt.org**

bone densitometry The science of measuring the mass of bone per unit of volume. This is especially important in the prevention, diagnosis, and treatment of osteoporosis (loss of bone mass).

Boren Amendment See the *Omnibus Budget Reconciliation Act of 1981*.

BOS See *Bureau of Osteopathic Specialists*.

botanical product Defined by the Food and Drug Administration (FDA) as a finished, labeled product that contains as ingredients plant material or its constituents. This includes, but is not limited to, whole plants or any parts of plants, algae, macroscopic fungi, etc., or combinations thereof, whether processed or unprocessed. The definitions of botanicals and plant materials do not include yeast, bacteria, or other microscopic organisms previously approved for drug use or accepted for food use in the United States, or homeopathic products that may be derived from botanical sources.

bottom-up planning See *strategic planning*.

bounty hunter See *recovery audit contractor*.

boutique medicine See *concierge physician practice*.

bovine spongiform encephalopathy (BSE) See *mad cow disease*.

BPHC See *Bureau of Primary Health Care*.

BPPA Bipartisan Patient Protection Act of 2001. See *Patient's Bill of Rights*.

brachytherapy Radiation treatment in which the source of radiation is placed close to the tissue to be treated. Radium therapy to the cervix of the uterus and the prostate are examples, as are new techniques for applying the radiation within the blood vessels of the heart following certain types of surgery in order to prevent restenosis (narrowing again) of the blood vessels that have been treated.

break-even analysis An analytical technique for studying the relation among fixed costs and variable costs (see *cost*), volume or level of activity (sales), and profits.

break-even chart A chart graphically presenting the results of a break-even analysis.

break-even point The volume of activity (for example, sales) where revenues and expenses are exactly equal, that is, the level of activity where there is neither a gain nor a loss from operations. Activity above the break-even point produces profits; activity below it results in losses.

breastfeeding nursing The area of nursing focusing on the special needs of breastfeeding mothers and their babies.

Breaux-Thomas Medicare Reform Proposal See *National Bipartisan Commission on the Future of Medicare*.

BRFSS See *Behavioral Risk Factor Surveillance System*.

bribe Any money or equivalent of money that is offered to induce some action. See also *Anti-kickback Statute* and *fraud and abuse*.

Bridges to Excellence (BTE) A nonprofit organization whose mission is to encourage "significant leaps" in healthcare quality by recognizing and rewarding healthcare providers who demonstrate that they deliver safe, timely, effective, efficient, and patient-centered care. The primary method is pay-for-performance. BTE began its program with three initiatives: Diabetes Care Link (DCL) and Cardiac Care Link (CCL), both of which reward patients as well as physicians for meeting goals, and Physician Office Link (POL), which rewards physician offices that implement specific processes to reduce errors and increase quality.

BTE is a multi-state, multi-employer coalition. Participants include groups affiliated with the National Business Coalition on Health, large employers, health plans, the National Committee for Quality Assurance, the American Board of Internal Medicine, and several quality improvement organizations. **www.bridgestoexcellence.org**

brown bag program A program to improve medication usage in which employees or plan members are encouraged to empty their medicine cabinets into brown bags and bring them to their pharmacist for review. Potential problems, including drug-interaction issues, can be identified and rectified. See *polypharmacy*.

BRS-CL See *Board Recognized Specialist in Child Language* under *speech-language pathologist*.

BRS-FD See *Board Recognized Specialist in Fluency Disorders* under *speech-language pathologist*.

BRS-S See *Board Recognized Specialist in Swallowing and Swallowing Disorders* under *speech-language pathologist*.

BS See Blue Cross and *Blue Shield*.

BSC Benefit Security Card. See *Electronic Benefits Transfer*.

BSE Bovine spongiform encephalopathy. See *mad cow disease*.

BSN See *Bachelor of Science in Nursing*.

BT See *bodywork therapy*.

BTE See *Bridges to Excellence*.

BTW By the way.

bubba Sometimes pronunciation of BBA. See *Balanced Budget Act of 1997*.

budget neutrality A term that came into use as part of the prospective payment system (PPS) to mean that the new payment system may not pay hospitals, in the aggregate, any more or less for Medicare patients than the hospitals would have been paid under the previous system. More generally, a budget may be said to be "neutral" if, in total, it is neither larger than nor smaller than the previous budget.

budget reconciliation A part of the legislative budgeting process that defines federal programs in such a manner that program costs are consistent with Congress's decision as to how much money is to be spent for the program in question.

building code A set of regulations that owners must meet in the construction, use, and maintenance of buildings. Building codes are promulgated and enforced by government agencies and are designed to ensure that buildings are durable and safe. See also *Life Safety Code*.

bundle A small, straightforward set of practices—generally three to five—that, when performed collectively and reliably, have been proven to improve patient outcomes. Each step is essential, and all must be done. Someone must be responsible—either an individual or a team—to carry out the practices. A bundle differs from a checklist in that the bundle is limited, all items are necessary and sufficient (not just nice to do), and all have been scientifically established. The key is to do the bundle every time, on every patient for whom it applies. The concept was developed by the Institute for Healthcare Improvement (IHI) as a structured way of improving the processes of care and patient outcomes.

An example is the "Ventilator Bundle." Ventilator-associated pneumonia (VAP) is a serious lung infection that can afflict patients on a ventilator. The Ventilator Bundle has four care steps: (1) raising the head of the patient's bed between 30 and 40 degrees, (2) giving the patient medication to prevent stomach ulcers, (3) preventing blood clots when the patient is inactive, and (4) seeing if the patient can breathe on his or her own without a ventilator.

bundling Grouping things together into a package. See also *global fee* and *unbundling*.

outpatient bundling A requirement of hospitals to "bundle" into the bill to Medicare all diagnostic procedures or tests that are provided to a registered outpatient related to a single encounter (outpatient visit), even if a service is not provided by the hospital (for example, a blood test performed by an independent laboratory). Sometimes called "rebundling," if the practice had formerly been to bill separately.

Bureau of Health Professions (BHPr) One of the key program areas of the Health Resources and Services Administration (HRSA) whose charge is to ensure access to quality healthcare professionals in all geographic areas and to all segments of society. **bhpr.hrsa.gov**

Bureau of Narcotics and Dangerous Drugs (BNDD) See *Drug Enforcement Administration*.

Bureau of Osteopathic Specialists (BOS) A branch of the American Osteopathic Association (AOA) that is charged with establishing and maintaining standards in the various medical specialties for osteopathic physicians. There are eighteen specialty boards under its umbrella, each of which is titled "American Osteopathic Board of (Specialty)." **www.do-online.org**

Bureau of Primary Health Care (BPHC) One of the key program areas of the Health Resources and Services Administration (HRSA) whose commitment is to ensure that underserved and vulnerable people get the health care they need. According to a recent census, about 15% of the population—over 43 million people—in the United States lacked access to primary health care. See also *Federally Qualified Health Center*. **bphc.hrsa.gov**

burn care unit A special unit of the hospital set up to give intensive care to burn patients. It is a specialized intensive care unit.

burn center A highly specialized facility in a tertiary care center, set up with specially trained physicians, nurses, and allied health professionals, and with special equipment, to care for severely burned individuals. Only a handful of burn centers are found in the United States, and the practice is to transfer severely burned patients to them. Burn centers have proven superior to less specialized units in saving the lives of burn patients and restoring them to optimal function.

business associate Under the *Privacy Rule*, a person to whom a *covered entity* discloses *protected health information (PHI)* so that the business associate can perform some service for the covered entity. This would include consultants, lawyers, third-party administrators, or even other covered entities. Employees of the covered entity are specifically excluded from the definition of a business associate for this purpose. Earlier regulations under *HIPAA* had used the term "business partner" in place of "business associate." See also *business associate agreement*. 45 C.F.R. § 160.103 (October 1, 2006).

business associate agreement (BAA) Under the *Privacy Rule*, any agreement made between a *covered entity* and a *business associate* (or other covered entity). To achieve HIPAA compliance, the parties to the agreement must specifically agree to safeguard the treatment of any *protected health information (PHI)* that they might exchange. Note that the use of the term "agreement" here is not limited to written contracts. 45 C.F.R. § 164.502 (October 1, 2006).

business judgment rule A legal doctrine that protects the officers and directors of a corporation from liability for mistakes in judgment. It provides that courts will not second guess the decisions of a corporate officer or director if those decisions are within their authority, have an arguably rational basis, and are made in good faith even if those decisions turn out to cause harm.

business partner See *business associate*.

business partner agreement See *business associate agreement*.

business record The information kept by a healthcare provider that relates to maintaining itself as a business, and generally distinguished from the medical record, although some information may exist in both. Although the definition of "business record" is not as strict as that of the "medical record," it is generally accepted that the business record includes books of account, canceled checks, payroll information, records of sales, and correspondence. Federal law does not define what a healthcare business record is, and very few state laws do either. However, many laws do exist that specify a retention period (the length of time a business record must be kept), and these periods vary greatly.

A healthcare provider generally maintains business records for at least three reasons: (1) to comply with legal requirements; (2) to allow it to accomplish its purpose, which includes getting paid for the services it provides; and (3) to protect itself in the event of litigation. For the purposes of evidence in litigation, a legal business record must be kept in the regular course of business, made at or near the time of the matter recorded, and made by the person within the business with knowledge of the facts, opinions, or events recorded. In this sense, a medical record can be a business record; see *legal medical record* under *medical record*.

Federal agencies that require healthcare providers to maintain business records include the Department of Labor (DOL), Equal Employment Opportunity Commission (EEOC), Occupational Safety and Health Administration (OSHA), Food and Drug Administration (FDA), and Department of Health and Human Services (HHS).

Business Roundtable An association of chief executive officers (CEOs) of leading U.S. corporations, formed in 1972 to advocate public policies that foster vigorous economic growth, a dynamic global economy, and a well-trained and productive U.S. workforce. It has a number of initiatives, including a task force on health policy. See also *Leapfrog Group*. **www.businessroundtable.org**

buy-in See *Medicaid buy-in*.

bylaws A document adopted by a corporation or association that governs its business conduct and the rights and duties of its members. Bylaws may also authorize the separate issuance of rules and regulations to govern specific activities. The process for changing the rules and regulations is less cumbersome than that for changing the bylaws themselves.

hospital bylaws The bylaws of the hospital corporation, which cover such matters as how directors will be elected to the board of directors (governing body), their terms, how often they will meet, and so forth.

medical staff bylaws The portion of the bylaws of the hospital pertaining to the rights and duties of physicians and others as members of the medical staff of the hospital. The medical staff bylaws cover medical staff governance, membership, privileges, discipline, and the like. Typically the bylaws are drafted and proposed by the medical staff, but they are approved and adopted by the hospital governing body, and their force stems from this governing body action. Serious consideration is being given to separating the traditional medical staff bylaws; the plan is to retain organizational matters within the medical staff bylaws, but to create a separate policy on credentials matters (appointment, reappointment, and privileges) so that the separate documents may be more easily amended, if necessary, and to minimize potential legal problems (such as antitrust allegations, which may charge that the medical staff has too much control over credentials decisions if the process is entirely within the medical staff bylaws).

C

C (initial) See *Chemistry Technologist* under *clinical laboratory technologist*.

c(3) See *501(c)(3)* under *501(c)(*)*.

c(4) See *501(c)(4)* under *501(c)(*)*.

c(6) See *501(c)(6)* under *501(c)(*)*.

CA See *certification authority* and *clinical alert*.

CAC See *computer-assisted coding*.

cafeteria plan Also referred to as a "flexible benefit plan," it allows participating employees to choose from a cafeteria-type menu of different healthcare coverage and provider options. If the cafeteria plan qualifies under Section 125 of the Internal Revenue Code (IRC), employees may also choose between nontaxable benefits and taxable cash. The advantages of one of these plans for employers is lower FICA (Federal Insurance Contributions Act) and FUTA (Federal Unemployment Tax Act) taxes. The advantages for employees are being allowed to pick and choose benefits, and to pay for the benefits with before-tax dollars. See also *Zero Balance Reimbursement Account*.

CAH Critical Access Hospital; see *Critical Access Hospital Program*.

CAHEA Committee on Allied Health Education and Accreditation. Now the *Commission on Accreditation of Allied Health Education Programs (CAAHEP)*.

CAHIIM See *Commission on Accreditation for Health Informatics and Information Management Education*.

CAHPS See *Consumer Assessment of Healthcare Providers and Systems*.

CAHPS Hospital Survey See *Hospital Consumer Assessment of Healthcare Providers and Systems*.

calcium entry blockers (CEBs) A class of drugs that block the entry of calcium to certain tissues.

California Public Employees' Retirement System (CalPERS) A California state agency first created in 1932 to provide retirement benefits for state employees that has since expanded to other public entities. In 1962, CalPERS was authorized to provide health coverage as well. In 2007 CalPERS had more than 1.5 million members, including active workers and retirees, their families and beneficiaries, and their employers. **www.calpers.ca.gov**

California Wellness Foundation, The (TCWF) An independent, private foundation created in 1992 by an endowment from Health Net, one of California's largest health maintenance organizations, when Health Net became for-profit (see *conversion foundation*). TCWF provides grants for health promotion, wellness education, and disease prevention. **www.tcwf.org**

call See *on call*.

call center nursing See *telephone nursing practice*.

CalPERS See *California Public Employees' Retirement System*.

CAM See *complementary and alternative medicine*.

CAMH See *Comprehensive Accreditation Manual for Hospitals*.

Canadian Council on Health Facilities Accreditation (CCHFA) The former name of the *Canadian Council on Health Services Accreditation (CCHSA)*.

Canadian Council on Health Services Accreditation (CCHSA) The Canadian counterpart to the Joint Commission on Accreditation of Healthcare Organizations (JCAHO) in the United States. It was formerly called the Canadian Council on Hospital Accreditation (CCHA) and later the Canadian Council on Health Facilities Accreditation (CCHFA). Both CCHSA and JCAHO are voluntary bodies concerned with the quality of hospitals and other healthcare facilities. Originally JCAH (JCAHO's former name) performed its functions for hospitals in both the United States and Canada, but in 1955 CCHA was formed for Canadian hospitals. **www.cchsa.ca**

Canadian Council on Hospital Accreditation (CCHA) A former name of the *Canadian Council on Health Services Accreditation (CCHSA)*.

Canadian Healthcare Association (CHA) The national association of hospitals and healthcare organizations in Canada, the counterpart of the American Hospital Association (AHA) in the United States. Formerly called the Canadian Hospital Association. **www.cha.ca**

Canadian Institute for Health Information (CIHI) A national, independent, nonprofit organization that tracks data and provides analysis and reports on Canada's health system and the health of Canadians. Information is supplied to CIHI by hospitals, regional health authorities, medical practitioners, governments, and other sources regarding healthcare services, health spending, health human resources, and population health. Also known as Institut canadien d'information sur la santé. **www.cihi.ca**

Canadian Medical Association (CMA) The national voluntary professional association of Canadian physicians. Founded in 1867, it advocates on behalf of its members and the public for high-quality health care, and provides leadership and guidance for physicians. CMA's members include more than 60,000 physicians, medical residents, and medical students. CMA includes twelve provincial and territorial divisions. It also participates in an accreditation process that assesses educational programs in fifteen health science professions to ensure that national standards are met. **www.cma.ca**

Canadian-style system This phrase is often used to describe a single-payer, nationalized or socialized healthcare system. Actually, Canada has a system consisting of national health insurance and twelve separate single-payer systems—the ten provinces plus two territories— each with a global budget (see *global budget*). Most physicians are self-employed and reimbursed under a negotiated fee schedule. Patients choose their own physicians. About half of the hospitals are government-owned; the rest are nonprofits that are reimbursed in lump sums. The provinces approve investments in facilities and technologies.

There are five key and indispensable principles of the Canadian system:

- Universality
- Comprehensiveness
- Accessibility
- Portability
- Public administration

Proponents of this plan contend that the absence of paperwork (compared with the United States) would save enough money to virtually eliminate the cost crisis, that physicians are free from interference in their decisions about patient care, that patients have freedom of choice, and that both physicians and patients like the system.

cancer A general term for any tumor (growth) that is malignant; that is, which is subject to unlimited growth and extension or dispersal within the body. See *oncology*.

Cancer Genome Atlas See *The Cancer Genome Atlas*.

cap A limit on the amount of money that may be spent for a given purpose. A global budget for health care for a community would be such a cap.

out-of-pocket cap A maximum amount that an individual will be required to pay for health care in the form of copayments or deductibles in a given time period.

CAPA See *Certified Ambulatory Perianesthesia Nurse* under *perianesthesia nursing*.

CAPC See *Clinical Audit Professional, Certified* under *clinical auditor*.

capital Usually, the long-term assets of the organization that are not bought and sold in the course of its operation. These assets are primarily fixed assets such as land, equipment, and buildings.

working capital The difference between current assets and current liabilities.

capital budgeting The process of planning expenditures on capital items, that is, assets whose useful life is expected to extend beyond one year: property, plant, and equipment.

capital cost See under *cost*.

capital expenditure An expenditure (chargeable to an asset account) made to acquire an asset that has an estimated life in excess of one year and is not intended for sale in the ordinary course of business. It is also known as a capital expense. Expenses for operation (including maintenance) of the asset are not capital expenditures, but operating expenses.

capital expenditure review (CER) See under *review*.

capital financing Obtaining funds for building or renovation, that is, for additions to capital, as opposed to the financing of operations. For the most part, operations are financed by fees for services rendered.

capital leverage See *financial leverage* under *leverage*.

capital pass-through Costs, such as depreciation and interest, that are "passed through." In other words, these costs are not included in the DRG prices, but are paid directly to the hospital in the prospective payment system (PPS).

capital rationing A situation where a constraint is placed on the total size of capital investment during a particular period.

capital structure The permanent long-term financing of an organization or institution represented by long-term debt, preferred stock, and net worth. Capital structure is distinguished from financial structure, which includes short-term debt plus all reserve accounts.

capitation Capitation is a flat periodic payment to a healthcare provider per person cared for—"per capita" (per head). The provider assumes the risk that the payment will cover the costs for whatever the patient needs. Careful actuarial study beforehand in determining the amount of the fee makes this far less of a gamble than might be thought. Capitation has probably the lowest administrative cost of any payment mechanism.

Managed care plans commonly utilize this method of payment. Opponents allege that capitation offers too great a temptation to skimp on care in order to enhance profits. Proponents respond that avoiding this problem is one reason to emphasize quality measurements and adequate supervision of the system.

Capitation may vary according to *who* is covered, what *services* are provided, the *amount* of the capitation payment, and the *allocation* of those funds to providers.

Who may be a geographic population, an enrolled (subscribed) population, or a subset of either. **Global capitation** covers an entire geographic population.

Services may be comprehensive or limited. **Full-risk capitation** provides all healthcare services, including outpatient care, hospitalization, preventive care, prescription drugs, and home care (and sometimes dental care, mental health services, and substance abuse treatment), to its enrolled population.

In traditional capitation, all covered individuals are capitated for the same *amount* (i.e., the physician or institution receives the same amount for every individual, regardless of age or initial medical condition). In **risk-adjusted capitation**, individuals with known highly expensive medical problems, who are predicted to cost more, are capitated at a higher amount than normal individuals. For example, a physician with a specialized practice involving diabetes and heart disease would see fewer patients and would receive a higher capitation than a physician with an average practice.

Age- and sex-specific capitation is sometimes used in primary care, with payments adjusted for the demographic distribution by age and sex of the practice. A different demand as to frequency and nature of care is placed on a pediatric practice as compared with one specializing in care of the elderly.

Capitation payments often need to be divided (*allocated*) among individual providers or groups. The payment itself is often called the **capitation pool**.

Contact capitation is a way to pay specialists according to the number of patients they are managing. A capitation rate is developed for the specialty for the insured population. When a primary care physician refers a patient to a specialist, the patient is credited to the specialist upon initial "contact" with that specialist. The specialist's pro rata share of the capitation pool is based upon the number of such contacts (during a specified period of time).

capitation pool See *capitation*.

captain of the ship doctrine A concept that says the physician is completely in charge of the care—his or her word is law and, conversely, everything that happens is the physician's responsibility. It has been used most often in the operating room, where it is important that decisions be made surely and swiftly, just as on a ship. It is sometimes used in legal cases to determine and/or assign liability. This doctrine is not nearly as strong as it once was. Generally today, each person is held accountable for his or her own actions, and may not be excused by the claim that he or she was "just following orders." See also *respondeat superior*.

captive insurance company An insurance company formed to underwrite (insure) the risks of its owner(s). Hospitals and other healthcare providers sometimes form or buy their own insurance companies, either alone or with other providers.

CAQ See *certificate of added qualification*.

carcinogen A substance that induces cancer.

cardiac Referring to the heart. Words developed with this adjective usually take the form "cardio-," for example, cardiology. See also *coronary*.

cardiac arrest The cessation of circulation with the disappearance of blood pressure. Cardiac arrest may be caused either by the heartbeat going from its normal rhythm to an abnormal, ineffective rhythm or by the heart stopping its beat altogether.

cardiac care unit (CCU) A specialized kind of intensive care unit with cardiac monitoring abilities for inpatients having, or suspected of having, acute cardiac (heart) conditions. Synonyms: coronary care unit, cardiac surveillance unit.

cardiac catheterization See *catheterization*.

cardiac massage See *closed-chest cardiac massage*.

cardiac rehabilitation nursing See *cardiac/vascular nursing*.

    Certified Cardiac Rehabilitation Nurse The former certification for a certified cardiac/vascular nurse.

cardiac rescue technician An emergency medical technician (EMT) with special training in the care of cardiac (heart) emergencies, and authorization from the appropriate authority (such as a state agency) to use the title and carry out the measures required. Synonym: cardiac technician.

cardiac surveillance unit See *cardiac care unit*.

cardiac technician See *cardiac rescue technician* and *cardiovascular technologist*.

cardiac/vascular nursing The nursing specialty that provides "comprehensive care to individuals diagnosed with cardiac/vascular disease as well as those identified at risk for cardiac/vascular events." Previously called cardiac rehabilitation nursing.

    Board Certified Cardiac/Vascular Nurse A registered nurse with a Bachelor of Science in Nursing (BSN) degree who is qualified in cardiac/vascular nursing and has passed an examination of the American Nurses Credentialing Center (ANCC) (**nursingworld.org/ancc**). The credential is RN,BC (Registered Nurse, Board Certified).

    Certified Cardiac/Vascular Nurse A registered nurse with an associate degree or diploma who is qualified in cardiac/vascular nursing and has passed an examination of the American Nurses Credentialing Center (ANCC) (**nursingworld.org/ancc**). The credential is RN,C (Registered Nurse, Certified).

cardiologist A physician specializing in diseases and disorders of the heart and circulatory system.

cardiology The study of diseases and disorders of the heart and the circulatory system.

cardiopulmonary resuscitation (CPR) The restoration of heart output and breathing after cardiac arrest (stopping of the heart) and stopping of breathing. The technique requires artificial respiration and *closed-chest cardiac massage*. More heroic measures to restore heart function and breathing are employed in hospitals and by trained and equipped emergency medical personnel. The American Heart Association offers training in CPR for both professionals and laypersons. Synonym: resuscitation. See also *life support*.

cardiovascular Pertaining to the heart (cardio) and circulatory system (vascular).

cardiovascular disease (CVD) Disease of the heart and blood vessels. In 2007, it was the leading cause of death and serious illness in the United States, its incidence having increased steadily throughout the 20th century. CVD is a primary focus for the National Heart, Lung and Blood Institute (NHLBI).

cardiovascular-interventional radiography The use of an iodinated contrast medium to help visualize the heart and blood vessels during a radiographic examination. The medium is injected into the circulatory system, and then radiation is used to view the movement of the medium through the system. This procedure is commonly called an angiogram or angiography.

> **Registered Technologist—Cardiac-Interventional Radiography (RT(CI))** A *Registered Technologist (RT)* (see under *radiologic technologist*) with advanced qualifications in cardiac radiography from the American Registry of Radiologic Technologists (ARRT). **www.arrt.org**

> **Registered Technologist—Cardiovascular-Interventional Radiography (RT(CV))** A *Registered Technologist (RT)* (see under *radiologic technologist*) with advanced qualifications in cardiovascular-interventional radiography (formerly technology) from the American Registry of Radiologic Technologists (ARRT). **www.arrt.org**

> **Registered Technologist—Vascular-Interventional Radiography (RT(VI))** A *Registered Technologist (RT)* (see under *radiologic technologist*) with advanced qualifications in vascular radiography from the American Registry of Radiologic Technologists (ARRT). **www.arrt.org**

cardiovascular technologist A health professional who performs invasive and/or noninvasive tests (cardiac catheterization, echocardiography, stress tests, etc.) at the request of a physician. See also *diagnostic medical sonographer*.

> **Certified Cardiographic Technician (CCT)** A cardiovascular technologist who specializes in electrocardiography, cardiac stress testing, and Holter monitors, and has met the requirements for certification of Cardiovascular Credentialing International (CCI). **www.cci-online.org**

> **Registered Cardiovascular Invasive Specialist (RCIS)** A cardiovascular technologist who has met the certification requirements in invasive/cardiac catheterization of Cardiovascular Credentialing International (CCI). **www.cci-online.org**

> **Registered Vascular Specialist (RVS)** A cardiovascular technologist who has met the certification requirements in vascular technology/vascular ultrasound of Cardiovascular Credentialing International (CCI) (**www.cci-online.org**). Formerly registered cardiovascular technologist (RCVT) with specialization in vascular.

cardioversion See *defibrillator*.

care The treatment, accommodations, and other services provided to a patient. Care is often described according to the needs of the patient; for example, neonatal care describes the care given newborns, and respiratory care describes the care provided for patients with respiratory (breathing) difficulties. Care may also be described according to its intensity (see *level of care*), urgency ("emergency care"), or the facility required ("rest home care"). See also *assisted living*, *home health care*, *long-term care*, *managed care*, and *nursing care*.

CARE Act See *Ryan White CARE (Comprehensive AIDS Resources Emergency Care) Act*.

care delivery organization (CDO) A provider of healthcare services, such as a hospital or physician's office. This term is sometimes used in the context of electronic health records (EHRs), with the CDO being the legal "owner" of the electronic medical record (EMR) (although the patient presumably still owns the information, as with paper medical records). The CDO is also spoken of as one component of the Nationwide Health Information Network (NHIN).

caregiver A term applied to any individual who provides care to another, from physician to friend.

care management The application of systems, science, incentives, and information to improve medical practice and help patients manage their medical conditions more effectively. The goal of care management is to improve patient health status and reduce the need for expensive medical services. Some use "care management" to incorporate utilization management, discharge planning, case management, disease management, population management, and wellness management. Sometimes used interchangeably with *case management* and *disease management*.

care manager A health professional specializing in *care management*. See also *case manager* and *gatekeeper (health care)*.

Care Manager, Certified (CMC) A credential for long-term care managers, offered by the National Academy of Certified Care Managers (NACCM). **www.naccm.net**

care plan See *nursing care plan*.

care plan oversight (CPO) The ongoing supervision by a physician of complex or multidisciplinary care modalities required by a patient. The term is used by CMS in the context of reimbursement under Medicare.

CARN See *Certified Addictions Registered Nurse* under *addictions nursing*.

CARN-AP See *Certified Addictions Registered Nurse—Advanced Practice* under *addictions nursing*.

carrier (disease) An individual who carries, and can transmit, a contagious disease without showing symptoms or signs of the disease.

carrier (genetics) An apparently unaffected individual who possesses a single copy of a recessive gene that is obscured by an alternative form of that gene.

carrier (insurance) An entity that carries the risk in an insurance contract or health plan. A carrier may be an insurance company, a prepayment plan, a managed care organization, or a government agency. The carrier may handle and pay claims of beneficiaries for services received, or provide those services directly, or both. Also called insurer.

   In the context of Medicare, a carrier previously was a private company that had contracted with CMS to process Medicare Part B claims. See *Medicare Administrative Contractor*.

carve-out Services not available in a basic health plan, but that may be purchased separately. See also *carving out* and *managed behavioral healthcare organization*.

carving out A practice by insurers of providing group coverage only to healthy individuals in a small business, while permitting sicker co-workers to purchase only expensive high risk pool coverage. Carving out is a method of avoiding adverse selection. The practice is questionable and sometimes illegal. See also *carve-out*.

CAS See *complex adaptive system*.

C(ASCP) See *Chemistry Technologist* under *clinical laboratory technologist*.

case (health care) A patient and his or her medical problem. Used alone, the term "patient" does not indicate whether the individual is ill or well. However, the term "case" denotes that the patient is ill, injured, or otherwise presents a problem to the healthcare provider. With a modifier or additional information, "case" describes the patient's problem, as, for example, a "case of influenza."

case (legal) A controversy that is contested in a court of law. In common usage, a legal "case" refers to the particular facts of the controversy and the legal theories, allegations, and defenses being applied to those facts.

   When a case concerns the interpretation to be given a particular statute (legislation), or another legal case in a lower court, the conclusions reached in the case are generally referred to as "case law." Over time, the entire collection of legal cases (referred to as case law generally), comprises a major source for the definitions of various legal rights and duties. See *common law*.

case abstract See *discharge abstract* under *abstract*.

case law See *case (legal)*.

case management The centralizing, in one person (the *case manager*), of the planning, arranging, and follow-up of care needed by an individual either for a single episode or for ongoing care. Case management may involve wellness (following members of a health plan, for example), acute disease or injury (dealing with the patient's needs from onset through treatment and recovery or rehabilitation), or chronic disease or disability. See also *care management*.

case manager A health professional specializing in *case management*. The case manager is the patient's advocate, seeing that the patient gets everything he or she needs to get and/or stay healthy, with acceptable quality, in the most effective manner and appropriate setting, at the best price.

The case manager works as a resource, educator, and facilitator. The tasks include assessment of the patient (or client) to identify needs; creation of a care plan; arranging for medical, home-health, rehabilitation, and other services; making referrals to community programs or resources; working with the patient and family to make good decisions; and making sure that payment is obtained for the care. The goal is to assist the individual through the maze of the healthcare system, ensuring continuity of care, follow-up, and the best result possible.

The case manager is a clinician rather than a bureaucrat. Currently, about 90% are nurses; most of the others are social workers, rehabilitation counselors, psychologists, therapists, and MDs. Specialists are evolving in long-term care, workers' compensation, catastrophic head injuries, burn care, behavioral disorders, special needs, and so forth. There are now many types of certification available:

Case Management Administrator Certification (CMAC) A credential for administrators of case management programs, offered by the Center for Case Management (CCM). **cfcm.com**

Case Manager Certified (CMC) A credential for health professionals (physicians, nurses, executives, respiratory therapists, social workers, pharmacists, etc.) who qualify in case management, offered by the American Institute of Outcomes Care Management (AIOCM). **www.aiocm.com**

Certified Case Manager (CCM) A health professional specializing in case management who has met the requirements of the Commission for Case Manager Certification (CCMC). **www.ccmcertification.org**

Certified Nursing Case Manager A registered nurse with an associate degree or diploma, or a Bachelor of Science in Nursing or higher degree, who is qualified in case management and has passed an examination of the American Nurses Credentialing Center (ANCC) (**nursingworld.org/ancc**). The credential is RN,C (Registered Nurse, Certified).

Certified Occupational Health Nurse/Case Manager (COHN/CM) A *Certified Occupational Health Nurse* (see under *occupational health nursing*) who has passed an examination in case management given by the American Board for Occupational Health Nurses (ABOHN). **www.abohn.org**

Certified Occupational Health Nurse—Specialist/Case Manager (COHN-S/CM) A *Certified Occupational Health Nurse—Specialist* (see under *occupational health nursing*) who has passed an examination in case management given by the American Board for Occupational Health Nurses (ABOHN). **www.abohn.org**

Continuity of Care Certification, Advanced (A-CCC) A credential offered by the National Board for Certification in Continuity of Care (NBCCC). **nbccc.net**

case mix The mix of cases, defined by age, sex, diagnoses, treatments, severity of illness, and so on, handled by a practitioner or hospital. Case mix is defined by: (1) grouping patients (classification) according to these factors, and then (2) determining the proportion of the total falling into each group. At present, the most widely used classification for this purpose is the DRG system. Sometimes the term "case mix" is used, inaccurately, to mean the grouping system itself (DRG, for example).

In the Medicare prospective payment system (PPS), which sets a price for each DRG, the total revenue for the hospital for its Medicare patients depends on how many "items" it "sells," and of what kind, that is, the number of patients cared for and the DRG of each. The revenue, therefore, is dependent upon the hospital's case mix.

case mix complexity A phrase used to convey the idea that hospitals (and physicians) differ in the variety of patients they serve. A specialized hospital would have a less complex mix of patients than a general hospital. The complexity is sometimes described quantitatively by the use of a case mix index.

Case-Mix Group (CMG) See *inpatient rehabilitation facility prospective payment system* under *prospective payment system*.

case mix index (CMI) A term used in the prospective payment system (PPS) to indicate the "expected costliness," per patient, of treating a given hospital's mix of cases. CMI is scaled so that a hospital whose mix is like that in base data would have a CMI of 1.0. The base data for a CMI usually come from a broad sector of inpatients, often the Medicare patients, discharged from the nation's hospitals during a base year.

For calculating CMIs, a classification (scheme) of patients is used, in which each category (class) is assigned a "weight" that is proportional to the average cost of treating a patient in that class. These weights are calculated from the base data. A hospital's CMI for a given time period may be calculated as follows: (1) for each patient, identify his or her class and note the associated weight; (2) take the average of these weights.

case mix management information system (case mix MIS) See under *information system*.

case mix severity A term referring, as yet without a single definition, to the degree of illness of a given group of patients. For example, one hospital's (or one time-period's) group of diabetes patients (or a specific DRG) may be much more severely ill than another's. Various "severity of illness" index methods are under development to quantify this fact.

case mix system Usually, an information system in which clinical and financial data are merged, patient by patient, in such a manner that analyses can be made as to the profitability of a given type of patient (DRG category, for example), clinical department, physician, or other aspect of the hospital.

case shifting See *dumping*.

case summary A summary of the medical record of a patient, prepared by a physician, nurse, or other qualified individual, which condenses the essential elements of history, physical examination, other diagnostic findings, treatment, and recommendations. Although similar to a case abstract (see *discharge abstract* under *abstract*), a case summary (1) reflects the individual case rather than carrying predefined data elements, uniform for all patients; (2) is written out rather than coded, as is the case abstract; and (3) may also contain the summarizer's interpretations, rather than being required to transfer the data exactly as recorded.

CASP Certified Aging Services Professional; see *American Association of Homes and Services for the Aging*.

CAT Computed axial tomography. See *computed tomography*.

catalyst A substance that accelerates a chemical reaction but is not itself changed by the reaction. An enzyme is a specific kind of biological catalyst.

catalyst therapy See *tailored drug/catalyst therapy*.

catastrophic illness An illness that requires very costly treatment that is catastrophic to the patient's or family's finances. The illness may be either acute or chronic, and it may run its course quickly or over a protracted period.

catastrophic insurance See under *insurance*.

catchment area See *service area*.

category A pigeonhole ("class") of a *classification (scheme)*. For each category there is a definition and an explicit list of all the entities to be placed under (within) the category in question. The label of a category is called its rubric (although "rubric" sometimes is used interchangeably with "category"). For example, "pickup trucks" would be the rubric (label) for a category in a classification of motor vehicles. There would be a definition of what distinguishes a pickup truck from other vehicles, and a list of all the vehicles (for a given model year, for example) that were "officially" to be classified as pickup trucks. A category may be designed to contain only a single item (entity) and thus be a "single-entity category," or it may be designed to contain a variety of related entities.

combination category A category containing items from two or more universes. The resulting combination coding is an obsolete scheme for handling information that, in other contexts, has been replaced by the "relational database" (see *database management system*) approach, which puts the items together as needed. Examples of combination categories:

- Sex is one universe, age another. A system using combination categories might have categories for (1) male + age and (2) female + age. To find all persons age 20, one would have to look in both the male and female categories for that age.
- Disorders are one universe, anatomical sites another. Combination categories could be constructed for fractures, for example, as (1) fracture, right arm; (2) fracture, left arm; (3) fracture, right leg; (4) fracture, left leg; and so on. Another category, for "laceration," following the same scheme would have (1) laceration, right arm; (2) laceration, left arm; and so on for other types of injuries or ailments. To find all persons with anything wrong with the right arm, one would have to look in all the categories where the site has been combined with some sort of condition.

The coding process for combination categories is cumbersome, and the retrieval process complicated. And both coding and retrieval are exceptionally error prone.

single-diagnosis category A category in a classification of diagnoses, such as DRGs or ICD-9-CM, which contains only one diagnosis.

category coding See under *coding (process)*.

catheter A thin tube to be inserted into the body, via a natural opening or an incision into a blood vessel or other structure, for the purpose of putting something into the body or taking something out. For example, radiopaque drugs used in x-ray examinations may be introduced, or blood or urine may be removed by catheter.

catheterization Insertion of a tube into a body orifice or structure in order to put something in or take something out. Cardiac catheterization is the insertion of a tube into the heart, via a blood vessel, in order to permit chemical determinations on heart blood, or to introduce dyes or radioactive materials to be detected in diagnostic tests or imaging. More common catheterizations include insertion of a tube into a blood vessel to permit intravenous feeding, and insertion of a tube into the urinary tract to relieve an obstruction to the flow of urine or to obtain a clean specimen of urine.

cardiac catheterization The insertion of a tube (catheter) into the heart via an artery or vein for diagnostic purposes, for example, to measure the blood pressures in the heart, to take samples of blood for analysis, or to introduce radiopaque drugs (drugs that are visible by x-ray). Information can also be obtained by watching, via fluoroscope, the passage of the catheter as it is inserted.

Catholic Health Association of the United States (CHA) A national organization of Catholic healthcare sponsors, systems, facilities, and related organizations. In 2007, Catholic hospitals constituted the largest single group of the nation's nonprofit hospitals, over 12% of the nation's total community hospitals. There is a counterpart Canadian organization called the Catholic Health Association of Canada. Founded in 1915, CHA unites members to advance issues of interest to its members. Its mission includes advocating for a just healthcare system, convening leaders to share ideas and foster collaboration, and uniting the Catholic ministry issues critical to it. Formerly called the Catholic *Hospital* Association. **www.chausa.org**

CAT scanner See *CT scanner*.

cause The thing that effected the result. The law distinguishes intervening cause and proximate cause:

intervening cause Something that happens after an act of negligence and that causes the resulting injury. If the intervening cause is significant, it may relieve the person who was originally negligent of legal liability; in this case, it is usually called a "superceding" cause. May also be called intervening force or intervening act.

proximate cause A legal term describing the direct cause of an injury. The proximate cause is that which in a natural sequence, unbroken by intervening factors, produced the injury, and without which the injury would not have happened. A negligent person's liability is usually limited to those injuries proximately caused by the negligence.

cause of action Legal grounds upon which to base a lawsuit. A cause of action may be based upon breach of a contract, commission of a tort, violation of a statute, or violation of a constitutional right.

cause of death See under *death*.

CBC Center for Beneficiary Choices. See *CMS*.

CBE See *charting by exception*.

CBER See *Center for Biologics Evaluation and Research*.

CBET See *Certified Biomedical Equipment Technician* under *biomedical instrumentation technologist*.

CBO See *Congressional Budget Office*.

CBP Comprehensive benefit package. See *benefit package*.

CBPP See *commons-based peer production*.

CBRN Chemical, biological, radiological, nuclear. See *weapons of mass destruction*.

CBSPD Certification See under *sterile processing and distribution*.

CC *Complications* and *comorbidities* (see under *morbidity*). See also *Clinical Center* under *National Institutes of Health*.

CCA See *Certified Coding Associate* under *coding specialist*.

CCBH See *Connecting Communities for Better Health*.

CCC See *Certified Clinical Coder* (under *coding specialist*), *Clinical Care Classification*, and *Council on Clinical Classifications*. Also means certificate of clinical competence; see *audiologist* and *speech-language pathologist*.

CCC-A See *Certificate of Clinical Competence in Audiology* under *audiologist*.

CCCN See *Certified Continence Care Nurse* under *wound, ostomy, and continence nursing*.

CCC-SLP See *Certificate of Clinical Competence in Speech-Language Pathology* under *speech-language pathologist*.

CCE See *Certified Clinical Engineer* under *clinical engineer*.

CCEHIP See *Coordinating Center for Environmental Health and Injury Prevention* under *Centers for Disease Control and Prevention*.

CCHA See *Canadian Council on Hospital Accreditation*.

CCHFA See *Canadian Council on Health Facilities Accreditation*.

CCHIS See *Coordinating Center for Health Information Service* under *Centers for Disease Control and Prevention*.

CCHIT See *Certification Commission for Health Information Technology*.

CCHSA See *Canadian Council on Health Services Accreditation*.

CCHT See *Certified Clinical Hemodialysis Technician* under *hemodialysis technician*.

CCI Correct Coding Initiative. A system of edits made to the *CPT* codes, issued quarterly by CMS. The edits, developed under contract by AdminaStar Federal, Inc., a Medicare carrier in Indiana, are based on CPT code descriptors, CPT coding instructions and guidelines, local Medicare carrier and national edits, and Medicare billing history. Fiscal intermediaries use the CCI system when determining payments to physicians.

CCID See *Coordinating Center for Infectious Diseases* under *Centers for Disease Control and Prevention*.

CCLS See *Certified Child Life Specialist* under *child life specialist*.

CCM See *Certified Case Manager* (under *case manager*) and *Clinical Context Management Specification*.

CCMHC See *Certified Clinical Mental Health Counselor* under *mental health counselor*.

CCMM See *Certifying Commission in Medical Management*.

CCN See *Certified Clinical Nutritionist* (under *nutritionist*) and *community care network*.

CCNS See *Acute and Critical Care Clinical Nurse Specialist* under *critical care nursing*.

CCOA See *Corporate Certified Ophthalmic Assistant* under *ophthalmic medical assistant*.

CCOW See under *Clinical Context Management Specification (CCM)*.

CCP See *Certified Clinical Perfusionist* (under *perfusionist*).

CCR See *Continuity of Care Record* (under *data set*) and *cost-to-charge ratio* (under *ratio*).

CCRC See *continuing care retirement community*.

CCRN See *Critical Care Nurse* under *critical care nursing*.

CCS See *Cardiovascular and Pulmonary Certified Specialist* under *physical therapist*. See also *Certified Coding Specialist* under *coding specialist*.

CCS-P See *Certified Coding Specialist—Physician-based* under *coding specialist*.

CCT See *Certified Cardiographic Technician* under *cardiovascular technologist*.

CCU See *cardiac care unit*.

CD See *chemical dependency*.

CDA See *Certified Dental Assistant* under *dental assistant*, or the discussion of "Clinical Document Architecture" under *clinical document*.

CDAC See *Clinical Data Abstraction Center*.

CDC See *Centers for Disease Control and Prevention*. Also CERT Documentation Contractor; see *Comprehensive Error Rate Testing*.

CDDN See *Certified Developmental Disabilities Nurse* under *developmental disabilities nursing*.

CD(DONA) See *Certified Doula* under *doula*.

CDE See *Certified Diabetes Educator* (under *diabetes educator*) and *Certified Disability Examiner* (under *disability examiner*).

CDER See *Center for Drug Evaluation and Research*.

CDHA Consumer-driven health arrangement; see *consumer-driven health plan*.

CDHC Consumer-driven health care or consumer-directed health care; see *healthcare consumerism*.

CDHP See *consumer-driven health plan*.

CDIRT See *Classification of Death and Injury Resulting from Terrorism*.

CDISC See *Clinical Data Interchange Standards Consortium*.

CDM See *charge description master*.

CDMS See *Certified Disability Management Specialist* under *disability management*.

CDN See *Certified Dialysis Nurse* under *dialysis nursing*.

CDO See *care delivery organization*.

CDONA See *Certified Director of Nursing Administration* under *nursing administration*.

CDRH See *Center for Devices and Radiological Health*.

CDSS See *clinical decision support system* and *decision-support software*.

CDT See *Code on Dental Procedures and Nomenclature*. See also *Certified Dental Technician* under *dental laboratory technician*.

CE See *clinical engineer, continuing education*, and *covered entity*.

CEA See *Certified Ergonomics Associate* under *ergonomist*; also *cost-effectiveness analysis* under *cost-analysis*.

CEBs See *calcium entry blockers*.

CEBT See *Certified Eye Bank Technician* under *eye bank technician*.

CEC See *Committee on Energy and Commerce*.

ceding company See *reinsurance* under *insurance*.

CEFACT United Nations Centre for Facilitation of Procedures and Practices for Administration, Commerce and Transport. The Centre's mission is to improve the ability of business, trade, and administrative organizations—whether from developed, developing, or transitional economies—to exchange products and relevant services effectively and so contribute to the growth of global commerce. CEFACT works toward this through the simplification and harmonization of processes, procedures, and information flows. **www.unece.org/cefact**

cell A small plant or animal structure that forms the building block (the structural unit) of a tissue. A cell contains two components known as nuclear material and cytoplasmic material, and is enclosed by a membrane. In the human body, all cells fall into one of five general types according to the tissues they form: epithelial (surface and lining tissues), connective and supporting (bones and cartilages), muscle, nerve, and blood and lymph.

CEN (nursing) See *Certified Emergency Nurse* under *emergency nursing*.

CEN (organization) Comité Européen de Normalisation. In English, it's the European Committee for Standardization; in German, the Europäisches Komitee für Normung. CEN is the key *standards development organization (SDO)* in Europe, with participant countries including the European community and allied countries. There are also associate members from the chemical industry, the construction industry, consumers, environmentalists, the machine tools industry, the medical technology industry, small- and medium-sized enterprises, and trade unions.

CEN is the European analogue of ANSI, but the analogy is imperfect. CEN develops standards itself, whereas ANSI confines itself to coordinating standards activities, approving and publishing standards, and approving the standards developers. Voting in CEN is by countries, whereas in the United States all interested parties may vote. In the United States, standards are developed voluntarily by the industry and interested users, and participants fund themselves. CEN often funds the development of standards directly. The CEN Management Centre is in Brussels, Belgium. See also *COPANT*. **www.cen.eu**

census The number of patients in a hospital at a given time.

average daily census (ADC) The average number of inpatients (see *patient*) in a hospital (or unit of the hospital, such as a patient care unit) each day for a given period of time. Newborns (born in the hospital) are not included in the inpatient count for calculation of this statistic.

boarder census The number of boarders (nonpatients residing temporarily) in a hospital.

CEN TC 251 CEN develops standards by way of Technical Committees (TCs); the one responsible for health informatics standards is TC 251. It has funded more than thirty project teams with tasks including the registration of code book identifiers and clinical reporting. These teams have done an enormous amount of very thoughtful work, particularly regarding data modeling, the development of the concept of an abstract message, a conceptual model for a medical record, and many categories of clinical vocabulary. TC 251 presently has four Working Groups (WGs):

WG I.   Information Models
WG II.   Terminology and Knowledge Representation
WG III.   Security, Safety and Quality
WG IV.   Technology for Interoperability

TC 251 is working with HL7 to develop technically identical and interchangeable U.S. and European standards. The Secretariat for CEN TC 251 is in Stockholm, Sweden. **www.centc251.org**

Center for Biologics Evaluation and Research (CBER) The division of the Food and Drug Administration (FDA) that regulates biological and related products including the nation's blood supply, vaccines, human tissue, allergenics, anti-toxins, and biological therapeutics. **www.fda.gov/cber**

Center for Devices and Radiological Health (CDRH) A component of the Food and Drug Administration (FDA) responsible for ensuring the safety and effectiveness of medical devices and eliminating unnecessary human exposure to man-made radiation from medical, occupational, and consumer products. Examples of medical devices are heart pacemakers and contact lenses. Radiation-emitting products regulated by the FDA include microwave ovens, video display terminals (VDTs), and medical ultrasound and x-ray machines. **www.fda.gov/cdrh**

Center for Drug Evaluation and Research (CDER) The division of the Food and Drug Administration (FDA) with the responsibility to make sure that drugs (both prescription and over-the-counter) are safe and effective. See also *National Drug Code*. **www.fda.gov/cder**

Center for Food Safety and Applied Nutrition (CFSAN) The division of the Food and Drug Administration (FDA) that regulates the nation's food supply to ensure that it is safe, sanitary, wholesome, and honestly labeled, and also that cosmetic products are safe and properly labeled. **www.cfsan.fda.gov**

Center for Healthcare Industry Performance Studies (CHIPS) See *CHIPS*.

Center for Healthcare Information Management (CHIM) A national, nonprofit, health information technology (HIT) trade association founded in 1986 within the structure of the *Healthcare Information and Management Systems Society (HIMSS)*, which at that time was connected to the American Hospital Association (AHA). In 1990 the two organizations became independent of each other, but maintained collaborative relations through operating agreements. CHIM reunited with HIMSS in 2002.

Center for Health Transformation (CHT) A collaboration of private and public sector leaders committed to "creating a 21st century intelligent health system in which knowledge saves lives and saves money for all Americans." Members are stakeholders, including providers, employers, vendors, trade associations, disease groups, think tanks, and government leaders at both the state and federal level. **www.healthtransformation.net**

Center for Information Technology (CIT) See under *National Institutes of Health*.

Center for Scientific Review (CSR) See under *National Institutes of Health*.

Center for Veterinary Medicine (CVM) The division of the Food and Drug Administration (FDA) that regulates the manufacture and distribution of food additives and drugs that will be given to animals, including animals from which human foods are derived, as well as food additives and drugs for companion animals. **www.fda.gov/cvm**

center of excellence (COE) A healthcare facility or department that has gained a reputation for superior quality in a special area (or areas) of care. Such a facility can bring in patients from great distances, and so can increase its expertise in its specialty while lowering the cost of care. A COE can also be used as a marketing tool to distinguish between providers.

Centers for Disease Control and Prevention (CDC) An agency within the Department of Health and Human Services (HHS) that is responsible for monitoring and studying diseases that are controllable by public health measures. New diseases that appear to occur in epidemics are investigated, as are those due to environmental problems. Here, for example, is the government's center for monitoring and research on acquired immunodeficiency syndrome (AIDS), toxic shock syndrome, Legionnaire's disease, and health problems related to smoking. The CDC works with local governments in responding to environmental, chemical, and radiation emergencies. Originally called the Communicable Disease Center, the CDC's concerns have expanded to include chronic disease, global health, bioterrorism, injury, disability, occupational health, and environmental health. The CDC also performs many administrative functions for its "sister" agency, the Agency for Toxic Substances and Disease Registry (ATSDR). Headquartered in Atlanta, Georgia. **www.cdc.gov**

The CDC has the following major components:

Coordinating Center for Environmental Health and Injury Prevention (CCEHIP) A center of the Centers for Disease Control and Prevention (CDC) that coordinates efforts in the areas of environmental and occupational health and injury prevention, including oversight of the following centers:

National Center for Environmental Health/Agency for Toxic Substances and Disease Registry (NCEH-ATSDR) A division of the Centers for Disease Control and Prevention (CDC) that promotes health and quality of life by preventing or controlling those diseases, birth defects, disabilities, or deaths that result from interactions between people and their environment. It has programs concerning birth defects, child development, disability and health (including ongoing surveillance systems), emergency and environmental health services (including response to technologic disasters such as radiation, chemical, or biological releases, and to natural disasters), and environmental hazards and health effects (such as toxic waste, pesticides, lead poisoning, and second-hand smoke). It also works with states and other federal agencies to prevent exposures to hazardous substances from waste sites, unplanned releases, and other sources of environmental pollution.

NCEH has three divisions: Emergency and Environmental Health Services, Environmental Hazards and Health Effects, and Laboratory Sciences. ATSDR has four: Health Assessment and Consultation, Health Studies, Regional Operations, and Toxicology and Environmental Medicine. **www.cdc.gov/nceh** and **www.atsdr.cdc.gov**

National Center for Injury Prevention and Control (NCIPC) A division of the Centers for Disease Control and Prevention (CDC) established in 1992 to reduce morbidity, disability, mortality, and costs associated with injuries outside the workplace. Its main areas of activity are violence prevention (youth violence, family and intimate violence, suicide, and firearm injuries), unintentional injury prevention (focusing on motor vehicle–related injuries and home- and recreation-related injuries), and acute care, rehabilitation research, and disability prevention. NCIPC has three divisions: Violence Prevention, Unintentional Injury Prevention, and Injury Response. **www.cdc.gov/ncipc**

Coordinating Center for Health Information Service (CCHIS) A center of the Centers for Disease Control and Prevention (CDC) that coordinates efforts in the areas of health information technology, informatics, and statistics, including oversight of the following centers:

National Center for Health Marketing (NCHM) The center within the Centers for Disease Control and Prevention (CDC) that provides national leadership in health marketing science and its application to public health. The CDC defines health marketing as "creating, communicating, and delivering health information and interventions using customer-centered and science-based strategies to protect and promote the health of diverse populations." NCHM has four divisions: Creative Services, Health Communication and Marketing Strategy, Health Information Dissemination, and Partnerships and Strategic Alliances. **www.cdc.gov/healthmarketing**

National Center for Health Statistics (NCHS) The center within the Centers for Disease Control and Prevention (CDC) that serves as the nation's principal vital and health statistics agency. Current initiatives include Trends in Health and Aging, Classifications of Diseases and Functioning and Disability, Healthy People 2010, and Injury Data and Resources. NCHS makes numerous data surveys and reports publicly available from its web site. **www.cdc.gov/nchs**

National Center for Public Health Informatics (NCPHI) A division of the Centers for Disease Control and Prevention (CDC) established in 2005 to provide leadership in the application of information and computer science and technology to public health practice, research, and learning. The center includes five divisions: Alliance Management and Consultation, Emergency Preparedness and Response, Shared Services, Integrated Surveillance Systems and Services, and Knowledge Management. **www.cdc.gov/ncphi**

Coordinating Center for Health Promotion (CoCHP) A center of the Centers for Disease Control and Prevention (CDC) that coordinates efforts in the areas of health promotion. Its mission is to "[i]ncrease the potential for full, satisfying, and productive living across the lifespan for all people, in all communities." **www.cdc.gov/cochp**. CoCHP oversees the following centers:

National Center for Chronic Disease Prevention and Health Promotion (NCCD-PHP) A center in the Centers for Disease Control and Prevention (CDC) whose charge is to reduce the harm caused by chronic diseases such as diabetes, cancer, and cardiovascular (heart) problems. It includes divisions for Adult and Community Health, Adolescent and School Health, Cancer Prevention and Control, Diabetes Translation, Nutrition and Physical Activity, Oral Health, Reproductive Health, Smoking and Health, Genomics and Disease Prevention, and Heart Disease and Stroke Prevention. **www.cdc.gov/nccdphp**

National Center on Birth Defects and Developmental Disabilities (NCBDDD) A division of the Centers for Disease Control and Prevention (CDC) established in 2001 and charged with improving the health of children and adults by preventing birth defects and developmental disabilities, promoting optimal child development, and promoting health and wellness among children and adults living with disabilities. It assumed the mission of the former Division of Birth Defects, Child Development, and Disability and Health, which was in the National Center for Environmental Health. **www.cdc.gov/ncbddd**

National Office of Public Health Genomics (NOPHG) A division of the Centers for Disease Control and Prevention (CDC) dedicated to using genomic information to improve population health and prevent disease. Programs include: Family History Public Health Initiative, Evaluations of Genomic Applications in Practice and Prevention (EGAPP), Integrating Genomics into Public Health Investigations, Integrating Genomics into Chronic Disease Prevention Programs, and Developing a Knowledge Base on Genomics and Population Health. Formerly the Office of Genetics and Disease Prevention, then the Office of Genomics and Disease Prevention. **www.cdc.gov/genomics**

Office of Genetics and Disease Prevention (OGDP) See *National Office of Public Health Genomics*, above.

Coordinating Center for Infectious Diseases (CCID) A center of the Centers for Disease Control and Prevention (CDC) that coordinates efforts in the area of infectious diseases, including oversight of the following centers:

National Center for HIV/AIDS, Viral Hepatitis, STD, and TB Prevention (NCHH-STP) An interdisciplinary program within the Centers for Disease Control and Prevention (CDC) that integrates epidemiology, laboratory science, and intervention and prevention initiatives related to infectious diseases such as HIV/AIDS, viral hepatitis, sexually transmitted diseases (STDs), and tuberculosis (TB). **www.cdc.gov/nchstp/od/nchstp.html**

National Center for Immunization and Respiratory Diseases (NCIRD) A program within the Centers for Disease Control and Prevention (CDC) that brings together vaccine-preventable disease science and research with immunization program activities. Its divisions include Influenza, Viral Diseases, Bacterial Diseases, Global, and Immunization Services. See also *Vaccines for Children*. **www.cdc.gov/nip**

National Center for Preparedness, Detection, and Control of Infectious Diseases (NCPDCID) The division within the Centers for Disease Control and Prevention (CDC) charged with improving preparedness and response capacity for new and complex infectious disease outbreaks.

National Center for Zoonotic, Vector-Borne and Enteric Diseases (NCZVED) The division within the Centers for Disease Control and Prevention (CDC) charged with prevention and control of diseases that pass from animals to humans. It is estimated that 75% of newly emerging infectious diseases are caused by microorganisms in animals, and that livestock are a major source of pathogens. One focus of the center is disease control in livestock populations. See also *zoonosis*, *vector (epidemiology)*, and *enteric disease*.

Coordinating Office for Global Health (COGH) The office within the Centers for Disease Control and Prevention (CDC) that provides national leadership, coordination, and support for the CDC's global health activities in collaboration with its global health partners. The CDC's worldwide efforts include health promotion (sharing knowledge, tools, and other resources with people and partners around the world), health protection (protecting Americans at home and abroad from health threats through a transnational prevention, detection, and response network), and health diplomacy (being a trusted and effective resource for health development and health protection around the globe). **www.cdc.gov/cogh**

Coordinating Office for Terrorism Preparedness and Emergency Response (COTPER) The office within the Centers for Disease Control and Prevention (CDC) that provides strategic direction for and manages CDC-wide terrorism preparedness and emergency response programs, including maintaining the Strategic National Stockpile (SNS). Focus areas on the COTPER web site include Bioterrorism, Chemical Emergencies, Radiation Emergencies, Mass Casualties, Natural Disasters and Severe Weather, and Recent Outbreaks and Incidents. **www.bt.cdc.gov**

National Institute for Occupational Safety and Health (NIOSH) A division of the Centers for Disease Control and Prevention (CDC) charged with conducting research and making recommendations for the prevention of work-related disease and injury. Examples of programs include prevention of needlestick injuries in healthcare settings, mining health and safety, fire-fighter fatality investigation and prevention, and study of noise-induced hearing loss. NIOSH divisions include Health Effects Laboratory; Education and Information; Compensation Analysis and Support; Applied Research and Technology; Respiratory Disease Studies; Safety Research; and Surveillance, Hazard Evaluations, and Field Studies. NIOSH was created by the Occupational Safety and Health Act of 1970, along with the Occupational Safety and Health Administration (OSHA). **www.cdc.gov/niosh**

Office of the Director (CDC OD) Serves as Director of the Centers for Disease Control and Prevention (CDC) and as the Administrator of the Agency for Toxic Substances and Disease Registry (ATSDR). **www.cdc.gov/od**

Centers for Education and Research on Therapeutics (CERTs) A research program administered by the Agency for Healthcare Research and Quality (AHRQ), in consultation with the Food and Drug Administration (FDA). Its mission is to conduct research and provide education that will advance the optimal use of drugs, medical devices, and biological products. **www.certs.hhs.gov**

Centers for Medicare and Medicaid Services (CMS) See *CMS*.

centralized services Services that are carried out from a single location, in an effort to improve efficiency, reduce cost, or both. See also *decentralized services*.

central processing In hospital administration, a term that refers to the recycling of reusable items used in patient care (surgical instruments, for example), their collection, cleaning, sterilization, and repackaging. These are functions of the central service department (CS).

central service department (CS) The hospital department that provides sterile medical and surgical instruments and supplies. The pharmacy is not a part of CS. Synonym: central supply department.

CEO See *chief executive officer*.

CER See *capital expenditure review* under *review*.

CERT See *Comprehensive Error Rate Testing*.

certificate A document verifying that someone or something has fulfilled specific requirements.

certificate authority (CA) A public or private company or organization that issues *digital certificates* to others as part of a *public key infrastructure (PKI)*. To be really useful, the CA needs to be a trusted organization, which increasingly means regulated by one or more governmental agencies. Also called a "certification authority."

certificate of added qualification (CAQ) A credential granted by some specialty boards to health professionals who are already specialists and have obtained additional qualifications (usually including an examination) in a subspecialty or special focus area. See also *advanced qualifications*.

certificate of authority (COA) A license issued by a state to a health maintenance organization or insurance company permitting it to do business in that state.

certificate of clinical competence (CCC) See *audiologist* and *speech-language pathologist*.

certificate of insurance (COI) A document issued by an insurance company to verify that a particular person or institution is in fact insured for a certain type of risk, during a specific period of time. The dollar limits of the insurance are shown. A hospital may require a COI from each medical staff member, for example, to assure that the member has adequate malpractice insurance coverage.

certificate of need (CON) A certificate, issued by a governmental or planning agency, that approves the hospital's contention that it needs a given facility or service (for example, open heart surgery). A certificate of need is required under many regulatory situations in order to obtain approval to build, purchase, or institute the service in question.

certification (credential) The issuance of a "certificate" that gives evidence that its recipient (an individual, facility, or device) meets certain standards against which testing has been done by the certifying body. A certificate thus issued is a credential, and the recipient is said to be certified. Most certifying bodies require continuing education or renewal to maintain certification.

States with certification laws limit the use of particular titles (e.g., dietitian or nutritionist) to persons meeting specific requirements of the state; however, persons not certified can still practice. Consumers in these states who are seeking nutrition therapy assistance, for example, need to be cautious and aware of the actual qualifications of the provider they choose.

certification (software) Formal recognition by a certifying body that software meets specified criteria. See *Certification Commission for Health Information Technology*.

certification authority (CA) See *certificate authority*. See also *public key infrastructure*.

Certification Commission for Health Information Technology (CCHIT) An independent, private-sector, voluntary organization whose mission is to accelerate adoption of health information technology. CCHIT, the first *Recognized Certification Body (RCB)*, has developed over 300 criteria for certification of ambulatory electronic health record (EHR) products, and is developing criteria for inpatient EHRs. CCHIT certification indicates that a product has met baseline standards of functionality, interoperability, and security. Certification lasts for three years. CCHIT was founded in 2004 with support from the American Health Information Management Association (AHIMA), Healthcare Information and Management Systems Society (HIMSS), and National Alliance for Health Information Technology (NAHIT). **www.cchit.org**

certification examination An examination given for the purpose of determining the applicant's qualification for the certification sought.

certification manual A book setting out the criteria for certification. For example, in 2007, the Joint Commission on Accreditation of Healthcare Organizations (JCAHO) published two certification manuals:

Disease-Specific Care Certification Manual, 2nd Edition
Health Care Staffing Services Certification Manual

certified A term applied to an individual, facility, or device after a certifying body has conducted its testing and declared that the subject has met the standards, and is entitled to certification. Being certified provides a credential.

certified nurse A registered nurse who has met certain eligibility requirements and passed an examination in a specialty area of nursing. The American Nurses Credentialing Center (ANCC) (**nursingworld.org/ancc**) offers three levels:

Certified (RN,C) Nurses holding associate degrees or diplomas may be awarded certification.

Board Certified (RN,BC) Nurses with bachelor's degrees or higher may obtain board certification.

Advanced Practice Registered Nurse, Board Certified (APRN,BC) Advanced practice nurses with graduate degrees may obtain this designation.

In addition, the National Certification Corporation (NCC) (**www.nccnet.org**) offers the credential **Registered Nurse, Certified (RNC)** to qualified nurses who pass examinations in any of a number of specialty areas.

There are a number of other organizations providing certification to nurses in their areas of specialty; the credential designation varies according to the credentialing organization.

For a list of specialty areas, see *nursing specialty*. See also *advanced practice nurse*, *clinical nurse specialist*, and *nurse practitioner*.

Certifying Commission in Medical Management (CCMM) A board that certifies physicians specializing in *medical management*. See *physician executive*. **ccmm.org**

CERTs See *Centers for Education and Research on Therapeutics*.

CETN Certified Enterostomal Therapy Nurse. See *Certified Wound, Ostomy, and Continence Nurse* under *wound, ostomy, and continence nursing*.

CFA See *Certified First Assistant* under *first assistant*.

CFO See *chief financial officer*.

CFR See *Code of Federal Regulations*.

CFRN See *Certified Flight Registered Nurse* under *flight nursing*.

CFSAN See *Center for Food Safety and Applied Nutrition*.

CGC See *Certified Genetic Counselor* under *genetic counselor*.

CGN See *Certified Gastroenterology Nurse* under *gastroenterology nursing*.

CGRN See *Certified Gastroenterology Registered Nurse* under *gastroenterology nursing*.

CHA See *Canadian Healthcare Association* and *Catholic Health Association of the United States*.

chain organization See *multihospital system*.

chairman of service See *chief of service*.

CHAMPUS See *TRICARE*.

CHAMPVA Civilian Health and Medical Program of the Department of Veterans Affairs. The federal program, administered by the Defense Department for the Veterans Administration (VA), that provides care for the dependents of totally disabled veterans. Care is given by civilian providers. See also *TRICARE* (originally CHAMPUS). **www.va.gov/hac/forbeneficiaries/champva/**

channeling A term used in long-term care in which efforts are made to avoid institutionalization of patients by having them directed ("channeled") to community-based long-term care services. From 1980 to 1985, HCFA (now CMS) and other federal agencies financed a demonstration of the concept, which used comprehensive case management, but ended the demonstration when a study showed no lowering of cost. More recently, reports suggest that when a *gatekeeper (health care)* participates in the financial planning as well as the healthcare decisions, significant savings may be realized.

CHAP See *Community Health Accreditation Program*.

chaplain A member of the clergy whose duty is to provide pastoral services to patients and their families, and to the hospital staff.

Board Certified Chaplain (BCC) A chaplain who has been certified by the Association of Professional Chaplains (APC) (**www.professionalchaplains.org**). Qualified chaplains of all faiths and cultures are eligible.

HCMA Professional Certified Chaplain (PCC) A chaplain who has been certified by the Healthcare Chaplains Ministry Association (HCMA) (formerly Hospital Chaplains' Ministry of America). **www.hcmachaplains.org**

charge The dollar amount asked for a service by a healthcare provider. It is contrasted with the cost, which is the dollar amount the provider incurs in furnishing the service. It is difficult to determine precise costs for many services, and in such cases charges are substituted for costs in many reimbursement and payment formulas (often with the stipulation that the hospital's bookkeeping follow certain rules). Synonym: fee. See also *contractuals*.

allowable charge See *covered charge*, below.

covered charge An item of service that, when billed to a third-party payer, will be paid, because it is for a benefit provided under the contract. The charges for television and meals for visitors, for example, are not ordinarily covered charges. Synonym: allowable charge.

daily service charge Same as "room rate"; see *room rate* under *rate (charge)*.

normal charge See *contractuals*.

charge compression The tendency for hospitals to mark up the charges for high cost items to a lesser extent than they mark up low cost items.

charge description master (CDM) A comprehensive "master" list of everything (services, supplies, medical devices, medications) that a healthcare facility provides to its patients and would also like to bill ("charge") them for. Each line item on the list contains detailed information, including at minimum a description of the item and its price. The CDM is the "lookup table" used by the facilities when they generate the bill (invoice) for each patient or for third-party payers. Because the CDM for even a small healthcare provider is likely to contain thousands of line items, most CDMs are computerized databases that are linked to the provider's billing and accounting systems.

Patient bills generated by the provider for third-party payers (such as insurance companies and the federal government) frequently have very specific coding requirements, so the provider's CDM must also be kept in compliance with these payers' reimbursement requirements. Under some plans, including the federal government's prospective payment system (PPS) as used for Medicare, reimbursement is based on the DRG (Diagnosis Related Group) for inpatients and the APC (Ambulatory Patient Category) for outpatients. This means that each line item in the CDM may need to be linked to corresponding CPT, HCPCS, or ICD codes, because a noncompliant bill is less likely to be reimbursed.

As might be predicted, the CDM has resulted in quite an industry, which involves helping the provider (1) construct the CDM in compliance with the rules of what can and can't be "bundled" with the charge for the given item, (2) periodically review the CDM and see that it complies with the rules, and (3) make sure everything is captured that can be defended (i.e., optimizing the CDM). Synonym: chargemaster.

chargemaster See *charge description master*.

charitable purpose Section 501(c)(3) of the Internal Revenue Code provides that one test of the qualification of an organization for tax-exemption under that section of the code is that it serve a "charitable purpose." The term is defined administratively by the Internal Revenue Service, and current regulations should be consulted.

charity allowance A reduction of a charge (a discount) to a patient because that patient is indigent or medically indigent.

charity care Healthcare services provided free of charge to those who are uninsured or otherwise unable to pay for care. Although the U.S. Constitution does not guarantee a right to health care, the federal government has linked a duty to treat people unable to pay with government-financed healthcare programs. See also *medically indigent* under *indigent*, *Emergency Medical Treatment and Labor Act*, *Hill-Burton Act*, and *501(c)(3)* under *501(c)(*)*.

chart See *medical record*.

charting The process of creating a medical record for a patient. It includes the writing of nurses' and doctors' notes, and addition of test results and other documentation relevant to the patient's stay and progress in the hospital. There are various methods adopted by hospitals; for examples, see *charting by exception*, *Focus charting*, *PIE charting*, and *problem centered charting*.

charting by exception (CBE) A charting system developed to eliminate lengthy narrative notes (which can bury abnormal data within normal data), decrease charting errors, and minimize documentation time. CBE relies on the assumption that, unless there is documentation to the contrary, all (clearly defined) standards and protocols were followed and all assessment values were within accepted limits—only exceptions will be noted.

During the nursing assessment, for example, a form is completed that defines all normal parameters for each body system. If the patient meets these, the nurse enters only a check mark on the form for each item. Notes are written only for abnormal findings. A care plan is created and written in longhand, using the SOAPIER format: S = subjective data, O = objective data, A = assessment, P = plan, I = interventions, E = evaluation, and R = revisions. Care plan problems are numbered and followed. Day-to-day care is documented on forms, using check marks, and shorthand notes are used for treatments and other nursing or physician orders. Only exceptions are charted in narrative form. The system was developed in 1983 at St. Luke's Medical Center in Milwaukee, Wisconsin.

Charting by exception is acceptable if used properly. However, CBE was found, in one malpractice case, to be negligence, and to violate a health department regulation that nurses' notes be qualitative for each nursing shift. The jury concluded that more complete documentation would have alerted doctors to the presence of an infection. "Intermittent charting failed to provide the sort of continuous danger signals that would be the most likely to spur early intervention by a physician," the appellate court noted. *Lama v. Borras*, 16 F.3d 473 PR (1st Cir. 1994).

CHC See *Certified Healthcare Consultant* under *healthcare consultant*. Also means Community Health Center; see *Federally Qualified Health Center*.

CHE See *Certified Healthcare Executive* under *healthcare executive*.

CHEC See *Consumer Health Education Council*.

chemical dependency (CD) The generic term covering alcoholism and addiction to other drugs, both legal drugs (prescribed by a physician or available over the counter) and illegal drugs.

chemical pathology The study of the biochemical basis of disease.

chemical substance A substance produced by chemistry, as distinguished from a biological substance, which is produced by a living organism. Both chemical and biological substances are used in diagnostic procedures and the treatment of disease.

chemistry The study of the molecular and atomic structure of matter.

Chemistry Technologist (C) See under *clinical laboratory technologist*.

chemotherapy Treatment by the application of chemical reagents that have a specific and toxic effect upon the microorganism that causes the disease. A "reagent" is a substance involved in a chemical reaction.

cherry picking A practice by insurers of selling policies only to people who do not need medical care, then dropping them once they do. Any Medicare provider paid under a risk (capitated) plan, for instance, has an incentive to pursue this form of favorable selection. Some efforts to do this are illegal (such as asking Medicare HMO enrollees about their health status prior to joining), but it is apparently not illegal for HMOs to have their offices up one flight of stairs to discourage some potential enrollees, or to affirmatively market the HMO plan in environments frequented by the healthier retirees. Synonym: cream skimming.

CHESS Comprehensive Health Enhancement Support System. A "computer-based system of integrated services designed to help individuals cope with a health crisis or medical concern." CHESS uses an ordinary personal computer and the Internet (or software) to provide current information and communication to individual patients for a growing number of topics, including HIV/AIDS, breast cancer, sexual assault, and stress management. The technique has also been employed for students in academic crisis. The user has instantly available a tutorial about the system and the topic, a library about the topic, a referral directory, a computer support group, personal stories, decision aid tools, and a "pop-up" dictionary. The system may be used in the individual's own setting.

CHESS is developed by a team of decision, information, education, and communication scientists at the University of Wisconsin-Madison's Center for Health Systems Research and Analysis (CHSRA), and is copyrighted and licensed by CHSRA and the Wisconsin Alumni Research Foundation. **chess.chsra.wisc.edu**

CHFP See *Certified Healthcare Finance Professional*, under *healthcare finance professional*, and *Certified Human Factors Professional*, under *ergonomist*.

CHI See *Consolidated Health Informatics*.

chief engineer See *administrative engineer*.

chief executive officer (CEO) The person appointed by the governing body to direct the overall management of the hospital (or other organization). The CEO is the *board in residence*. Synonym: executive director.

chief financial officer (CFO) The corporate treasurer. Sometimes the term is also applied to the controller of the organization (the person in charge of the ongoing financial administration, including billing, accounting, budget management, and the like). Synonym: financial director.

chief information officer (CIO) The title often given to the person in charge of the organization's management information system (MIS) (see *information system*). Also, a company's chief *information technology (IT)* officer. Sometimes also called CKO, for chief knowledge officer.

chief knowledge officer (CKO) See *chief information officer*.

chief medical information officer (CMIO) A physician with expertise in informatics who is employed by a hospital or other organization to oversee planning for, implementing, and operating electronic health record (EHR) and other clinical information systems.

chief medical officer (CMO) The person (usually a physician) responsible for the medical affairs of a corporation or organization. The actual duties will vary widely depending upon the context. Synonym: chief medical director. See also *chief of staff*.

chief of nursing See *nursing service administrator*.

chief of service A medical staff officer responsible for the management of a clinical department, such as internal medicine or surgery. Synonym: chairman of service.

chief of staff The physician designated by the governing body, usually after nomination by the medical staff, to be responsible for management of the medical staff and for carrying out policy promulgated by the board. The term "chief of staff" or "president of the medical staff" usually refers to an unpaid person, whereas a paid physician with either of these same duties is likely to be called the "medical director," "vice president for medical affairs (VPMA)," "director of medical affairs (DMA)," or some like title.

There is some ambiguity in the duties and titles, because there really are two duties involved "at the top of the medical staff": (1) to provide management for the medical staff as a component of the hospital, and for this duty, the title "chief of staff" seems appropriate; and (2) to act as the "spokesperson" for the medical staff members, and for this duty, the title "president" seems more apt.

Many hospitals have two separate positions: a president (often unpaid), elected by the medical staff (and approved by the governing body) to represent the medical staff, and a director of medical affairs (or similar title), employed by the hospital, to manage medical staff affairs.

chief operating officer (COO) The person in charge of the internal operation of the organization, for example, a hospital. The chief executive officer (CEO), while responsible for the internal operation of the organization, also has external responsibilities with the governing body, with the community, with other institutions, and so on. Often a single individual is made responsible for "inside" affairs, under the CEO. This person would be the COO, whether or not he or she is given that title.

chief privacy officer (CPO) See *privacy officer*.

chief technology officer (CTO) The person in an organization who is responsible for administering and advising other senior management on the use of technology in the organization. Typically the focus is on information technology (IT), and the CTO may be the same person who is the head of "the IT department" or who is the manager of information systems (MIS).

chi kung See *qi gong*.

Child Abuse Amendments Amendments, enacted in 1984, to the federal Child Abuse Prevention and Treatment Act concerning medical treatment decisions for seriously ill newborns. The amendments added the phrase "withholding of medically indicated treatment" to the statutory definition of child neglect; this is now often referred to as "medical neglect." The law was passed in response to the *Baby Doe case*, and makes it a form of neglect to fail to treat correctable, life-threatening conditions in a child unless in the physician's "reasonable medical judgment" (1) the child is irreversibly comatose; (2) treatment would be futile in saving the child's life; or (3) the treatment would be virtually futile and inhumane under the circumstances. States must require hospitals to report cases of suspected medical neglect to the child protective service agencies, and provide procedures for appropriate intervention. Synonym: Baby Doe law. The amendments are codified at 42 U.S.C. §§ 5101–5106h (2004).

childbirth center A facility, either a part of a hospital or free-standing, that provides prenatal care for the mother, delivery, and postnatal care. Typically a facility with this name involves the family rather than just the mother and baby; it permits the father's attendance at the delivery and his assistance in caring for the baby, and so on. Synonym: birthing center.

childbirth educator A health professional specializing in guiding women and their families through pregnancy and childbirth.

Lamaze Certified Childbirth Educator (LCCE) A childbirth educator who has been certified by Lamaze International. **www.lamaze.org**

child life specialist A health professional with special training to help children and their families deal with stressful experiences, including health care and hospitalization.

Certified Child Life Specialist (CCLS) A child life specialist with a bachelor's or master's degree and who has qualified to be certified by the Child Life Council (CLC). **www.childlife.org**

child neurology See *neurology*.

Child Nutrition Database (CN) Previously referred to as the National Nutrient Database for Child Nutrition Programs (NNDCNP), this U.S. Department of Agriculture (USDA) database serves the National School Lunch and Breakfast programs as part of the School Meals Initiative for Healthy Children. The CN is maintained by the USDA's Food and Nutrition Service (FNS) as part of the *USDA National Nutrient Database for Standard Reference*.

child psychiatry See *psychiatry*.

Children's Health Insurance Program (CHIP) See *State Children's Health Insurance Program*.

CHIM See *Center for Healthcare Information Management*.

CHIME See *College of Healthcare Information Management Executives*.

CHIMIS See *community health integrated management information system* under *information system*.

CHIN Community health information network. See *community health integrated management information system* under *information system*.

CHIP Children's Health Insurance Program. See *State Children's Health Insurance Program*. See also *Community Health Intervention Partnership*.

CHIPS Center for Healthcare Industry Performance Studies. CHIPS, a Division of St. Anthony Publishing, Inc., originally published the *Almanac of Hospital Financial and Operating Indicators* (sometimes referred to as "CHIPS indicators"). Data used in preparing the *Almanac* come from three sources: (1) audited hospital financial statements, (2) strategic hospital operating data submitted by hospitals, and (3) Medicare cost reports. The *Almanac* presents some thirty-three financial indicators, presented as ratios placed in five categories: profitability, liquidity, capital structure, asset efficiency, and other. It also presents forty-three operating indicators that relate to profitability, in seven categories: profitability, price, volume, length of stay, intensity of service, efficiency, and unit cost of inputs. The *Almanac of Hospital Financial and Operating Indicators* is now published by Ingenix and subtitled, *A Comprehensive Benchmark of the Nation's Hospitals*. Also available on CD-ROM. **www.ingenixonline.com**

chiropody See *podiatry*.

chiropractic See under *medicine (system)*.

chiropractor A practitioner of *chiropractic* (see under *medicine (system)*). In order to practice, the chiropractor must be licensed by the state. The chiropractor has the degree doctor of chiropractic (DC).

Board Certified Chiropractic Neurologist A chiropractor who has completed specialty training in neurology and been certified by the American Chiropractic Neurology Board (ACNB). **www.acnb.org**

CHIS See *community-wide health information system*.

CHM See *Consumer Health Manager*.

CHN See *Certified Hemodialysis Nurse* under *dialysis nursing*. Also community health network, see *Federally Qualified Health Center*; and community health nursing, see *public health nursing*.

CHP See *Certified Health Physicist* under *health physicist*, under *physicist*. See also *Certified in Healthcare Privacy*, under *privacy and security professionals*, and *comprehensive health planning*, under *planning*. Also community health plan; see *Hospital Health Plan*.

CHPLN See *Certified Hospice and Palliative Licensed Nurse* under *hospice and palliative nursing*.

CHPN See *Certified Hospice and Palliative Nurse* under *hospice and palliative nursing*.

CHPNA See *Certified Hospice and Palliative Nursing Assistant* under *hospice and palliative nursing*.

CHPS See *Certified in Healthcare Privacy and Security* under *privacy and security professionals*.

Christian Science A religious group that prohibits all forms of medical care and relies solely on spiritual healing. Similar to the "Peculiar People," who have presented the courts in England with the same questions as Christian Scientists have presented in the United States. Although adults can refuse medical treatment, courts routinely allow medical authorities to treat children against the wishes of the parent, even when these wishes are based on religious beliefs. Although some states have adopted statutes that provide that children are not being abused if treated only by spiritual healing (these statutes were the result of lobbying by the Christian Scientists), these statutes apply only to "recognized" churches. However, it is argued that these statutes are unconstitutional because they violate the Establishment clause of the U.S. Constitution in requiring the state to determine which churches are "recognized" and which are not, which improperly advances religion and entangles church and state. Also known as the "Church of Christ, Scientist."

CHRN See *Certified Hyperbaric Registered Nurse* under *baromedical nursing*.

chromosome A microscopic unit containing a set of genes within the nucleus of a cell. Most human cells contain two sets of chromosomes, one set given by each parent. Each set has twenty-three single chromosomes. See also *allele*.

autosome Any chromosome other than a sex chromosome.

sex chromosome The X and Y chromosomes, which determine the sex of an individual. Females require two X chromosomes; males require both an X and a Y.

chronic An illness that lasts for a long time, and usually without prospect of immediate change for either the better or the worse. It is contrasted with acute, which refers to having a short course, which often is relatively severe. "Chronic" is also used for the portion or portions of an illness, ordinarily in its later stages, in which symptoms are less severe and the patient may be at relatively low risk.

chronobiology The branch of biology dealing with circadian biological rhythms (rhythms in a cycle of about a day, about twenty-four hours). For example, shifting work hours, which require an individual to change his or her pattern of sleep and wakefulness, create serious health problems for many individuals; studies have shown increases in errors in performance, and in accidents, during the periods of the circadian rhythm when neural functions are at their lowest ebb—for individuals "working the day shift," this is between 2 am and 7 am, and between 2 pm and 5 pm. See also *patient safety*.

chronohygiene That branch of the science of health dealing with the problems associated with changes in the individual's sleep and wakefulness cycle, such as "jet lag" and the shifting of work hours for nurses. See also *patient safety*.

CHS See *Certified in Healthcare Security* under *privacy and security professionals*.

CHSR See *Coalition for Health Services Research*.

CHT See *Center for Health Transformation*, and *Certified Hemodialysis Technologist/ Technician* under *hemodialysis technician*, and *Certified Hyperbaric Technologist* under *hyperbaric technologist*.

churning The practice of discharge of a patient from the hospital and readmission of the same patient for what is really a single episode of care in order to be able to charge for two or more hospitalizations. Only the last discharge is "real" from a medical standpoint—except for the financial benefit of being paid for two or more hospitalizations under the prospective payment system (PPS), there would have been no intermediate discharges.

price churning See *predatory pricing*.

churning the books See *predatory pricing*.

CIA See *complementary, integrative, or alternative practitioner*. Also *corporate integrity agreement*, and *cost-identification analysis* under *cost-analysis*.

CIC See *Certified in Infection Control* under *infection control professional*.

CIHI See *Canadian Institute for Health Information*.

CIMT See *constraint-induced-movement therapy*.

CINAHL See *Cumulative Index to Nursing and Allied Health Literature*.

CIO See *chief information officer*.

CIOMS See *Council for International Organizations of Medical Sciences*.

circadian Pertaining to biological rhythms that occur in a cycle of about twenty-four hours. See also *chronobiology*.

circulator A health professional who is the "nonsterile" member of the operating room team. Duties may include responding to the needs of the scrubbed members, keeping a written account of the surgical procedure, assisting the anesthesiologist, and helping account for sponges, needles, and instruments before, during, and after surgery. The circulator may be a *registered nurse (RN)* (see under *nurse*), a *surgical technologist*, or another qualified professional.

CISTERN Clinical Information Systems Interoperability Network. CISTERN is a multi-vendor project begun in May 2000 to define and demonstrate XML-based methods for exchanging healthcare data securely between applications using the Internet. The project uses open standards such as XML, HL7, and PKI to facilitate the interoperability of different healthcare information systems (HIS).

CIT See *Center for Information Technology* (under *National Institutes of Health*).

Citizens Health Portal (myNDMA) See under *portal*.

Civilian Health and Medical Program of the Uniformed Services (CHAMPUS) See *TRICARE*.

Civilian Health and Medical Program of the Veterans Administration (CHAMPVA) See *CHAMPVA*.

civil monetary penalty A fine. "Civil" pertains to legal matters that are not criminal, but "penalty" means that the money to be paid is for punishment of the wrongdoer, rather than as compensation to the injured. Synonym: civil money penalty. See also **punitive damages** under **damages**.

Civil Rights Act of 1964 Title VI: Federal legislation prohibiting *programs that receive federal funding* from discriminating against program participants on the basis of race, color, or national origin. Generally, Title VI has not been applied to credentialing, but a claim of staff privileges discrimination might succeed if the plaintiff were the actual intended beneficiary of the funding from the federal government. 42 U.S.C. §§ 2000d–2000d-4 (2004).

Title VII: Federal legislation prohibiting discrimination in *employment practices* based on race, color, religion, sex, or national origin. Title VII applies to every institution, regardless of whether they receive federal funding or not. Some courts have found an employment relationship between physicians and hospitals and some have not, depending on the degree of control the hospital maintains over the physician. See also **employee** and **independent contractor**. 42 U.S.C. § 2000e (2004).

CKO Chief knowledge officer. See **chief information officer**.

clade A group of descendants from a single biological organism, that is, having a common ancestor, along with that ancestor.

It has been suggested that the concept could be used to depict graphically other phenomena—for example, the situation with HIV infections. The usual illustration is that HIV infections are like an iceberg, with the visible portion consisting of the proportion of the persons who are clinically ill with AIDS, in contrast with the submerged portion consisting of the number who are infected, but clinically well at any given time. The iceberg analogy is flawed because an iceberg melts and disappears, whereas the clade (and HIV infection) is a constantly growing number. See the illustration below, which depicts the growing number of persons infected with HIV but without symptoms ("silent" cases), along with the growing number of diagnosed ("visible") cases.

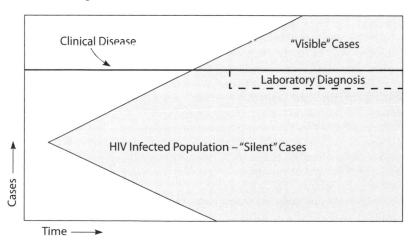

HIV Infection – Viewed as a clade (shaded area)

cladistics A method of organizing "creation"—biological entities—according to their parentage and heredity.

cladogram A tree-like diagram showing the evolution of an organism. The tips of the branches represent species, showing where they have diverged from a common ancestor.

claim (insurance) A request for payment of insurance benefits to be paid to or on behalf of a beneficiary.

claim (legal) An allegation of legal liability and an accompanying demand for damages (money) or other rights due. The term is sometimes used in health care to refer to a medical malpractice lawsuit, or to an allegation of malpractice (which allegation may or may not result in a lawsuit).

> **open claim** A claim for damages, usually involving professional liability (see *liability (legal)*), in which a decision has not been reached, either by settlement out of court or by court decision.
>
> When an individual believes that she or he has been injured by the hospital or a physician, a claim may be made for damages. The claim may eventually be withdrawn. Claims not withdrawn may be settled, either by negotiation or by court decision. Before the settlement, the claim is open (pending); after settlement it is closed.
>
> **closed claim** A claim for which the issues of liability and damages (who owes what to whom) have been decided, either by settlement out of court or by court decision.
>
> Closed claims are discussed in health care because they are the basis for analysis of the liability (malpractice) "problem" (i.e., the costs in the healthcare industry of malpractice insurance, judgments, and settlements, and related costs both monetary and otherwise; for example, the practice of "defensive medicine"). But although closed claim studies may be carefully done, at best they only display a part of the liability picture. This is so because: (1) the only claims certain to be available for analysis are those closed claims in which a court decision has been rendered, because these are in the public domain; (2) claims may be pending for years, and pending claims are kept confidential; (3) claims settled by negotiation (out of court) need not be made public; and (4) although a number of institutions and insurance companies do contribute data on their settled claims to bona fide research institutions for confidential use in statistical analysis, not all closed claims are submitted, so published analyses of closed claims are always an understatement of the liability problem.

claim form See *insurance claim form*.

claims filing service A service offered by private entrepreneurs to Medicare beneficiaries and others with health insurance. The service offers to "file, follow-up, and manage" claims (see *claim (insurance)*). Often the service charges a "registration" fee plus monthly fees. Such a service, which costs perhaps $100 per beneficiary per year, adds to the cost of health care by that amount and, equally importantly, decreases the individual's benefits by that amount.

claims-made coverage See under *insurance coverage*.

claims processing The procedure by which claims for payment for services are reviewed in order to determine whether they should be paid, and for what amount (see *claim (insurance)*). The review includes verifying that an authorized provider is submitting the claim, that the person served is a beneficiary, that the services are medically reasonable and are for available benefits, and the amount to be paid.

claims review See under *review*.

CLAS See *culturally and linguistically appropriate services*.

class See *category*.

classification (process) Derived from the verb "to classify." The process of placing an entity (item) of a universe into its category (pigeonhole) within a classification (scheme). This is a specialized function that requires a "judgment call" as to which category a given entity falls into in cases where the entity is described in a term or terms that are not found in the classification as printed (or its index). Classification requires expert knowledge of the universe of objects to be classified. Compare *coding (process)*.

classification (scheme) A scheme for grouping the entities (items) making up a universe into categories (see *category*). A classification is a systematic scheme of organization of information in which a whole body of things—for example, automobiles, houses, hospitals, or procedures—have been grouped (classified) into categories (classes or "pigeonholes") so that the groups can be compared, studied, analyzed, or otherwise processed. Classifications are used in health care to organize patient (and patient care) information for such purposes as studying diseases, assessing quality of care, and determining charges to be made for healthcare services. Confusion results when the word "classification" (the whole schema) is used when "class" or "the classification process" are intended.

The purpose of the classification determines its organization or grouping system. A classification to describe the body of hospitalized patients requires different groupings than one for general office practice. For example, patients with the common cold are so rarely hospitalized that, in a hospital diagnosis classification, the common cold is grouped with miscellaneous respiratory conditions, whereas in general office practice the common cold may be seen so frequently that it deserves a category of its own. See also *taxonomy*.

Classification of Death and Injury Resulting from Terrorism (CDIRT) A set of codes within the framework of ICD-10 and ICD-9-CM to permit classifying deaths and injuries that result from terrorism. The existing classifications did not have a way to identify terrorism as a cause, so the National Center for Health Statistics (NCHS) developed CDIRT.

For mortality, the codes developed include *U01–*U02 for terrorism involving an assault (homicide) and *U03 for terrorism involving intentional self-harm (suicide). The asterisk preceding each code indicates that the code was introduced by the United States but is not officially part of the ICD. Codes from the "U" chapter of ICD-10 were selected because this chapter was reserved specifically for "future additions and changes and for possible interim classifications to solve difficulties arising at the national and international levels between revisions." To maintain international comparability in reporting homicide and suicide rates, deaths coded to *U01–*U02 are included in general tabulations with other homicides (X85–Y09 and Y87.1), and deaths coded to *U03 are included with other suicides (X60–X84 and Y87.0). Implementation of the codes developed for mortality classification were effective beginning with 2001 mortality data.

For injuries associated with terrorism not resulting in death, the codes developed include E979 and E999.1. E979 was unused previously in ICD-9-CM. E999, which was used previously to denote the late effects of war operations, was modified to include the late effects of terrorism. E999.0 was created to classify the late effects of war operations, and E999.1 was created for the late effects of terrorism. For statistical purposes, codes E979 and E999.1 are tabulated with other assaults (E960–E969). No plans exist to create a parallel category for self-inflicted injury. Codes developed for morbidity were implemented effective October 1, 2002.

For the terrorism codes to be used for the classification of deaths and injuries, the incident in question must be designated as a terrorist act by the U.S. Federal Bureau of Investigation (FBI), which has jurisdiction over the investigation and tracking of terrorism in the United States. The FBI defines a terrorism-related injury as one resulting from the "unlawful use of force or violence against persons or property to intimidate or coerce a government, the civilian population, or any segment thereof, in furtherance of political or social objectives." The codes may not be used based on individual judgments made by medical examiners, coroners, medical coders, nosologists, or hospital staff. If the FBI labels the incident as a terrorist act before the completion of the death certificate or the filing of the medical record, it may be so described on the certificate and/or medical record. If the incident is labeled as terrorism later, the medical record and/or death certificate can be amended.

classifier A person who classifies, that is, who does classification (process).

classifying Making the decisions necessary for placing an entity (item) into a category of a classification (scheme).

Clayton Act One of the primary federal antitrust laws. The Clayton Act specifically prohibits price discrimination (selling to different buyers at different, discriminatory prices) (Section 2(a), as amended by the Robinson-Patman Act), tying arrangements, exclusive dealing, and corporate expansion if these activities substantially lessen competition or create a monopoly. It also prohibits interlocking corporate directorships where the corporations are competitors; no individual may simultaneously serve on the boards of directors of two or more competing corporations, if one of the corporations has assets over $1 million. 15 U.S.C. § 12 et seq. (2005).

CLCP See *Certified Life Care Planner* (under *life care planning*) and *Clinical Laboratory Compliance Professional* (under *clinical laboratory compliance*).

CLDir See *Clinical Laboratory Director* under *clinical laboratory manager*.

clean room A room (which may be a "room within a room") with environmental controls that prevent bacteria and dirt from coming in or going out. This is accomplished by using a filtered air supply and by providing methods for manipulating the patient without direct contact. Ports in the room permit persons wearing sleeved rubber gloves or using special devices to perform tasks within the room.

CLES See *Certified Laboratory Equipment Specialist* under *biomedical instrumentation technologist*.

CLI Clinical and laboratory immunology. See *medical specialty*.

CLIA See *Clinical Laboratory Improvement Amendments*.

CLICKS Medical Information System See under *information system*.

client A person who receives professional services. In health care, a client may or may not be sick. See also *patient*.

CLIMS Clinical laboratory information management system. See *laboratory information management system*.

clinhaven See *cybermedicine*.

clinic (education) An instructional session, such as a prenatal clinic where expectant mothers are instructed in their own care and prepared for the care of their babies. In medical education, a clinic is where students are taught by demonstration with actual patients.

clinic (facility) A facility for ambulatory patients.

> **free clinic** A facility that provides free care, primarily to the working poor. The first of this generation in the United States was the Haight-Ashbury Free Clinic, established in San Francisco in 1967. Free clinics usually offer medical care in the form of physical examinations, prenatal care, family planning, and primary care for their clientele. Some may also provide dental health care and mental health services, while others offer social and legal services. Financing is usually by donations. A great deal of the staff are volunteers. Supplies are often provided at a discount, and space may be donated (e.g., by churches). See also *Volunteers in Medicine Clinic*.

clinic (practice) A group of physicians practicing together, either all of one specialty (single specialty) or with various specialties (multispecialty). Such a clinic may or may not have inpatient facilities.

clinical A term referring to direct contact with or information from patients and to the course of illness; "things" medical about a patient. Thus personal (bedside) contact with the patient is clinical contact, a laboratory that examines blood and other specimens from patients is a clinical laboratory, the patient's medical record is a clinical record, research involving patients is clinical research, and a nurse taking care of patients is a clinical nurse.

clinical alert (CA) Guidance as to possible problems with certain medications, procedures, and other proposed care. Usually found in the context of an electronic notice given at the point of entry of an order (see *computerized physician order entry*).

For example, medication clinical alerts can identify (1) drug-drug interactions, (2) drug-food incompatibilities, (3) laboratory values that could influence drug dosages, (4) drugs contraindicated in pregnancy, (5) drugs contraindicated in certain medical conditions, (6) drug duplication, and (7) advice on pediatric drug dosage.

Clinical and Translational Science Awards (CTSA) A consortium of academic health centers (AHCs) developed to promote clinical and translational research, with the aim of providing new treatments for patients more quickly and efficiently. Begun in 2006 with twelve AHCs, the goal is to reach sixty AHCs nationwide by 2012. The consortium is funded by the National Center for Research Resources, a part of the National Institutes of Health. **ctsaweb.org**

clinical auditor A health professional who performs the *clinical audit (reimbursement)* (see under *audit*). Some have special training, and certification is available (see below). Sometimes called clinical chart auditor.

Certified Clinical Auditor A clinical auditor who is also a clinical health professional (for example, a physician, physician's assistant, physical therapist, or paramedic), other than a registered nurse, who has completed the Clinical Auditing Certification examination of the American Association of Clinical Coders and Auditors, Inc. (AACCA). **www.aacca.net**

Clinical Audit Professional, Certified (CAPC) A clinical auditor who has been certified by the American Institute of Outcomes Case Management (AIOCM). **www.aiocm.com**

RN-Auditor A clinical auditor, who is also a registered nurse, who has completed the Clinical Auditing Certification examination of the American Association of Clinical Coders and Auditors, Inc. (AACCA). **www.aacca.net**

Clinical Care Classification (CCC) A standardized framework and coding structure of nursing diagnoses and interventions used for assessing, documenting, and classifying home health and ambulatory care services. The CCC is used to track and measure patient care "holistically" over time and across care settings, population groups, and geographic locations. Formerly the Home Health Care Classification (HHCC). **www.sabacare.com**

clinical care path See *clinical path*.

Clinical Center (CC) See under *National Institutes of Health*.

clinical chart audit See *clinical audit (reimbursement)* under *audit*.

clinical chart auditor See *clinical auditor*.

clinical chemist See *biochemist*.

clinical clerk A student in a medical or dental school who carries out certain tasks with patients (clinical tasks) under supervision as part of her or his training. The training period is called a clinical clerkship.

clinical clerkship A training experience, involving actual care and treatment of patients (clinical experience) under medical or dental supervision, provided by a hospital to a medical or dental student. The trainee is called a clinical clerk.

Clinical Context Management Specification (CCM) A set of guidelines that helps different software applications, from different vendors, share common data and information in the clinical healthcare setting, at the point of use ("on the desktop"). CCM Version 1.0, concerned with visual integration in healthcare IT systems, became an ANSI standard in 1999, while version 1.3 was approved as a standard in 2001. The new version of the standard adds, among other things, capabilities relating to the security of patient information as required under HIPAA. This standard is also known as CCOW (pronounced "sea cow"), which originally was an acronym for the Clinical Context Object Workgroup, an independent organization working on visual integration standards at the clinical desktop level. CCOW then joined *HL7*, at which point it was referred to as the Special Interest Group for Visual Integration (SIGVI), before going back to the CCOW name to identify this standards effort.

Clinical Data Abstraction Center (CDAC) An organization that provides data collection and data monitoring tasks for CMS.

Clinical Data Interchange Standards Consortium (CDISC) An open, multidisciplinary, nonprofit organization whose mission is to establish global, vendor-neutral, platform-independent standards for the electronic acquisition, exchange, submission, and archiving of clinical trials data and metadata for medical and biopharmaceutical research and product development. Its sponsors and members include academia, biopharmaceutical companies, technology and service providers, institutional review boards, and other organizations interested in streamlining biopharmaceutical product development and clinical data quality. **www.cdisc.org**

clinical data repository (CDR) A database that collects clinical information, usually in the form of online transactions, in a healthcare setting. It is usually part of a larger software system to help make patient information available where and when it's needed. It may be linked to and be part of an electronic health record (EHR) system.

clinical data set See *data set*.

clinical decision support system (CDSS) An information system used by healthcare providers in a clinical setting to assist in providing the right care at the right time. Several key components to any CDSS are an appropriate repository of knowledge (knowledgebase), a set of rules that spell out what consequences flow from what causes, and a collection of events (triggers) that cause one or more of the foregoing rules to be processed.

    Clinical decision support systems are frequently computer based, and are commercially marketed under their respective trade names by a variety of vendors. A CDSS as used by a healthcare provider may be built using different components from different vendors, but these components must communicate with each other using a standardized language, or "messages." See also *decision-support software*, *HL7*, and *Arden Syntax*.

clinical document A term describing any of a variety of written or printed reports, notes, correspondence, or pictures typically found in a medical record. The standards group *HL7*, in its Clinical Document Architecture (CDA), states that a "clinical document" is defined by the following five characteristics:
1. *Persistence.* It continues to exist in an unaltered state, for a time period defined by local and regulatory requirement.
2. *Stewardship.* It is maintained by a person or organization entrusted with its care.
3. *Potential for authentication.* It is an assemblage of information that is intended to be legally authenticated.
4. *Wholeness.* Authentication of a clinical document applies to the whole and does not apply to portions of the document without the full context of the document.
5. *Human readability.* It can be read by a human.

Clinical Document Architecture (CDA) See discussion under *clinical document*.

clinical engineer (CE) A health professional who specializes in the technology of biomedical equipment. The CE is responsible for advising healthcare providers on acquisition of equipment, user training, safe and efficient use, quality assurance, and problem solving. The American College of Clinical Engineering (ACCE) (**www.acce-htf.org**) defines clinical engineer as "a professional who supports and advances patient care by applying engineering and managerial skills to healthcare technology." See also *biomedical instrumentation technologist*.

    Certified Clinical Engineer (CCE) A clinical engineer who has passed a certification examination and met other requirements of the Healthcare Technology Certification Commission (HTCC) (**www.acce-htf.org**). This credential was formerly offered by the International Certification Commission for Clinical Engineering and Biomedical Technology (ICC) (**accenet.org**).

clinical engineering department See *biomedical engineering department*.

clinical genetics See under *genetics*.

clinical investigator See *investigator*.

clinical knowledge worker See *informationist*.

clinical laboratory compliance The task of ensuring that a clinical laboratory meets the requirements of the Clinical Laboratory Improvement Amendments (CLIA), as well as other federal, state, and quality standards. See also *Qualification in Laboratory Compliance* under *clinical laboratory qualification*.

    Clinical Laboratory Compliance Professional (CLCP) A clinical laboratory compliance professional who has met the certification requirements of the National Credentialing Agency for Laboratory Personnel (NCA). **www.nca-info.org**

Clinical Laboratory Improvement Amendments (CLIA) An act passed by Congress in 1988 with the goal of improving office laboratory quality. Office laboratory procedures were classified by level of complexity and regulations were established for each level—the more complicated the test, the more stringent the requirements. Under the act, a laboratory is defined as "any facility which performs laboratory testing on specimens derived from humans for the purpose of providing information for the diagnosis, prevention, treatment of disease, or impairment of, or assessment of health." CMS is charged with the implementation of CLIA, while the Centers for Disease Control and Prevention (CDC) is responsible for test categorization and the CLIA studies. These amendments were made to the Clinical Laboratories Improvement Act of 1967 (CLIA-67) (Pub. L. No. 90-174, 81 Stat. 533). Pub. L. No. 100-578, 102 Stat. 2903 (1988).

clinical laboratory manager A health professional who manages, supervises, directs, or administers one or more clinical laboratories.

Clinical Laboratory Director (CLDir) A clinical laboratory manager who meets the qualifications for Clinical Laboratory Supervisor and has additional management experience, and has been certified by the National Credentialing Agency for Laboratory Personnel (NCA). **www.nca-info.org**

Clinical Laboratory Supervisor (CLSup) A clinical laboratory manager, certified as a clinical laboratory technologist or specialist, who has been certified by the National Credentialing Agency for Laboratory Personnel (NCA). **www.nca-info.org**

Diplomate in Laboratory Management (DLM(ASCP)) A credential offered by the American Society for Clinical Pathology Board of Registry (ASCP/BOR) for clinical laboratory management professionals with advanced education and experience. **www.ascp.org/bor**

clinical laboratory qualification A credential offered by the American Society for Clinical Pathology (ASCP) to certify that a clinical laboratory professional has met certain requirements. **www.ascp.org/bor**

Point of Care Testing Evaluator Program (POCTE) A clinical laboratory qualification given to persons who are trained by the American Society for Clinical Pathology (ASCP) in evaluating the quality of testing done at the point of care. The POCTE program provides standardized criteria, evaluations, and documentation to assist in compliance with CMS, JCAHO, and other regulatory requirements.

Qualification in Cytometry (QCYM) A clinical laboratory qualification granted when a clinical laboratory professional has demonstrated proficiency in counting and measuring cells.

Qualification in Immunohistochemistry (QIHC) A clinical laboratory qualification granted to a clinical laboratory professional who demonstrates proficiency in the technical application of immunohistochemical techniques, such as DNA probes and antigen retrieval.

Qualification in Laboratory Compliance (QLC) A clinical laboratory qualification granted to a clinical laboratory professional trained and experienced in *clinical laboratory compliance*.

Qualification in Laboratory Informatics (QLI) A clinical laboratory qualification granted to a clinical laboratory professional specializing in laboratory informatics.

clinical laboratory specialist A clinical laboratory professional with advanced education, training, and experience, who has been certified as a specialist in a specific area by a certifying agency.

Clinical Laboratory Specialist in Cytogenetics (CLSp(CG)) A clinical laboratory professional who specializes in the chromosomal analysis of tissue samples, and has been certified by the National Credentialing Agency for Laboratory Personnel (NCA). **www.nca-info.org**

Certified Laboratory Specialist in Molecular Biology (CLSp(MB)) A clinical laboratory professional who specializes in molecular biology, and has been certified by the National Credentialing Agency for Laboratory Personnel (NCA). **www.nca-info.org**

Hemapheresis Practitioner (HP) A specialist in hemapheresis is involved in either the procurement of blood components (donor selection, extraction, preparation and storage of components, returning blood to donor) or their therapeutic use, or both. HP(ASCP) designates certification by the American Society for Clinical Pathology (ASCP). **www.ascp.org/bor**

Specialist in Blood Banking (SBB) A specialist in blood banking will perform procedures such as blood typing, antibody detection, and cross matching; select, prepare, and collect blood from donors; and process and store blood for transfusions. SBB(ASCP) designates certification by the American Society for Clinical Pathology (ASCP). **www.ascp.org/bor**

Specialist in Chemistry (SC) A specialist in chemistry performs procedures such as blood gases, electrolytes, enzymes, hormones, therapeutic drug monitoring, and toxicology. SC(ASCP) designates certification by the American Society for Clinical Pathology (ASCP). **www.ascp.org/bor**

Specialist in Cytotechnology (SCT) A specialist in cytotechnology examines cells for early signs of cancer and other diseases. SCT(ASCP) designates certification by the American Society for Clinical Pathology (ASCP). **www.ascp.org/bor**

Specialist in Hematology (SH) A specialist in hematology performs a full range of blood procedures, from complete blood count and coagulation tests to bone marrow evaluation and platelet function studies. SH(ASCP) designates certification by the American Society for Clinical Pathology (ASCP). **www.ascp.org/bor**

Specialist in Laboratory Safety (SLS) A specialist in making and keeping the clinical laboratory safe will be knowledgeable about standard procedures, chemical safety, biohazard control, physical environment, operations management, and what is required to meet regulatory requirements for lab safety. SLS(ASCP) designates certification by the American Society for Clinical Pathology (ASCP). **www.ascp.org/bor**

Specialist in Microbiology (SM) A specialist in microbiology studies microorganisms, including bacteria, fungi, parasites, and viruses. SM(ASCP) designates certification by the American Society for Clinical Pathology (ASCP). **www.ascp.org/bor**

Specialist in Virology (SV) A specialist in virology studies viruses with cell cultures, antigen detection, immunoassay, immunomicroscopy, molecular techniques, and viral serology. SV(ASCP) designates certification by the American Society for Clinical Pathology (ASCP). **www.ascp.org/bor**

clinical laboratory technician A health professional who performs specific test procedures in a clinical laboratory, under the supervision of a clinical laboratory technologist.

Apheresis Technician (AT) A clinical laboratory technician who is trained in apheresis techniques. AT(ASCP) designates certification by the American Society for Clinical Pathology (ASCP). **www.ascp.org/bor**

Certified Office Laboratory Technician (COLT) A clinical laboratory technician who is trained in the procedures typical of a physician's office practice, and is certified by the American Medical Technologists (AMT). **www.amt1.com**

Clinical Laboratory Technician (CLT) A clinical laboratory technician qualified to perform most medical laboratory tests. CLT(NCA) designates certification by the National Credentialing Agency for Laboratory Personnel (NCA). **www.nca-info.org**

Histotechnician (HT) A clinical laboratory technician who prepares very thin sections of body tissues for microscopic examination by a pathologist. HT(ASCP) designates certification by the American Society for Clinical Pathology (ASCP). **www.ascp.org/bor**

Medical Laboratory Technician (MLT) A clinical laboratory technician qualified to perform general tests in all laboratory areas, including blood banking, chemistry, hematology, immunology, and microbiology. An MLT performs tests that are less complicated than those performed by a Medical Technologist or Clinical Laboratory Technologist. MLT(ASCP) designates certification by the American Society for Clinical Pathology (ASCP) (**www.ascp.org/bor**). MLT(AMT) designates certification by the American Medical Technologists (AMT) (**www.amt1.com**).

Phlebotomy Technician (PBT) A clinical laboratory technician who draws blood from the patient for testing. Also called a phlebotomist. PBT(ASCP) designates certification by the American Society for Clinical Pathology (ASCP). **www.ascp.org/bor**

Clinical Laboratory Phlebotomist (CLPlb) A Phlebotomy Technician who has been certified by the National Credentialing Agency for Laboratory Personnel (NCA). **www.nca-info.org**

Donor Phlebotomy Technician (DPT) A clinical laboratory technician who draws blood from donors. DPT(ASCP) designates certification by the American Society for Clinical Pathology (ASCP). **www.ascp.org/bor**

Registered Phlebotomy Technician (RPT) A Phlebotomy Technician who has received this credential from the American Medical Technologists (AMT). **www.amt1.com**

clinical laboratory technologist A person who performs clinical laboratory tests, confirms the accuracy of the results, and reports the findings to the physician.

Blood Banking Technologist (BB) A clinical laboratory technologist specializing in testing, preparing, and storing blood. BB(ASCP) designates certification by the American Society for Clinical Pathology (ASCP). **www.ascp.org/bor**

Chemistry Technologist (C) A clinical laboratory technologist who specializes in chemical processes. C(ASCP) designates certification by the American Society for Clinical Pathology (ASCP). **www.ascp.org/bor**

Clinical Laboratory Scientist (CLS) A clinical laboratory technologist qualified to perform most medical laboratory tests. CLS(NCA) designates certification by the National Credentialing Agency for Laboratory Personnel (NCA). A CLS may be certified as a "Generalist," or as a "Categorical" in Chemistry/Urinalysis, Hematology, Immunohematology, and Microbiology. **www.nca-info.org**

Cytotechnologist (CT) A clinical laboratory technologist who specializes in the examination of cells. CT(ASCP) designates certification by the American Society for Clinical Pathology (ASCP). **www.ascp.org/bor**

Hematology Technologist (H) A clinical laboratory technologist specializing in hematology (blood testing). H(ASCP) designates certification by the American Society for Clinical Pathology (ASCP). **www.ascp.org/bor**

Histotechnologist (HTL) A clinical laboratory technologist who specializes in the preparation and examination of tissue. Also called histologic technologist. HTL(ASCP) designates certification by the American Society for Clinical Pathology (ASCP). **www.ascp.org/bor**

Medical Technologist (MT) A clinical laboratory technologist qualified to perform most medical laboratory tests. MT(ASCP) designates certification by the American Society for Clinical Pathology (ASCP) (**www.ascp.org/bor**). MT(AMT) designates certification by the American Medical Technologists (AMT) (**www.amt1.com**).

Microbiology Technologist (M) A clinical laboratory technologist who specializes in microorganisms. M(ASCP) designates certification by the American Society for Clinical Pathology (ASCP). **www.ascp.org/bor**

Molecular Pathology Technologist (MP) A clinical laboratory technologist who specializes in molecular pathology. MP(ASCP) designates certification by the American Society for Clinical Pathology (ASCP). **www.ascp.org/bor**

clinical librarian See *clinical medical librarian*.

clinical medical librarian (CML) A specialized librarian in a teaching hospital who participates in teaching activities (including those at the bedside), making notes of questions and then obtaining relevant literature. Synonym: clinical librarian. See also *health science librarian* and *informationist*.

clinical nurse specialist (CNS) A registered nurse with advanced education, training, and experience who has completed the requirements for clinical nurse specialist of the American Nurses Credentialing Center (ANCC) (**nursingworld.org/ancc**), or another credentialing organization, in a *nursing specialty*. See also *advanced practice nurse* and *nurse practitioner*.

clinical path A statement of what steps and procedures should be carried out for the diagnostic evaluation of a patient or for the management (treatment) of a given diagnosis or problem, and the optimum sequence in which they should be carried out. The method was derived from the Critical Path Method (CPM), which is similar to the **program evaluation and review technique (PERT)**, first described in connection with project management procedures developed during World War II.

A major influence toward the use of CPM in medical care was the emergence of teams for taking care of patients, and the communication problems that ensued. (There was less need for coordination when medical care involved only the one physician.) The goal of clinical paths is to ensure that (only) the indicated steps are taken, that they are taken in the correct sequence, and that they are distributed over the shortest time consonant with high quality of care. As a result, the quality of care should be optimal and the cost minimal.

Because resources vary from hospital to hospital, clinical paths are usually produced locally, in contrast with **clinical practice guidelines** (see under **guidelines**), which generally come from authoritative bodies. Synonyms: clinical care paths, clinical pathways.

clinical practice guidelines (CPGs) See under **guidelines**.

clinical practice plan See **medical practice plan**.

clinical prediction rule A rule that uses specified clinical findings to make predictions (decisions) about the diagnostic or management course to be used for a specific patient. With the increased use of computers, the numbers of such rules appearing in the literature are increasing rapidly. Synonym: decision rule.

clinical privileges See under **privileges**.

clinical quality indicator (CQI) See **quality indicator** under **indicator**.

clinical record See **medical record**.

clinical service A division of the medical staff according to clinical specialty, such as surgery, specialties of surgery, internal medicine, specialties of internal medicine, obstetrics and gynecology, pediatrics, neurology, and the like. In some hospitals, clinical services are called departments; for example, the "surgical service" may mean the same thing as the "surgical department." In other instances, a service may be a subdivision of a department; for example, the "orthopedics service" may be part of the larger "department of surgery."

clinical specialist See **clinical nurse specialist**.

Clinical Terms Version 3 (CTV3) The Read Codes. In 1982, a British physician named James Read, then a full-time General Practitioner, developed a simple set of mnemonic codes for his first practice computer to record those conditions that presented commonly in his practice. Over the next few years, the number of codes and the sophistication of the file structure increased to produce one of the leading coding systems for the recording of clinical care. This was the "Read Clinical Classification System," most often called simply the "Read Codes." In 1990, the United Kingdom National Health Service (NHS) acquired the system, and the Read Codes became the recommended standard in U.K. General Practice, with the name changed to the "NHS Codes" (later NHS "Clinical Terms"). In the early 2000s, the latest version, CTV3, was merged into SNOMED Clinical Terms.

clinical trial A systematic experiment on humans designed to evaluate the safety, efficacy, and effectiveness of a drug, biological, medical device, procedure, or other clinical intervention. Synonyms: clinical study, research study.

clinic clerk A person who carries out clerical functions in an outpatient (clinic) setting.

clinician A person who uses a recognized scientific knowledge base and has the authority to direct the provision of personal health services to patients. An Institute of Medicine (IOM) report recommends the use of the term "clinician" as defined here over the term "provider," limiting the use of provider to systems of health care rather than individual health professionals.

clinic without walls (CWW) A legally organized business entity consisting of independent group practices and/or solo practitioners at multiple sites, who combine for centralized management and other services, and to share administrative, purchasing, and billing costs. Synonym: group practice without walls (GPWW).

Clivus Multrum See *composting toilet*.

clone A group of genes, cells, or organisms produced from a common ancestor. Because there is no combining of genetic material (as in sexual reproduction), the members of the clone are genetically identical with the one parent.

cloning The process of producing offspring that are genetically exactly the same as the parent; the process of producing clones.

closed account See under *account*.

closed-chest cardiac massage A technique for stimulating the heart (and producing some circulation of the blood) by compressing the heart between the spine and the breast bone. Pressure is applied by the hands pressing on the front of the chest with the patient lying on his or her back. The technique is a part of cardiopulmonary resuscitation (CPR). Synonym: external cardiac massage.

closed-door pharmacy A pharmacy that can only fill prescriptions for those who are clearly defined as beneficiaries of the client organization or health plan. This type of pharmacy is commonly found in employer-sponsored health-care arrangements.

closed medical staff See under *medical staff*.

closed staff See *medical staff*.

CLPlb See *Clinical Laboratory Phlebotomist* under *Phlebotomy Technician*, under *clinical laboratory technician*.

CLS See *Clinical Laboratory Scientist* under *clinical laboratory technologist*.

CLSp(CG) See *Clinical Laboratory Specialist in Cytogenetics* under *clinical laboratory specialist*.

CLSp(MB) See *Certified Laboratory Specialist in Molecular Biology* under *clinical laboratory specialist*.

CLSup See *Clinical Laboratory Supervisor* under *clinical laboratory manager*.

CLT See *Clinical Laboratory Technician* under *clinical laboratory technician*.

CLVT See *Certified Low Vision Therapist* under *low vision therapist*.

CM See *Certified Midwife* under *midwifery*.

CMA See *Canadian Medical Association* and *Certified Medical Assistant* (under *medical assistant*).

CMAC See *Case Management Administrator Certification* under *case manager*.

CMAS See *Certified Medical Administrative Specialist* under *medical administrative specialist*.

CMC See *Care Manager, Certified* under *care manager*, and *Case Manager Certified* under *case manager*.

CMC-A See *Case Manager Certified—Associate* under *case manager*.

CMCN See *Certified Managed Care Nurse* under *managed care nursing*.

CMD See *Certified Medical Dosimetrist* under *medical dosimetrist*.

CME See *continuing medical education* under *continuing education*.

CMF See *Certified Mastectomy Fitter* under *mastectomy fitter*.

CMG Case-Mix Group. See *inpatient rehabilitation facility prospective payment system* under *prospective payment system*.

CMHC Community mental health center. See *community mental health service program*.

CMHS Center for Mental Health Services. See *Substance Abuse and Mental Health Services Administration*.

CMI See *case mix index* and *Certified Medical Illustrator* (under *medical illustrator*).

CMIO See *chief medical information officer*.

CML See *clinical medical librarian*.

CMM Center for Medicare Management. See *CMS*.

CMO See *chief medical officer*.

CMP See *Certified Medical Physicist* (under *medical physicist*, under *physicist*) and *competitive medical plan*.

CMPE See *Certified Medical Practice Executive* under *medical practice management*.

CMQ Certified in Medical Quality; see *American College of Medical Quality*.

CMR See *computerized medical record* under *electronic health record*.

CMS Centers for Medicare and Medicaid Services. The agency within the Department of Health and Human Services (HHS) that administers Medicare, Medicaid, and the State Children's Health Insurance Program (SCHIP). CMS has three "business centers":

The **Center for Medicare Management (CMM)** manages the traditional fee-for-service Medicare program, including development and implementation of payment policy and management of the Medicare carriers and fiscal intermediaries.

The **Center for Beneficiary Choices (CBC)** provides consumer education to help Medicare beneficiaries make their healthcare decisions. The CBC also manages the Medicare Advantage program, consumer research and demonstrations, and grievance and appeals.

The **Center for Medicaid and State Operations (CMSO)** manages programs administered by the states, including Medicaid, the State Children's Health Insurance Program, private insurance, survey and certification, and the Clinical Laboratory Improvement Amendments (CLIA).

Prior to 2001, CMS was called the Health Care Financing Administration (HCFA). **cms.hhs.gov**

CMS 1450 See *UB-04*.

CMS Common Procedure Coding System See *HCPCS*.

CMSO Center for Medicaid and State Operations. See *CMS*.

CMSRN See *Certified Medical-Surgical Registered Nurse* under *medical-surgical nursing*.

CMSS See *Council of Medical Specialty Societies*.

CMT See *Certified Medical Transcriptionist* under *medical transcriptionist*.

CMTPT See *Certified Myofascial Trigger Point Therapist* under *myofascial trigger point therapist*.

CMV See *cytomegalovirus*.

CN See *Certified Nutritionist* under *nutritionist*.

CNA See *Board Certified Nursing Administrator*, under *nursing administration*, and *Certified Nursing Assistant*, under *nursing assistant*.

CNAA See *Board Certified Nursing Administrator, Advanced* under *nursing administration*.

CNE See *continuing nursing education* under *continuing education*.

CNIM See *Certified Neurophysiologic Intraoperative Monitoring Technologist* under *intraoperative monitoring technologist*.

CNLCP See *Certified Nurse Life Care Planner* under *life care planning*.

CNM See *Certified Nurse-Midwife* under *midwifery*.

CNMT See *Certified Nuclear Medicine Technologist* under *nuclear medicine technologist*.

CNN See *Certified Nephrology Nurse* under *nephrology nursing*.

CNN-NP See *Certified Nephrology Nurse—Nurse Practitioner* under *nephrology nursing*.

CNOR See *Certified Perioperative Nurse* under *perioperative nursing*.

CNRN See *Certified Neuroscience Registered Nurse* under *neuroscience nursing*.

CNS See *Certified Nutrition Specialist*, under *nutritionist*, and *clinical nurse specialist*.

CNSD See *Certified Nutrition Support Dietitian* under *nutrition support*.

CNSN See *Certified Nutrition Support Nurse* under *nutrition support*.

CNSP See *Certified Nutrition Support Physician* under *nutrition support*.

CO See *Certified Orthoptist*, under *orthoptist*, and *Certified Orthotist*, under *orthotist*.

COA See *certificate of authority*, and *Certified Ophthalmic Assistant* (under *ophthalmic medical assistant*).

Coalition for Health Services Research (CHSR) The "advocacy arm" of *AcademyHealth*, which works to enhance funding for health services research. **www.chsr.org**

COB See *coordination of benefits*.

COBRA See *Consolidated Omnibus Budget Reconciliation Act of 1985*.

CoCHP See *Coordinating Center for Health Promotion* under *Centers for Disease Control and Prevention*.

Cochrane Collaboration An international network of individuals and institutions committed to preparing, maintaining, and disseminating systematic reviews of the effects of health care. It was founded in 1993 in England and named in honor of Archie Cochrane, the eminent physician-epidemiologist. The first such reviews, relating to pregnancy and childbirth, were the prototype studies that led to the decision to form the collaboration and extend systematic reviews to all interventions in clinical medicine. Reviews, which emphasize meta-analyses, are based on randomized controlled trials (RTC) whenever available. In their absence, the next best studies are used.

Topics for review are selected by groups with special interests in the topics; thus the collection of reviews grows from the bottom up, which ensures that each review is developed by people with special motivation. Wide dissemination of information about reviews in progress is expected to expand collaboration and prevent duplication of topics. The protocol for each review must pass peer review before it can be registered, and the reviews themselves are also peer reviewed. Review groups are registered, and formal training in review methodology is provided.

The project has been compared in ambition to the Human Genome Project. It plans to discover and include studies in all languages, thousands of which have not previously been electronically indexed. The collaboration has two organizational units. The first are **Cochrane Centers**: Australasian, Brazilian, Canadian, Chinese, Dutch, German, Iberoamerican, Italian, Nordic, South African, United Kingdom, and the United States. The second organizational units are *Cochrane Review groups*. **www.cochrane.org**

Cochrane Database of Systematic Reviews An electronic journal that is updated quarterly reporting systematic reviews (see *Cochrane Review group*) of the effects of health care. Available via the Internet at the Cochrane Library. **www.thecochranelibrary.com**

Cochrane Review group A group of collaborating authors who review the literature of the effects of health care, using explicitly defined procedures in order to reduce the effects of bias in the reviews. The groups are expected to develop the reviews and to maintain them (i.e., to keep abreast of the literature and to modify the reviews as new information warrants). Input from the users of the reviews is sought, and the authoring review group is expected to respond to such input, including publishing the inputs and the responses to them. The reviews are published in the *Cochrane Database of Systematic Reviews*, issued several times each year. See also *Cochrane Collaboration*.

Cockpit Resource Management (CRM) See *Crew Resource Management*.

COCN See *Certified Ostomy Care Nurse* under *wound, ostomy, and continence nursing*.

codable diagnosis See under *diagnosis*.

code (data) A unique symbol (usually alphanumeric) having a one-to-one correspondence with a term or a rubric (label of a category). Codes may be used on the patient's bill, for example, to indicate the service for which the charge is shown. Diagnoses and procedures are commonly coded for ease of manipulation by computer (see *coding*).

code (jargon) A shorthand representation for something. Hospitals often use colors or numbers to indicate urgent situations. For example, "code blue" often is used to mean that a patient needs resuscitation; "code 2" may signal a disruptive (violent) patient or visitor; "Dr. Red" might mean a fire. A "code purple" in some hospitals means that a "VIP" (very important person) has arrived as an inpatient or at the emergency department (ED). The codes are spoken over the public address system, usually along with information about the location of the situation; for example, "code 7, ICU" (intensive care unit). These codes give the people who need to know (and respond) concise information, without unnecessarily upsetting patients and visitors. See also *code blue* and *coded (jargon)*.

show code A situation where a code blue (call for resuscitation) is made on a patient whose heart has stopped, but where the healthcare providers really do not believe that resuscitation is appropriate. The "code" is thus for "show," because authentic resuscitation efforts are not made. Show codes were sometimes done in the past if no clear decision had been made regarding whether the patient should be resuscitated in case of cardiac arrest, or where a physician was uncertain whether to document the decision. These days, most hospitals require an actual resuscitation attempt unless a do not resuscitate (DNR) order has been written on the patient's chart by the physician. Synonyms: slow code, code gray, code pink.

slow code See *show code*.

code blue Perhaps the most common code used in hospitals for signaling a cardiac (heart) emergency, meaning that someone is in need of cardiopulmonary resuscitation (CPR). (Some hospitals will have a different code; for example, "Code 7" or "Code Yellow.") Those individuals who are expected to respond know who they are, what it means, and what their response is expected to be. It is sometimes said that a patient has been "coded" when a code blue alarm has been sent. See also *show code* under *code (jargon)*.

code creep See *DRG creep*.

coded (data) When data or information has been replaced by a code, it is said to have been coded (i.e., the coding process has been carried out).

coded (jargon) Hospital jargon referring to a patient for whom a code blue signal has been sent, indicating the occurrence of a cardiac (heart) emergency. Similarly, when a do not resuscitate (DNR) order has been recorded for a patient, that patient, in hospital jargon, is "not to be coded" (resuscitated).

code gray See *show code* under *code (jargon)*.

Code of Federal Regulations (CFR) A federal government publication containing the rules and regulations issued by various federal agencies as a result of laws enacted by the legislature. Federal laws will frequently contain provisions that authorize a particular federal agency to "promulgate" regulations that help carry out the letter and spirit of the law. One reason for doing this is to prevent the law itself from becoming bogged down in unnecessary administrative details. Although the enacted law itself may set the public policy goals and objectives to be achieved, the regulations often implement the law in a day-to-day setting. The body of these rules and regulations is often referred to as "administrative law," to distinguish it from the law found in legislation, or "judicial law," which is the law found in court decisions. Administrative law has grown tremendously in the last several decades.

The CFR is subdivided into fifty separate titles, according to the administrative agency and subject matter covered. CMS regulations, for instance, would be found in Title 42 of the CFR. Generally, before regulations become effective they must be published in the *Federal Register*. **www.gpoaccess.gov/cfr**

Code on Dental Procedures and Nomenclature (CDT) A publication of the American Dental Association (ADA) containing its classification of dental procedures. It is the dental equivalent of the CPT (codes for other-than-dental procedures). Hence the ADA's choice of the official abbreviation CDT rather than CDPN. The CDT is generally updated every two years.

code pink See *show code* under *code (jargon)*.

coder A person who does coding. See also *coding specialist*.

Code Set See *Transactions and Code Sets*.

coding (billing) Adding a code or codes (typically alphanumeric) to a patient's medical record. The codes identify (1) the diagnosis or diagnoses for which services were provided (these are usually ICD-9-CM codes), and (2) procedures performed and other services or supplies provided (ICD-9-CM, CPT, and/or HCPCS codes). In some cases, the code identifies both the diagnosis and the services (DRGs, Ambulatory Patient Groups). This is an integral part of the billing process, for the codes determine the charge. Computer programs are commercially available to assist providers in obtaining **optimal coding** and avoiding **undercoding** and **overcoding** (see below). See also **gaming**.

downcoding A practice of insurance companies (and other payers) of recoding the service or procedure on a bill to a lower reimbursement category, so that the insurer pays less to the provider than would otherwise be required.

optimal coding Coding to qualify for the highest reimbursement possible, yet avoid any suggestion to the payer's audit system that an attempt is being made to obtain unjustified reimbursement (i.e., to avoid interpretation of the bill as "overcoded").

overcoding Coding that suggests to the payer's audit system that an attempt is being made to obtain a higher reimbursement than was probably justified. An audit of the coding and billing is likely to be triggered by such coding.

undercoding Coding that will result in a smaller reimbursement than the patient's condition and the care rendered would actually justify.

upcoding Changing the coding of a patient's diagnoses (and perhaps operations) in order to obtain a higher payment for the services rendered. More accurately called "upclassifying." Upcoding may result in liability for false claims or fraud.

coding (process) The process of substituting a symbol (code), usually a numeric or alphanumeric string of characters, for a term, such as a diagnosis or procedure. Of course, every term coded can be decoded (i.e., the code can be looked up and one can find precisely the term that it represents).

Coding ordinarily has three purposes: (1) to compress the information from a string of letters or words into a compact, usually uniform, space; (2) to facilitate handling the information by mechanical (computer) methods; and (3) to introduce precision (reduce ambiguity), because numbers are not subject to spelling errors and it is easier to make an exact check of a number than of a word. (Inventories are controlled, for example, by code numbers rather than narrative descriptions of their contents.)

Coding should only require substituting a code for the term to be coded. However, in many circumstances, the term to be coded will not be found in the coder's reference material, and a judgment will have to be made. In this case, the coder must know both the meaning of the term and also the way the coding system works, so that proper coding can be done. Under such circumstances, the task is really one of **classification (process)** rather than coding.

There are two basic ways to code: (1) assigning to each individual entity (term) its own unique code (number); and (2) assigning to each term a code that represents a category, which category may include one or more individual entities (terms). The first technique is called **entity coding**; the second is **category coding** (see below).

See also **cryptography** and **transforming**.

category coding Coding in which each code (number, character string) represents (the rubric of) a category rather than an individual term being coded. Category coding is designed to achieve grouping to established classification "pigeonholes" in a single step that combines coding and classifying.

Category coding is the method presently used by hospitals and physicians for coding diagnoses and procedures. This coding is done for the indexing of medical records for retrieval and research, and in the submission of discharge abstracts for billing (see **coding (billing)**). Each diagnosis and procedure is given the code for the category of diagnoses or procedures to which it belongs, rather than a unique code ("entity code") that represents the diagnosis or procedure itself.

Except for "single-diagnosis categories," the diagnosis of the case cannot be retrieved precisely because decoding retrieves the rubric (label) of the category rather than the specific diagnosis or procedure that was coded. For example, a specific new condition such as AIDS (acquired immunodeficiency syndrome), which had not been foreseen and had no category or pigeonhole of its own, for several years was placed into various categories, such as the "wastebasket" category labeled "other immune deficiency disorders." Such a system makes it impossible, without going back to the original medical records, to determine the exact number of AIDS cases or to retrieve them by themselves; all cases of "other immune deficiency disorders" are retrieved and counted together.

In the coding system now in use in the United States, which is a category coding system (ICD-9-CM), over 100,000 diagnostic terms are forced into about 11,000 groups or classes; further detail is lost when these categories, in turn, go into the 468 **DRGs**.

entity coding Coding in which each code represents an individual entity (term) rather than a category (group) of terms. In entity coding, each entity (specific term) to be coded (for example, a diagnosis or procedure) is exchanged for a code (number) that, when decoded, yields exactly the same words (term) that were coded (see decoding). No detail is lost as is the case in category coding; entity coding achieves one of the major purposes of coding, the elimination of ambiguity in the information in order to increase its precision, because numbers are not subject to spelling errors and it is easier to make an exact check of a number than of a word. In the special case in which the original term is transformed into a standardized language, each term of which has its own termcode, as in SNOMED, the coding is entity coding, but decoding will only retrieve the transformed term, not the original.

The principle behind entity coding is that classification should be a two-step process: in the first step, information is coded so that it can be manipulated (usually by a computer); in the second step, the coded information is then classified according to the needs of the particular user or the demands of a particular classification (scheme) system. In entity coding, the integrity of the items of information remains intact, and the system can meet the needs of any number of classification systems. For example, a person investigating the frequency of office visits for various medical problems would need to have a discrete class for the common cold because of its frequency in that setting. Because common colds seldom require hospitalization, however, placing the cold in a category of "other respiratory diseases" or "other infectious diseases" might meet the needs of a hospital studying reasons for admission.

coding specialist A health professional who classifies clinical data from patient records, assigning code numbers to diagnoses and procedures for billing and other health information purposes.

Certified Clinical Coder (CCC) A coding specialist who is also a clinical health professional (for example, a physician, physician's assistant, physical therapist, or paramedic), other than a registered nurse, who has completed the Clinical Coding Certification examination of the American Association of Clinical Coders and Auditors, Inc. (AACCA). **www.aacca.net**

Certified Coding Associate (CCA) An entry-level credential offered by the American Health Information Management Association (AHIMA). Coding specialists who have a U.S. high school diploma or equivalent and pass the requisite CCA examination can obtain this credential.

Certified Coding Specialist (CCS) A coding specialist, usually based in the hospital, who has met the requirements of the Council on Certification (COC) of the American Health Information Management Association (AHIMA). **www.ahima.org**

Certified Coding Specialist—Physician-based (CCS-P) A certified coding specialist with expertise in physicians' offices, group practices, clinics, and specialty centers, who has passed an examination in this area given by the Council on Certification (COC) of the American Health Information Management Association (AHIMA). **www.ahima.org**

Certified Professional Coder (CPC) A coding specialist in physician practices who has met the certification requirements of the American Academy of Professional Coders (AAPC). **www.aapc.com**

Certified Professional Coder—Hospital (CPC-H) A coding specialist in outpatient facilities who has met the certification requirements of the American Academy of Professional Coders (AAPC). **www.aapc.com**

Certified Professional Coder—Payer (CPC-P) A coding specialist who works in the payer industry, who has met the certification requirements of the American Academy of Professional Coders (AAPC). **www.aapc.com**

Radiology Certified Coder (RCC) A coding specialist who specializes in radiology coding and has been certified by the Radiology Coding Certification Board (RCCB). **www.rccb.org**

RN-Coder A coding specialist, who is also a registered nurse, who has completed the Clinical Coding Certification examination of the American Association of Clinical Coders and Auditors (AACCA). **www.aacca.net**

coding summary form See *physician query form*.

Codman Award An award created in 1996 by the Joint Commission on Accreditation of Healthcare Organizations (JCAHO) to recognize achievement in "the use of process and outcomes measures to improve organization performance and, ultimately, the quality of care provided to the public." JCAHO named the award for Ernest A. Codman, "the father of outcomes measurement."

codon See under *DNA*.

COGH See *Coordinating Office for Global Health* under *Centers for Disease Control and Prevention*.

COGME See *Council on Graduate Medical Education*.

cognitive Pertaining to knowledge.

cognitive dissonance When two sets of information are not compatible with each other.

cognitive rehabilitation See under *rehabilitation*.

cognitive services A term applied to all the activities of a physician (or other professional) other than the performance of *procedures*. The charges of physicians are relatively easy to explain in surgery and other instances where "something is done" to the patient. High charges for, say, diagnostic evaluations, patient and family counseling, and the care of patients with infectious diseases are much harder to explain, and thus charges are considerably lower.

"Cognitive services" require as much time and skill as surgery. However, much of this effort and skill is simply not seen by the patient or payer. Nonetheless, an education as long and arduous as the surgeon's may be required, as well as unseen time in the library and informal consultation with colleagues. Efforts to overcome the resulting perceived inequities in payment have led to the labeling of nonprocedural services as cognitive (intellectual). No term for "noncognitive" services seems to have appeared.

cognome See *Human Cognome Project*.

COHN See *Certified Occupational Health Nurse* under *occupational health nursing*.

COHN/CM See *Certified Occupational Health Nurse/Case Manager* under *case manager*.

COHN-S See *Certified Occupational Health Nurse—Specialist* under *occupational health nursing*.

COHN-S/CM See *Certified Occupational Health Nurse—Specialist/Case Manager* under *case manager*.

COI See *certificate of insurance*.

coinsurance A percentage to be paid by a health plan enrollee (beneficiary) of the cost of healthcare services. For example, if an enrollee has a 50% coinsurance contract, this requires the enrollee to pay 50% of the charge amount that has been approved for that service by the plan. The health plan pays its portion of the charge (50% in this case) and sends the enrollee an "explanation of benefits," which shows the amount owed by the enrollee. The enrollee sends payment directly to the provider of the service. This is a method of cost-sharing between the enrollee and the plan, and serves as an incentive for the enrollee to stay healthy and to use healthcare resources wisely, thus helping to contain healthcare costs. See also *copayment* and *deductible*.

collaborative care See *managed care*.

collaboratory A word made from the combination of "collaboration" and "laboratory." A collaboratory is two or more laboratories collaborating with each other via a telecommunications network. A report on collaboratories prepared on behalf of the National Research Council described a collaboratory as a ". . . center without walls in which the nation's researchers can perform research without regard to geographical location, interacting with colleagues, accessing instrumentation, sharing data and computational resources, and accessing information from digital libraries." The rise of the Internet will likely result in collaboratories playing a greater role in health care in the future.

collateral source rule A legal rule of evidence that prohibits the jury from considering the fact that the plaintiff has been compensated from any source other than the defendant. The practical result is that a medical malpractice defendant may have to pay the full amount of the plaintiff patient's medical and other expenses, even if the patient has already received reimbursement for those expenses from another source, such as medical insurance.

collective bargaining The process of negotiation regarding compensation, working conditions, benefits, and other matters, between an employer and an organization representing the employees. In collective bargaining, the employees may be represented by a union or by some other form of association.

college health nursing The nursing specialty focusing on the health needs of college and university students.

Certified College Health Nurse A specialist in college health nursing who has met the requirements of the American Nurses Credentialing Center (ANCC). The certification examination was eliminated in 2005. **nursingworld.org/ancc**

College of American Pathologists (CAP) The principal organization of board-certified pathologists, which represents the interests of patients, the public, and pathologists. It encourages excellence in the practice of pathology and laboratory medicine worldwide. Founded in 1946, it had nearly 16,000 physician members by the year 2007, and is the world's largest association composed exclusively of pathologists. CAP was also responsible for developing and maintaining *SNOMED*. **www.cap.org**

College of Healthcare Information Management Executives (CHIME) An organization dedicated to the professional development needs of healthcare chief information officers (CIOs) and to advocating the more effective use of information management within health care. **www.cio-chime.org**

collegial The sharing of power or authority equally among a number of colleagues. In a truly collegial environment, no one individual can be held accountable because no one individual is in charge.

colon and rectal surgery A *medical specialty*.

COLT See *Certified Office Laboratory Technician* under *clinical laboratory technician*.

coma A state of deep unconsciousness.

COMAH Clinical Outcome Measure Amended HEDIS Strategy. See *Health Plan Employer Data and Information Set* under *data set*.

comfort animal See *service animal*.

comfort care Medical or other health care whose sole or primary purpose is the comfort of the patient. In the Oregon Health Plan, comfort care is defined to exclude health services that are diagnostic, curative, or focused on active treatment of the primary condition and intended to prolong life. Examples of comfort care include pain medication, hospice services, medical equipment and supplies (beds, wheelchairs, etc.), and services for symptom relief (e.g., radiation therapy). See also *palliative care*.

Comité Européen de Normalisation (CEN) See *CEN (organization)*.

Commission on Accreditation for Health Informatics and Information Management Education (CAHIIM) The accrediting organization for degree-granting programs in health informatics and information management. The standards for accreditation are set by the

American Health Information Management Association (AHIMA) in cooperation with the commission. **www.cahiim.org**

Commission on Accreditation of Allied Health Education Programs (CAAHEP) A non-profit organization whose purpose is to accredit certain health science education programs. It is the largest such organization in the United States, accrediting more than 2,000 programs in nineteen health science disciplines. Formerly the Committee on Allied Health Education and Accreditation (CAHEA). **www.caahep.org**

Commission on Professional and Hospital Activities (CPHA) An independent nonprofit organization dedicated to the improvement of healthcare quality through the use of comparative data. It was formed in 1955 with the national sponsorship of the American College of Physicians (ACP), the American College of Surgeons (ACS), and the American Hospital Association (AHA), with a founding grant from the W.K. Kellogg Foundation. CPHA provided certain shared clinical and management information services (MIS) data processing, performed interpretive research services for hospitals and other healthcare institutions, and disseminated information to the healthcare field. Its largest and oldest program was the prototype hospital discharge abstract system, the *Professional Activity Study (PAS)*. CPHA has been incorporated into the facilities of the University of North Carolina at Chapel Hill. **www.shepscenter.unc.edu/research_programs/health_care**

commitment The legal process by which a court orders the admission of an individual to a psychiatric facility or unit. The procedure may be criminal or civil, and voluntary or involuntary. See also *assisted outpatient treatment*.

involuntary commitment The admission of a person to a mental healthcare facility against that person's will. Involuntary commitment is the result of a court proceeding. In most jurisdictions, mental illness alone is insufficient for an involuntary commitment. Usually, at least one of the following factors must also be present: (1) the person is incapable of taking care of him- or herself; (2) he or she is likely to injure him- or herself (intentionally or unintentionally); or (3) he or she is likely to injure another (intentionally or unintentionally).

committee A group of people set up for a specific purpose: to consider or investigate a matter, to report on a matter, or to carry out certain duties. Committees can be self-appointed, but in the healthcare setting, they are ordinarily appointed, and their scope and powers derive from the authority that appointed them. The term "committee" is more often applied to a standing body than it is to an ad hoc (one-time) body set up to carry out a specific task and then be dissolved. The latter is more appropriately termed a "task force."

committee of the incompetent See *guardian*.

Committee on Allied Health Education and Accreditation (CAHEA) Former name of the *Commission on Accreditation of Allied Health Education Programs (CAAHEP)*.

Committee on Energy and Commerce (CEC) The oldest legislative standing committee in the U.S. House of Representatives. It includes six subcommittees: Health; Energy and Air Quality; Environment and Hazardous Materials; Commerce, Trade and Consumer Protection; Oversight and Investigations; and Telecommunications and the Internet. The CEC periodically publishes a compilation of federal health laws, including the Public Health Service Act (PHSA). **energycommerce.house.gov**

Committee on Health, Education, Labor, and Pensions (HELP) The legislative standing committee in the U.S. Senate that deals with issues on health. Its Subcommittee on Bioterrorism and Public Health Preparedness focuses on ensuring that the United States is prepared for public health emergencies, whether deliberate, accidental, or natural. The subcommittee has jurisdiction over a wide range of bioterrorism and public health issues including Project BioShield, the Centers for Disease Control and Prevention (CDC), immunizations, infectious diseases, pandemic flu, and vaccines. **help.senate.gov**

Committee on Health Informatics See *ASTM E31 Committee on Health Informatics*.

common law Law that has been created by the courts, through decisions of judges, rather than by the legislature (statutory law). Synonyms: case law, judicial law. See also *case (legal)*.

commons-based peer production (CBPP) A recently recognized mode of economic production using wide-spread collaboration, which supplements and competes with the traditional modes: (1) done by employees in firms, following the directions of management; and (2) done by individuals, following price signals in markets. CBPP has appeared in software development, where it is called *Open Source* software and is typified by the operating system Linux, and in the open online encyclopedia Wikipedia (**www.wikipedia.org**). Thousands, even tens of thousands, of programmers or contributors collaborate freely on projects of their own choice and the product is, in turn, available to those who wish to use it. The term was coined by Yochai Benkler in his article, "Coase's Penguin, or, Linux and the Nature of the Firm" (*Yale Law Journal*, 2002;112:369).

Commonwealth Fund A philanthropic foundation created in 1918 by Anna M. Harkness to "enhance the common good." The fund supports programs in the areas of improving healthcare services and the well-being of minority Americans, people with low incomes, the elderly, the uninsured, and young children. The fund emphasizes promotion of healthy behavior and prevention of illness, and also conducts independent research in the areas of health and social policy issues. In 1986, the fund was given the assets of the James Picker Foundation, in support of Picker programs to advance the fund's mission. One project was the Picker/Commonwealth Program for Patient-Centered Care; see *Picker Institute*. **www.cmwf.org**

community benefit See *community consent* under *informed consent*.

community care network (CCN) A demonstration program for delivering health care in the local community. The National Community Care Network Demonstration Program, begun in 1994, was a collaborative effort of the American Hospital Association, Catholic Health Association of the United States (CHA), and VHA Inc., and received funds from the W.K. Kellogg Foundation, Duke Endowment, Robert Wood Johnson Foundation, California Wellness Foundation, and the Health Resources and Services Administration (HRSA) of the Department of Health and Human Services (HHS).

Twenty-five sites were selected from throughout the United States to represent urban, rural, and suburban areas. Communities in each site formed partnerships to focus "on achieving better accountability, aligning resources with social needs, and improving the health of the population." CCNs included healthcare providers, human service agencies, businesses, government agencies, schools, religious organizations, and individual members of the community. Phase II of the program, which began in 1999, focused on "institutionalization and dissemination of the CCN vision."

community consultation See *community consent* under *informed consent*.

community counselor A counselor who works in community agencies or institutions; also called a service agency counselor.

Community Health Accreditation Program (CHAP) An independent, nonprofit accrediting body for community-based healthcare organizations, including home health agencies and programs, hospice services, and other community-based programs. CHAP has standards pertaining to planning, finance, service delivery, operations, human resources, evaluation, and outcomes of care. Those programs meeting the standards of CHAP are given accreditation. CHAP also has authority to determine whether organizations meet the Medicare conditions of participation (COPs).

Created in 1965 as a joint venture between the American Public Health Association (APHA) and the National League for Nursing (NLN), CHAP was for a time a subsidiary of NLN but spun off as an independent entity in 2001. **www.chapinc.org**

Community Health Center (CHC) A federal program to provide healthcare services to Medically Underserved Areas and Medically Underserved Populations; see *Federally Qualified Health Center*.

community health information network (CHIN) See *community health integrated management information system (CHIMIS)* under *information system*.

community health integrated management information system (CHIMIS) See under *information system*.

Community Health Intervention Partnership (CHIP) A program designed to help hospitals and health systems work with community development corporations to assess local health needs, identify major community health problems, and develop plans to address them. A project of the Hospital Research and Educational Trust (HRET) of the American Hospital Association (AHA) under a grant from the Robert Wood Johnson Foundation.

community health network (CHN) A term sometimes employed as a label for a municipally operated system of providing health care for the poor. See also *community care network*.

community health nursing See *public health nursing*.

community health plan (CHP) See *Hospital Health Plan*.

community health services A term that encompasses preventive procedures, diagnosis, and treatment for residents of a community. It does not imply any organizational structure.

community health worker (CHW) A community member who serves as a connector between healthcare providers and healthcare consumers. Most of the work is done in the community setting among groups that have traditionally been underserved. The CHW identifies community health problems, develops innovative solutions, and translates the solutions into practice. Sometimes called a "lay health provider."

community living facility See *halfway house*.

community mental health center (CMHC) See *community mental health service program*.

community mental health service program An organization set up to provide mental health services to a defined community. Synonym: community mental health center (CMHC).

Community of Science (COS) An organization providing information resources to researchers, scholars, and other professionals. Services include expert databases, information about funding opportunities, a collaborative online authoring system, and access to a number of professional reference databases including U.S. Patents, MEDLINE, AGRICOLA, GeoRef, and others. **www.cos.com**

community rating See under *rating*.

community residential facility See *intermediate care facility for the mentally retarded*.

community resource management (CRM) The concept, in health care, that the unit that should be considered in the allocation of resources is the entire community rather than each of its component organizations.

community-wide health information system (CWHIS) An undefined term used in a *Stark II* "safe harbor" regulation. The Stark law prohibits physicians from referring Medicare patients to any healthcare facility with which they have a financial relationship. The development of electronic health information systems to share information between the hospital and its physicians is sometimes hindered by the physicians' lack of the necessary hardware, software, training, and support to participate in the exchange of information, including e-prescribing. Hospitals sometimes donate (or subsidize) these ingredients to facilitate participation by physicians. This arguably violates the Stark law, so CMS issued a regulation to provide a safe harbor for hospitals and physicians who participate in such an arrangement. The regulation, entitled "Medicare Program; Physicians' Referrals to Health Care Entities With Which They Have Financial Relationships; Exceptions for Certain Electronic Prescribing and Electronic Health Records Arrangements" (42 C.F.R. § 411.357 (October 1, 2006)) states:

Exceptions to the referral prohibition related to compensation arrangements.

For purposes of Sec. 411.353, the following compensation arrangements do not constitute a financial relationship:

. . .

   (u) Community-wide health information systems. Items or services of information technology provided by an entity to a physician that allow access to, and sharing of, electronic health care records and any complementary drug information systems, general health information, medical alerts, and related information for patients served by community providers and practitioners, in order to enhance the community's overall health. . . .

The items or services must be necessary to enable the physician to participate in the community-wide health information system, be used principally for that purpose, and not be provided in a way that takes into account the volume or value of the physician's referrals. The CWHIS itself must be "available to all providers, practitioners, and residents of the community who desire to participate." In addition, the arrangement must not violate the **Antikickback Statute** or other federal or state law or regulation governing billing or claims submission. The regulation does not further define "community-wide health information system." Synonym: CHIS. See also *regional health information organization*.

comorbidity See under *morbidity*.

comparability See *data comparability*.

Compassion & Choices A nonprofit organization promoting choice and care at the end of life, including comprehensive pain control and palliative care, and legal aid in dying if suffering is unbearable. Created in 2005 by the unification of Compassion in Dying and End-of Life Choices. (Both of these came after, and had some connection with, the Hemlock Society.) **www.compassionandchoices.org**

compassionate use Approval by the Food and Drug Administration (FDA) to use an experimental drug or therapy, before final FDA approval, in the case of a very sick individual for whom other treatments have failed, or for whom there are no other treatment options. See also *Emergency Use Authorization*.

compensable Something for which the law allows money to be awarded to make amends or restore someone to their prior position. Not all types of injury (for example, mental distress suffered by an unusually sensitive person) are compensable. See *damages*.

   In workers' compensation law, "compensable" describes an injury or illness that is work-related, and therefore covered by the workers' compensation system.

compensation In addition to the common meaning of payment for work done, compensation covers systems to make reparation for damage or injury done. Traditionally, patients who have been injured by the healthcare system, either by malpractice or otherwise, have sought compensation by filing a claim—which usually results in a lawsuit—against the healthcare provider. This system is lengthy and costly, and does not always provide a fair result. Thus, alternatives are being proposed. See also *deferred compensation*.

neo-no-fault compensation See *patients' compensation* below.

no-fault compensation A system of compensation for persons who have been injured or adversely affected, without the need to prove fault or wrongdoing. No-fault systems are presently in use to compensate auto and industrial accident victims (see *workers' compensation* below). Several no-fault (or no-fault-like) plans have been suggested for the healthcare arena; see, for example, *patients' compensation* below.

patients' compensation A no-fault system for compensating patients who suffer harm as a result of some aspect of medical or hospital care, proposed as an alternative to malpractice litigation. Synonym: neo-no-fault compensation. See also *early offer*.

workers' compensation (WC) A system of compensating workers for on-the-job injuries, developed as an alternative to lawsuits by injured employees. The typical workers' compensation law compensates workers who suffer work-related injuries (regardless of fault), and provides that workers' compensation benefits are the "exclusive remedy," the only means of receiving compensation for work-related injuries and illnesses. Workers may therefore not sue their employers (but see also *dual injury doctrine*). Workers' compensation was formerly called workmen's compensation.

competent A legal term describing a person whom the law considers capable of making decisions. Competency is relative, and standards of competency vary according to the type of decision to be made. This concept is discussed further under *incompetent (legal capacity)*.

competitive medical plan (CMP) A health plan, licensed by the state, that provides healthcare services to enrolled members on a prepaid, capitated basis. Most often used to refer to an entity that has met certain requirements of the federal government to be designated as a competitive medical plan (see 42 C.F.R. § 417.407 (October 1, 2005)). A federally designated CMP is eligible for a risk contract with CMS to provide services to Medicare beneficiaries. The requirements for CMP designation are not as strict as those for becoming a federally qualified HMO (FQHMO).

complementary and alternative medicine (CAM) Healthcare practices traditionally outside the mainstream U.S. healthcare system. The National Center for Complementary and Alternative Medicine (NCCAM) defines complementary and alternative medicine (CAM) as "a group of diverse medical and health care systems, practices, and products that are not presently considered to be part of conventional medicine." "Alternative" referred to therapies used instead of mainstream care, and "complementary" to therapies serving a supporting role. Hospitals are now offering some of these therapies, and health insurance sometimes covers care previously considered unconventional. Physicians and other health professionals are obtaining formal credentials in practices formerly considered alternative, such as acupuncture. The term "**integrative medicine**" is coming into use to describe a broader philosophy that seeks to evaluate and incorporate methods that are useful, regardless of "category." Some use "blended medicine" in a similar sense.

   CAM, in the meantime, covers a very broad range of health philosophies and practices, some with well-established education, training, and credentialing programs, and others that are as-yet difficult to pin down and/or be accepted. NCCAM categorizes CAM into five **major domains**:

alternative medical systems These "involve complete systems of theory and practice that have evolved independent of and often prior to the conventional biomedical approach. Many are traditional systems of medicine that are practiced by individual cultures throughout the world, including a number of venerable Asian approaches." (See *medicine (system)*.)

mind-body interventions Techniques to facilitate the mind's capacity to affect the body, such as hypnosis, creative arts therapies, prayer, and mental healing.

biological-based therapies Use of agents that affect the body's biological processes. Examples include herbal medicine, biological therapies, special diets, and orthomolecular therapies.

manipulative and body-based methods Techniques to improve health through manipulation or movement of the body, such as chiropractic and osteopathic manipulation and massage.

energy therapies Techniques focusing on energy fields, either those originating within the body (biofields) or those coming from exterior sources (such as electromagnetic fields). Examples include qi gong, Reiki, and bioelectromagnetic therapy.

   A 2001 article in *Annals of Internal Medicine* placed CAM into five slightly different classes: (1) professional systems, (2) popular health reform, (3) New Age healing, (4) mind-body, and (5) non-normative scientific enterprises. See *unconventional healing practices*.

complementary, integrative, or alternative practitioner (CIA) A collective term for practitioners of *complementary and alternative medicine (CAM)*.

complementary medicine See *complementary and alternative medicine*.

complex adaptive system (CAS) A collection of individual "agents" (components) that have the freedom to act in ways that are not always predictable and whose actions are interconnected, such that one agent's actions change the context for other agents. This is in contrast with a mechanical system in which the various agents always act in the same manner—a thermostat always sends a signal when it reaches the temperature for which it has been set. An adaptive system does not always respond to the same stimulus in the same way—a physician and patient may react to each other quite differently at different times. An increasing amount of research is going into CAS as a science itself and in biology, medicine, and organizational behavior. A section of the Institute of Medicine's 2001 report *Crossing the Quality Chasm* was devoted to the implications of CAS theory to the redesign of health care.

compliance Meeting the statutory or regulatory requirements set out for a particular activity in providing health care. Although many such requirements are based on legislation of one kind or another, some are based on private or voluntary efforts and are similar in some ways to accreditation and licensure. A failure to comply with certain legal requirements can result in serious consequences, including criminal penalties.

Many healthcare providers have begun to formalize this under the concept of assessing their **compliance risk** and implementing a **corporate compliance program**, headed by a corporate **compliance officer**. Typically such a program also includes a corporate **compliance policy** that has the approval of the governing board, the corporate officers, and the medical staff. This policy will discuss standards of conduct for individuals acting on behalf of the corporation, including such areas as conflict of interest, political activity, acceptance of gifts from vendors, confidentiality, dealing with competitors, and physician recruitment.

complication A disease or injury that develops during the course of treatment for another disease or injury. As used in the prospective payment system (PPS), a complication is a diagnosis occurring during hospitalization that is thought to extend the hospital stay at least one day for roughly 75% or more of the patients. The occurrence of a complication is determined in the PPS by the presence, as a secondary ICD-9-CM diagnosis code in the patient's bill, of a condition defined by PPS as a complication. See also *comorbidity* under *morbidity*.

composting toilet A system for handling human wastes and food scraps by composting them without added water, thus producing a safe, rich humus resembling garden soil and a liquid high-nitrogen fertilizer. Among keys to the success of the process are (1) providing properly designed composters that direct air flow over the composting material, (2) using waterless or ultra-low-flush toilets, (3) periodic addition of small amounts of high-carbon material such as sawdust to the composter, and (4) separating the wash water, "greywater," from baths, lavatories, sinks, dishwashers, and laundries into a separate waste system and subjecting this water to separate treatment, with later use for irrigation.

The system is promoted as ecologically sound, offering substantial reduction in water use and resulting in decreased need for public water supplies and sewage systems and sewage treatment plants. The earliest composter reported is the "Clivus Multrum," which has been in use since 1939, and bears the National Sanitation Foundation Seal of Approval. Installations have been successful in private homes and also in such sites as highway washrooms, parks, resorts, schools, community centers, libraries, clinics, and restaurants.

Comprehensive Accreditation Manual for Hospitals (CAMH) A publication of the Joint Commission on Accreditation of Healthcare Organizations (JCAHO), updated quarterly, which specifies the standards that must be met for a hospital to be accredited. It includes standards, intent statements, scoring, aggregation rules, decision rules, and accreditation policies and procedures. Nearly every hospital will have a current edition of *CAMH*.

comprehensive benefit package (CBP) See *benefit package*.

Comprehensive Error Rate Testing (CERT) A program established by CMS in 2002 to calculate the *payment error rate* for claims submitted to Medicare Administrative Contractors

(MACs) (formerly carriers, fiscal intermediaries, and durable medical equipment regional carriers, collectively referred to as "affiliated contractors" (ACs)). Of the 2 billion claims processed per year, CERT randomly selects a statistical sample for review to determine whether the claims were properly paid or denied. CERT activities are performed by two contractors: the **CERT Review Contractor (CRC)** and the **CERT Documentation Contractor (CDC)**. The CRC performs the review function, while the CDC is responsible for obtaining documentation of claims from the providers. Claims submitted for acute care inpatient hospital stays are reviewed by the *Hospital Payment Monitoring Program* (*HPMP*).

comprehensive health care Services that are intended to meet all the healthcare needs of a patient: outpatient, inpatient, home care, and other.

comprehensive healthcare delivery system A healthcare delivery system that includes both facilities and professionals, and that is set up to provide comprehensive health care to a defined population.

Comprehensive Health Enhancement Support System (CHESS) See *CHESS*.

comprehensive health planning (CHP) See under *planning*.

comprehensive outpatient rehabilitation facility (CORF) An outpatient facility that provides, at a single fixed location, diagnostic, therapeutic, and restorative services for the rehabilitation of injured, disabled, or sick persons, by or under the supervision of a physician. Physical therapy, occupational therapy, and speech-language pathology services may be provided off-site.

Comprehensive Severity Index (CSI) A severity of illness measurement method that uses objective data—for example, a patient's laboratory, radiology, and diagnostic test results; vital signs; and history and physical exam—in addition to diagnosis to determine the patient's condition. The severity level for each disease diagnosed is measured on a 1 to 4 scale (mild, moderate, severe, life threatening). For example, in a pneumonia patient, a fever below 100.4°F is considered a level 1 severity finding, whereas fever greater than 104° is a level 4. In order for a diagnosis to be considered at a particular severity level, it must have at least two factors at that level. Thus, a high fever alone would not make a patient a level 3 pneumonia. There must also be at least one other level 3 finding present, such as a chest x-ray showing infiltrate or consolidation in two lobes.

In addition to CSI scores for each diagnosis, the patient receives an overall severity score based on all diagnoses and their interaction with each other. For example, a pneumonia patient with a secondary diagnosis of a broken toe would receive a lower overall score than a pneumonia patient with a secondary diagnosis of congestive heart failure (CHF).

The CSI includes disease-specific, setting-specific, and age-specific criteria and weighting systems to measure severity for inpatients, ambulatory patients, hospice, rehabilitation, and long-term care patients, for all diagnoses and all ages of patients. It can be used for patients with any ICD-9-CM diagnostic or procedure codes and includes severity criteria for all diagnoses. CSI can be used to predict any severity-dependent outcome, including mortality, morbidity, complications, cost, length of stay, and admission to a critical care area.

CSI was originally developed by a research team at Johns Hopkins University led by Dr. Susan Horn for use with intensive care inpatients (it was then called the Computerized Severity Index). It is available from International Severity Information Systems, Inc. (ISIS). www.isisicor.com

compression of morbidity See under *morbidity*.

comptroller See *controller*.

computational biology The National Institutes of Health (NIH) defines computational biology as the "development and application of data-analytical and theoretical methods, mathematical modeling and computational simulation techniques to the study of biological, behavioral, and social systems." See also *bioinformatics*.

computed axial tomography (CAT) See *computed tomography*.

computed tomography (CT) An imaging technique carried out by using radiation (*x-rays*) and analyzing and displaying the absorption (or transmission) of the radiation by the tissues. The key to this technology is a microcomputer within the machine. CT was formerly called "computed axial tomography" (CAT). The machine that creates the image is a CT (or CAT) scanner.

computed tomography technologist A health professional trained to do computed tomography procedures.

Registered Technologist—Computed Tomography (RT(CT)) A *Registered Technologist (RT)* (see under *radiologic technologist*) with advanced qualifications in computed tomography from the American Registry of Radiologic Technologists (ARRT). **www.arrt.org**

computer-assisted coding (CAC) A process in which a person (coder) is assisted by a computer in the process of coding. The coder, using a computer keyboard, enters the words of the diagnosis (or other item to be coded) and the computer identifies the correct code. The better systems are "interactive" in that they "prompt" the coder to enter more detailed information, more exact terminology, or additional information in order to find the most precise term and its code. When used for diagnosis or procedure coding in the hospital, the prompting insists on careful study of the medical record, and considerably improves precision over manual coding. For example, "myocardial infarction" is a valid term to label a disease process involving the heart; a more precise term tells which part of the heart is involved, for example, "anterior (front) myocardial infarction." Each of these two terms has its own code, but the more precise code is preferred; the interactive system prompts the coder to seek the detail (which almost certainly is in the record) needed to use the detailed term rather than the more general term.

computer-based patient record (CPR) See under *electronic health record*.

Computer-based Patient Record Institute (CPRI) See *CPRI-HOST*.

computer decision support system (CDSS) See *decision-support software*.

computer hardware See *hardware*.

computerized patient record (CPR) See *computer-based patient record* under *electronic health record*.

Computerized Patient Record System (CPRS) See *VistA*.

computerized physician order entry (CPOE) A computer application that allows physicians to order tests, medications, and other services electronically. A major advantage is in providing legibility. Such an application has been shown to reduce adverse drug events (ADE), decrease medication errors, decrease cost, and improve patient care. At the time of entering a prescription, for example, the physician is typically guided by menus that list the medications available on the formulary and offered guidance as to suggested dosages, recommended duration of therapy, and patient information. (Comparative costs of proprietary and generic products may also be shown.)

The system can trigger clinical alerts, track patients on each medication, provide automatic renewals, and permit printing and faxing. The prescription can also be placed in the electronic health record, reported to the billing system, and used to update pharmacy inventory records.

Because some allied health professionals (AHPs) write orders for medication and other services, CPOE is sometimes interpreted as care provider order entry or computerized provider order entry. See also *e-prescribing*.

Computerized Severity Index (CSI) See *Comprehensive Severity Index*.

computerized thermography An imaging technique in which computer image processing technology is used to display the distribution of temperatures on the skin surfaces of patients. This method is used in neurology, surgery, orthopedic surgery, physiotherapy, emergency and trauma medicine, dermatology, and oncology.

computer-mediated communications (CMC) The generic term for the technology employed by all computer networks, such as CompuServe, America Online (AOL), the Internet, and others.

computer modeling The use of computers to design and test real-world structures and processes, relying on the computers' ability to process vast amounts of data and perform complex mathematical calculations. In AIDS research, for instance, computer modeling could be used to study the effect of the virus on a variety of genetic structures that might be impossible to produce in the laboratory.

COMS See *Certified Orientation and Mobility Specialist* under *orientation and mobility specialist*.

COMT See *Certified Ophthalmic Medical Technologist* under *ophthalmic medical technologist*.

CON See *certificate of need*.

concierge physician practice An arrangement between a physician or other caregiver (or organization) and a patient under which the patient is provided, for a retainer fee (reported to range from about $1,000 to $20,000 per year) a special class of care and services. The services usually include immediate twenty-four-hour access to the physician in person and by phone, fax, or email; more leisurely personal time with the physician; special help with prescriptions and referrals; medical services while traveling; and often a private reception area at the physician's office. They may include preventive and wellness services. The practice is usually limited to a specific number of concierge patients (for example, 500). Reported attractions are that physicians like the ability to spend more time with individual patients, who, in turn, appreciate the personalized, unhurried attention. The care under concierge practice is often called "boutique care" or "**boutique medicine**."

Questions have been raised, however, regarding both the legal and ethical aspects of the practice. Legally, for example, there is concern that the practice might double bill (both the patient and the insurance company) for the same services. For Medicare, it is illegal to bill a patient for services that are provided by Medicare. Ethically, there is concern that boutique medicine will reduce care available for those unable to pay the annual fee, and reduce the number of available physicians generally. There is also concern that the quality of care will vary according to ability to pay.

The American Medical Association has issued a policy (E-8.055 Retainer Practices), which finds that concierge practices are "consistent with pluralism in the delivery and financing of health care" but raise ethical concerns, and so provides guidelines. Among the recommendations are that the same level of care should be provided to both member and nonmember patients, that patients not be pressured into joining, that the physician facilitate the transfer out of her or his practice of nonparticipating patients, that patients should be able to opt out of the program at any time without penalty, and that the physician should provide urgent care to patients without regard to membership or ability to pay.

concurrent review See under *review*.

condition See *patient condition*.

condition of participation (COP) Something required by CMS of a healthcare provider in order for that provider to be eligible for reimbursement in Medicare, Medicaid, or another federal program.

confidentiality The aura of protection given medical records and other patient care information to protect personal, private information about the patient and the patient's care. The ethics (see *ethics (professional)*) of the healthcare profession require that patient confidences not be disclosed except where necessary to treat the patient, or with the patient's permission. The law provides a privilege (legal protection) for patient information, and requires that such information not be disclosed without the patient's permission or a proper court order. Improper disclosure of confidential patient information can result in legal liability. This has been greatly expanded under HIPAA for what is referred to as *protected health information (PHI)*. See also *informed consent*, *privileged communication*, and *privacy*.

confined to the home See *homebound*.

conflict of interest A situation where a person (or organization) has two separate and distinct duties owed concerning, or interests in, the same thing, and therefore cannot act completely impartially with respect to that thing. It is like one servant trying to serve two masters. For example, a hospital trustee has a legal duty to act in the best interests of the hospital. If that trustee owns real estate that the hospital wishes to buy, the trustee has a personal interest in obtaining the highest price, but as a trustee he has an interest in obtaining the lowest price. Because such a conflict of interest may cloud his judgment, the trustee is obligated to inform the hospital board about his personal interest, and usually will excuse himself from participating in the purchase negotiations. Even if there is no real conflict, or if the trustee is capable of making the right decision for the hospital, he would be wise to excuse himself so that the transaction will not appear to be tainted with impropriety, and so that no one can challenge it as such. Most corporate bylaws address conflict of interest situations.

institutional conflict of interest Conflict of interest is ordinarily thought of as involving individuals, but it can also arise when an institution has a financial stake in the research conducted in its laboratories or clinics. Because most such research involves a compound, process, or therapy that requires approval by the Food and Drug Administration (FDA), it has been suggested that the FDA regulations for individual conflicts of interest be augmented by regulations for institutional conflicts of interest as well. One approach would be to make research involving institutional conflict of interest inadmissible as evidence for FDA approval of the drug or device unless there was sufficient reason to admit the evidence, and sufficient safeguards were in place.

Congressional Budget Office (CBO) A federal agency that assists the House and Senate Budget Committees, and the Congress, in the budget process by preparing objective reports and impartial analyses on proposed budgets. **www.cbo.gov**

Congressional Research Service (CRS) An agency within the Library of Congress that performs public policy research for members of Congress, their committees, and staff. **www.loc.gov/crsinfo**

Connecting Communities for Better Health (CCBH) A program to provide seed funding and technical support to state, regional, and community-based health information organizations and initiatives across the country. CCBH is conducted by eHealth Initiative in cooperation with the Department of Health and Human Services (HHS). See also *regional health information organization*.

Connecting for Health (U.K.) An agency of the National Health Service (NHS) in the United Kingdom that is responsible for the National Programme for IT (NPfIT), a ten-year effort initiated in 2005. NPfIT aims to "give healthcare professionals access to patient information safely, securely and easily, whenever and wherever it is needed." It plans to connect over 30,000 general practitioners (GPs) in England to almost 300 hospitals and give patients access to their personal health and care information. **www.connectingforhealth.nhs.uk**

Connecting for Health (U.S.) A public-private collaborative in the United States of more than 100 organizations committed to realizing "the full potential of information technology in health and health care, while protecting patient privacy and the security of personal health information." One of its achievements was broad consensus on a "Roadmap" for attaining electronic connectivity in health care. Connecting for Health was created in 2001 by the Markle Foundation. It is funded by both Markle and the Robert Wood Johnson Foundation (RWJF). **www.connectingforhealth.org**

conscience clause A law (or portion of a law) that allows individuals (or institutions) the right to refuse to do something that is contrary to their moral or religious beliefs. For example, some state laws regulating abortion specifically state that no hospital, physician, or hospital employee may be compelled to participate in an abortion. The employee would have to state the refusal in writing, and could not be disciplined or sued for refusing to participate.

Consensus Development Program See *National Institutes of Health Consensus Development Program*.

consent See *informed consent*.

conservation medicine A scientific discipline that focuses on the health inter-relationships of humans, animals, and the environment. It is interdisciplinary, involving physicians, veterinarians, ecologists, microbiologists, pathologists, marine biologists, toxicologists, epidemiologists, climate biologists, anthropologists, economists, political scientists, and others. The term was first used in the mid-1990s, as it was becoming clear that the crossover of diseases from animals to humans (see *zoonosis*) was increasing, and that changes in the ecosystem often had something to do with this. See also *medical geology*.

conservator A person who has the legal authority and duty to protect the assets of another, "protected person" (a minor or incompetent). A conservator is appointed by a court, in the same way that a guardian is appointed, but he or she can only make decisions about property, not about medical care or other decisions personal to the protected person. A guardian may have authority over personal matters only, over property matters only, or over both, depending on what authority the court has granted. The guardianship papers describe the authority given.

Consolidated Health Informatics (CHI) A collaborative effort within the federal government to adopt health information interoperability standards, particularly health vocabulary and messaging standards, for implementation in federal government systems. About twenty departments and agencies, including the Department of Health and Human Services (HHS), the Department of Defense (DoD), and the Department of Veterans Affairs (VA), are active in the CHI governance process. CHI is an integral part of the Federal Health Architecture (FHA) initiative. See also *Patient Medical Record Information*. **www.hhs.gov/healthit/chi.html**

Consolidated Omnibus Budget Reconciliation Act of 1985 (COBRA) A federal law that requires (among other things) that employers of twenty or more workers must continue former employees' health insurance coverage (at the former employees' expense) for up to three years for qualified beneficiaries. Qualified beneficiaries include widows and divorced and separated spouses of former employees, as well as their dependents (even dependents who lost their dependent status). The law amends the Internal Revenue Code of 1954. COBRA also included the "anti-dumping law," *Emergency Medical Treatment and Labor Act (EMTALA)*. Pub. L. No. 99-272 (1986).

consolidation The formal union of two or more corporations (such as hospitals) into a single corporation. In a consolidation, all of the corporations that unite cease to exist, and a new corporation is formed with its own new identity. The new corporation acquires the assets and assumes the liabilities of the former corporations. See also *merger*.

consortium (alliance) An alliance between two or more parties (for example, hospitals) to achieve a specific purpose.

consortium (companionship) The right of a husband or wife to the companionship, comfort, and aid—including sexual relationships—of his or her spouse. In a malpractice case, for example, if the husband has been injured, the wife may join as a plaintiff to recover for her loss of consortium.

conspiracy of silence The supposed tacit agreement among physicians (or other professionals) not to testify against one another in malpractice lawsuits. It is sometimes said that malpractice plaintiffs are not able to obtain a fair trial of their cases because the only way to prove the case is by expert testimony, and because of the so-called "conspiracy of silence," it is difficult to find experts (namely, physicians) willing to testify.

constraint-induced-movement therapy (CIMT) Therapy for persons with brain injuries, especially those that are the result of strokes, in which the portion of the body not involved is constrained and the patient is thus forced to use the affected counterpart. To use CIMT, patients must be able to extend their wrists and move their arm and fingers. If the right arm is affected, for example, the "good" left arm is restrained and for periods of about six hours per day, the patient is "forced" to use the affected arm for normal tasks. Such therapy usually is continued for three weeks or more. CIMT differs from traditional physical therapy, which concentrates on improving the skills of the "good" arm for doing tasks "one-handed."

Research has shown marked improvement with the use of CIMT, even when used for patients several years after the stroke or injury. CIMT was developed by Dr. Edward Taub, a professor of psychology at the University of Alabama in Birmingham. He noted that after a stroke, the survivor tries unsuccessfully to use the affected side, and so gives up. Dr. Taub calls this "learned non-use." CIMT forces the patient to relearn to use the affected side.

constructed beds See under *bed capacity*.

consultation (management) Advice from an expert, given after a study of a situation or problem presented by the individual obtaining the consultation. In the healthcare field, such consultation often concerns organization, management, strategic planning, personnel policies, and the like.

consultation (medical) A review of a patient's problem by a second individual, namely a physician or other healthcare provider (for example, a clinical psychologist), and the rendering of an opinion and advice to the referring physician. The review in most instances involves the independent examination of the patient by the consultant. In a consultation some evidence, such as x-rays, may not need to be repeated if it is made available to the consultant. The consultant's opinion and advice are not binding on the referring physician. See also *second opinion*.

consumer An individual who does or may receive healthcare services. In the context of healthcare programs or legislation, a consumer is not a provider. See also *customer*.

Consumer Assessment of Healthcare Providers and Systems (CAHPS) A program of the Agency for Healthcare Research and Quality (AHRQ) to develop and support the use of standardized surveys that ask consumers and patients to report on and evaluate their experiences with health care. The original name was Consumer Assessment of Health Plans Study. See also *Hospital Consumer Assessment of Healthcare Providers and Systems*. **www.cahps .ahrq.gov**

consumer-centric Focused primarily on the needs of the patient (the consumer) rather than the needs of the provider or third-party payer. Synonym: patient-centric.

consumer choice A 1993 reform approach that would get individuals to purchase health insurance by making it mandatory but providing a tax break; the poor would get a tax refund. Companies providing insurance would not get a tax break. Also called the "market-based approach." See also *individual mandate* under *mandate*.

consumer-driven health care (CDHC) See *healthcare consumerism*.

consumer-driven health plan (CDHP) A health plan option designed not only to control costs, but also to educate plan participants (the "consumers") and influence their behavior. CDHPs typically offer a cost-sharing health plan in conjunction with discretionary healthcare dollars—for example, a high-deductible health plan (HDHP) combined with a health reimbursement account (HRA) or Health Savings Account (HSA). Often, tools and resources—such as health and wellness, disease management, and case management programs—are provided to help participants increase health and keep medical conditions under control. Consumers, using more of their own money to pay for health care, presumably become more involved in healthcare decision making and make better choices, based on cost, quality, and treatment options. Also called consumer-directed health plan, consumer-directed health arrangement (CDHA), consumer-choice, or self-directed health plan (SDHP).

Consumer Health Education Council (CHEC) A group whose goal is health insurance coverage expansion through education of workers and employers. Members include the Employee Benefit Research Institute, the Association of American Medical Colleges, the American Hospital Association, and the Milbank Memorial Fund. Also on its policy board are the Blue Cross and Blue Shield Association, AARP, the Health Resources and Services Administration, the Agency for Healthcare Research and Quality, and the U.S. Department of Labor.

consumer health informatics Making health information directly available to consumers by electronic methods. Includes data banks ready to be installed on one's own computer, such as reference material from the Mayo Clinic, computer networks, use of voice mail systems, web sites—any electronic method.

Consumer Health Manager (CHM) A chip or specification that permits mobile communications devices such as cell phones to be the basis for a number of consumer health–related functions. For example, with CHM the device could store personal health information (such as the *Continuity of Care Record* (CCR), see under *data set*), communicate with providers, serve as the platform for consumer health–related software such as wellness and disease management programs, and facilitate Internet access to allow the consumer to look up information about medications, symptoms, and so forth. Proposed in 2005 by the Mobile Healthcare Alliance (MoHCA).

consumerism See *healthcare consumerism*.

consumer price index (CPI) See under *index (numerical)*.

Consumer-Purchaser Disclosure Project (CPDP) A group of leading employer, consumer, and labor organizations working to ensure that all Americans have access to publicly reported healthcare performance information. Its vision is that consumers will be able to select hospitals, physicians, and treatments based on nationally standardized measures for clinical quality, consumer experience, equity, and efficiency. **healthcaredisclosure.org**

contact capitation See *capitation*.

contact lens technician A health professional trained in the fitting and dispensing of contact lenses.

Board Certified Contact Lens Technician (NCLC) The credential NCLC shows that the contact lens technician has passed a certifying examination of the National Contact Lens Examiners. **www.ncleabo.org**

Board Certified Contact Lens Technician—Advanced Certification (NCLC-AC) The credential NCLC-AC designates advanced certification obtained by a contact lens technician with several years of experience who has met the requirements of the National Contact Lens Examiners. **www.ncleabo.org**

contagious Transmissible by direct contact with an infected person or fresh secretions or excretions.

containment Keeping a dangerous or potentially harmful substance or element from the possibility of actually doing harm. In the clinical laboratory environment, for example, containment is used to describe the safe methods for handling and managing infectious materials. In the political context, containment usually means limiting or controlling the flow of information.

contaminate To transfer bacteria or other infectious agents or harmful substances.

contingency fee A fee that is paid to an attorney only if the client wins. Contingency-fee arrangements are commonly used in malpractice cases, where the attorney receives a portion (usually about one third) of the amount awarded the plaintiff by the court or in an out-of-court settlement. If the plaintiff receives nothing, the attorney receives nothing (except reimbursement of expenses).

contingent worker A person who works less than thirty-five hours a week (or in some usages, less than twelve months a year). Such individuals typically have lower earnings, less job security, and fewer promotions than full-time employees. Contingent workers are often without health insurance. Synonyms: peripheral workers, marginal workers.

continued stay denial notice (CSDN) See *hospital-issued notice of noncoverage*.

continued stay review See under *review*.

continuing care Care provided over an extended period of time. The term may cover care during both wellness and illness, and varying levels of care, from intensive care to rest home care. It may also be provided in various settings.

continuing care retirement community (CCRC) A retirement community that offers lifetime independent living and various healthcare services to residents.

continuing education (CE) Learning that takes place after formal education (such as postgraduate school) is completed. Most health professionals are required to acquire a specific number of hours or credits of CE each year in order to retain licensure or certification.

continuing medical education (CME) The education of practicing physicians through refresher courses, medical journals and texts, attendance at regularly scheduled teaching programs, approved self-study courses (both traditional and computer-assisted), and so forth. CME programs are provided by medical schools, professional organizations, publishing companies, educational organizations, and hospitals. The necessity for continuing education is well accepted by the medical profession. In some states, CME is required for continued licensure.

continuing nursing education (CNE) The education of practicing nurses in order to update or advance their knowledge and skills. CNE is required in most areas of the profession to maintain licensure or certification.

> **Nursing Continuing Education/Staff Development** A certificate available to registered nurses who pass an examination in continuing nursing education and staff development given by the American Nurses Credentialing Center (ANCC). **nursingworld.org/ancc**

continuity of care The degree to which the care of a patient from the onset of illness until its completion is continuous, that is, without interruption. Interruptions occur sometimes because the patient does not follow through, sometimes because the system has gaps, often because of lack of facilities or because of financial impediments (absence of benefits, for example, which cover certain services). The term "continuity of care" is sometimes used to refer to a longer span of time than the single episode of illness, and to the patient's health care during both wellness and illness. See also *continuum of care*.

Continuity of Care Certification, Advanced (A-CCC) See under *case manager*.

Continuity of Care Record (CCR) See under *data set*.

Continuous Operational Assessment and Response (COAR) System A system designed to monitor the functioning of basic quality control processes and to respond quickly when they are found to be failing to operate properly.

continuous quality improvement (CQI) See under *quality improvement*.

continuum of care A term defined by the Department of Health and Human Services (HHS) as the "entire spectrum of specialized health, rehabilitative, and residential services available to the frail and chronically ill. The services focus on the social, residential, rehabilitative and supportive needs of individuals as well as needs that are essentially medical in nature." See also *continuity of care*.

contract An agreement between two or more parties that gives legally enforceable rights and duties to both. A contract need not be in writing to be enforceable, unless it is a certain kind of agreement, such as one for the sale of real estate. A state law called the "Statute of Frauds" specifies which contracts must be supported by written evidence (must be in writing).

adhesion contract A contract that has not been negotiated, but rather has been entirely written by one party, and presented to the other on a "take it or leave it" basis. Usually, there is great inequality of bargaining power, and the contract of adhesion strongly favors its author, while strongly disfavoring the rights of the other party. Because of this disparity, courts will not always enforce adhesion contracts in their entirety. Also called "contract of adhesion."

cost-plus contract A type of agreement, often used in construction, in which the owner agrees to pay for all costs incurred by the contractor in executing the plans and specifications, "plus" an additional amount (fixed sum, percentage, or other arrangement) as a fee or profit.

direct contract An agreement between an employer (or health plan or insurer) and a healthcare provider for the provision of healthcare services to the employees (beneficiaries). This is sometimes called a "direct provider agreement (DPA)."

When this term is used in the context of a Medicare beneficiary contracting with a health-care provider, it is more commonly referred to as a *private contract* (see below).

exclusive contract A term that, in the hospital, usually refers to a written agreement under which a given physician or physician group is given the exclusive right to furnish certain, specified administrative or clinical services in the hospital. During the life of the exclusive contract, other physicians are precluded from the same activities in that hospital. Exclusive contracts have raised antitrust issues for hospitals; see *Rule of Reason*.

indemnity contract A healthcare insurance contract in which the benefits are money (cash) rather than service.

private contract An agreement for the provision of health care made between a person who is eligible for Medicare ("beneficiary") and a healthcare provider, typically a physician. The beneficiary agrees to pay the provider on a direct fee-for-service (FFS) basis, instead of having the provider submit a claim under Medicare. This is sometimes also referred to as a "direct contract," and is subject to strict federal regulation, including provisions contained in the Balanced Budget Act of 1997 (BBA). See also *Kyl-Archer Amendment*.

risk contract A contract under which a provider agrees to furnish a given service for a pre-arranged fee, and thus assumes the risk (financial) that the fee will cover its costs for providing the service. A health maintenance organization (HMO) that operates under a capitation method of payment is a risk contractor.

service contract A healthcare insurance contract in which the benefits are the actual services rather than money.

contract management See under *management*.

contractor See *independent contractor*.

contract provider organization (CPO) See *preferred provider organization*.

contract research organization (CRO) An independent organization that contracts with the sponsor of a clinical trial and assumes some of the responsibilities of the sponsor. The CRO is subject to federal regulation of clinical trials. See also *site management organization*.

contract service A service purchased from a person or another organization. If a hospital does not operate its own laundry or laboratory, for example, these may be obtained as contract services. Similarly, the physician services for an emergency department may be obtained by contract with an organization set up to furnish such services.

contractual adjustment See *contractuals*.

contractuals Short for "contractual adjustments," a bookkeeping procedure that has to be made by a hospital because it must, under contracts with third-party payers (including Medicare and Medicaid), give the payers discounts on hospital charges.

The aggregate effect of all contractual adjustments on the hospital's total income must be calculated before it can establish what the hospital's "normal charge" will be for its services. **Normal charge** is defined as the charge to a nondiscounted patient (i.e., to a private pay patient or to an insurance company without a contract).

For example, a third-party payer (TPP) may contract to pay the hospital's normal charge, less 25%. If the hospital needs $4,000 per patient day to remain solvent, and the TPP pays only $3,000 ($4,000 – 25%), the hospital will not receive enough to cover its costs. So to determine what the normal charge must be, the hospital takes into account the predicted effects of all discounted TPP contracts and the total number of anticipated patient days expected under each contract, including private pay patients. The normal charge is then set so that the total received from all payers will recover the hospital's costs. (Physicians also enter into contracts that give them the same problem as the hospital.)

The hospital's net revenue, after all contractual adjustments (discounts), must be sufficient to meet the revenue needs of the hospital. The tables below illustrate the process and its effects.

Effect of Contractual Adjustments on Hospital Revenue

Annual Totals as Shown on Financial Statement	Amount
Net patient revenue: Actual patient revenue required to keep hospital solvent	$27,000,000
Contractual adjustments ("contractuals," which must be added to net patient revenue to create gross patient revenue or gross charges)	$13,000,000
Gross patient revenue (the result of normal charges)	$40,000,000[a]

a. Net, contractuals, and gross revenue approximate those of an actual hospital in 2001.

Calculation of Normal Charge

Average Charges per Day, Assuming 10,000 Patient Days of Care Per Year	
Net: actually received (charged)	$2,700
Contractual deduction (add to create normal charge)	$1,300
Normal charge	$4,000

Effects of Contractual Discounts on Payers

Payer	Number of Patient Days[a]	Discount[b]	Expected Payment Per Patient Day[c]	Hospital Revenue
Medicare	5,000	38%	$2,480	$12,400,000
Medicaid	3,000	38%	$2,480	$7,440,000
Other contracts	1,500	14%	$3,440	$5,160,000
Noncontract payers	500	0%	$4,000	$2,000,000
Overall total	10,000	32.5%	$2,700	$27,000,000

a. Distribution of patient days is assumed, but reasonable.
b. Discount percentages assumed.
c. The charge in all cases is $4,000 per day.

contraindication A known reason for not using a given treatment, usually a drug. Some contraindications are drug interactions, and thus depend on the use of a conflicting drug. Some relate to foods that should be avoided. Others depend on the patient's condition; for example, nasal decongestants typically tend to raise patients' blood pressure, and thus are contraindicated in a patient who already has high blood pressure. "High blood pressure" appears on the label in a warning statement that it is a contraindication to the use of the product. See also *indicated* and *indication*.

contribution A defendant who is sued in tort is entitled to recover money (damages) from any others who contributed to the plaintiff's injury and who were liable to the plaintiff. For example if, for whatever reason, not all of the possible defendants are brought into the lawsuit, one defendant may have to pay the entire damage award. That defendant can then seek "contribution" (reimbursement) from any other liable parties.

control (experiment) A term used in research that refers to comparing an experimental situation with another situation, the control situation, which is as nearly like the experimental situation as possible except for the factor being tested in the experiment. For example, the benefits of a drug may be tested by giving it to the experimental group of patients, while it is not given to the control group, and the results are then compared. Statistical methods are employed to determine whether any differences between the fates of the two groups are significant.

control (organization) The term used by the American Hospital Association (AHA) in its listing of hospitals in the *AHA Guide to the Health Care Field* to indicate the kind of organization or institution responsible for operating the hospital. Some twenty-four categories are used. In the nonfederal sector, the grouping is quite general, such as "church-operated" and "investor-owned (for-profit), partnership." In the federal sector, however, classification is much more specific; for example "Army" hospitals are separated from "Navy" hospitals.

controlled substance A drug listed as being subject to federal regulation under the Controlled Substances Act (CSA) (21 U.S.C. § 801 et seq. (2005)). Such drugs require a prescription, and the physician must have a *DEA number* from the federal government to prescribe them. See also *prescription drug* (under *drug*).

controlled substance analogue See *designer drug* under *drug*.

controlled vocabulary See *vocabulary*.

controller The person who is in charge of the hospital's ongoing financial administration, including billing, accounting, budget management, and the like. A controller may or may not be the chief financial officer (CFO) (treasurer). "Controller" is sometimes spelled "comptroller."

convalescence The period of time after the acute phase of an illness before the patient is back to "normal."

convenience clinic A healthcare facility to provide nonemergency, ambulatory care services, typically for more hours than a regular physician's office (evenings and weekends, for example). Convenience clinics may be staffed by licensed independent practitioners (LIPs) rather than physicians, and are appearing in malls, drug stores, and supermarkets, as well as being free-standing. In addition to convenience for the patient, they are designed to cut healthcare costs and reduce overuse of the emergency room.

conversion (corporate) Changing from a nonprofit to a for-profit corporation or organization. A number of nonprofit hospitals and health plans are converting to for-profit status, and the change has legal ramifications. Conversions take place by sale, merger, joint ventures, or restructuring within the corporation. See also *conversion foundation*.

conversion (insurance) Retaining health insurance when changing employers without having to be reevaluated as to insurability. An employee retiring or otherwise ineligible to remain in a group usually converts to an individual health insurance policy. The privilege to convert in this manner is guaranteed in many circumstances by the Consolidated Omnibus Budget Reconciliation Act of 1985 (COBRA).

conversion factor A dollar amount for one base unit in the *relative value scale (RVS)*. The price to be paid to the provider for a given service equals the relative value of the service multiplied by the dollar amount of the conversion factor. For example, a blood sugar determination might have a relative value of 5.0, and the conversion factor might be $5.00. The "price" of the blood sugar determination would therefore be $25.00.

conversion foundation A philanthropic organization created as a "byproduct" of **conversion (corporate)**. In some states, when a nonprofit corporation converts to for-profit, it is required to transfer a significant amount of its assets to a charitable foundation. See, for example, **California Wellness Foundation**.

converter Federal terminology for the conversion factor used in the prospective payment system (PPS).

COO See **chief operating officer**.

cooperative care Care provided by family and friends, as in earlier times. These caregivers must work together cooperatively to ensure that the needs of the patient are met at all times. For example, family members may reside with the patient and handle much of the care; friends and neighbors may take turns giving needed therapies and providing relief for the primary caregivers.

Cost savings of 30–40% in labor and similar savings in capital, as well as shorter institutional stays, are reported for patients who receive cooperative care (when appropriate). Fewer falls and fewer medication errors, as well as greater patient satisfaction, have been reported compared with traditional inpatient care. Cooperative care can be appropriate for both acute bedfast and ambulatory inpatients, with such conditions as hysterectomy, laparoscopy, arthroscopy, cosmetic surgery, and medical problems. Homebound patients may also receive such care, such as those with chronic or terminal conditions.

Cooperative Research and Development Agreement (CRADA) A written agreement between a private company and a federal government agency to work together on a project.

cooperative services See **shared services**.

coordinated care See **managed care**.

Coordinating Center for Environmental Health and Injury Prevention (CCEHIP) See under **Centers for Disease Control and Prevention**.

Coordinating Center for Health Information and Service (CoCHIS) See under **Centers for Disease Control and Prevention**.

Coordinating Center for Health Promotion (CoCHP) See under **Centers for Disease Control and Prevention**.

Coordinating Center for Infectious Diseases (CCID) See under **Centers for Disease Control and Prevention**.

Coordinating Office for Global Health (COGH) See under **Centers for Disease Control and Prevention**.

Coordinating Office for Terrorism Preparedness and Emergency Response (COTPER) See under **Centers for Disease Control and Prevention**.

coordination of benefits (COB) An insurance claims review process used when a beneficiary is insured by two or more carriers (see **claim (insurance)**). The process determines the liability of each carrier in order to eliminate duplication of payments. For example, benefits to which an individual is entitled under workers' compensation are not permitted to be duplicated by ordinary health insurance, even though the injury or illness would be covered were the problem not work-related.

COP Or CoP. See **condition of participation**.

COPANT A civil, nonprofit association that promotes the development of technical standardization and related activities among thirty or so Pan-American countries, which are represented by standards organizations (for example, the member from the United States is **ANSI**). COPANT's full name is Pan-American Standards Commission, the Regional Standardization Body of the Americas. See also **CEN (organization)** and **standards development organization**. www.copant.org

copayment A fixed amount of money paid by a health plan enrollee (beneficiary) at the time of service. For example, the enrollee may pay a $10 "copay" at every physician office visit, and $5 for each drug prescription filled. The health plan pays the remainder of the charge directly to the provider. This is a method of cost-sharing between the enrollee and the plan, and serves as an incentive for the enrollee to use healthcare resources wisely. An enrollee might be offered a lower price benefit package in return for a higher copayment. See also *coinsurance* and *deductible*.

copyright A form of legal protection for the specific "expression" of intellectual property. Applied to "works of authorship" including, for example, writings, pictures, and music, copyright protection is designed to protect against outright copying of a particular work. Copyright laws do not protect the "ideas" inherent in the work, so an imitation is not a copyright infringement if the expression of the same idea is different. This is a key point that distinguishes copyright protection from *patent* protection, which does protect the idea itself. Copyright protection lasts significantly longer than patent protection, however, being typically the life of the creator (author) plus seventy years. This term is even longer when the author created the intellectual property for his or her employer or under a "work for hire" agreement.

Recent changes in copyright law have made this form of protection easier to use. Work is "copyrighted" automatically when created, even if no copyright notice (©) is placed on the work. Appropriate copyright notices should, however, be properly placed on all published work to gain other advantages, such as international protection. It is not necessary to formally "register" a copyright with the U.S. Copyright Office unless you are a U.S. copyright owner and wish to enforce your copyright against an infringer. However, as with placing a copyright notice, there are significant advantages that come with registration of a copyright. See also *patent*.

core measure See *performance measure*.

core services Those services that must be provided by an institution if it is to be accepted by the American Hospital Association (AHA) as an institution eligible for registration with AHA and inclusion in the annual *AHA Guide to the Health Care Field*. These services include an organized medical staff, a nursing service with registered nurse (RN) supervision, food service, pharmacy, and maintenance of medical records.

CORF See *comprehensive outpatient rehabilitation facility*.

CORLN See *Certified Otorhinolaryngology and Head-Neck Nurse* under *otorhinolaryngology and head-neck nursing*.

coronary "Crown-like" or "relating to a crown," or "encircling." In healthcare usage, coronary refers to the blood vessels of the heart, which encircle the heart and are called coronary vessels. A cardiac care unit is often called a coronary care unit, because most of the patients treated there suffer from problems of the circulation serving the heart muscle.

coronary care unit See *cardiac care unit*.

coroner A public official, usually elected, whose duty it is to investigate sudden, suspicious, or violent death as prescribed by law and to determine the cause of death. A coroner may or may not be a physician. In some states the office of coroner has been replaced by that of *medical examiner*.

corporate compliance See *compliance*.

corporate integrity agreement (CIA) A formal settlement between the Department of Health and Human Services (HHS) Office of Inspector General (OIG) and a healthcare provider who has been investigated by the OIG under false claim and related laws. There is no finding of fault (or admission of guilt), but rather the provider agrees to specified obligations, and in exchange the OIG agrees not to exclude the provider from participation in Medicare, Medicaid, and other federal programs. A typical CIA lasts five years, and requires, for example, that the provider hire a compliance officer (or appoint a compliance committee), develop written standards and policies, implement employee training programs, audit billings to federal payers, submit reports to the OIG, and so forth. The compliance officer may have a title such as "Organizational Responsibility Officer (ORO)," and administer a program referred to as an "Organizational Responsibility Program (ORP)."

corporate liability See under *liability*.

corporate planning See under *planning*.

corporate practice of medicine doctrine Prohibits corporations and business entities from practicing medicine. The doctrine, usually embodied by a state in a statute or licensing requirement, attempts to prohibit businesspeople and lay people without medical licenses from practicing medicine and to prevent doctors from avoiding liability by incorporating. This doctrine bars companies from hiring doctors to treat their employees and also bars doctors and health professionals from incorporating.

However, there are many exceptions to the doctrine (for example, statutes enacted removing HMOs from the reach of the doctrine), and doctors are allowed to form *professional corporations (PCs)* (see under *corporation*, below). The doctrine has been mostly ignored since the 1920s, and many say that it needs to be reexamined in light of the changes to the healthcare delivery systems across the country. Because of the increasing use of managed care, this doctrine may well become more common as the question of who ultimately controls medical decision making and use of resources gets more attention.

corporation A legal entity that exists separately, for all legal purposes, from the people or organizations that own it. To take advantage of legal advantages (limitation of liability and tax benefits, for example), a corporation must observe certain "formalities" required by law, such as meetings, minutes, and filing of annual reports and tax returns.

for-profit corporation A corporation whose profits (excess of income over expenses) are distributed, as dividends, to shareholders who own the corporation (in contrast to a nonprofit corporation, in which the profits go to corporate purposes rather than to individual shareholders).

medical staff corporation Sometimes a medical staff incorporates itself, and the matters that are ordinarily the subject of the medical staff bylaws are then handled by contract between the medical staff corporation and the hospital corporation, much as an emergency services corporation could be contracted with to provide emergency department services.

nonprofit corporation A corporation whose profits (excess of income over expenses) are used for corporate purposes rather than returned to shareholders or investors (owners) as dividends. To qualify for tax exemption, no portion of the profits of the corporation may "inure" to the benefit of an individual. See *inurement*. "Nonprofit" does not necessarily mean "tax-exempt." See also *501(c)(3)* under *501(c)(*)*.

parent corporation A corporation that owns at least a majority of the shares of (controls) one or more subsidiary corporations.

professional corporation (PC) A corporation in which all of the shareholders (owners) are members of a given profession, such as physicians. In some respects, a professional corporation is not the same as other corporations. One difference is that persons who are not members of the profession forming the corporation may not be shareholders (for example, physicians may not be shareholders of a legal PC). Another difference is that unlike a normal business corporation, the liability of a PC is not limited; in other words, its owners can be held personally liable for the PC's debts. The ethical dilemma confronting the state in allowing professionals to incorporate is that it is good policy to protect professionals by limiting liability, but professional accountability is just as vital. A PC may also be called a "professional service corporation," "professional association," or "service corporation."

service corporation (SC) See *professional corporation* above.

sibling corporation (SC) Two or more corporations owned by the same shareholders. Also known as "brother sister corporations."

subchapter C corporation The traditional corporate format, with limited liability and double taxation (taxed at the corporate level and the dividend level). The subchapter reference is to the Internal Revenue Code.

subchapter S corporation An optional election for a closely held corporation for favorable tax treatment. The subchapter reference is to the Internal Revenue Code. If the corporation meets certain requirements (among others: less than thirty-five shareholders, all shareholders are U.S. citizens, and the corporation has only one class of voting stock) and "elects" to operate under "sub S" status, the corporation is taxed much like a partnership (characterized by flow through or conduit taxation).

subsidiary corporation A corporation of which another corporation (the "parent corporation") owns at least a majority of the shares.

Corps, The See *National Health Service Corps*.

Correct Coding Initiative (CCI) See *CCI*.

correctional nursing The nursing specialty focused on the health needs of inmates of jails, prisons, and other correctional facilities.

corrective therapy See *kinesiotherapy*.

COS See *Community of Science*.

COSA See *Certified Ophthalmic Surgical Assistant* under *ophthalmic surgical assistant*.

cost The expense incurred in providing a product or service.

allowable cost Items of service that are contractually included in the benefits of an insurance or payment plan, similar to "covered charges" (see *charge*). The charges for television and meals for visitors are not ordinarily allowable costs.

capital cost The cost of developing or acquiring new equipment, facilities, or services; that is, the investment cost to the institution of such growth.

direct cost A cost that can be identified directly with any part of the hospital organization that the hospital designates as a cost center. In fact, cost centers are defined as such because they are segments of the hospital, such as the operating rooms, to which direct costs can be assigned rather clearly. To the direct costs of each cost center are added, on the basis of some accounting formula, allocated proportions of the hospital's indirect costs (costs, such as for heat and housekeeping, that are not easily allocated to specific cost centers).

fixed cost A cost that is entirely independent of the volume of activity. If no charges are made for individual local calls, the cost of local telephone service is a fixed cost; on the other hand, long distance service, which depends as it does on the number and length of calls made, is a variable cost (however, an unlimited WATS line would be a fixed cost).

indirect cost There are two kinds of indirect costs in a hospital. The first kind is costs that must be incurred by any organization furnishing services, but that cannot be exactly identified with any specific service rendered or support department. For example, the cost of having a chief executive officer (CEO) is necessary, but it cannot be charged directly to, for example, the operating room as can the salaries of operating room nurses. The second kind of indirect costs is the costs of "support activities," the costs of which can be determined, but which do not produce revenue. Such activities (for example, a hospital's medical record department) have clear direct costs, and must bear their share of the indirect costs of the first type above. But, because these activities do not produce revenue, their costs—both direct and indirect—become indirect costs for the revenue-producing departments and services.

Accountants have developed a variety of formulas for "cost allocation." Cost allocation means assigning appropriate portions of the indirect costs to the various cost centers and then further allocating the costs of non-revenue-producing cost centers to the revenue-producing cost centers, where they influence the charges.

marginal cost The addition to total cost resulting from the production of an additional unit of service or product. This cost varies with the volume of the operation. A hospital, for example, has a high cost for its first meal served. Subsequent meals have much lower costs each (marginal costs) until the volume is so large as to require changes in facilities, supervision, and the like. At this point the marginal cost will usually rise until a new equilibrium ("optimum output level") is established.

pass-through cost A term with a specific definition in the prospective payment system (PPS). It refers to hospital costs, such as for medical education, that are not incorporated in the

DRG prices. Funds are provided to the hospital directly, that is, outside the per-case payments for patient care; the costs are simply passed through (or outside of) the DRG mechanism.

reasonable cost A term with a specific definition given by the federal government for use in Medicare and Medicaid. It is used only in connection with services in institutions that are exempt from the prospective payment system (PPS) and for beneficiaries who are not inpatients.

semi-variable cost A cost that is partly a variable cost and partly a fixed cost in its behavior in response to changes in volume. Automobile rental is typically a semi-variable cost, with a fixed charge per day and a variable charge depending on miles driven.

variable cost A cost that is entirely dependent on the volume of activity, as opposed to a fixed cost, which is not affected by volume. In a typical telephone billing system, for example, long distance calls represent a variable cost whereas local calls represent a fixed cost.

cost allocation An accounting procedure by which costs that cannot be clearly identified with any specific cost center are distributed among cost centers, and by which the costs of support services are distributed among revenue-producing services so as to be recovered in the charges.

cost-analysis A group of analyses from the discipline of economics that can be applied to a variety of healthcare interventions. See also *discounting*.

cost-benefit analysis (CBA) An economic analysis done to determine whether money was well spent or not. It is a comparison between the dollar value of the benefits realized and the dollar cost of the resources expended to obtain those benefits. The goal is to develop a **cost-benefit ratio (CBR)**, which is the mathematical result of dividing the benefits value by the cost value. If the ratio is greater than 1.0, the benefits more than outweigh the costs (good); if the ratio is less than 1.0, the costs are greater than the benefits (bad). This analysis is difficult to use in health care where the benefits are frequently not assigned a dollar value, such as those relating to quality of life (QOL).

cost-effectiveness analysis (CEA) The comparison of the cost-benefit ratios, or net effectiveness, for the same benefits derived from different services, therapies, or interventions (clinical). Effectiveness is defined as the degree to which the desired benefits are obtained from the particular service, therapy, or intervention being analyzed. No effort is made to quantify benefits in dollar units. Benefits might be described as adding one year to a patient's life expectancy or reducing her blood pressure by twenty points.

cost-identification analysis (CIA) The comparison of the costs where the benefits are assumed to be equal. Synonym: cost-minimization analysis.

cost-utility analysis (CUA) Frequently used when comparing alternative drug therapies where benefits are measured not in dollar values but in units such as *quality-adjusted life-years (QALYs)*. See also *pharmacoeconomics*.

cost center An area of activity of the hospital with which direct costs can be identified. Accounting practice is to assign direct costs to such cost centers, and to allocate to each cost center its proportionate share of indirect costs, in order to give management a tool for cost control (or pricing). When a cost center is also revenue-producing, that is, an area for which charges are made (for example, an operating room), the allocation of direct and indirect costs, along with data about the services rendered, permits the charge for each service to be sufficient to cover the cost of that service.

Some other cost centers, over which management wants to maintain control, do not produce revenue. An example is the medical record department. The costs of such departments (direct plus indirect costs) are reallocated as indirect costs to the revenue-producing cost centers.

cost containment Efforts to prevent increase in cost or to restrict its rate of increase. Cost containment is rarely addressed at reducing cost.

cost control A term usually applied to an external constraint of costs (or charges), such as legislation or the actions of a regulatory agency.

cost-effective Providing a service at a "reasonable" cost (which might not necessarily be the lowest cost). See also *cost-effectiveness analysis* under *cost-analysis*.

cost-effectiveness analysis (CEA) See under *cost-analysis*.

cost-per-case management The method (philosophy) of hospital management in which hospitals try to control the costs for each kind of case so that the revenue for that case will cover the cost. Cost-per-case management is a style of management that was developed when hospital revenue changed from reimbursement for services rendered to prospectively determined prices for various kinds of services. This change in reimbursement, in turn, came from the adoption of the prospective payment system (PPS) in the Medicare program. Previously, hospitals simply had to ensure that the aggregate of income covered the aggregate of costs.

cost-plus contract See under *contract*.

cost-sharing Out-of-pocket payment by patients for part of the cost of benefits of an insurance plan. The term is not properly applied to sharing in the cost of the insurance premium; it applies only to deductibles, coinsurance, and copayments.

cost-shifting Increasing the charges to one group of patients (such as private pay patients, who presumably have the ability to pay) when the payment for another group of patients will not cover the costs for that group. If the government pays too little for its beneficiaries, for example, through the prospective payment system (PPS), it is clear that the cost will be shifted to other payers.

cost-to-charge ratio (CCR) See under *ratio*.

COT See *Certified Ophthalmic Technician* under *ophthalmic technician*.

COTA See *Certified Occupational Therapy Assistant* under *occupational therapy assistant*.

COTPER See *Coordinating Office for Terrorism Preparedness and Emergency Response* under *Centers for Disease Control and Prevention*.

Council for International Organizations of Medical Sciences (CIOMS) An organization founded in 1949 under the auspices of the World Health Organization (WHO) and the United Nations Educational, Scientific and Cultural Organization (UNESCO), which serves to promote international activities in the field of medical sciences and bioethics. **www.cioms.ch**

Council of Medical Specialty Societies (CMSS) A nonprofit organization representing twenty-three national medical specialty organizations. **www.cmss.org**

Council on Accreditation (COA) See *Commission on Accreditation for Health Informatics and Information Management Education*.

Council on Clinical Classifications (CCC) A nonprofit organization formed in 1975 to prepare the North American adaptation of the *International Classification of Diseases, 9th Revision* (ICD-9) (World Health Organization, Geneva, 1975). Its product was the *International Classification of Diseases, 9th Revision, Clinical Modification* (ICD-9-CM) (1978). CCC was sponsored by the American Academy of Pediatrics (AAP), the American College of Obstetricians and Gynecologists (ACOG), the American College of Physicians (ACP), the American College of Surgeons (ACS), the American Psychiatric Association (APA), and the Commission on Professional and Hospital Activities (CPHA).

Council on Graduate Medical Education (COGME) An organization authorized by Congress (originally in 1986) to provide an ongoing assessment of physician workforce trends and needs in the United States, and to make recommendations to the Secretary of the Department of Health and Human Services (HHS); the Senate Committee on Health, Education, Labor and Pensions (HELP); and the House of Representatives Committee on Commerce. **www.cogme.gov**

counselor A health professional (usually with at least a master's degree) who assists individuals by providing advice, guidance, and other services. Most states require licensure or certification. Counselors may be called therapists; in some states, the title is regulated by law. See also *addiction counselor*, *alcoholism counselor*, *community counselor*, *gambling counselor*, *genetic counselor*, *marriage and family counselor*, *mental health counselor*, *rehabilitation counselor*, *school counselor*, *student affairs practitioner*, *substance abuse counselor*, and *vocational rehabilitation counselor* (under *rehabilitation counselor*).

National Certified Counselor (NCC) A counselor who has met the certification requirements of the National Board for Certified Counselors, Inc. (NBCC). **www.nbcc.org**

countermeasure See *medical countermeasure*.

coupler See *Problem Knowledge Couplers (PKCouplers)*.

courtesy staff See *courtesy medical staff* under *medical staff member*.

covenant not to compete A clause of an employment contract that prohibits the employee from competing with the employer in their field of work, during and/or after the contract. Generally, a covenant not to compete will be enforced if it is (1) ancillary to a lawful contract, (2) supported by consideration (such as salary), (3) is reasonable, and (4) does not impose undue hardship. For example, if the clause prohibited the employee from working in the same field as the employer forever, the clause would not be reasonable and would not be enforced. These clauses are becoming more important in the healthcare field as competition is increasing and physicians are working with more than one hospital. Hospitals are trying to get more control over the care within their service areas. Some states have laws governing these covenants. Also called a noncompete clause or restrictive covenant.

coverage In healthcare reform discussions, "coverage" is most often used to describe the group of people for whom health insurance is available, rather than the particular services paid for (see *benefits* and *insurance coverage*). For example, coverage may be for senior citizens (as a part of Medicare), for employees of a given company, and so on.

covered entity (CE) Under the *Privacy Rule*, any entity that is a health plan, a healthcare clearinghouse, or a *healthcare provider* (see under *provider*) that electronically transmits or maintains *protected health information (PHI)*. Employers, life/casualty insurance companies, government agencies, or researchers may be deemed not to be a "covered entity," unless they are also a covered health plan or provider. A person or organization, not otherwise a covered entity, may nevertheless be subject to the Privacy Rule if they are a *business associate* of another covered entity. The Department of Health and Human Services (HHS) maintains a web site on this topic at **aspe.os.dhhs.gov/admnsimp**. 45 C.F.R. § 160.103 (October 1, 2006).

covered person See *enrollee*.

CP See *Certified Prosthetist* under *prosthetist*. Also corporate portal; see *portal*.

CPA See *Certified Public Accountant* under *accountant*.

CPAN See *Certified Post Anesthesia Nurse* under *post anesthesia nursing*.

CPC See *Certified Professional Coder* under *coding specialist*.

CPC-H See *Certified Professional Coder—Hospital* under *coding specialist*.

CPC-P See *Certified Professional Coder—Payer* under *coding specialist*.

CPCS See *Certified Provider Credentialing Specialist* under *provider credentialing specialist*.

CPDM See *Certified Professional in Disability Management* under *disability management*.

CPDN See *Certified Peritoneal Dialysis Nurse* under *dialysis nursing*.

CPDP See *Consumer-Purchaser Disclosure Project*.

CPE See *Certified Physician Executive*, under *physician executive*, and *Certified Professional Ergonomist*, under *ergonomist*.

C.Ped See *Certified Pedorthist* under *pedorthist*.

CPFT See *Certified Pulmonary Function Technologist* under *pulmonary function technologist*.

CPGs See *clinical practice guidelines* under *guidelines*.

CPHA See *Commission on Professional and Hospital Activities*.

CPHIMS See *Certified Professional in Healthcare Information and Management Systems* under *health information management professional*.

CPHQ See *Certified Professional in Healthcare Quality* under *quality management professional*.

CPHRM See *Certified Professional in Healthcare Risk Management* under *risk management professional*.

CPhT See *Certified Pharmacy Technician* under *pharmacy technician*.

CPI See *Certified Physician Investigator* under *physician investigator* (under *investigator*), and *consumer price index* under *index (numerical)*.

CPM See *Certified Professional Midwife* under *midwifery*. Also means Critical Path Method; see *clinical path*.

CPMSM See *Certified Professional Medical Services Management* under *medical staff services professional*.

CPN See *Certified Pediatric Nurse* under *pediatric nursing*.

CPNP See *Certified Pediatric Nurse Practitioner* under *pediatric nursing*.

CPO See *care plan oversight*, *Certified Prosthetist-Orthotist* under *orthotist*, and chief *privacy officer*. Also contract provider organization; see *preferred provider organization*.

CPOE See *computerized physician order entry*.

CPON See *Certified Pediatric Oncology Nurse* under *oncology nursing*.

CPP See *Credentialed Pain Practitioner* under *pain management*.

CPQA See *Certified Professional in Quality Assurance* under *quality management professional*.

CPR See *cardiopulmonary resuscitation*, *computer-based patient record* (under *electronic health record*), and *customary, prevailing, reasonable charge (or fee)*.

CPRI Computer-based Patient Record Institute. See *CPRI-HOST*.

CPRI-HOST A 2000 consolidation of the Computer-based Patient Record Institute (CPRI) and Healthcare Open Systems and Trials (HOST). CPRI was formed in 1991 to establish routine use of a *computer-based patient record (CPR)* (see under *electronic health record*) system in all healthcare settings. Its formation was recommended in the *Computer-Based Patient Record*, a study by the Institute of Medicine (IOM), which called for fully automated medical records in hospitals by the end of the decade. CPRI was formed by a coalition of about thirty-five interested groups, which included the American Medical Association (AMA), the American Health Information Management Association (AHIMA), and the U.S. Chamber of Commerce. HOST was created in 1994 by CPRI and Microelectronics and Computer Technology Corporation to "accelerate the deployment of open, interoperable and integrated information systems in health care though education of health and technology professionals, research, development and testing of appropriate technologies in real-world community health settings."

CPRI-HOST described itself as "a neutral forum for bringing diverse interests together to raise issues, exchange ideas, and develop common solutions for management of health information." In 2002, promising to create the "definitive information resource" on electronic information systems and computer-based patient records (CPR), CPRI-HOST united with *Healthcare Information and Management Systems Society (HIMSS)*.

CPRS Computerized Patient Record System. See *VistA*.

CPS See *Current Population Survey*.

CPSN See *Certified Plastic Surgical Nurse* under *plastic surgical nursing*.

CPT *Current Procedural Terminology*. A publication of the American Medical Association (AMA) containing its classification of procedures and services, primarily those carried out by physicians. It is widely used for coding in billing and payment for physicians' services, including HCPCS. Each "package" of physician services (for example, care for a fracture—including diagnosis, setting the fracture, and putting on and removing the splint) is given one code number and commands one fee for the package. In contrast to *CPT*, ICD-9-CM, the classification used for hospital coding of diagnoses and procedures, has separate codes for each of the four factors: diagnosis, setting the fracture, applying the cast, and removing the cast.

CPT is similar in theory to DRGs (which apply to hospital—not physician—care) in that both are built on the "one code, one fee" basis. Although the fourth edition of *CPT* appeared in 1977 (at which time it was called "CPT-4"), it has been revised repeatedly since then, and now the volume is labeled annually. The 2006 edition, *CPT 2006*, contained over 7,000 codes and descriptors. A CPT code can be recognized as a five-digit number falling into the range of 00100 to 99499. See also **modifier**. Compare to **ABC Codes**, which are used in alternative medicine.

CPUM See *Certified Professional Utilization Management* under *utilization manager*.

CPUR See *Certified Professional Utilization Review* under *utilization review*.

CQI See *continuous quality improvement* under *quality improvement*. Also means clinical quality indicator; see *quality indicator* under *indicator*.

CRA See *Certified Retinal Angiographer* under *retinal angiography*.

CRADA See *Cooperative Research and Development Agreement*.

crazy cow disease See *mad cow disease*.

CRC See *Certified Rehabilitation Counselor* under *rehabilitation counselor*. Also CERT Review Contractor; see *Comprehensive Error Rate Testing*.

cream skimming See *cherry picking*.

creative arts therapies Use of creative arts to restore, maintain, or improve an individual's physical, mental, emotional, or social functioning. See *art therapy*, *dance/movement therapy*, *drama therapy*, *manual arts therapy*, and *music therapy*.

credential An individual's right to a certain claim, for example, as to education. Usually a credential is supported by an official document: the physician's medical school diploma, state license, and specialty certification certificate are examples. Credentials, once attained, tend to be fixed, although in some instances they expire, and renewal or recertification may be required. In other instances, credentials may be withdrawn by the issuing body. And, of course, the individual may acquire additional credentials. See also *credentials*.

Credentialed Pain Practitioner (CPP) See under *pain management*.

credential examination An examination given for the purpose of determining the applicant's qualification for the credential sought.

credentialing A term used to describe the process of determining eligibility for hospital medical staff membership and/or *privileges* to be granted to physicians and allied health professionals (AHPs) in the light of their academic preparation, licensing, training, and performance. A basic premise of credentialing is that the applicant always has the burden to prove that he or she is qualified and capable of performing the requested privileges according to applicable standards. This process is typically delegated by the governing body to a credentials committee and sometimes an allied health review committee (AHRC). (The administrative verification of credentials is usually handled by a *provider credentialing specialist*. This includes obtaining references, including statements from previous mentors and institutions, confirming that licensure is current, and so forth. The information obtained is then used by the credentials committee in its determinations.)

First, the credentials of the physician (or other practitioner) are examined to determine qualification for admission to the medical staff (if appropriate; some allied health professionals are granted clinical privileges, but not medical staff membership; this depends on the hospital's policy). Then a decision is made on privileges to be granted initially. Periodically, the person's credentials and performance are reviewed. Medical staff membership and/or privileges may under appropriate circumstances be denied, modified, or withdrawn. (The exact procedure for "credentialing" is delineated in the hospital or medical staff bylaws.) See also *allied health professional* and *investigation*.

centralized credentialing Credentialing of physicians by an organization outside a hospital, either nonprofit or private. A single application from a physician will serve for all the hospitals participating in the service. The hospitals also share disciplinary information.

economic credentialing A term sometimes used to describe decisions by a hospital about medical staff appointment and/or clinical privileges of a practitioner that take economic factors into account, such as patient lengths of stay, number of tests ordered, costs, or competition with the hospital.

credentials The formal education, training, licensure, certification, performance, experience, examination results, and other accomplishments of an individual that make him or her qualified to do something, such as practice medicine. In health care, "credentials" usually refers to those qualifications required by the law and the healthcare facility.

credentials committee A committee of the medical staff charged with reviewing the credentials and performance of physicians (and, in some hospitals, allied health professionals) and making recommendations as to medical staff membership and clinical privileges to be granted or modified. See also *allied health review committee* and *credentialing*.

creditor A business or individual to whom money is owed.

CRES See *Certified Radiology Equipment Specialist* under *biomedical instrumentation technologist*.

Crew Resource Management (CRM) A training program for flight crews to improve aviation safety by reducing human error. CRM is designed to help people work effectively in high stress, high risk situations. Emphasis is on safety, efficiency, and morale. Pilots and crew members learn about human limitations and the effects of fatigue, how to use all available resources to make decisions, how to develop contingency plans, and how to work effectively together by supporting and listening to each other, resolving conflicts, and communicating problems. Some healthcare providers are implementing aspects of this training to reduce errors in medical care, for example in anesthesia and intensive care units. Also called Cockpit Resource Management.

crib death See *sudden infant death syndrome*.

critical (condition) A term that, when used to describe *patient condition*, means that the condition is life-threatening. Of the terms commonly used to describe a patient's condition, "critical" indicates the greatest severity of illness.

critical (essential) Highly important or essential, as used in connection with systems or their components.

mission-critical A system whose failure is likely to result in failure to accomplish a given task. For example, a space-heating control system is primarily mission-critical; its failure will result in a cold or overheated house. A control system for a washing machine is mission-critical because its failure will result in dirty clothes.

safety-critical Systems whose failure can cause injury or death or damage to life-sustaining qualities of the earth. For example, a control system for radiation therapy dosage is a safety-critical system; its failure may result in radiation burns or death. A water heating control system is also safety-critical because its failure may result in a burned person.

Critical Access Hospital (CAH) Program The popular name of the Medicare Rural Hospital Flexibility Program, created by the Balanced Budget Act of 1997. The purpose is to help rural communities preserve access to primary care and emergency services by improving reimbursement and having different operating requirements for rural hospitals. To qualify for special treatment under the act, a hospital must be designated a **Critical Access Hospital (CAH)**. A CAH must participate in the Medicare program, be located in a rural area and at least thirty-five miles from another hospital (fifteen miles if the area is mountainous or limited to secondary roads), and meet a number of other requirements, including participation in a *rural health network (RHN)*. A CAH may receive federal funding to help it meet the needs of its community. See also *Medicare Dependent Hospital Program*.

critical care medicine A multidisciplinary specialty focusing on the treatment of patients with acute, life-threatening illness or injury. The site of care is not significant, although it will most commonly be provided at an accident scene or in an ambulance, emergency room, or intensive care unit. Physician subspecialty certification is available in anesthesiology, internal medicine, obstetrics and gynecology, and ophthalmology (see *medical specialty*). See also *critical care nursing*.

critical care nursing The area of nursing focusing on the needs of critically ill patients.

Acute and Critical Care Clinical Nurse Specialist (CCNS) A clinical nurse specialist in critical care nursing and acute care nursing who has met the requirements of the American Association of Critical-Care Nurses (AACN) Certification Corporation. **www.certcorp.org**

Critical Care Nurse (CCRN) A specialist in critical care nursing who has met the requirements of the American Association of Critical-Care Nurses (AACN) Certification Corporation. **www.certcorp.org**

critical care unit See *intensive care unit*.

critical path See *clinical path*.

Critical Path Method (CPM) See *clinical path*.

CRM See *community resource management* and *Crew Resource Management*.

CRN See *Certified Radiology Nurse* under *radiology nursing*.

CRNA See *Certified Registered Nurse Anesthetist* under *anesthetist*.

CRNFA See *Certified Registered Nurse First Assistant* under *first assistant*.

CRNH Certified Registered Nurse Hospice. Now *Certified Hospice and Palliative Nurse (CHPN)*; see under *hospice and palliative nursing*.

CRNI See *Certified Registered Nurse Infusion* under *infusion nursing*.

CRNO See *Certified Ophthalmic Registered Nurse* under *ophthalmic nursing*.

CRO See *contract research organization*.

cross-functional A term used in quality management teams to indicate that more than one department is involved. For example, if both nursing and pharmacy are involved in a team, it is a cross-functional team.

Crossing the Quality Chasm See *Institute of Medicine's Health Care Quality Initiative*.

cross-training Learning a new skill outside of one's primary area; see *upskilling*.

crosswalk Sometimes called a "conversion table." In connection with coding and classification, a table that gives the labels and the codes or category numbers for a given term under each of two or more systems. When two classifications represent the same universe, it would seem to be a simple matter of producing the new numbers for the same things. But two different classifications handle the universe in different manners, so crosswalks among classifications are, at best, approximations.

For example, in the *Crosswalk from ICD-9-CM to ICD-10-CM*, prepared for the U.S. National Center for Health Statistics (NCHS), about 13% of the entries, or nearly 5,000 of them, bear a symbol that " indicates the best match of one to many matches."

The original diagnosis rarely ends up in a class with the same *content* as the one in which it started. For example, "congenital absence of the ear lobe" is in class 744.21 in ICD-9-CM but is in Q17.8 in ICD-10-CM—"specified ear anomaly, not elsewhere classified." Code 744.21 represents a "single diagnosis" class, and it could always be decoded to the one, and only the one, diagnosis. Code Q17.8 is the home for "all other specified abnormalities," of which congenital absence of the ear lobe is only one. Decoding Q17.8 will never identify the absent ear lobe uniquely.

Because the code number is actually the equivalent of the *label* for the class, the crosswalk also often results in a change in *terminology* (the label). Code 5550 in ICD-9-CM was labeled "regional ileitis of the small intestine." The crosswalk leads to a number of codes, K50.–0–K50.04 plus K50.09, with labels for variations of "Crohn's disease of the small bowel." Thus the K50 codes will never decode to "regional ileitis."

Sometimes a radical *reclassification* of terms, and even of *meaning*, occurs, as when "persistent vomiting," which had been a stomach disorder in ICD-9-CM with code 536.2 was "converted" by the crosswalk to "projectile vomiting," a symptom (not "disorder") with code R11.2 in ICD-10-CM.

CRRN See *Certified Rehabilitation Registered Nurse* under *rehabilitation nursing*.

CRS See *Congressional Research Service*.

CRT See *Certified Respiratory Therapist* under *respiratory therapist*.

cryptography The science of information privacy. Individuals who practice this field are known as **cryptographers**. The word is derived from the Greek "kryptos," meaning hidden. Information is hidden by "encrypting" it, and revealed again by "decrypting" it. This process is also known as **enciphering** and **deciphering** information, using secret **ciphers**.

Although cryptography can be applied to almost any kind of information (pictures, movies, sounds), in the healthcare world today cryptography is most often associated with encrypting **plain text** (sometimes referred to as "clear text") into **ciphertext**, then decrypting it back again.

Earlier forms of cryptography used the same device or method ("**key**") to encrypt the information and to decrypt it, a form known as **symmetric cryptography**. The single key obviously had to be kept secret. More modern methods tend to use two different keys, one private as before, but also a **public key**. This is the method used in the public key infrastructure (PKI), the most common type of cryptography used in the healthcare environment.

Encryption involves processing information with a device or method so that its true meaning or content is completely hidden from unauthorized view. Modern encryption almost always involves computers and digital data, although information may be encrypted in other ways. It should be noted that encrypted information may still be intercepted and copied without authorization, but it would essentially be meaningless gibberish to anyone without the key to reverse ("**decrypt**") the process by which the information was encrypted.

Basically, cryptography as used in the healthcare context is concerned with four objectives:

1. *Privacy/confidentiality:* The information is effectively hidden from anyone who is not supposed to see it.
2. *Integrity:* The information can't be changed without authorization.
3. *Nonrepudiation:* The source of the information can't deny being the source.
4. *Authentication:* Everyone involved with the information can prove that they are who they claim to be.

Note that there is no mention of any objective to keep the encrypted information from falling into the wrong hands. The effectiveness of cryptography rests entirely on the information's resistance to being decrypted—a resistance that is not perfect. Given enough time and resources (typically massive quantities of computing power), any encrypted information is susceptible to being decrypted. However, you still lock your front door when you leave your house, even though you know a bulldozer can open it without a key.

With current efforts in health care to utilize the electronic health record (EHR), sometimes over large public networks like the Internet, cryptography becomes an important part of the plan used to keep protected health information (PHI) private.

CS See *central service department*.

CSA See *Certified Surgical Assistant* under *surgical assistant*.

CSAP Center for Substance Abuse Prevention. See *Substance Abuse and Mental Health Services Administration*.

CSAT Center for Substance Abuse Treatment. See *Substance Abuse and Mental Health Services Administration*.

CSDN Continued stay denial notice; see *hospital-issued notice of noncoverage*.

CS-DRG See *consolidated severity-adjusted DRG* under *DRG*.

CSI See *Comprehensive Severity Index*.

CSM/M See *Customer Satisfaction Measurement and Management*.

CSP Board Certified Specialist in Pediatric Nutrition; see *Registered Dietitian* under *dietitian*.

CSR See *Center for Scientific Review* under *National Institutes of Health*. Also Certified Specialist in Renal Nutrition; see *Registered Dietitian* under *dietitian*.

CSSD Board Certified Specialist in Sports Dietetics; see *Registered Dietitian* under *dietitian*.

CST See *Certified Surgical Technologist* under *surgical technologist*.

CST,CFA See *Certified First Assistant* under *first assistant*.

CT See *computed tomography* and *Cytotechnologist* (under *clinical laboratory technologist*).

CTO See *chief technology officer*.

CTRN See *Certified Transport Registered Nurse* under *transport nursing*.

CTRS See *Certified Therapeutic Recreation Specialist* under *therapeutic recreation specialist*.

CTSA See *Clinical and Translational Science Awards*.

CT scanner A machine that carries out *computed tomography*. Also called a "CAT scanner."

CTT See *computed tomography technologist*.

CTV3 See *Clinical Terms Version 3*.

CUA See *Certified Urologic Associate* under *urologic associate*.

CUCNS See *Certified Urologic Clinical Nurse Specialist* under *urologic nursing*.

cultural competence Possession of the knowledge, skills, and attitudes needed to provide effective health care for diverse populations, taking into account the culture, language, values, and reality of the patient and the patient's community.

For example, the Department of Health and Human Services (HHS) Center for Mental Health Services has developed cultural competence standards for managed care mental health services targeting four "underserved/underrepresented racial/ethnic groups": African Americans, Hispanics, Native Americans/Alaska Natives, and Asian/Pacific Islander Americans.

culturally and linguistically appropriate services (CLAS) Health services provided with sensitivity to the particular cultural and language needs of the patient. As the diversity of patient populations in the United States is becoming recognized, efforts are underway to accommodate specific needs to achieve better outcomes. The Department of Health and Human Services (HHS) Office of Minority Health has issued national standards on CLAS in health care. See also *cultural competence*.

Cumulative Index to Nursing and Allied Health Literature (CINAHL) A reference database providing access to nursing and allied health literature and information from 1982 to the present. **www.library.ucsf.edu/db/cinahl.html**

CUNP See *Certified Urologic Nurse Practitioner* under *urologic nursing*.

CUPA See *Certified Urologic Physician's Assistant* under *urologic physician's assistant*.

curbside consultation The practice by a physician of obtaining advice or information from another physician on the diagnosis or management of a particular case, informally (at the "curbside") rather than through formal channels. Also called curbstone consultation. The consulted physician is sometimes said to have been "curbsided" or "curbstoned."

CURN See *Certified Urologic Registered Nurse* under *urologic nursing*.

Current Population Survey (CPS) A survey that the U.S. Department of Commerce Census Bureau conducts monthly to gather information on the noninstitutionalized population of the United States. Every March, the CPS focuses on health-related information, including whether individuals have health insurance.

Current Procedural Terminology (CPT) See *CPT*.

current ratio See under *ratio*.

custodial Pertains to watching over and protecting, rather than, in the healthcare field, attempting to provide treatment.

custodial care See *rest home care* under *nursing care*.

custodial care facility See *rest home*.

customary fee See *customary, prevailing, reasonable charge (or fee)*.

customary, prevailing, reasonable charge (or fee) (CPR) The charge or "fee" (same as charge), usually of a physician, which has traditionally been defined as that charge which is the lowest of the following: the actual charge made for the service, the physician or supplier's "customary" (usual) charge for the service, or the fee "prevailing" in the community for the service. Such fees vary according to specialty, geographic area, and the physician's charge system. Increases in such fees are typically limited by economic indexes imposed by the paying agency. The definition of "reasonable and customary charge (or fee)" is under scrutiny by the federal government with the idea that the fees should be "inherently" reasonable, that is, related to some real worth of the service rather than a comparison. The Tax Equity and Fiscal Responsibility Act (TEFRA) and Medicare regulations both give specific formulas for calculating the "reasonable charges" limitation on physician fees. Synonyms: customary fee, prevailing fee, and Usual, Customary and Reasonable (UCR).

customer In health care, "customer" is often used to mean the person or entity buying the services. For example, an employer might be the customer of a health plan that enrolls the employees. In the context of quality management, the customer is the person (or department) for whom services are provided. For example, the customers of the clinical laboratory include not only the patient, but also the physician who receives the lab results, and perhaps the accounting department that must determine the charges. An important process in quality improvement is to determine who the customers are, what they need, and whether these needs are being met. See also *consumer*.

Customer Satisfaction Measurement and Management (CSM/M) Efforts undertaken by a healthcare provider to keep existing customers. Some research suggests that customers who say they are satisfied with their healthcare provider are just as likely to go to another provider as those who say they are dissatisfied. Because of this, CSM/M programs are typically not content to merely do surveys of customers to spot dissatisfaction, but go beyond into such issues as customer loyalty and perceived value.

CVD See *cardiovascular disease*.

CVM See *Center for Veterinary Medicine*.

CVRT See *Certified Vision Rehabilitation Therapist* under *vision rehabilitation therapist*.

CVT See *cardiovascular technologist*.

CWCN See *Certified Wound Care Nurse* under *wound, ostomy, and continence nursing*.

CWHIS See *community-wide health information system*.

CWOCN See *Certified Wound, Ostomy and Continence Nurse* under *wound, ostomy, and continence nursing*.

CWON See *Certified Wound and Ostomy Nurse* under *wound, ostomy, and continence nursing*.

CWS See *Certified Wound Specialist* under *wound specialist*.

CWW See *clinic without walls*.

cybercadaver A computer model of a body. The first two human cybercadavers were the "Visible Human Male" and the "Visible Human Female." They were produced by the University of Colorado's Center for Human Simulation for the $1.4 million Visible Human Project of the National Library of Medicine (NLM).

Radiographic and photographic techniques were used in a method that "sliced" the two human cadavers, creating digital images that were then used to "assemble" the databases. The male cybercadaver requires fifteen gigabytes of storage; the female, which was made later with improved techniques, takes up thirty-nine gigabytes, and displays the images with three times the resolution. Although these databases can be downloaded without charge from the Internet, be cautioned that fifteen gigabytes represents a massive amount of information, requiring enormous storage capability and bandwidth.

An increasingly wide range of uses is being made of the databases, ranging from animated programs for teaching anatomy in grade schools to training physicians in delicate procedures. **www.nlm.nih.gov/research/visible/visible_human.html**

cyberchondria A condition of anxiety brought on by the wealth of information—both legitimate and erroneous—available on the Internet. A person may surf the Internet to investigate his or her symptoms, and self-diagnose based on the information found, which may or may not be accurate. From "cyber" (referring to cyberspace) and "hypochondria" (excessive anxiety about one's health). Sometimes called Internet printout syndrome.

cybermedicine A term coined by Warner V. Slack, MD, and the title of his 1997 (revised and updated in 2001) book. Slack uses the term to describe a style of health and medical care in which clinical computing assists in patient diagnosis and assessment, physician and patient guidance and decision making, self-care, prevention, and patient empowerment. It emphasizes using the computer for tasks to which it is uniquely suited, such as (1) providing access to up-to-the-minute biomedical knowledge for both the physician and the patient via the Internet and other routes, (2) giving the patient the opportunity to put full details of his or her problems and history on a private and secure basis into his or her medical record, (3) communicating electronically among caregivers and patients, (4) making instructions for patients and caregivers available on the spot just when they're needed (e.g., diet, medication, procedures), (5) providing instant consolidation of all pertinent information about the patient (e.g., laboratory reports, consultations, and nurses' findings), (6) management of treatment as appropriate to the patient's response, and (7) simplification and reduced cost of care.

Slack argues persuasively that cybermedicine rehumanizes medical care, freeing the doctor to spend much more time with patients, and at the same time be assured that the fundamental patient care information system is more reliable and under better control than possible if left to human memory and to traditional paper-based methods.

In this book, Slack also coins the term "clinhaven" for a clinical facility of the future. The clinhaven would be small and decentralized, located within walking distance of many patients (although it would also have plentiful parking). It would be able to perform even complex diagnostic and therapeutic procedures on an ambulatory basis. The clinhaven would be staffed and run by humanistic clinicians, who would be able to offer high-quality medical care at lower cost, taking full advantage of current and future technological developments.

Other subjects included in medical informatics, such as control of laboratory equipment and the necessary details of message transfer and the like, are not included in Slack's "cybermedicine" concept.

cybernaut See *cyberspace*.

cyberspace Computer-generated space, in which the traveler is called a **cybernaut**. The term was coined by science fiction author William Gibson in 1984. It is now also being applied to computer conferencing, computer bulletin boards, and other innovative communication activities and applications of information technology (IT), particularly in education and health care. For example, a college course may be said to be conducted in cyberspace when it is carried out primarily or largely with an electronic network rather than in a classroom (this is called an "online" course). Students in such a course may be employed in widely separated sites, and the faculty member may address them informally in the electronic network from wherever she or he happens to be. The reference library is, of course, electronic. Questions, answers, and student and faculty discussion may be posted on the class's computer bulletin board at any time by students or faculty. In addition, scheduled interactive "class periods" for the dispersed faculty and students may be held. See also *e-learning* and *telehealth*.

cybertherapy Obtaining psychological advice or other counseling via the Internet. The number of online therapy services is rising. Included are professional psychologists, advice-column-type counselors, support groups, and so forth. Some give advice free, whereas others charge a fee.

cyto- Pertaining to cells.

cytogenetics See under *genetics*.

cytology The study of the cell (cyto-): its formation, biology, chemistry, physiology, structure, function, and diseases.

cytomegalovirus (CMV) A virus that infects 50% to 85% of adults in the United States by the age of forty. CMV is related to the herpes virus. The infection is often transmitted to infants before birth. Transmission is from person to person; it can be transmitted sexually and by breast milk, organ transplantation, and blood transfusion. For most healthy people, there are no symptoms or long-term health consequences. However, CMV infection is of special concern with unborn babies, people who work with children, and those who are immunocompromised, such as recipients of organ transplants and AIDS patients. See also *leukoreduction*.

cytosine (C) See *DNA*.

Cytotechnologist (CT) See under *clinical laboratory technologist*.

D

DABHP Diplomate of the American Board of Health Physics. See *Certified Health Physicist* under *health physicist*, under *physicist*.

DABMA See *Diplomate of the American Board of Medical Acupuncture* under *acupuncturist*.

daily service charge Same as *room rate*; see under *rate (charge)*.

damages A legal term describing the money to be paid to a plaintiff by the defendant when the defendant is found to be liable. The term "damages" is sometimes used more restrictively to describe the monetary value of the plaintiff's injuries, property loss, and the like.

actual damages Money paid to compensate actual loss by the plaintiff, such as medical expenses, loss of earnings (or value of services, such as homemaking), pain and suffering, and (rarely) emotional distress. Synonym: compensatory damages.

compensatory damages See *actual damages*, above.

exemplary damages See *punitive damages*, below.

liquidated damages An amount of money decided on by the parties to a contract at the time of contracting, which will be paid to one party upon default of the other. Such damages are permitted only if the actual amount of damages is very difficult to ascertain, and if the amount is reasonable.

nominal damages A token sum (usually one dollar) paid to the plaintiff where legal liability is proven but there are no actual damages.

punitive damages Damages allowed in a tort action that are not calculated from the actual damages (medical expenses, property damages) incurred by the plaintiff, but rather used as punishment for the wrongdoing of the defendant. Punitive damages are like the fine imposed for criminal behavior, except that the money is paid to the plaintiff instead of the state. Most states have enacted caps on these damages in products liability cases as part of tort reform. The federal government has attempted to cap punitive damages by considering an FDA defense. See *FDA defense*. Synonym: exemplary damages.

treble damages Three times the damages (monetary compensation) the plaintiff would otherwise be entitled to. Certain laws permit treble damages as a punitive measure, to discourage certain types of conduct and to encourage injured parties to enforce those laws as "private attorneys general" (or as qui tam claimants). For example, federal antitrust laws provide for treble damages; the jury's (or judge's) award to a successful plaintiff is tripled. See *False Claims Act*.

dance/movement therapy The use of movement and dance to further a person's emotional, cognitive, social, and physical integration.

dance therapist A health professional skilled in dance/movement therapy. Also called dance/movement therapist.

Dance Therapists Registered (DTR) This credential denotes a dance therapist with at least a master's degree, qualified to work as part of a professional healthcare team, under supervision, by the American Dance Therapy Association (ADTA). **www.adta.org**

Academy of Dance Therapists Registered (ADTR) This credential denotes a Dance Therapist Registered with advanced training and experience who is qualified to work independently, teach, and supervise, by the American Dance Therapy Association (ADTA). **www.adta.org**

D&O See *Directors' and Officers' insurance* under *insurance*.

DAO See *decedent affairs office*.

Darling case A landmark hospital law case that established that the hospital is responsible for care provided to patients, and that the medical staff must be accountable to the hospital for the care provided by medical staff members. The case involved a young man named Darling who was brought to a hospital with a leg fracture suffered while playing football. Through a series of events (notably, lack of communication among nurses, doctors, and hospital, and failure by the hospital and medical staff to enforce their own bylaws) the patient's leg became gangrenous and was eventually lost. *Darling v. Charleston Community Memorial Hospital*, 33 Ill.2d 326, 211 N.E.2d 253 (1965), cert. denied, 383 U.S. 946 (1966).

DARPA See *Defense Advanced Research Projects Agency*.

Dartmouth Atlas of Health Care The first national study on regional differences in health-care delivery. The work is an outgrowth of a number of years of study of regional variations in healthcare practices by John Wennberg, MD, and his group. Included are data on resources available, including hospital beds and hospital employees; physician specialties; physician practice patterns, such as solo and group practice; resource use; and Medicare inpatient reimbursement for acute short-stay care.

The Dartmouth Atlas project is a funded research effort of the faculty of the Center for the Evaluative Clinical Sciences at Dartmouth Medical School. Current atlases—including national, state, specialty, and regional editions—can be viewed or ordered from their web site, as can other related information and reports. **www.dartmouthatlas.org**

dashboard A visual display of key information needed to make decisions. The term, which commonly describes the instrument panel in an automobile, has been adopted by hospitals to describe a type of report on the hospital's activities.

An automobile dashboard is really a collection of gauges, "idiot lights," and other displays of critical conditions (speed, engine temperature, fuel supply) and events (failed headlight, elapsed miles). The information is provided instantly, in real time, so that the driver can react immediately if necessary. In an airplane this collection is called an instrument panel and includes additional gauges, such as an altimeter. A Hobbs meter measures elapsed time (for example, since the engine was last overhauled).

The hospital's adaptation of the dashboard is a printed report, provided to the governing body periodically, that may show financial conditions, clinical performance, patient incidents, lawsuits filed, employee turnover, patient satisfaction, construction progress, and so forth. Although these factors may be constantly variable, they are frozen in the published dashboard report, which by its nature can only be a "snapshot" of the hospital's condition. It is thus, no matter how recent, a historical document, so the term "dashboard"—which was created to describe real-time monitoring—is misleading; "**performance panel**" is a more appropriate term for this report.

Management, meanwhile, is increasingly obtaining actual "dashboard"-type information showing current hospital conditions and events, with appropriate gauges and displays fueled by hospital information systems. This display can be provided via computer screen rather than paper, so much of it is contemporaneous—in real time—resulting in virtually no lag time between events and the ability to respond.

Construction of the governing board's dashboard (performance panel) is a forbidding task. To serve its function, it should meet at least the following criteria:

1. Report on key elements of the hospital's operation—finance, operations, clinical performance, satisfaction (patients, employees, physicians), and other items.
2. Give a limited, manageable number of indicators.
3. Tell the hospital's target for every indicator—should the performance be above, below, or at the given target, or within a stated range.
4. Tell the hospital's performance with reference to each target
5. Be supported by reference material that
   — Tells why each indicator is important.
   — Tells the source of each target.
   — Tells the source of each element of the hospital's performance information.
6. Use appropriate presentation methods, preferably graphic.

7. Transmit information "instantly."
8. Change with the hospital's needs. For example, during a building program, it could give progress against a schedule; during a fund-raising effort, it could report progress toward the financial goal.

A performance monitor, however, can never present *all* the information a trustee should know. Avoid the trap of implying that if all the items presented are OK, everything is OK. See also **benchmark** and **indicator**.

clinical quality dashboard Dashboards containing clinical quality indicators (CQIs) are developed for and by physicians, nurses, and other clinical professionals. See *quality indicator* under *indicator*.

management dashboard A number of standard indicators, developed over many years and taken from the business world, are being utilized for the management dashboard. Examples, some unique to health care, include:

Net revenue
Full-time equivalent (FTE) employees per bed
Net income
Employee turnover
Patient satisfaction
Employee satisfaction
Bed occupancy percentage
Admissions per clinical service

data Material, facts, or figures on which discussion is held or from which inferences are drawn or decisions made. A distinction is sometimes made between "data" and "information"; generally, data have to be somehow "digested" (manipulated, summarized, organized, or interpreted) in order to become information. No rigid standardization in terminology has appeared in this regard, although generally the term "information" is rarely applied to material that is "raw." The Joint Commission on Accreditation of Healthcare Organizations (JCAHO) defines data as "uninterpreted material, facts, or clinical observations." See also *information*.

qualitative data Data that are not expressed in numbers. This type of data may be expressed in natural language, images, audio, and other forms.

quantitative data Data that are expressed in numbers.

data accountability Identification of the party (for example, patient, physician, hospital, organization) or agent (software, device, instrument, monitor) responsible for data origination, amendment, verification, translation, stewardship, access and use, disclosure, and transmission and receipt. In other words, the who, what, when, where, how, under what conditions, and in what context of health information.

data bank See *data warehouse*.

Data Bank (NPDB) See *National Practitioner Data Bank*.

database Any collection of data or information organized with some type of structure, such as records (rows) and fields (columns). A collection of records, all sharing the same structure, may be referred to as a table. A database record, or a single row in a table, is a group of information items logically related in some fashion (e.g., name, address, phone number of one individual). Rows are typically subdivided into columns—smaller units of data known as data elements or "fields." For example, a telephone book is a database (table), each person or company listing being one row. Each row in the telephone book is further subdivided into three data elements or columns: name, address, and telephone number. Although today it seems that databases only exist in computers, it should be remembered that people have created and managed databases since long before the advent of computers.

The word "database" also describes a type of software application or language used to store and manipulate such data on computer systems. In this context, it is more appropriately referred to as a *database management system (DBMS)*.

clinical database The array of information about a patient that is collected by the physician and others caring for the patient in order to make a diagnosis and to be able to detect changes in the patient's condition during treatment.

knowledge database (KDB) See *knowledgebase.*

online database A system providing access for many users to a computer-stored database. Users gain access via their own computers (or terminals), using telephone lines or network connections to receive data. The Medical Literature Analysis and Retrieval System (MED-LARS), for example, is an online database providing access to the National Library of Medicine (NLM). The explosive growth of the Internet in the mid 1990s resulted in an equivalent growth in the number of online databases available.

relational database See *database management system.*

statistical database A compilation of data about a number of events (illnesses, for example) or objects (patients, for example) that has as its purpose the description of the group of events or objects. For example, a statistical database consisting of identical items of information about many patients who smoke gives a statistical description of smokers, and is used to estimate the risk of smoking, an element in health risk appraisal.

database management system (DBMS) A computer program used to manage a database. In its simplest form, it is a computerized filing system. In more elaborate forms, it relates information from different files together to produce new files, reports, and detailed analyses. Different DBMSs also tend to have their own languages with which they can be programmed for specific purposes, such as automatically performing certain functions ("triggers") when certain types of data are entered. The actual DBMS is frequently hidden from the user by a "user-friendly interface" that prompts and guides the user every step of the way.

Most DBMSs use the "relational" database model. It is characterized by having two or more "tables," each of which is "related" to one or more of the other tables by means of primary and (optionally) secondary "keys." The keys are simply columns of the same information that appear in all the tables that are related to each other, and thus allow one row in one table to be linked to a companion row in another table. As you might guess, when selecting a key you need to choose a column whose values are unique (no duplicates allowed). In a hospital's database, for instance, a unique patient identifier number (PatientID) is likely to be used as a primary key, as would a unique physician identifier number (PhysicianID).

Like a phone book, one table might contain all of that hospital's patients—one row per patient. Another table may contain all of the physicians who are on the hospital's staff. The patient table would include one column for PatientID and probably at least one column for PhysicianID, allowing a "relation" between each patient and at least one physician. This DBMS would be able to answer the question, "Who is Mr. Jones's doctor?" as well as "Who are Dr. Smith's patients?"

A major advantage to a DBMS that uses relational database technology is the elimination of duplicate data. If correctly designed ("normalized"), a relational DBMS will contain only one copy of any data element, such as a patient's address. Any other table that needs the patient's address will simply be linked to it via a key common to both tables. Changing a patient's address requires a change in only one place. In real life, of course, design and normalization of a relational database can become quite complex, but the idea behind it has been fairly constant since this technology's invention in the 1970s.

data comparability A feature of data that permits them to have precisely the same meaning to all parties with whom they are shared. Lack of comparable data can have a negative effect on patient care. For example, physical therapists use a pain scale that ranges from 1 to 4, whereas nurses use one ranging from 1 to 10. Pain designated as "level 3" would have very different meanings to these two groups. See also *interoperability.*

data element See *data set.*

Data Elements for Emergency Department Systems (DEEDS) See under *data set.*

data integrity A feature of data that keeps them from being altered or destroyed in an unauthorized manner or by unauthorized users, or even by accident.

Data Interchange Standards Association (DISA) A nonprofit organization that facilitates development of standards for international exchange of information. Its mission is to
promote development of and facilitate the application of electronic commerce technology
across industries and around the world. Representing e-commerce ("EC") professionals from
around the world, DISA's affiliation with EC User Groups, ANSI ASC X12N, and many others facilitates an interchange of e-commerce topics hitting the global market. In the international arena, DISA and ANSI ASC X12N serve as the entry point for the United States into
the United Nations *EDIFACT* (Electronic Data Interchange for Administration, Commerce
and Transport) process. **www.disa.org**

data mart A repository of data, gathered from operational data or from a data warehouse,
that is designed to serve a particular community of end users. Unlike the data warehouse, the
data mart's emphasis is on meeting the specific needs of specific users, presenting the data in
terms that are familiar to that particular group. A data mart is generally more accessible to
end users than the ***data warehouse***.

data mining Extracting previously unknown information from existing data using an artificial intelligence computer program that employs statistical and visualization techniques. The
existing data frequently reside in a data warehouse. Data mining is often distinguished from
online analytical processing (OLAP), which generally assumes that you already know the
questions you want to ask of your data. Data mining looks for relationships in data, including the following: sequences or associations (one event related to another event), classifications (pattern recognition), and clustering (finding groups of facts not previously known).
This type of analysis, if correctly done, is capable of discovering patterns in raw data that can
assist in forecasting (making predictions about the future). The implications of this capability
for health research are immense.

One recent example of data mining involved its use to uncover fraud and abuse by healthcare providers. Using a data mining software program developed by IBM, a New York health
insurance company discovered an ear-nose-and-throat doctor from Long Island, New York,
who claimed he was giving patients bronchoscopies as often as once a week. This invasive test
is usually needed once or twice in a lifetime, if at all. The insurance company paid the doctor
more than $800,000 before investigating his case and turning it over to the FBI. The doctor
pled guilty to insurance fraud, punishable by a maximum three-year federal prison sentence
and $3 million in fines.

See also ***knowledge discovery in databases***.

data processing department See ***information management department***.

data quality A feature of data that ensures that they are accurate and complete and convey
the intended meaning, unambiguously. See also ***data comparability***.

data record See ***database***.

data repository See ***data warehouse***.

data set A specified set of items of information. The data set for a person's address, for example, may be street address, city, state, and ZIP code. Each item is called a **data element**. In
the hospital, the term "data set" would be applied, for example, to a discharge abstract (see
under ***abstract***) and to a patient's bill. In this illustration, the nucleus of both data sets is, at a
minimum, the Uniform Hospital Discharge Data Set (UHDDS) specified by the federal government (see below).

Data sets used in healthcare information systems describe a group of data elements to be
collected in a standardized manner for a specific purpose. A number of formal data sets are
described below. See also ***Patient Medical Record Information***.

Continuity of Care Record (CCR) An ASTM standard specification for a core data set
of the most relevant administrative, demographic, and clinical information facts about a

patient's health care, covering one or more healthcare encounters. The CCR is to be created (or updated) by a provider whenever a patient is referred, transferred, or otherwise changes to a different clinic, hospital, or provider. The next provider will then have instant access to critical information about the patient, thus contributing to continuity of care. The goal is to reduce medical errors, achieve higher efficiency, and increase quality of care.

The CCR provides a "snapshot in time" of the patient. It includes patient and provider information, insurance information, advance directives, the patient's health status (e.g., allergies, medications, vital signs, diagnoses, recent procedures), recent care provided, recommendations for future care (i.e., a care plan), and the reason for referral or transfer. The CCR may be prepared, displayed, and transmitted on paper or electronically, provided the information required by the specification is included.

The CCR specification was developed by the ASTM E31 Committee on Health Informatics, with support from the Massachusetts Medical Society (MMS), Healthcare Information and Management Systems Society (HIMSS), American Academy of Family Physicians (AAFP), American Academy of Pediatrics (AAP), American Medical Association (AMA), Patient Safety Institute (PSI), American Health Care Association (AHCA), National Association for the Support of Long Term Care (NASL), Mobile Healthcare Alliance (MoHCA), Medical Group Management Association (MGMA), and American College of Osteopathic Family Physicians (ACOFP). The origins of the CCR stem from a Massachusetts Department of Public Health three-page, NCR paper–based Patient Care Referral Form that has been in widespread use over many years in Massachusetts. Synonym: patient care referral data set (PCRDS).

Data Elements for Emergency Department Systems (DEEDS) The data set recommended by the Centers for Disease Control and Prevention (CDC) for use in the emergency department (ED). Although ED data can be used for a variety of purposes (including statistical studies and bioterrorism surveillance), DEEDS was designed based on the principle that the primary function of an ED record system is to store clinical data and facilitate their retrieval during direct patient care. Thus, it focuses on data elements in current clinical use, and its 156 data elements are organized in the approximate sequence of data acquisition during an ED encounter. Standards used include HL7 Version 2.3, U.S. Bureau of the Census industry and occupation codes, Office of Management and Budget standards for classifying race and ethnicity, the X12 healthcare provider taxonomy, Logical Observation Identifiers Names and Codes (LOINC) for laboratory result types, and the ICD-9-CM external cause of injury and condition codes. In addition, DEEDS includes its own code set for mode of transport to the ED (ground ambulance, helicopter ambulance, etc.) and patient acuity (requires immediate evaluation or treatment, requires prompt evaluation or treatment, etc.). DEEDS 1.0 was released in 1997 by the National Center for Injury Prevention and Control (NCIPC).

Health Plan Employer Data and Information Set (HEDIS) A set of information about a managed care plan (MCP) designed to serve as a "report card" for the plan. HEDIS has measures of quality, access and patient satisfaction, membership and utilization, finance, and plant management. It was developed by the National Committee for Quality Assurance (NCQA). HEDIS is a registered trademark. **www.ncqa.org/Programs/HEDIS**

In the 1990s, Washington State's Quality Improvement Implementation Task Force, university research centers, clinics, and the Washington State Department of Health developed **Clinical Outcome Measure Amended HEDIS Strategy (COMAH)**, which goes beyond performance measurement by adding measurements of clinical outcomes.

International Nursing Minimum Data Set (i-NMDS) An international version of the *Nursing Minimum Data Set* (see below). Its development is a collaborative effort of the International Medical Informatics Association, Nursing Informatics Special Interest Group (IMIA NI-SIG), and the International Council of Nurses (ICN), and is being coordinated at the University of Iowa.

Minimum Data Set (MDS) See *Resident Assessment Instrument*.

National Uniform Claim Committee Data Set (NUCC-DS) A standardized data set intended for use by noninstitutional (physician and other nonhospital) healthcare providers, to transmit claim and coordination of benefits (COB) transactions to and from all third-party payers. Developed by the National Uniform Claim Committee, the NUCC-DS is aimed for use in an electronic environment, but is applicable to traditional paper forms as well. The NUCC works towards data content standardization as well as reducing the number of attachments required to process a claim and improving their handling. To help assure that data sets for institutional and noninstitutional claims are compatible, the NUCC works closely with the National Uniform Billing Committee (NUBC).

Nursing Management Minimum Data Set (NMMDS) A minimum data set for reporting nursing services information to support nursing executive decision making, including the environment (type of nursing delivery unit, patient/client population, method of care delivery, etc.), nurse resources (staffing, satisfaction), and financial resources (payment source, budget, etc.). Developed collaboratively by the University of Iowa and the American Organization of Nurse Executives (AONE).

Nursing Minimum Data Set (NMDS) A minimum set of nursing data elements. The NMDS was the first effort (begun in the 1980s) to standardize the collection of essential nursing information. It includes nursing care elements (nursing diagnoses, interventions, outcomes, intensity), patient demographics (personal identification, age, sex, etc.), and service elements (facility/provider, nurse, date of encounter or admission, discharge/disposition, expected source of payment, etc.). Some elements are also included in the Uniform Hospital Discharge Data Set (UHDDS). The NMDS is maintained and updated by the USA Nursing Minimum Data Set Consortium at the University of Iowa. See also *International Nursing Minimum Data Set*, above.

Outcome and Assessment Information Set (OASIS) A data set developed for use in monitoring outcomes of adult home healthcare patients, required for Medicare-certified home health agencies. The system of outcome measures was developed by HCFA (now CMS) with support from the Robert Wood Johnson Foundation over a ten-year period. **www.cms.hhs.gov/OASIS**

Patient Care Data Set (PCDS) A nursing data set containing a data dictionary and sets of terms and codes representing specific values of patient problems, patient care goals, and patient care orders. PCDS was initially developed by Judy Ozbolt at the University of Virginia, in collaboration with member institutions of the University HealthSystem Consortium, and was revised at Vanderbilt University Medical Center (VUMC). The PCDS was subsumed as integrated content within the clinical database of *Logical Observation Identifiers Names and Codes (LOINC)*.

Perioperative Nursing Data Set (PNDS) A standardized nursing vocabulary that serves as a minimum data set for nursing services in the perioperative area. Developed by the Association of Perioperative Registered Nurses (AORN) (**www.aorn.org**). According to AORN, "[a]s a nursing language, it is parsimonious, validated, reliable, and useful for clinical practice."

Uniform Ambulatory Care Data Set (UACDS) A standard minimum data set for ambulatory health care, developed by the National Committee on Vital and Health Statistics (NCVHS).

Uniform Clinical Data Set (UCDS) A system developed by HCFA (now CMS) during the early 1990s to facilitate standardized review of the quality of care delivered by hospitals treating Medicare patients. The UCDS automated system collected a standard set of data to make peer review organization (PRO) reviews more consistent from state to state, and to more uniformly monitor the care provided by the Medicare program.

Uniform Hospital Discharge Data Set (UHDDS) The items of medical record information required by CMS as the medical content of the patient's bill under Medicare. Assignment to a

DRG is made from this data set by the fiscal intermediary. The data set contains patient age, sex, and multiple diagnoses and procedures, as well as other information. Both diagnoses and procedures are expressed not in words but in the numerical category codes of ICD-9-CM. The UHDDS is the nucleus of the Uniform Billing Code of 1992; see **UB-92**. Its origin was in the case abstract developed by the **Professional Activity Study**.

data standards Standards (see **standard (norm)**) including methods, protocols, and terminologies for data, to allow disparate information systems to operate successfully with one another. For example, under the administrative simplification provisions of HIPAA, data standards for health information, issued by the Department of Health and Human Services, cover:

- Unique **identifier** numbers for individuals, employers, health plans, and healthcare providers
- Code sets for data elements of the **electronic transactions standards**
- **Security**, **electronic signatures**
- **Coordination of benefits**

Detailed information can be found at **aspe.os.dhhs.gov/admnsimp**. See also **Patient Medical Record Information**.

data structure See **data record**.

data warehouse A computer-based data repository used for storing integrated data in such a way that querying and analysis is more efficient than if the same data were kept in a simple database. Data are extracted from one or more sources as they are generated or updated, and then may be transformed and "cleaned up" before being stored in the data warehouse. The data warehouse makes data more readily available for answering management questions about the organization and its activities.

In the hospital, transactions such as patient billing, collecting insurance payments, giving services to patients, purchasing, and others are going on continuously, and access to this flowing stream of data "online" in order to obtain management information is awkward and costly. An "offline" data warehouse system:

1. takes periodic (daily, weekly, monthly) "snapshots" of the computer records coming from these transactions,
2. retains only the data elements of each transaction that are needed for management information (to reduce the bulk of the data and speed the access to it),
3. formats the data in such a fashion that the data from different sources can be handled by the computer as though they were from a single source,
4. stores the data with an eye to ease of access, and
5. provides tools (computer systems) by which the data can be interrogated.

A data warehouse would probably be classified as a "value-added" component of a data system, because it stores and transfers data. The resulting database (or set of relational databases) may be within the hospital or off-site, if the data warehouse operation serves a number of hospitals. A multihospital data warehouse not only may offer economies of scale, but also offers a unique opportunity for exchange of information—governed, of course, by strict security measures for the preservation of confidentiality as to patients, physicians, and institutions. Synonym: data repository. See related terms **data mart**, **knowledgebase**, and **database management system**.

Daubert test A standard for determining the admissibility of expert testimony in court. The judge, serving as "gatekeeper," must determine whether the evidence is both relevant and reliable before it is offered to the jury. To be relevant, the evidence must assist the jury in determining a material fact at issue in the trial. To be reliable, the expert opinion must be based on sound scientific theory or technique. The judge should consider at least:

1. Whether the theory or technique has been scientifically tested.
2. Whether it has been subjected to peer review or publication.

3. The known or potential error rate of the technique used.
4. The existence and maintenance of standards controlling the technique's operation.
5. Whether there is widespread acceptance of the theory or technique in the relevant scientific community.

This test was first stated in *Daubert v. Merrell Dow Pharmaceuticals, Inc.*, 509 U.S. 579 (1993). In that case, the U.S. Supreme Court was interpreting Rule 702 of the Federal Rules of Evidence, so the ruling applies to federal cases only. However, the test has been applied by courts in a number of states, and has influenced decisions in others. There are also many variations of the test.

The *Daubert* case notably overturned the standard established in 1923 in *Frye v. United States*, 293 F. 1013 (D.C. Circuit 1923). In *Frye*, expert testimony was permitted if based on a theory or method that was "generally accepted" in the scientific community. The *Daubert* test more readily permits new or novel theories and methodologies (note that there does not have to be widespread acceptance), but it generally subjects expert testimony to greater scrutiny than under the old standard. See also *gatekeeping history*.

DAW Dispense as written. See *generic equivalent*.

day Typically, a day is an overnight stay in the hospital or other facility (but see also *day patient*). The term is used in hospital statistics and claims for payment.

adjusted inpatient service days See *inpatient day equivalents*, below.

bed day See *inpatient service day*, below.

charity care day An inpatient service day for which the hospital makes no charge. See also *charity care*.

inpatient day equivalents The total number of inpatient service days, plus the volume of outpatient services expressed as (converted to) an estimate of inpatient service days. This computation has to use some sort of relative value unit (RVU) approach to convert outpatient services into inpatient service days. Synonym: adjusted inpatient service days.

inpatient service day A day of inpatient care; one person in the hospital one day is one inpatient service day. An inpatient day requires an overnight stay in the facility. Usually the day of admission is counted as a day but the day of discharge is not. Synonyms: bed day, patient day. See also *patient days* (under "P").

partial hospitalization day The services provided to a partial hospitalization patient in one twenty-four-hour period.

patient day See *inpatient service day*, above; see also the separate listing for *patient days* under "P."

resident day The services provided to one resident in a long-term care institution during one twenty-four-hour period.

day care Care, provided by an institution, that does not include an overnight stay; patients reside at night at home or in some other facility.

adult day care Care, provided during the day, that will permit a patient to function in the home. The care may include a wide range of services—medical, social, nutritional, psychological, and the like.

child day care Care provided for children. Child day care does not usually provide care for sick children.

day healthcare services See *adult day health services*.

day patient An *outpatient*. The term is typically used for those outpatients who spend some time at the facility (for example, coming in every weekday for therapy; a *day care* patient) or for ambulatory surgery patients, who come in for treatment in the morning and leave later in the day, without staying overnight. See also *day* and *inpatient*.

DC Doctor of Chiropractic; see *chiropractor*. Also *defined contribution*.

DCGs See *diagnostic cost groups*.

DD See *developmental disability* under *disability*.

DDC See *Developmental Disabilities Certified* under *developmental disabilities nursing*.

DDS Doctor of Dental Surgery (or Science). See *dentist*.

DEA See *Drug Enforcement Administration*.

deal breaker An issue arising, during negotiations toward an agreement, that is absolutely unacceptable to one of the parties. For example, permitting or prohibiting abortions in a facility may prevent a merger between hospitals with different philosophies.

DEA number The number assigned by the federal government indicating that an individual (a physician, a pharmacist, a hospital, a pharmacy, or some other qualified "business activity") registered with the Drug Enforcement Administration (DEA) is authorized to dispense or prescribe *controlled substances*. The former agency with this authority was the Bureau of Narcotics and Dangerous Drugs (BNDD); the DEA number formerly was known as the BNDD number.

death The cessation of life. Until recent years, death meant the cessation of respiration and circulation; however, with mechanical respirators and other medical devices, life as previously defined may be continued indefinitely. A new definition of death therefore became necessary so that decisions to terminate life support systems and to remove organs for transplant could be made appropriately. Thus death is defined in most states, for most purposes, as either the irreversible cessation of circulatory and respiratory function, or brain death (absence of all measurable or identifiable electrical or other brain functioning for more than twenty-four hours). See *Uniform Determination of Death Act*.

cause of death For statistical purposes, this typically means the single "underlying" condition that caused the death, as stated on the official death certificate. It may also mean, however, the "immediate" cause of death, which is the last event or condition that resulted in the death. The U.S. National Center for Health Statistics, which regularly reports the leading causes of death in the United States, uses the *International Classification of Disease, Ninth Revision, Clinical Modification* (ICD-9-CM) for defining the underlying conditions used in its reports. Similar reporting is done on a worldwide scale by the World Health Organization (WHO), which uses compatible rules for classifying the causes of death.

fetal death The death of a baby before birth.

infant death Death within the first year of life (after birth).

maternal death In public health (vital) statistical usage, a death of a pregnant woman or of a woman within a specified time period after delivery (the time period ranges from forty-two days, as defined by the World Health Organization, to one year in some jurisdictions). Maternal deaths are sometimes classified as direct (due to some element of the pregnancy, labor, or immediate recovery period), indirect (due to some disease not related to obstetric causes but aggravated by the pregnancy), and as nonmaternal (for example, from unrelated accidents). See also *maternal death rate* under *death rate*.

death certificate The official record of a person's death. State law governs the death certificate's content, which includes the deceased person's name, age, sex, and the date, time, and cause of death. State law also specifies the person (for example, a physician, coroner, or medical examiner) who is authorized to sign a death certificate. The certificate is filed with the registrar (vital records) for the local unit of government, who in turn files a copy with the state office of vital statistics.

death rate The number of deaths divided by the number of patients at risk. The death rate is usually multiplied by 100, so as to be expressed as a percentage. One death in 100 patients undergoing gallbladder removal (cholecystectomy), for example, would be expressed as a "cholecystectomy death rate of 1%." A death rate may be calculated for any group of patients (for example, all patients, for the hospital overall death rate; or newborns, for the hospital newborn death rate). For rare events, the death rate may use a different base, for example, per 10,000, and will be expressed not as a percentage, but as "per 10,000." Synonym: mortality rate.

disease-specific death rate The number of deaths attributed to a given disease in a specified population, expressed as a proportion. This rate is more likely given per 100,000 than as a percentage. Synonym: disease-specific mortality rate.

fetal death rate The number of fetal deaths (deaths of babies before birth) as a proportion of total births, with total births defined as live births plus fetal deaths. The rate is usually expressed per 1,000 total births. When computed in a hospital, it should be called the "hospital fetal death rate" and refer only to births in the hospital. Synonyms: fetal mortality rate, stillbirth rate.

   hospital fetal death rate The number of fetal deaths in the hospital (deaths of babies before birth) as a proportion of total births in the hospital for the same time period, with total births defined as live births plus fetal deaths. The rate is usually expressed per 1,000 total births.

hospital death rate The number of deaths in the hospital as a proportion of the number of discharges, both alive and by death, during the same time period. Newborn deaths are excluded from the numerator and babies born in the hospital are excluded from the denominator. The figure is usually given as a percentage (per 100). Synonym: hospital mortality rate.

hospital obstetric death rate The more accurate term for *hospital maternal death rate* (under *maternal death rate*, below).

infant death rate The number of infant deaths (deaths of children under one year old) in a given time period as a proportion of the number of live births in the same population in the same time period. It is usually expressed per 1,000. Synonym: infant mortality rate.

maternal death rate A vital statistic (a public health rather than hospital statistic; see *hospital maternal death rate*, below). For the computation, the number of "maternal deaths" (see *maternal death*, under *death*) is the numerator, and the number of live births during the same time period (as a proxy for pregnant women) is the denominator. Because maternal deaths are relatively rare, the rate is usually expressed per 1,000 or per 100,000 live births. Synonym: maternal mortality rate.

   hospital maternal death rate A bad label for a statistic computed in hospitals as the number of deaths of maternity patients in a hospital in a given time period, as a proportion of the number of maternity patients discharged from the hospital alive or by death during the same time period.

   The hospital maternal death rate should not be confused with the public health term "maternal death rate," which pertains to all deaths of pregnant women and women within a specified time period after delivery from whatever cause, and which uses live births as the denominator. A maternal death rate thus defined cannot be calculated from hospital data for a number of reasons; for example, hospital data do not have information about what happens to patients after discharge, nor would a hospital record as a "maternal death" the death of a pregnant woman if pregnancy were incidental to the patient's cause of hospitalization.

   What is called here the "hospital maternal death rate" should be called the "hospital obstetric death rate."

neonatal death rate A vital statistic (a public health rather than hospital statistic; see *hospital neonatal death rate*, below), calculated with the number of deaths within the first twenty-eight days of life (the "neonatal" period) as the numerator and the number of live births in the same period, usually a year, as the denominator. It is usually expressed per 1,000 live births. Synonym: neonatal mortality rate.

   hospital neonatal death rate The number of newborn deaths in the first twenty-eight days of life occurring in the hospital in a given period of time, as a proportion of the number of newborns discharged during that time period, both alive and by death. This rate is usually given as a percentage (per 100).

   The hospital neonatal death rate cannot be compared to the public health neonatal death rate because the hospital counts only those deaths that occur before the newborn is discharged; a baby may leave the hospital before it is twenty-eight days old, and yet still die within the twenty-eight days. The hospital has no way to count those neonatal deaths. Synonym: hospital neonatal mortality rate.

perinatal death rate In vital (public health) statistics from developed countries, the numerator for computing this rate is deaths of fetuses after twenty-eight weeks of gestation plus deaths within the first week after delivery; the denominator is these same deaths plus live births. For less developed countries, the denominator of the formula is different in that only live births are used in the denominator, on the basis that these countries do not keep adequate records of the late fetal deaths. This difference in definitions makes comparisons between the health conditions in the two types of areas invalid. The rate is usually expressed per 1,000. Synonym: perinatal mortality rate.

> **hospital perinatal death rate** A statistic that can be calculated from hospital data, with the numerator being deaths in the hospital of fetuses after the twenty-eighth week of gestation plus those dying in the hospital within one week after delivery, and the denominator being these same deaths plus live births in the hospital in the same time period. The rate is usually expressed as per 1,000. As with the hospital neonatal death rate (see discussion above), the hospital has no way to count those newborns who leave the hospital before they are one week old, yet die within that week. Synonym: hospital perinatal mortality rate.

total death rate The number of deaths, of all ages, in a given population in a specified time period as a proportion of the population. The rate is usually expressed as per 1,000. Synonym: total mortality rate.

death spiral The practice of steeply raising premiums for health insurance as the beneficiary becomes sicker and incurs increasing healthcare costs. This eventually makes the insurance unaffordable, and the beneficiary loses coverage just when it is most needed.

death with dignity A movement supporting an individual's right to be allowed to die without the use of "heroic measures" (see *extraordinary treatment* under *treatment*). The meaning has more recently expanded from passive to active death; see *Oregon Death with Dignity Act*. See also *right to die*.

debenture A bond or long-term loan (more than one year) that is not secured by a mortgage on specific property.

debt An obligation (duty) to pay, whether in cash, services, or goods.

long-term debt Debt that does not have to be paid within one year.

short-term debt Debt to be paid within one year.

debt ratio See under *ratio*.

Decade of Health Information Technology (DHIT) See *Strategic Framework*.

decedent affairs office (DAO) A centralized service in a hospital (sometimes within a pathology department) that is established to help the family of a deceased patient make decisions about autopsy and organ and other anatomy donation on the basis of valid information, and to assist in obtaining autopsies and organ donations.

Decentralized Hospital Computer Program (DHCP) The predecessor to *VistA*.

decentralized services Services that are carried out from several locations in an effort to improve efficiency, reduce cost, or both. A given type of service is usually under a single management division in an institution although, when decentralized, it may be under several managements.

decision rule See *clinical prediction rule*.

decision-support software (DSS) A special class of computer software designed to make relevant knowledge accessible to decision makers. In health care, DSS falls into three classes, depending on who is the intended decision maker:

> **Reference DSS** For physicians and other professionals, there are indexing tools that significantly improve access to published literature and the information it contains. Literature is typically organized around diseases, injuries, and procedures rather than the

problems presented by patients, so these tools facilitate the traditional practice of medicine in which the professional is the authority and the patient is the passive recipient of care. They may also cite probabilities for various diagnoses and the success of various treatments for the *typical*, rather than *specific*, patient.

Lay education DSS For consumers, there is a fast-growing array of popular software and there are numerous informal networks on the Internet.

Guidance DSS For joint use by the professional caregiver and the patient, there is DSS that presents the current information from the literature in a manner understandable by both professionals and laypersons. The goal of this software is the elimination of knowledge asymmetry between the two. It reduces the necessity for the professional to rely on memorized information, ensures completeness of knowledge, and provides guidance for shared decision making (SDM) and truly informed consent. Synonyms: decision-support system, computer decision support software. See also *clinical decision support system*.

decoding The process of translating a code (usually a number) back into the term that the code represents. With many coding systems used in health care, which are really category coding systems, the original term is not retrievable because the categories of the classification are designed to hold groups of similar things (see *category*). For example, in category coding, hospitals are coded as being under "church" or some other "control." When all one knows about a hospital is this code, all that can be retrieved about a given church hospital by decoding is the fact that it is a church hospital; whether the church is Catholic or Methodist cannot be determined by decoding from the category coding. See *coding (process)*.

decrypt See *cryptography*.

deductible The amount of money an insured person must pay "at the front end" before the insurer will pay. In automobile collision insurance with a $100 deductible, the insured must pay any damage under $100 in its entirety, and the first $100 when the total is over that amount. The reason for introducing this concept into healthcare coverage is primarily to discourage "unnecessary" use of services, and also to reduce insurance premiums, because all claims have a minimum amount that the insurer will be spared on every claim. Health plans have developed two other types of "front end" payments; see *coinsurance* and *copayment*.

DEEDS See *Data Elements for Emergency Department Systems* under *data set*.

deep pockets An individual or institution that has a lot of money. The phrase is frequently used in the context of deciding whom a plaintiff is going to sue for some perceived wrongdoing. Lawyers typically advise their clients that even if they are "legally" right (likely to win), it still only makes economic sense to sue someone who can pay the judgment. This, for instance, frequently accounts for why employers are sued when it is clear that the employee is responsible for the wrongdoing. Favorite deep pockets include insurance companies and large corporations.

Another factor involved is that deep pockets are perceived to be in a better position to pay than others, and juries are more likely to make the deep pockets pay just because they can, especially in cases where serious harm has occurred, and none of the parties involved seems particularly blameworthy. This phenomenon can be so powerful that some jurisdictions forbid any testimony about ability to pay to reach the jury. Contrast with *judgment proof*. See also *malpractice crisis*.

defamation The publication of a statement that injures the reputation of another. "Publication" means that the statement is communicated to a third person (someone other than the "defamer" and the "defamed"); if no one else hears or reads the statement, it is not defamation. Written defamation is called "libel"; oral defamation is "slander." Both libel and slander are torts for which the defamer may face liability.

Some kinds of statements are considered defamatory "per se" (by themselves); that is, if the plaintiff (person defamed) can prove the words were spoken or written to a third party, she does not have to prove actual injury. Criticizing another's professional knowledge, expertise, or performance is defamatory per se. Thus, if one physician criticizes the performance of another, the critical physician may be liable for defamation. That physician may be protected, however, in one of two ways: (1) truth is always a defense to a defamation action (in other words, a statement is not defamatory if it is true); and (2) there are now a number of laws granting immunity (legal protection from suit) to physicians evaluating quality of care who act in good faith (without malice or bad motive).

defendant The person (or organization) against whom a lawsuit is brought. Commonly, the defendant in a lawsuit is the alleged wrongdoer who has injured the plaintiff (the person bringing the suit).

Defense Advanced Research Projects Agency (DARPA) An agency of the U.S. Department of Defense established in the 1960s, staffed by computer programmers and electronics engineers, to redesign how computers were operated. They developed interactive computing to replace (for some purposes) the previous method in which punch cards provided input to the computer, and printouts on paper the output. These were replaced in interactive computing with a keyboard (and now mice and other devices) for input and a cathode ray tube screen (and now other devices) for output. The human could then interact directly with the computer, and almost immediately the computer became a communication device as well as a data processing and computing device.

DARPA developed the first computer network, ARPANET, so that its scientists could operate various computers in its system remotely. ARPANET quickly became a vehicle for communication among people, and was part of the foundation on which the Internet was built from 1969 through 1990. Sometimes referred to as ARPA. **www.darpa.mil**

defensive medicine The obtaining of services, mainly diagnostic procedures, in anticipation of defending against a possible lawsuit by the person treated alleging malpractice. The primary reasons for obtaining the services are to avoid having to defend against a contention that omission of a test was negligent medical care, and to show the jury in a malpractice trial documented evidence that other possibilities were "ruled out" by the tests.

Ordinarily, diagnostic tests are obtained because the physician honestly needs the information they provide. In defensive medicine, however, the tests have little or no medical value. For example, a physician may be quite satisfied that a sprained ankle is just that; nevertheless, because of the threat of a malpractice suit, the physician may still obtain an x-ray in order to have evidence that he or she did not overlook a fracture.

deferred compensation A method of paying in the future for services provided today. Typically, an amount of money is put aside by an employer into a trust and not taxed to the employee until the employee actually receives the money, perhaps five or ten years later (or at retirement). The deferred compensation arrangement has been blended into a patent-pending process to solve the problem of compensation for physicians who take emergency room (ER) call (see **on call**). In this process, called the "Call Pay Solution," the hospital funds a "Rabbi trust" (so called because the first ruling of the IRS on this arrangement involved a rabbi and his synagogue) and the physician can direct how it is to be invested. However, the arrangement is subject to a personal services agreement, and the physician may forfeit the money if he or she fails in his or her part of the bargain. Some hospitals have included in their personal services agreements forfeiture for not taking ER call, dropping out of Medicare or Medicaid, refusing to treat charity cases, and so forth. The concept uses the tax deferral provisions of Section 457(f) of the Internal Revenue Code. It was developed by MaxWorth Consulting Group, LLC, in Charlotte, North Carolina.

defibrillation Stopping the fibrillation (a certain type of abnormal contractions) of the heart muscle and restoring the normal heartbeat. The procedure usually is carried out by the use of an electrical shock.

defibrillator An electrical system for correcting disturbances of the rhythm of the heart by sending electrical shocks to the heart, a process called cardioversion. It does not treat an underlying heart condition.

external defibrillator A defibrillator operated by placing electrical contacts on the skin of the patient's chest.

> **automated external defibrillator (AED)** A portable, self-contained device for use in an emergency cardiac arrest. "Paddle" electrodes are placed on the patient's chest. These are connected to a box containing a computer that "reads" the patient's heart condition as detected by the electrodes and sends strong electric shocks to the paddles. AEDs are extremely easy to operate, with clear, simple, legible directions on the case. Efforts are being made to provide AEDs (costing about $3,000 each) in airplanes, auditoriums, ambulances, public buildings, police and other emergency vehicles, physicians' offices, and even in the home. AEDs first appeared around 1995.

implantable cardioverter-defibrillator (ICD) An internal defibrillator with a tiny computer that continuously monitors the heart rate and rhythm and, when a disruption of the rhythm is sensed, "instantly" sends a corrective impulse (shock) back down the lead to restore normal rhythm. Similar to a *pacemaker* system, an ICD has three parts. Two are inside the body: a small metal case containing the defibrillator itself, which is implanted under the skin, and an insulated wire ("lead") connecting the defibrillator to the heart. The third part is external, the programmer, a special computer that communicates wirelessly with the defibrillator, and is used by the physician periodically to make sure the battery is properly charged, to monitor the stored information about the patient's heart rhythm and any disturbances that may have occurred, and to give the defibrillator necessary instructions. The ICD is used most often to correct abnormally fast heart rates, but some are dual function devices that can also serve as pacemakers, correcting rates that are abnormally slow. ICDs have been in use since about 1985.

Deficit Reduction Act of 2005 (DRA) A federal law to reduce spending, which included major changes to the Medicaid program. For the first time, states can charge premiums to Medicaid beneficiaries, and the cost-sharing amounts can be increased. States are permitted to offer benefit packages other than that previously mandated by CMS. As of July 1, 2006, new Medicaid applicants, and current beneficiaries at redetermination, have to document their U.S. citizenship. One provision of the act, called the **Family Opportunity Act (FOA)**, allows families with disabled children to "buy in" to the Medicaid program for their children if the family income is less than 300% of the federal poverty level. Another provision calls for a demonstration program for a **Health Opportunity Account (HOA)** to pay for medical services, similar to a Health Savings Account (HSA). The DRA required healthcare organizations that receive at least $5 million a year from Medicaid to educate all employees and officers on how to detect fraud, waste, and abuse. The act also included changes to the Medicaid long-term care policies, provider reimbursement, and other provisions. Pub. L. No. 109-171, 120 Stat. 4 (2006).

defined benefit A type of health insurance in which specific benefits are promised (defined). If the benefits are held constant, and the costs of health care increase, of course the premium will also increase. Employers are increasingly offering *defined contribution* plans, instead, in order to stabilize costs.

defined care A model of healthcare financing that gives the consumer direct decision-making power over what health plan, benefits, and/or services she or he will purchase, using dollars allocated by his or her employer. The term encompasses a wide variety of arrangements; see, for example, *cafeteria plan* and *defined contribution*.

defined contribution (DC) A type of health insurance in which the purchaser of the insurance (e.g., an employer) agrees to spend a specific (defined) amount (contribution) for the insurance. Under such a plan, if the costs of health care increase, and the contribution is held constant, the benefits purchased will decrease. Defined contribution plans enable an employer to predict its health insurance costs. Such plans are often coupled with arrangements under which the employee is given a choice among insurance products, can decide which product best meets his or her needs, and can supplement the employer's contribution in order to buy the insurance he or she wants. See also **defined benefit**.

definitive care A level of therapeutic intervention capable of providing comprehensive healthcare services for a specific condition.

degree program in nursing A nursing education program operated by an educational institution that confers a degree (usually, Bachelor of Science in Nursing (BSN)) upon successful completion. The term is sometimes used in connection with a program that confers an associate degree (AD). A degree program is contrasted with a diploma program, which is conducted by a hospital that confers a diploma rather than a degree.

de-identification Removing elements from healthcare data so as to render it anonymous (i.e., no longer person-identifiable). The HIPAA **Privacy Rule** contains a "safe harbor" provision that states **health information** may be considered "de-identified" if all of the following elements have been removed:

1. Names
2. All geographic subdivisions smaller than a state, including street address, city, county, precinct, ZIP code, and their equivalent geocodes, except for the initial three digits of a ZIP code if, according to the current publicly available data from the Bureau of the Census: (1) the geographic unit formed by combining all ZIP codes with the same three initial digits contains more than 20,000 people; and (2) the initial three digits of a ZIP code for all such geographic units containing 20,000 or fewer people is changed to 000
3. All elements of dates (except year) for dates directly related to an individual, including birth date, admission date, discharge date, date of death, and all ages over eighty-nine and all elements of dates (including year) indicative of such age, except that such ages and elements may be aggregated into a single category of age ninety or older
4. Telephone numbers
5. Fax numbers
6. Electronic mail addresses
7. Social Security numbers
8. Medical record numbers
9. Health plan beneficiary numbers
10. Account numbers
11. Certificate/license numbers
12. Vehicle identifiers and serial numbers, including license plate numbers
13. Device identifiers and serial numbers
14. Web universal resource locators (URLs)
15. Internet Protocol (IP) address numbers
16. Biometric identifiers, including finger and voice prints
17. Full face photographic images and any comparable images
18. Any other unique identifying number, characteristic, or code

In addition to the above specifics, the Privacy Rule requires that one "does not have actual knowledge that the information could be used alone or in combination with other information to identify an individual who is the subject of the information." This means that even if the eighteen specifically defined elements were removed, if there is a way the remaining information can be used to identify an individual, then the information is not considered de-identified. Synonym: anonymization. 45 C.F.R. § 164.514(b)(2) (October 1, 2006).

deinstitutionalization The discharge of mental patients from mental institutions, with continued care to be provided in the community. This movement was made possible by the development of psychotropic drugs, which modify a patient's behavior to such an extent that she or he is considered able to function within the community.

delegated practice See under **practice (action)**.

delivery room A room equipped for giving care to the obstetric patient during delivery, and for first care to the newborn infant.

Delta Society An organization that studies the health benefits of animals for humans and promotes and provides training for *animal-assisted activities* and *animal-assisted therapy*. **www.deltasociety.org**

demand management An emerging strategy in managed care for influencing the demands placed on healthcare providers by consumers. The intent is to lower consumer demand for health care, with the result of fewer healthcare services required and a lower cost. One method used is to provide consumers with more information about health problems, allowing them to make decisions that waste fewer healthcare resources. See also *health promotion*.

demarketing Efforts to persuade individuals not to buy, or to go elsewhere. A hospital has a serious problem when the price set for a given DRG under the prospective payment system (PPS) is lower than the lowest cost the hospital can achieve for care for a patient with that DRG and still maintain quality. Under those circumstances, the hospital may elect to discontinue caring for such patients (for example, pediatrics). Alternatively, it may develop some more subtle strategy to discourage patients with a problem that falls into the DRG from coming to that hospital, or to discourage physicians from bringing such patients. The latter efforts have been labeled "demarketing."

democratization A process of putting more decision making into the hands of the individual. A system of health care in which persons collaborate in the decisions about their health and health care is a democratized system.

demographic data The class of information about a person that includes such items as age, sex, race, income, marital status, and education. Demographic data are important for proper patient care, and are also used as the data with which to compile certain statistics (demographics) on a population, for example, in the study of the distribution of certain types of injuries and illnesses.

demographics Descriptions of patient populations or service area populations in such terms as age, sex, race, educational level, income, family size, and ethnic background.

dental assistant A health professional who assists a dentist in patient care, and may perform other functions in the dental office or laboratory. Most dental assistants complete a training program in a community college or technical school; some are trained on the job.

　　Certified Dental Assistant (CDA) A dental assistant who has met the requirements of the Dental Assisting National Board (DANB). The DANB also offers the credentials Certified Orthodontic Assistant (COA) and Certified Dental Practice Management Administrator (CDPMA). **www.danb.org**

　　Registered Dental Assistant (RDA) A dental assistant who has met the requirements of the American Medical Technologists (AMT). **www.amt1.com**

dental hygienist A health professional who cleans teeth, takes x-rays, does prophylactic procedures, teaches oral health, and, in some states, may administer anesthetics, fill cavities, remove sutures, and so forth. Must have an associate or bachelor's degree in dental hygiene, pass a national examination administered by the American Dental Association (**www.ada .org**), and be licensed by the state.

　　Registered Dental Hygienist (RDH) A state-licensed dental hygienist.

dental laboratory technician A health professional who makes dental prostheses, dentures, orthodontic devices, crowns, and other items according to a dentist's prescription. Most complete at least a two-year program in dental technology, although some are trained on the job. Synonym: dental technician.

　　Certified Dental Technician (CDT) A dental laboratory technician who has become certified by the National Board for Certification in Dental Laboratory Technology (NBCDLT) (**www.nadl.org**). A CDT may specialize in one or more areas: complete dentures, partial dentures, crown and bridge, ceramics, or orthodontics.

dental technician See *dental laboratory technician*.

dentist A person whose profession is the care of the teeth and surrounding tissues. A dentist requires a state license. The degree held by the practitioner is Doctor of Dental Surgery (or Science) (DDS) or Doctor of Dental Medicine (DDM).

dentistry The healing art concerned with the diagnosis and treatment of diseases of the mouth, teeth, and associated structures, and with the restoration of function. Synonym: odontology.

Dent v. West Virginia A U.S. Supreme Court landmark case (1888) applying medical licensure requirements (educational and knowledge) equally on all applicants.

deoxyribonucleic acid (DNA) See *DNA*.

department A term with two major meanings in the hospital. When the term "department" is used without a modifier, in some contexts it is impossible to tell which of the two following meanings is intended:

clinical department A division of the medical staff according to clinical specialty, such as surgery, specialties of surgery, internal medicine, specialties of internal medicine, obstetrics and gynecology, pediatrics, and the like. In some hospitals, clinical departments are called services; for example, the surgical service may mean the same thing as the surgical department. In other hospitals, a service may be a subdivision of a department; for example, in a given hospital the orthopaedics service may be a part of the larger department of surgery.

hospital department A major organizational unit of the hospital, such as the nursing service, the pharmacy, housekeeping, dietary, and the like. The medical staff, which in some respects functions as a department, is not classified as one. On the other hand, the radiology department and the emergency department, although both employ members of the medical staff, are both termed hospital departments. Sometimes called hospital service instead of department.

Department of Agriculture (USDA) The department of the executive branch of the federal government in charge of a variety of programs dealing with the environment, food production, and natural resource use and preservation. In addition to the foregoing, the USDA is somewhat unique among the federal agencies in that it is also charged with the mission of coordinating federal assistance to rural America through its Rural Development (RD) agency. Specific health-related agencies within the USDA include the Animal and Plant Health Inspection Service (APHIS), Center for Nutrition Policy and Promotion (CNPP), Food and Nutrition Service (FNS), and Food Safety and Inspection Service (FSIS). **www.usda.gov**

Department of Commerce (DOC) The department of the executive branch of the federal government in charge of the business and economic sector. It also is responsible for such other issues as weather reports and the census, and includes the National Technical Information Service (NTIS). **www.commerce.gov**

Department of Defense (DoD) The department of the executive branch of the federal government in charge of the military and national defense. **www.defenselink.mil**

Department of Education (ED) The department of the executive branch of the federal government in charge of educational policy. The ED was derived from the Department of Health, Education, and Welfare (DHEW). **www.ed.gov**

Department of Energy (DOE) The department of the executive branch of the federal government in charge of energy policy. Its mission is to advance the national, economic, and energy security of the United States by promoting scientific and technological innovation, and to ensure the environmental cleanup of the national nuclear weapons complex. **www.energy.gov**

Office of Science (OS) A division of the Department of Energy (DOE) that includes the Office of Advanced Scientific Computing Research and the Office of Biological and Environmental Research. One of its projects is *Genomics:GTL*. **www.er.doe.gov**

Department of Health and Human Services (HHS) The department of the executive branch of the federal government responsible for the federal health programs in the civilian sector. Sometimes referred to as DHHS. **www.hhs.gov**

The following agencies are under the direction of the *Office of the Secretary of Health and Human Services (OS)*:

Administration for Children and Families (ACF)
Administration on Aging (AOA)
Agency for Healthcare Research and Quality (AHRQ)
Agency for Toxic Substances and Disease Registry (ATSDR)
Centers for Disease Control and Prevention (CDC)
Centers for Medicare and Medicaid Services (CMS)
Food and Drug Administration (FDA)
Health Resources and Services Administration (HRSA)
Indian Health Service (IHS)
National Institutes of Health (NIH)
Substance Abuse and Mental Health Services Administration (SAMHSA)

Department of Health, Education, and Welfare (DHEW) The antecedent of the Department of Health and Human Services (HHS) in the executive branch of the federal government. HHS was formed when the separate Department of Education was established. DHEW was sometimes referred to as HEW. It replaced the Federal Security Agency in 1953.

Department of Homeland Security (DHS) The department of the executive branch of the federal government responsible for protecting the United States against terrorist attacks and other hazards. Among its many components are the Federal Emergency Management Agency (FEMA), Coast Guard, Citizenship and Immigration Services (CIS), Customs and Border Protection (CBP), and Secret Service. **www.dhs.gov**

Department of Justice (DOJ) The department of the executive branch of the federal government that enforces certain federal laws, such as antitrust laws. The Department of Justice is headed by the U.S. Attorney General. **www.usdoj.gov**

Department of Labor (DOL) The department of the executive branch of the federal government in charge of administering federal employer/employee policies and regulations. It has a number of programs concerning health issues, including education of consumers and employers on health plans. **www.dol.gov**

Department of Transportation (DOT) The department in the executive branch of the federal government concerned with transportation. Formed in 1967, the DOT consists of a number of organizations including, among others, the Federal Aviation Administration (FAA), Federal Highway Administration, and National Highway Traffic Safety Administration (NHTSA). **www.dot.gov**

Department of Veterans Affairs (VA) The federal agency responsible for administering healthcare programs and facilities (and other benefits) for U.S. military veterans and their families. Up until 1989 it was called the Veterans Administration. See also *CHAMPVA* and *VistA*. **www.va.gov**

dependent practitioner (DP) See under *allied health professional*.

deposition During a lawsuit but outside of the courtroom, the questioning under oath of a party or witness by the attorney for the adverse party, with attorneys for both sides and a court reporter (stenographer) present. Although the deposition is used to obtain information for trial, part or all of it may itself be admissible (allowed as evidence) at the trial. The term "deposition" may refer either to the actual questioning or to the written record produced by the court reporter.

depreciation A technique used in accounting to recognize the fact that certain kinds of property (assets), such as equipment, depreciate (lose their value) over time; assets may wear out or be made obsolete by new inventions, materials, or techniques. Depreciated property must be replaced with the same or more modern equipment, or be abandoned as items no longer needed. Money must be spent on replacement, and a variety of accounting techniques have been developed to determine how much to allow for this purpose each year for each item.

Simply stated, the allowance is equal to the initial cost (or sometimes the future replacement cost) divided by the estimated life of the property. The total allowance for depreciation is shown on the balance sheet as a deduction from the initial value of the assets. This allowance may be "funded," that is, actually set aside in a savings account from which to draw to pay for replacement, or may be "unfunded," in which case no savings account is set up, and the organization must find the money elsewhere when it is needed. In either case, however, the depreciation entry is the same.

dermatologist A physician specializing in diagnosis and treatment of disorders of the skin.

dermatology The study of the skin and its disorders.

deselection A euphemism for "getting rid of." The term is being used, for example, when a physician is not kept as a member of a managed care organization. Such deselection may occur because the care provided by that physician is regarded as too costly by the organization, or because the outcome of the care is not considered satisfactory as determined from the physician's profile.

designated record set (DRS) Under the *Privacy Rule*, the "container" for an individual's *protected health information (PHI)*, which that individual has the right to access and amend if necessary. The following text is the entire definition, taken from Part 160 (General Administrative Requirements) of the final rule:

Designated record set means:

(1) A group of records maintained by or for a covered entity that is:

   (i) The medical records and billing records about individuals maintained by or for a covered health care provider;

   (ii) The enrollment, payment, claims adjudication, and case or medical management record systems maintained by or for a health plan; or

   (iii) Used, in whole or in part, by or for the covered entity to make decisions about individuals.

(2) For purposes of this paragraph, the term record means any item, collection, or grouping of information that includes protected health information and is maintained, collected, used, or disseminated by or for a covered entity. (45 C.F.R. § 164.501 (October 1, 2006))

It is clear that more than the traditional medical record is involved here. Also, there is no limitation about where the records are kept, or what media they are stored on (paper or digital, for instance). What the DRS does not include are the administrative and operational records kept by the covered entity on its own behalf. Presumably a patient cannot inspect a hospital's utility bills or phone records, for instance. Also specifically excluded from the DRS as part of the "health care operations" category are the covered entity's quality improvement, peer review, fraud and abuse detection, compliance, and credentialing activities, as well as a number of others specifically mentioned. On the other hand, the inclusion of an individual's billing records in the DRS, as well as the rather catchall "records . . . used . . . to make decisions about" them, appears to significantly broaden the scope of information that will be made available to individuals. The Privacy Rule, however, does not specify when, where, or how the DRS should be made available to an individual requesting access.

Designated Standard Maintenance Organization (DSMO) A type of organization established as a result of the final HIPAA rule entitled "Standards for Electronic Transactions," which provides that the Secretary of the Department of Health and Human Services (HHS) may designate as DSMOs those organizations that agree to maintain the standards adopted by the Secretary. It also establishes criteria for the processes to be used in such maintenance. Several data content committees (DCCs) and standard setting organizations (SSOs) have agreed to maintain those standards designated as national standards in the final rule. These include:

Accredited Standards Committee (ASC) X12 (ASC X12N)

Health Level Seven (HL7)

National Council for Prescription Drug Programs (NCPDP)
National Uniform Billing Committee (NUBC)
National Uniform Claim Committee (NUCC)
Dental Content Committee of the American Dental Association
See also *standards development organization*.

desmoteric Prison-associated, of or pertaining to the prison. Similar to "nosocomial," meaning hospital-associated.

detailing The process by which pharmaceutical sales representatives promote drugs to doctors in one-on-one meetings. This involves giving the physician information about the drug, samples, and in some instances, gifts and other perks. See also *e-detailing*.

development See *fund-raising*.

developmental disabilities nursing The area of nursing serving the needs of individuals who have a *developmental disability* (see under *disability*).

Certified Developmental Disabilities Nurse (CDDN) A specialist in developmental disabilities nursing who has passed an examination of the Developmental Disabilities Nurses Association (DDNA). **www.ddna.org**

Developmental Disabilities Certified (DDC) A credential available to qualified licensed practical or vocational nurses who pass an examination of the Developmental Disabilities Nurses Association (DDNA). **www.ddna.org**

developmental disability (DD) See under *disability*.

device See *medical device*.

DGME See *direct graduate medical education* under *medical education*, under *education*.

DHCP See *Decentralized Hospital Computer Program*.

DHEW See *Department of Health, Education, and Welfare*.

DHHS See *Department of Health and Human Services*.

DHIT Decade of Health Information Technology. See *Strategic Framework*.

DHR Digital health record; see *electronic medical record* under *electronic health record*.

DHS See *Department of Homeland Security*.

diabetes A condition in which too much glucose (sugar) builds up in the blood. This can result in body cells not receiving enough energy and, over time, cause damage to the eyes, kidneys, nerves, and heart.

type 1 diabetes (insulin-dependent diabetes) A disease in which the beta cells in the pancreas are damaged and cannot produce insulin, the hormone that helps cells take in glucose. Insulin shots are necessary to provide the missing hormone. Formerly called juvenile diabetes, although it is not limited to children.

type 2 diabetes A disease in which the pancreas does not produce enough insulin (the hormone that helps cells take in glucose) or the cells are not taking in glucose despite the insulin. This is the most common form of diabetes, and can usually be controlled with diet, exercise, and weight management.

diabetes educator A health professional with advanced education and training in the needs of people with diabetes, and who has acquired skills for passing on essential information to patients, their families, and the public.

Certified Diabetes Educator (CDE) A multidisciplinary credential for health professionals, offered by the National Certification Board for Diabetes Education (NCBDE). **www.ncbde.org**

diabetes management Health care focused on the needs of individuals with diabetes. Nurses, dietitians, pharmacists, and other health professionals may be involved.

Advanced Diabetes Management Certification (ADM) A credential jointly sponsored by the American Association of Diabetes Educators (AADE) (**www.aadenet.org**) and the American Nurses Credentialing Center (ANCC) (**nursingworld.org/ancc**). It is available to registered nurses, registered dietitians, and registered pharmacists with graduate degrees. Those who qualify and pass the examination receive the appropriate credential: nurse practitioners and clinical nurse specialists are designated **APRN,BC-ADM** (Advanced Practice Registered Nurse, Board Certified—Advanced Diabetes Management); dietitians are awarded **RD,BC-ADM** (Registered Dietitian, Board Certified—Advanced Diabetes Management); pharmacists are designated **RPh,BC-ADM** (Registered Pharmacist, Board Certified—Advanced Diabetes Management).

diabetes nursing The area of nursing concerned with the needs of individuals with diabetes and their families. See also diabetes management.

diabetic A person who has been diagnosed as having diabetes.

diagnose To apply a series of procedures for examining and gathering data about a patient in order to make a diagnosis.

diagnosis (Dx) In medicine, a diagnosis traditionally is a term, usually given by a physician, to the **symptoms** (disturbances of appearance or function or sensation of which the patient is or could be aware), **signs** (departures from the normal appearance or function of the patient, of which the patient may be unaware, but which may be detected by the physician or another observer), and **findings** (items of information about a patient elicited by laboratory, x-ray, or other diagnostic procedure, or by observation of the patient) that, taken together, explain an observed or detected condition of a patient. Examples are "diabetes," "fracture of the femur," "alcoholism," "lead poisoning," "avian influenza," "influenzal pneumonia," "[specified] chromosomal abnormality," or even "no disease."

The *International Classification of Diseases, Ninth Revision, Clinical Modification* (ICD-9-CM) is used in the United States for coding diagnoses, and all the terms that make up the category headings of the classification (as contrasted with the actual diagnostic terms that are listed as included under each heading) are often referred to as diagnoses, even though they are outside the traditional definition. ICD-9-CM contains, for example, a chapter called "External Causes of Injury and Poisoning" including causes such as "poisoning by barbiturate." "External causes" reflects the public health origin of the basic International Classification of Diseases (ICD) (from the World Health Organization (WHO)), because such information is a valid "axis" of a classification aimed at prevention.

Chapter XXI of the Tenth Revision of the *International Statistical Classification of Diseases and Health Related Problems* (ICD-10) added a chapter, "Factors Influencing Health Status and Contact with Health Services," which offers as diagnoses such conditions as "stressful work schedule" and "need for immunization against leishmaniasis." Thus, today a broad usage obtains for the term "diagnosis." Apparently, if it's in the book, it must be a diagnosis.

Note that a given diagnosis may essentially dictate therapy, but that a therapy is never a diagnosis. The terms "diagnosis" and "therapy" are often used improperly. For example, "hysterectomy" (removal of the uterus), although sometimes called a "diagnosis," is never a diagnosis, but rather a surgical procedure (therapy) done for a wide range of diagnoses, including tumors, infections, and other disorders.

The term "diagnosis" may be modified by a term indicating the way the physician arrived at the diagnosis. For example, a "laboratory diagnosis" is one established by the laboratory findings, a "clinical diagnosis" is one established by the patient's signs and symptoms, and a "physical diagnosis" is one established by physical examination of the patient.

See also *nursing diagnosis*.

admitting diagnosis The diagnosis provided by the physician at the time of the patient's admission to the hospital. At least one admitting diagnosis, that primarily responsible for the hospitalization, is expected. Although as much precision as possible is desired of the physician at the time of admission, the physician must not be required to be more exact than his clinical database justifies; complying with a rigid demand for a "codable diagnosis" at this time may, in fact, start the patient on an inappropriate course of treatment. Often the diagnosis recorded at the time of admission must be vague, because one of the functions of the hospitalization may be to add to the physician's information on the patient (for example, through observation by the nursing staff and others, diagnostic procedures, and response to treatment). As a result, the discharge diagnosis, benefiting as it does from these data sources, is often quite different from the admitting diagnosis.

One of the physician's first decisions regarding a patient is whether hospitalization is needed; if the decision is "yes," details on why hospitalization is necessary are often in part developed in the course of the care.

codable diagnosis A diagnosis for which a category has been provided in a given classification (scheme). As ordinarily used, however, the term means a diagnosis expressed in terminology that permits a coder to find it in the appropriate code book and affix its numeric code. In North America at this time, coding of hospital diagnoses is category coding (see under *coding (process)*) to the *International Classification of Disease, Ninth Revision, Clinical Modification* (ICD-9-CM).

Virtually all discharge diagnoses (see *discharge diagnosis*, below) likely to be used, except new terms, will be found in the ICD-9-CM; thus they are "codable" (actually "classifiable"). (With the use of "wastebasket categories"—for example, "Other diseases of the nervous system"—*all* diagnoses can be placed somewhere, although often improperly.)

Admitting diagnoses (see above) may necessarily at times be uncodable except to the most inexact categories; the patient's condition may be so vague as to defy terms that fit into the more specific categories of the classification, or they may be stated as "problems," many of which, due to the origin and purpose of the ICD-9-CM, cannot be accommodated. The *International Statistical Classification of Diseases and Related Health Problems* (ICD-10) has a new chapter (actually an expansion of an earlier "supplementary classification") entitled "Factors Influencing Health Status and Contact with Health Services" that will accommodate many more such "problems."

differential diagnosis A list, created by a physician early in the diagnostic process, of all the diagnoses that should be considered as explanations for the problems presented by a patient, and thus should be the subjects of investigation prior to a final decision. Similar to a *rule out list*, also created by a physician, but with the "flavor" that a given diagnosis is already seen as most likely, but that, just to be on the safe side, those other diagnoses on the list should be "proven" not to obtain.

discharge diagnosis A diagnosis supplied by the *attending physician* (see under *physician*) at the time of the discharge of the patient from the hospital. This diagnosis has the benefit of the clinical database developed up to the time of discharge, and is more accurate and also more exact than the *admitting diagnosis* (see above). The discharge diagnosis is likely to be the *principal diagnosis* (see below), but secondary diagnoses (see below) should also be recorded as appropriate. In virtually every case, the discharge diagnosis is a *codable diagnosis* (see above).

major diagnosis A term sometimes used to designate the diagnosis that is most responsible for the length of a given stay or the resource consumption (services provided) for a given patient's care. See also *principal diagnosis* (below).

possible diagnosis A diagnosis that, in the physician's opinion, must be considered as a possible cause of the patient's symptoms under the circumstances. See *rule out list*.

primary diagnosis A diagnosis (condition) that is an underlying cause for other diagnoses or symptoms. For example, diabetes would be the primary diagnosis for a patient with a diabetic ulcer of the skin or diabetic gangrene.

principal diagnosis A term defined in the *prospective payment system (PPS)* as "the condition established after study to be chiefly responsible for occasioning the admission of the patient to the hospital." Note that the term is specific to the cause of hospitalization; it may or may not be the *primary diagnosis* (see above) for which the patient is under care. For example, a patient with diabetes (the primary diagnosis) may be hospitalized because of a skin ulcer that needs hospital care, so the principal diagnosis would be the ulcer. The principal diagnosis is also not necessarily the reason for admission; see *admitting diagnosis* (above).

secondary diagnosis A diagnosis other than the principal diagnosis (patients often have more than one diagnosis). In the prospective payment system (PPS), the secondary diagnoses to be recorded are presumed to be those that affect the treatment rendered or the length of stay (LOS). Usual clinical practice, however, is to record in the medical record the complete array of diagnoses, including those that have no bearing on a given hospitalization. In the PPS, all diagnoses are given only as *International Classification of Diseases, Ninth Revision, Clinical Modification* (ICD-9-CM) codes (see *code (data)*).

suspected diagnosis A diagnosis that seems to the physician to be likely, but for which, at the time of suspicion, there is insufficient proof. Some of the usual signs, symptoms, or findings may not yet be present, or the patient may present evidence that is in conflict with that for the diagnosis suspected.

Diagnosis Related Group (DRG) See *DRG*.

diagnostic Done for the purpose of assisting in the making of a diagnosis.

Diagnostic and Statistical Manual of Mental Disorders, Fourth Edition See *DSM-IV*.

diagnostic cost groups (DCGs) A family of risk adjustment methods developed at Boston University and Harvard under contract from HCFA (now CMS) to be used in the Medicare program known as Medicare+Choice. The groups use clinical information, mainly the diagnoses as stated in ICD-9-CM codes, from claims to categorize patients according to their expected annual health expenditures. DCGs are not to be confused with *DRGs*, which use procedures, discharge status, and age, in addition to diagnoses, in the classification process, and were created for a different purpose.

diagnostic medical sonographer (DMS) A health professional who uses sonography to create images that are used by physicians for making medical diagnoses.

Advanced Practice Sonographer (APS) A diagnostic medical sonographer with advanced training, experience, and accomplishment. This credential is offered as a membership category of the Society of Diagnostic Medical Sonography (SDMS) (**www.sdms.org**). See also *ultrasound practitioner*.

Registered Cardiac Sonographer (RCS) A diagnostic medical sonographer who has met the certification requirements in sonography of Cardiovascular Credentialing International (CCI). **www.cci-online.org**

Registered Diagnostic Cardiac Sonographer (RDCS) A diagnostic medical sonographer who specializes in using sonography to observe the anatomy and hemodynamics (blood flow) of the heart, its valves, and related blood vessels, and has met the requirements of the American Registry of Diagnostic Medical Sonography (ARDMS) (**www.ardms.org**). Specialty areas for RDCSs include adult, pediatric, and fetal echocardiography.

Registered Diagnostic Medical Sonographer (RDMS) A diagnostic medical sonographer who has met the requirements for this credential awarded by the American Registry of Diagnostic Medical Sonography (ARDMS) (**www.ardms.org**). There are several specialty areas for RDMSs: abdomen, breast, neurosonology, obstetrics and gynecology, and fetal echocardiography.

Registered Physician in Vascular Interpretation (RPVI) A physician who has met the requirements for this credential awarded by the American Registry of Diagnostic Medical Sonography (ARDMS) (**www.ardms.org**). The RPVI is skilled in interpreting the vascular ultrasound images and physiologic tests required for making diagnoses in vascular disease.

Registered Technologist—Breast Sonography (RT(BS)) A *Registered Technologist (RT)* (see under *radiologic technologist*) with advanced qualifications in breast sonography from the American Registry of Radiologic Technologists (ARRT). **www.arrt.org**

Registered Technologist—Sonography (RT(S)) A *Registered Technologist (RT)* (see under *radiologic technologist*) with primary certification in sonography from the American

Registry of Radiologic Technologists (ARRT) (**www.arrt.org**). Advanced qualification certification is also available.

Registered Technologist—Vascular Sonography (RT(VS)) A *Registered Technologist (RT)* (see under *radiologic technologist*) with advanced qualifications in vascular sonography from the American Registry of Radiologic Technologists (ARRT). **www.arrt.org**

Registered Vascular Technologist (RVT) A diagnostic medical sonographer who specializes in using sonography to observe the hemodynamics (blood flow) of peripheral and abdominal blood vessels, and has met the requirements of the American Registry of Diagnostic Medical Sonography (ARDMS). **www.ardms.org**

diagnostic product A chemical or other material used in diagnostic testing.

diagnostic screens Batteries of diagnostic tests. See *screening (diagnostic)*.

diagnostic services Services aimed at determining the nature and cause of the patient's problem, rather than providing treatment. Diagnostic services include laboratory, x-ray, special testing such as stress testing, and the like.

dialysis Selective filtering of chemicals in a solution through a membrane, such as the wall of a tube made of special material.

hemodialysis A renal dialysis technique in which blood (hemo-) is passed through a tube made of a special material that permits some of the contents of the blood, such as certain waste products, to pass through the walls of the tubing and be removed from the blood. Other contents of the blood, which cannot pass through the tubing walls, are retained and returned to the body.

home hemodialysis The carrying out of hemodialysis in the home. Ordinarily, patients and their families are not trained in, nor is the home equipped for, this procedure except in cases of long-term illness such as end stage renal disease (ESRD).

peritoneal dialysis A renal dialysis technique that involves introducing a fluid into the person's abdomen (peritoneal cavity) where the waste materials pass from the body into the fluid, which is then removed. Peritoneal dialysis may be done either in an institution or on an ambulatory basis.

renal dialysis Removal by an artificial method of the waste materials that would be removed by the kidneys in a normally functioning individual. It is used for patients with kidney ("renal") failure. The techniques involve either hemodialysis or peritoneal dialysis. Renal dialysis may be used for long periods of time, in the hospital, in dialysis centers, and in the home. It is often a temporary measure preceding a kidney transplant. Renal dialysis is one of the costliest elements of the end stage renal disease (ESRD) program, a component of Medicare.

dialysis nursing The nursing specialty involving the care of dialysis patients, including performing dialysis procedures. See also *hemodialysis technician* and *nephrology nursing*.

Certified Dialysis Nurse (CDN) A dialysis nursing specialist who has passed an examination of the Nephrology Nursing Certification Commission (NNCC). **www.nncc-exam.org**

Certified Hemodialysis Nurse (CHN) A dialysis nursing specialist who has passed an examination in hemodialysis of the Board of Nephrology Examiners Nursing & Technology (BONENT). **www.bonent.org**

Certified Peritoneal Dialysis Nurse (CPDN) A dialysis nursing specialist who has passed an examination in peritoneal dialysis of the Board of Nephrology Examiners Nursing & Technology (BONENT). **www.bonent.org**

dialysis unit See *hemodialysis unit*.

DICOM Digital Imaging and Communications in Medicine. A standard for the transmission of medical images and other medical information. In development since 1985 by the American College of Radiology (ACR) in conjunction with the National Electrical Manufacturers Association (NEMA), this standard is designed so that all of the programs and hardware that conform to it will communicate accurately with each other. This standard is of particular importance in radiology due to the variety of digital imaging technologies in use, including

CT scanners, MRI, ultrasound, and nuclear medicine. The standard includes the definition of a "header" that is sent with the actual images that provides the necessary context for the image, such as how the image was made. DICOM is an open standard. **www.rsna.org**

diener A person who maintains a morgue and who assists in autopsies. See also *pathologist's assistant*.

diet Food and drink consumed by an individual. A particular set of nutrients may be prescribed for therapeutic purposes; see *medical nutrition therapy*.

modified diet A diet other than the regular (or "house") diet; one that is tailored to the individual's nutritional needs in terms of calories, food elements, or other factors.

special diet A scheme of food, drink, and nutrients designed to achieve a particular purpose, either under conventional medicine (this is more accurately called a modified diet) or some alternative theory of health and disease.

dietary assessment See under *nutrition assessment*.

dietary risk factors Eating patterns that increase the likelihood for developing disease or other adverse health effects. Examples are: eating a percentage of fat calories above 30% of total food calories increases one's risk for death from heart disease; being significantly overweight (obesity) is linked to heart disease, cancer, and diabetes; lack of adequate fluid intake puts many elderly persons at risk of dehydration.

dietary service See *food service*.

dietetics The science dealing with the relationships of foods and nutrition to human health (see also *nutrition* and *nutrition assessment*). Most states have laws regulating people working in this field, but the requirements for qualifications and restrictions on practice vary widely; see *health professional*. The titles of practitioners will vary as well; see *dietetic technician*, *dietitian*, and *nutritionist*.

dietetic technician (DT) A health professional who provides nutrition services. See also *dietitian*.

Dietetic Technician, Registered (DTR) A dietetic technician who has completed at least an associate degree, a dietetic technician program, and met other requirements of the Commission on Dietetic Registration (CDR). **www.cdrnet.org**

dietitian A health professional specializing in dietetics who assists the public in the modification and/or enhancement of its food-related behaviors. See also *dietetics*, *nutritionist*.

clinical dietitian A dietitian specializing in disease/nutrition relationships.

consulting dietitian A dietitian who works with food services, agencies, clinics, industry, and the general public on a fee-for-service basis. Synonym: consultant dietitian.

licensed dietitian A dietitian who is licensed by the state. Not all states require dietitians to be licensed.

Registered Dietitian (RD) A dietitian who has at least a bachelor's degree in food-related science and has met certain requirements of the Commission on Dietetic Registration (CDR). **www.cdrnet.org**

Board Certified Specialist in Gerontological Nutrition (CSG) A Registered Dietitian with practice experience who has passed a certification examination in gerontological nutrition given by the Commission on Dietetic Registration (CDR). **www.cdrnet.org**

Board Certified Specialist in Pediatric Nutrition (CSP) A Registered Dietitian with practice experience who has passed a certification examination in pediatric nutrition given by the Commission on Dietetic Registration (CDR). **www.cdrnet.org**

Board Certified Specialist in Renal Nutrition (CSR) A Registered Dietitian with practice experience who has passed a certification examination in renal nutrition given by the Commission on Dietetic Registration (CDR). **www.cdrnet.org**

Board Certified Specialist in Sports Dietetics (CSSD) A Registered Dietitian with practice experience who has passed a certification examination in sports dietetics given by the Commission on Dietetic Registration (CDR). **www.cdrnet.org**

Fellow of the American Dietetic Association (FADA) A Registered Dietitian who has at least eight years of work experience plus a master's or doctoral degree and who has met other requirements of the Commission on Dietetic Registration (CDR) (**www.cdrnet.org**). This credential is no longer offered.

differential diagnosis See under *diagnosis*.

digestion (genetics) The process of cutting DNA molecules using enzymes.

digital certificate Information issued by a certificate authority (CA) to another entity that includes that entity's public key and *electronic signature*. If read by a human, some of the information would resemble the following excerpts from an actual digital certificate: "1e:50:cf:82:d0:27:fc:a2:86:f1" and "ZXR3b3JraW5nMSkwJwYDVQQLE." Other information, including the identity of the CA, a serial number, and a time frame during which the certificate is valid, is represented in human-readable form. A digital certificate is one of the components of a *public key infrastructure (PKI)*, and is specifically designed to help prove an entity's electronic identity, thereby meeting the requirements of *authentication* and *nonrepudiation*.

digital health record (DHR) See *electronic medical record* under *electronic health record*.

Digital Imaging and Communications in Medicine (DICOM) See *DICOM*.

digital signature See *electronic signature*.

Dipl. Short for *diplomate*.

Dipl. A.B.T. See *Diplomate in Asian Bodywork Therapy* under *Asian bodywork therapy*, under *bodywork therapy*.

Dipl. Ac. See *Diplomate in Acupuncture* under *acupuncturist*.

Dipl. C.H. See *Diplomate of Chinese Herbology* under *herbologist*.

Dipl. O.M. See *Diplomate in Oriental Medicine* under *Oriental medicine*.

diploma program in nursing A nursing education program operated by a hospital school of nursing, which confers a diploma in nursing, rather than a degree. A degree in nursing is only awarded upon completion of a nursing program conducted by an educational institution.

diplomate A recipient of a diploma, which is a kind of certificate.

direct care provider An individual who is responsible for the care of an individual, as contrasted with a "consultant" who is responsible only for giving an opinion. However, the consultant may take over the care of the patient and become the direct care provider.

direct contract See under *contract*.

directive See *advance directive*.

director (governance) A member of the *governing body* when the official term for that body is "board of directors." When the governing body is called the "board of trustees," its members are individually "trustees."

director (management) An operating officer. The title "director" is used by many institutions for their officers and executives. The chief executive officer (CEO) may be called *the* director, and various subordinates may carry titles such as "director of development," "director of nursing," and the like.

director of buildings and grounds See *administrative engineer*.

director of education An individual responsible for arranging and coordinating employee training (on-the-job and continuing), employee orientation, and, in some circumstances, community health education programs and patient education programs. The director of education is not responsible for continuing medical education; that person is the director of medical education (DME). Synonym: in-service education coordinator.

director of medical affairs (DMA) The person designated by the governing body to be responsible for management of the medical staff and for carrying out policy for the medical staff as promulgated by the board. Ordinarily the DMA is a physician, and may be nominated by the medical staff. A physician with this title is ordinarily paid. This term is discussed further under *chief of staff*.

director of medical education (DME) The individual, ordinarily a physician, who is responsible for administering the educational program for physicians in training in the hospital. The actual training is provided by the clinical departments, for example, surgery, medicine, and so forth. However, the coordination of programs for both continuing and graduate medical education, such as collecting and giving primary review to applications for training, handling personnel matters for trainees (such as scheduling vacations), arranging conferences, and the like, is done by the DME. The DME may be either a physician or an educator.

director of nursing See *nursing service administrator*.

director of staff development A title often given to the individual responsible for *in-service training* of hospital employees (see under *training*).

director of volunteers A hospital employee who administers the hospital's volunteer services department.

Directors' and Officers' (D&O) See *Directors' and Officers' (D&O) insurance* under *insurance*.

direct provider agreement (DPA) See *direct contract* under *contract*.

direct-to-consumer (DTC) Advertising aimed at promoting healthcare goods and services directly to consumers, instead of to the providers of those goods and services. An example of DTC is a pharmaceutical manufacturer advertising the prescription drug Viagra on network television. The manufacturer aims the ad at consumers (patients), which encourages them to seek a prescription for this drug from their physicians. This differs from the more traditional manufacturer's promotion of the drug to physicians and other providers, who in turn then suggest and prescribe it for their patients.

disability The absence or loss of physical, mental, or emotional function and, sometimes, earning ability. May be temporary or permanent, total or partial. "Disability" will have a specific legal definition for a particular purpose; for example, Social Security or workers' compensation laws.

The *Americans with Disabilities Act (ADA)* defines disability as "(1) a physical or mental impairment that substantially limits one or more major life activities of an individual; (2) a record of such an impairment; or (3) being regarded as having such an impairment."

developmental disability (DD) A severe, chronic disability due to physical and/or mental impairment, which surfaces before the age of twenty-two and is likely to continue indefinitely.

disability examiner A health professional specially trained in evaluating individuals with disabilities, according to a specific set of rating guidelines. Sometimes called disability analyst.

Certified Disability Examiner (CDE) A disability examiner who has passed an examination of the Commission on Health Care Certification (CHCC). **www.cdec1.com**

disability management *Case management* for persons with short- or long-term disabilities.

Certified Disability Management Specialist (CDMS) A credential offered by the Certification of Disability Management Specialists Commission (CDMSC). **www.cdms.org**

Certified Professional in Disability Management (CPDM) A health professional who has completed a course of instruction in disability management offered by the Insurance Educational Association (IEA). **www.cpdm.org**

disaster A sudden natural or man-made event that causes extensive damage, destruction, or injury, and requires mobilization of emergency healthcare resources. Examples are fire, flood, earthquake, tornado, collapse of a building, nuclear accident, war, mine cave-in, or airplane crash.

mass disaster A disaster in which the local emergency medical services are overwhelmed or destroyed. See also *National Disaster Medical System*.

multicasualty accident A disaster that can be managed by local emergency medical services.

disaster drill A formal attempt to simulate a disaster as realistically as possible and to test as many elements as possible of a disaster preparedness plan under practice conditions. Such drills are carried out periodically by hospitals, communities, and other groups. The purposes of the disaster drill are to train personnel in execution of the plan and to discover flaws in the plan so that it can be improved.

Disaster Medical Assistance Team (DMAT) See under *National Disaster Medical System*.

disaster medicine Medical care organized to handle disasters.

Disaster Mortuary Operational Response Team (DMORT) See under *National Disaster Medical System*.

disaster plan See *disaster preparedness plan*.

Disaster Portable Morgue Unit (DPMU) See *Disaster Mortuary Operational Response Team* under *National Disaster Medical System*.

disaster preparedness plan A formal plan for coping with a disaster. An accredited hospital is expected to have both an external disaster plan and an internal disaster plan (see below). Often such plans have basic elements relating to any kind of disaster and dealing with such items as emergency communication, alerting of police and fire departments, mobilization of off-duty personnel, and the like. The basic plan also has supplements for various kinds of disasters; for example, a nuclear disaster would call for different procedures than a flood or a tornado. It is expected that the written plan will periodically be tested and modified on the basis of disaster drills. Synonym: disaster plan.

    external disaster plan A formal disaster preparedness plan for coping with a disaster in the community, or for which the hospital may be expected to provide healthcare services.

    internal disaster plan A formal disaster preparedness plan for coping with a disaster, such as a fire or hazardous materials, within the institution itself.

disbursement Paying money to take care of an expense or a debt.

discharge The formal release of a patient from a physician's care or from a hospital. (In Canada, a hospital discharge is called a "separation.") Sometimes called "signing out" the patient. A discharge terminates certain responsibilities on the part of the provider. There are several kinds of discharge:

    against medical advice (AMA) See *discharge against medical advice*, below.

    discharge against medical advice (discharge AMA) A type of discharge that occurs when the patient, contrary to the advice of the attending physician, refuses treatment and "signs herself out," thus releasing the hospital from liability for subsequent events.

    discharge by death A hospital discharge that occurs when a patient who has been admitted dies in the hospital. A patient who is "dead on arrival" cannot be a hospital discharge.

    discharge by transfer A discharge that occurs when the patient is transferred from one institution to another and responsibility for care is shifted to the receiving institution. Medicare has special rules for the payment to each of the two institutions for this kind of discharge.

    inpatient discharge The discharge of an inpatient (see *patient*) by release from the hospital. A special usage of this term occurs under Medicare, when transfer of the patient to another unit of the hospital for which Medicare does not provide benefits is also called an "inpatient discharge."

    outpatient discharge (OP discharge) The formal release of a patient receiving outpatient care; it occurs when the physician states that there is no need for the patient to return for more care.

discharge abstract See under *abstract*.

discharge abstract system See *hospital discharge abstract system*.

discharge coordinator See *discharge planner*.

discharge notice See *hospital-issued notice of non-coverage*.

discharge planner A person whose duties involve making arrangements so that patients who are being discharged have a place to go that is appropriate to their needs, with the necessary care available. These duties start early in hospitalization, so that discharge that is medically indicated will not be delayed because of the absence of needed medical or social resources. Synonym: discharge coordinator.

discharge planning The process of making sure that arrangements are made outside the hospital to receive the patient upon discharge and to provide the necessary continuity of care.

discharge summary A summary of the medical record, prepared at the end of hospitalization, giving the essentials of diagnosis, treatment, prognosis, and recommendations. Preparation of the discharge summary is the responsibility of the attending physician or dentist. A discharge summary must not be confused with a discharge abstract (see *abstract*), which is different in content, and the preparation of which is not the responsibility of the attending physician or dentist.

discipline A field of study, such as medicine or nursing.

disclosure See *release of information*.

discounting An adjustment made in the process of *cost-analysis* to account for the fact that current dollars are worth more than future dollars. For benefits that are likely to be realized only in the future, their dollar value is "discounted" by some annual factor (the amount of which is typically determined by rates of return on investments in the private sector).

discounting of accounts receivable See *pledging of accounts receivable*.

discoverable Information that may be legally obtained by a party to a lawsuit, from the adverse party. Not all such information is admissible during a trial, however; the rules concerning discoverable information are much broader than the rules of admissibility. Generally, information is discoverable if it may lead to admissible evidence.

discovery The process during a lawsuit, before trial, by which each party obtains information from the other party that may be used as evidence, or may lead to useful evidence, at the trial. Common methods of discovery include *interrogatories* (written questions), requests for documents, requests for admissions (see *admission (law)*), and *depositions* (verbal questions).

discovery period (insurance) The period of time after expiration of an insurance policy during which the beneficiary of the policy may report an event that occurred during the life of the policy.

discovery period (law) The period of time during the life of a lawsuit, after the suit is filed and prior to the trial, during which both parties may use discovery to find out as much as possible about the other side's case. There is a specific date, set by court rules and/or ordered by the judge, by which discovery must be completed.

discovery rule A provision in a state's *statute of limitations* that requires a plaintiff to file certain types of lawsuits within a specific period of time after she discovers (or should have discovered) her injury, rather than when her injury actually occurred.

disease An illness or disorder of the function of the body or of certain tissues, organs, or systems. Diseases differ from injuries in that injuries are the result of external physical or chemical agents.

    acute disease A disease that normally is of short duration—a rule of thumb is thirty days or less—and that ordinarily is confined to a single episode.

    chronic disease A disease that requires more than one episode of care, or is of long duration (more than thirty days, for example), or both.

disease management (DM) A philosophy of medical care under which the goal is to take care of the patient's entire continuum of needs for a specific disease, from the earliest possible moment for as long as the disease (or its threat) exists. Disease management pertains to chronic diseases, such as diabetes, asthma, chronic heart diseases, hypertension, Alzheimer's disease, cancer, and arthritis. Successful disease management reduces the disability from the disease, increases the quality of life of the patient, and is presumed to reduce the cost of care (although some fear that managed care organizations may exploit the cost containment potentials at the expense of quality of care).

    Ideally, disease management begins whenever it is suspected or known that an individual is a likely candidate for a given disease, even though the disease has not yet appeared. Such prior knowledge could come, for example, from genetic information, periodic health examination, family history, screening examinations, presence of risk factors, or possibility of exposure. In some instances, the warning information can result in care that prevents the development of active disease. In the absence of susceptibility information prior to symptoms, disease management begins with the first evidence of the disease itself. The care then is designed to minimize the effects of the disease and provide the best health for the individual. The disease management regimen includes encouragement of a suitable lifestyle, including essential medical evaluations and care, dietary assessment and advice, physical activity prescription, and other factors specific to the disease being managed and the values of the individual patient.

Disease management should be continuous (even if from different caregivers), and for this reason increasing attention is being given to a life-long medical record to replace the traditional episodic records (see *electronic health record*). Sometimes called disease state management (DSM).

Disease Management Association of America (DMAA) A nonprofit membership organization founded in 1999 dedicated to advancing population health improvement through *disease management*. www.dmaa.org

disease management organization (DMO) An organization that contracts with a health plan to provide coordination of care for all patients diagnosed with a specific disease through *disease management*. The DMO uses clinical practice guidelines and measures outcomes to ensure that patient care is of high quality, effective, and efficient.

Disease-Specific Care Certification (DSCC) A program of the Joint Commission on Accreditation of Healthcare Organizations (JCAHO) to evaluate disease management and chronic care services that are provided by health plans, disease management service companies, hospitals, and other care delivery settings. Certification is based on an assessment of compliance with relevant standards and criteria, the effective use of clinical guidelines, and measurement of outcomes.

disease staging See *staging (diseases)*.

disease state management (DSM) See *disease management*.

disincentive An undesirable "reward" for undesired behavior. For example, as part of efforts to reduce hospital and physician costs, patients are sometimes required to pay the first dollars for services; this payment may be a deductible, copayment, or coinsurance. The deductibles are a "disincentive" (a negative incentive) to seek the care, and thus an incentive to be frugal.

disintermediation The process of getting rid of the "middleman." The term came into use in the late 1990s, as the Internet began displacing traditional retailers—book sales is a good example. It is now being used in reference to "the traditional healthcare supply chain" as online pharmacies, information access, and so forth reduce the need for intermediaries between consumers and services. The trend toward greater consumer power in health care—see *healthcare consumerism*—is also contributing to disintermediation.

dispense See *drug dispensing*.

dispense as written (DAW) See *generic equivalent (drug)* and *drug dispensing*.

dispensing optician A health professional who fits eyeglasses upon the prescription of an optometrist or ophthalmologist. Dispensing opticians may learn their work on the job or as an apprentice, or through a formal one- or two-year program at a college or university. Many states require licensure.

Board Certified Dispensing Optician (ABOC) The credential ABOC shows that the dispensing optician has passed a national certification examination of the American Board of Opticianry. www.ncleabo.org

Board Certified Dispensing Optician—Advanced Certification (ABOC-AC) The credential ABOC-AC designates advanced certification obtained by a dispensing optician with several years of experience who has met the requirements of the American Board of Opticianry. www.ncleabo.org

Master in Ophthalmic Optics (ABOM) The credential ABOM denotes a dispensing optician who has written a technical thesis, passed an advanced examination, and met other requirements of the American Board of Opticianry. www.ncleabo.org

disproportionate share hospital (DSH) See under *hospital*.

dispute resolution See *alternative dispute resolution*.

disruptive innovation A new idea that "upsets" the status quo but in such a fashion that actual progress (e.g., better results or lower cost) is the end result.

disruptive physician A physician whose habitual behavior in the hospital, clinic, or other workplace is such that it interferes with patient care or the workflow of the institution. The doctor's disruptive behavior may upset the patient, family, colleagues, nurses, other health professionals, or administrators to the extent that the patient's response to treatment is affected or the function of the institution is impeded. The term may also be applied, unfairly (unless the behavior is also bad), to a physician who strongly disagrees with the hospital's policies or actions or other medical staff members in matters of patient care. The term is somewhat confusing because of the emergence of the term *disruptive innovation*, which uses "disruptive" in a positive, rather than negative, sense.

distance learning The use of telecommunications to make available and deliver educational content to anyone in the world who has been given access to the material. As telecommunications technology becomes more capable, distance learning is becoming increasingly interactive, with more frequent use of multimedia to convey knowledge. See also *e-learning* and *telehealth*.

distant healing Any method used for treatment of any medical condition that does not involve any type of physical contact with the patient. Includes, for example, prayer, mental healing, or spiritual healing. A review of published studies reported that approximately 57% of the randomized, placebo-controlled trials showed a positive treatment effect, and that therefore distant healing deserved further study.

distant site In the context of *telemedicine* services, the distant site is the place at the other end of the encounter from where the patient and/or the patient's physician is located (the *originating site*). Synonyms: hub site, specialty site, physician site, provider site, referral site.

distribution system In the hospital, a system for providing supplies such as linen, drugs, food, and equipment to patient care areas.

distributive justice Principles of *ethics (moral)* used to allocate resources that are in limited supply. The concept is extremely relevant to health care today, where costs continue to rise dramatically and not everyone has equal access to care, either physically or financially. There are many approaches—among the Western philosophies are egalitarianism (everyone gets an equal share), desert-based principles (those who deserve more get more), libertarianism (each person can have what they can legitimately get), the difference principle (those who are disadvantaged should get more), resource-based principles (people should not have to suffer for circumstances over which they have no control), and welfare-based principles (allocation should be made to best increase the welfare of the most people). See also *rationing*.

diver medic technician See *diving medical technician*.

diversification A term coming into use as hospitals enter lines of business other than care of the sick and injured in an effort to obtain revenue from a variety of sources and remain solvent. The hospital is typically restructured in the process of diversification, and foundations, holding companies, and the like may result. The new "businesses" may be other healthcare enterprises such as home care or neighborhood health centers; they may also be other activities, such as offering its collection or public relations services to other clients.

diversity action A lawsuit between citizens of different states. This is one basis of federal rather than state jurisdiction.

divestiture Getting rid of something, for example, to comply with a court order breaking up a monopoly. A corporate sale of a subsidiary corporation is said to be a divestiture.

divide and dump To separate high-risk from low-risk employees and "dump" (not insure) the high-risk employees.

divided standard of medical care See *standard of care (clinical)*.

dividend The distribution of the earnings of a company to its shareholders in proportion to the shares of stock held by each shareholder.

diving medical technician (DMT) A health professional trained as an undersea *First Responder* (see under *emergency medical technician*), with special training in *hyperbaric therapy*. Certification is available to qualified DMTs from the National Board of Diving and Hyperbaric Medical Technology (NBDHMT) (**www.nbdhmt.com**). Synonym: diver medic technician.

diving medicine See *undersea medicine*.

Division of Research Grants (DRG) The former name of the *Center for Scientific Review*; see under *National Institutes of Health*.

DLM(ASCP) See *Diplomate in Laboratory Management* under *clinical laboratory manager*.

DM See *disease management*.

DMA See *director of medical affairs*.

DMAA See *Disease Management Association of America*.

DMAT See *Disaster Medical Assistance Team* under *National Disaster Medical System*.

DMD Doctor of Dental Medicine, the professional degree held by some dentists. A minority of dental schools use this designation, which is the equivalent of DDS (Doctor of Dental Surgery (or Science)).

DME Direct medical education; see *direct graduate medical education* under *medical education*, under *education*. See also *director of medical education* and *durable medical equipment*.

DME MAC See *durable medical equipment* and *Medicare Administrative Contractor*. Formerly durable medical equipment regional carrier (DMERC).

DMEPOS Durable medical equipment, prosthetics, orthotics, and supplies.

DMERC See *durable medical equipment regional carrier*.

DMO See *disease management organization*.

DMORT See *Disaster Mortuary Operational Response Team* under *National Disaster Medical System*.

DMS See *diagnostic medical sonographer*.

DMT See *diving medical technician*.

DNA Deoxyribonucleic acid. The tightly coiled threads in the nucleus of a cell that contain the *genes*. The DNA molecule that carries genetic information consists of four chemicals called bases (adenine (A), thymine (T), guanine (G), and cytosine (C)) and a sugar-phosphate backbone, arranged in two connected threads to form a double helix. Each of the two connected threads is called a single strand.

anticodon A triplet sequence of ribonucleic acids (RNA) in transfer RNA that basepairs with its counterpart, a codon, in messenger RNA and thus receives the message carried by the codon.

base (genetics) Each of the four chemical units that, by their order in DNA molecules, control the genetic codes. The "bases" are the four amino acids: adenine (A), thymine (T), guanine (G), and cytosine (C).

base pair Two nucleotide bases on different strands of the DNA molecule that bond together. The bases can be paired only as follows:

Base pair 1: adenine with thymine (AT or TA)
Base pair 2: guanine with cytosine (GC or CG)

When used as a verb, it is written as "basepair" and means the act of joining together the different strands.

codon A sequence of three adjacent nucleotides that will identify a specific amino acid.

proteome All the proteins being made according to the instructions carried by the transcriptome.

purine The larger kind of base found in DNA, consisting of adenine (A) and guanine (G).

pyrimidine The smaller kind of base found in DNA, consisting of cytosine (C) and thymine (T).

recombinant DNA (rDNA) DNA formed by combining DNA from different types of organisms; a hybrid DNA.

ribonucleic acid (RNA) A chemical similar to DNA that functions primarily to carry genetic information from DNA to protein. RNA, like DNA, also contains adenine (A), thymine (T), guanine (G), and cytosine (C).

> **messenger ribonucleic acid (mRNA)** A specific type of RNA that carries messages to transfer RNA in the chemical process known as protein synthesis by using codons that have corresponding anticodons in the transfer RNA.

> **transfer ribonucleic acid (tRNA)** A specific type of RNA that receives messages from messenger RNA in the chemical process known as protein synthesis by using anticodons that have corresponding codons in the messenger RNA.

transcriptome The body of messenger ribonucleic acid (mRNA) being produced by a cell at any given time.

DNAR Do not attempt resuscitation. See *do not resuscitate*.

DNR See *do not resuscitate*.

DNSc Doctor of Nursing Science.

DO Doctor of Osteopathic Medicine. The degree awarded to an individual upon graduation from a school of osteopathic medicine. See *physician* and *osteopathy* (under *medicine (system)*). Note that "OD" refers to an optometrist, not to an osteopath.

DOC See *Department of Commerce*.

doc-in-a-box A slang term for any one of a growing variety of ambulatory care facilities: storefront physician's offices or clinics, walk-in outpatient facilities, or specialized offices for foot care, dietary advice, and the like. The term is less likely to be used for ambulatory surgical centers, sports medicine centers, and other similar facilities with more formal structure, and which offer continuity of care.

doctorate An advanced postgraduate academic degree, higher than the master's degree level.

Doctor Death A reference to Dr. Jack Kevorkian, the physician whose name is synonymous with "assisted suicide." Dr. Kevorkian publicized and used his "suicide machine" to assist seriously ill patients in committing suicide. Dr. Kevorkian chose to practice in Michigan because as of 1992 assisted suicide was not a crime in Michigan. In 1992, Michigan made assisting suicide a felony. In 1999, Dr. Kevorkian was convicted of second-degree murder in the poisoning of a 52-year-old man with Lou Gehrig's disease and sent to prison for a ten- to twenty-five-year term; he was paroled in June 2007. See *assisted suicide* under *suicide*.

doctor of medicine (MD) See *MD*.

doctor of osteopathic medicine (DO) See *DO*.

doctor-patient relationship A legal term for the relationship between a patient and healthcare provider that gives rise to legal obligations, including such issues as the standard of care and privileged communications. Such a relationship is usually a prerequisite for a dissatisfied patient to make a successful malpractice claim against the provider.

The details on when such a relationship arises and the obligations of the parties involved are governed by a number of sources, including the laws of the state concerned and previous court cases, as well as any agreement between the particular parties. Note that such a relationship may come into being even in situations where there was no express contract between the parties. For example, a routine preemployment physical may or may not create a legal doctor-patient relationship. Synonym: physician-patient relationship. See also *duty (legal)*.

doctor shopping The process of visiting more than one physician in order to obtain multiple prescriptions of the same drug during the same time period, usually of controlled substances. Sometimes used by drug addicts to get more than the medical dosage; the extra drugs are used or resold. In most places, it is illegal to obtain a prescription by misrepresentation, deception, or subterfuge—hence doctor shopping is usually a crime.

Doctor's Office Quality Project See *DOQ*.

doctor's order See *order (physician)*.

DoD See *Department of Defense*.

DOE See *Department of Energy*.

DOJ See *Department of Justice*.

DOL See *Department of Labor*.

dominant See *allele*.

DON Director of Nursing.

donated services The estimated monetary value of the services rendered by personnel who receive no monetary compensation or only partial monetary compensation for their services. The term is applied to services rendered by members of religious orders, societies, volunteers, and similar groups. Synonym: "in-kind" services.

donations In the context of Medicaid financing, donations are money that is "voluntarily" donated to the state government by hospitals and other health providers who receive payments from Medicaid. The money is used by the state for matching with the federal government Medicaid funds. On the average, nearly 60% of a state's Medicaid costs are picked up by the federal matching money, but in some states, the federal share is 80%. In states with 80% matching, $1 from the state draws $4 from the federal level, and thus $1 of donation from a hospital, for example, will bring the hospital back $5. In some states, a special tax is levied on providers, hospitals, and others, rather than asking for or permitting the voluntary donations. Both the donation programs and the special tax programs have been under scrutiny, and criticized as "scams." CMS has been working to regulate these practices.

donor (biological) The source, human or animal, of biological material, blood, organs, or tissues for transplantation to or implantation in a patient. The donor is labeled by the type of material for which he or she serves as a source:

blood donor A person who permits the removal of her blood for transfusion or other medical use.

professional blood donor A blood donor who is paid for the blood she donates to a blood bank. Professional blood donors are likely to be individuals with low incomes and economic levels, and who present a greater hazard with respect to the transmission of disease (such as hepatitis or AIDS) than voluntary blood donors who, generally speaking, come from a higher socioeconomic level, are generally healthier, and are less likely to carry the diseases transmissible by transfusion.

replacement blood donor A blood donor who gives her blood with the stipulation that it be used to replace the blood transfused to a specific individual. A blood bank typically levies charges for (1) the services it renders in processing, storing, and distributing blood; and (2) for the blood itself, with the understanding that for each unit of blood obtained on behalf of a given patient, the patient's charge for the blood itself will be offset one-for-one (one replacement unit would offset one unit transfused and its charge).

universal donor An individual whose blood type is O, Rh negative, and therefore may usually donate blood for anyone in the other ABO blood groups. Additional tests must be done, however, to ensure compatibility.

voluntary blood donor A blood donor who is not paid for her blood donated to a blood bank for transfusion or other use. A replacement blood donor is typically a voluntary blood donor.

organ donor An individual whose organ(s) are used for transplantation to an individual needing those organs. The organ donor may himself donate the organ, for example, in the case of a kidney, or the donation may be made by the donor's survivors. At other times, the donation may be made on the basis of a prior agreement by the donor that his organs will be available after death; often such an agreement is obtained at the time of driver's license renewals and recorded on the individual's driver's license. See also *United Network for Organ Sharing*.

tissue donor A person who donates a body tissue, other than blood or an entire organ, for transplantation into another human. A bone marrow donor would be a tissue donor, as would a donor from whom bone was obtained.

donor (financial) A person or organization that provides a gift of money or other item of value, such as equipment or property, to an institution.

do not attempt resuscitation (DNAR) See *do not resuscitate*.

do not code See *do not resuscitate*.

do not resuscitate (DNR) An order by the physician, with respect to a specific patient, to the effect that, should cardiac arrest or respiratory arrest occur, no attempt should be made to give cardiopulmonary resuscitation (CPR) to the patient (restart the heart or otherwise revive her). "Do not resuscitate" is sometimes translated into the jargon that the patient is "not to be coded," or "do not code this patient"; this means that a code blue signal should not be issued. A suggestion has been made that the term "do not resuscitate" be changed to "do not attempt resuscitation (DNAR)."

A DNR order may be issued for one or more of three reasons: (1) no medical benefit, (2) poor quality of life predicted after CPR, or (3) poor quality of life before CPR. Such an order also may be issued because a competent adult patient has asked not to be resuscitated. There is controversy about the circumstances under which a DNR order may be issued for an incompetent patient. The conservative approach is to obtain the consent of the patient's legal representative for any DNR order; however, some believe that no consent is required where there is no medical benefit, because CPR would not be medically indicated under these circumstances. (For example, consent is not required to "not perform" an appendectomy, if an appendectomy is not medically indicated.) Synonyms: not to be coded, do not code, no-code order, order not to resuscitate (ONTR), do not attempt resuscitation (DNAR).

Do Not Use List A list of abbreviations, acronyms, and symbols that should never be used by healthcare professionals because there is too much danger of confusion and error. For example, do not use "MS" because it could mean either morphine sulfate or magnesium sulfate. Instead, write out the full words. The list is published by the Joint Commission on Accreditation of Healthcare Organizations (JCAHO).

donut hole See *doughnut hole*.

DOQ Doctor's Office Quality Project, a project of CMS to develop a method to measure and improve the quality of care for chronic disease and preventive services in the physician's office.

DOQ-IT Doctor's Office Quality—Information Technology, a project of CMS to support the use of information technology and the electronic medical record (EMR) in small- and medium-sized physicians' offices to improve quality and safety for Medicare beneficiaries and "all Americans." DOQ-IT promotes the availability of high-quality, affordable technology and provides assistance to doctors' offices in implementing and using it.

dose The amount of medication or radiation to be given a patient at one time.

dosimetry The measurement of doses. See also *medical dosimetrist*.

DOT See *Department of Transportation*.

doughnut hole A gap in Medicare Part D prescription drug coverage. The standard benefit package includes a $250 deductible and a 25% copayment for the $2,000 beyond the deductible. When total prescription costs exceed $2,250 in a year, the beneficiary must pay 100% of drug costs out-of-pocket. This period is called the gap or "doughnut hole." Once total drug costs reach $5,100, the Medicare benefit kicks in again and pays 95%. The gap is $2,850 (2007 figures).

doula A health professional trained to provide emotional, physical, and informational support to patients and their families at the beginning and end of life. The doula does not perform clinical tasks, but rather focuses on the patient to help her have the kind of experience she wishes. "Doula" comes from the Greek word for servant.

birth doula A doula specializing in support of the mother during labor and delivery. Some birth doulas also provide support beginning in early pregnancy and/or after the mother goes home with her child.

Certified Doula (CD(DONA)) A *birth doula* who has met the education and training requirements of Doulas of North America (DONA) (**www.dona.com**). A CD must be a nurse with labor and delivery experience or a person with training in childbirth education or midwifery, and is required, among other things, to attend a DONA training workshop and provide support for at least three births and be evaluated by the doctors, nurses, and patients.

end-of-life doula A doula trained to support a patient and his family during life-threatening illness and at the end of life. Often volunteers trained by hospice care providers, end-of-life doulas teach families about the process of dying, from diagnosis through death, and provide emotional, physical, and spiritual comfort. Sometimes called death doula. See also *thanadoula*, below.

Postpartum Certified Doula (PCD(DONA)) A doula specializing in helping families during the postpartum period. Postpartum doulas "provide evidence-based information and support on infant feeding, emotional and physical recovery from childbirth, infant soothing and coping skills for new parents." The credential PCD(DONA) is offered by Doulas of North America (DONA). **www.dona.com**

thanadoula An *end-of-life doula* for people or their pets. "Thana" is Greek for death.

DoVA Department of Veterans Affairs; see *Department of Veterans Affairs*.

downcoding See under *coding (billing)*.

DP See *dependent practitioner* under *allied health professional*.

DPA Direct provider agreement. See *direct contract* under *contract*.

DPKC Diagnostic Problem Knowledge Coupler. See *Problem Knowledge Couplers*.

DPM Doctor of Podiatry; see *podiatry*.

DPMU Disaster Portable Morgue Unit. See *Disaster Mortuary Operational Response Team* under *National Disaster Medical System*.

DPT See *Donor Phlebotomy Technician* under *Phlebotomy Technician*, under *clinical laboratory technician*.

DRA See *Deficit Reduction Act of 2005*.

drama therapist A health professional trained in theater arts, psychology, and psychotherapy, qualified to provide drama therapy.

Board Certified Trainer (BCT) A Registered Drama Therapist (RDT) certified to train, guide, and mentor those aspiring to be RDTs by the National Association for Drama Therapists (NADT). **www.nadt.org**

Registered Drama Therapist (RDT) A drama therapist with at least a master's degree who has met the requirements of the National Association for Drama Therapists (NADT). **www.nadt.org**

drama therapy (DT) The use of theater and acting to help achieve symptom relief, emotional and physical integration, and personal growth.

DRG Diagnosis Related Group. A hospital patient classification system developed under federal grants at Yale University in the 1960s, initially for utilization review. In 1983, HCFA (now CMS) began using DRGs as the basis for Medicare payments. The current inpatient prospective payment system (IPPS) is based on the federal government's setting a predetermined price for the "package of care" in the hospital (exclusive of physicians' fees) required for each DRG. If the hospital can provide the care for less than the DRG price, it can keep the difference; if the care costs the hospital more than the price, the hospital has to absorb the difference. (The hospital may request higher payment by pleading that an extra-costly case is an *outlier*.)

Originally each DRG was intended to contain patients who were roughly the same kind of patients in a medical sense and who spent about the same amount of time in the hospital.

The groupings were subsequently redefined so that, in addition to medical similarity, resource consumption (ancillary services (see *service*) as well as inpatient service days) was approximately the same within a given group. In 2006 526 DRGs were identified on the basis of the following criteria: the *principal diagnosis* (the final diagnosis that, after study in the hospital, was determined to be chiefly responsible for the hospitalization), whether an *operating room procedure* (see under *procedure*) was performed, the patient's age and sex; *comorbidity* and *complications*, and discharge status.

A new rule issued in 2006 is aimed at improving the accuracy of payment rates for inpatient stays by basing the weights assigned to DRGs on hospital costs rather than charges, and by adjusting the DRGs for patient severity, possibly by replacing the current DRGs with 861 *consolidated severity-adjusted DRGs (CS-DRGs)* (see below).

Although DRGs were developed and are being used for payment, they are also widely used for other purposes, including hospital comparisons, evaluation of differences in mortality rates, clinical pathway development, quality improvement, strategic planning, and setting capitation rates. See also *prospective payment system*.

All Patient DRG (AP-DRG) Modified DRGs developed in the late 1980s by the New York State Department of Health (NYDH) and 3M Health Information Systems specifically to include non-Medicare patients. Two targeted groups were neonates and patients with human immunodeficiency virus (HIV) infections. The pediatric modifications adapted some of the Pediatric-Modified Diagnosis Related Groups (PM-DRGs) (see below). Modifications were also made for transplants, long-term mechanical ventilation patients, cystic fibrosis, nutritional disorders, high-risk obstetric care, acute leukemia, hemophilia, and sickle cell anemia. Medicare DRGs later adopted some of these changes.

All Patient Refined DRG (APR-DRG) A DRG classification system, based on the AP-DRG structure, that uses sophisticated clinical logic to adjust for severity of illness and risk of mortality. Patients are first assigned to an APR-DRG, then to a separate subclass for both severity of illness and risk of mortality. Severity of illness is defined as "the extent of physiologic decompensation or organ system loss of function experienced by the patient," which is classified as minor, moderate, major, or extreme. Risk of mortality is the "likelihood of dying," also classified as minor, moderate, major, or extreme. Developed in 1990 by 3M Health Information Systems. The pediatric portion was developed in collaboration with the National Association of Children's Hospitals and Related Institutions, Inc. (NACHRI).

All-Payer Severity-adjusted DRG (APS-DRG) A modification of DRGs to adjust for severity of illness in all patient populations, not just those whose care is paid for by Medicare. Developed by HSS, Inc.

CMS DRG Centers for Medicaid and Medicare Services DRG. See *Medicare DRG*, below.

consolidated severity-adjusted DRG (CS-DRG) A new type of DRG proposed by CMS in 2006 to be used in the inpatient prospective payment system (IPPS) to adjust for patient severity, to be based on the *All Patient Refined Diagnosis Related Groups (APR-DRGs)* (see above).

International-Refined DRG (IR-DRG) A system developed by 3M Health Information Systems to permit countries to develop local IR-DRGs using their own diagnosis and procedure codes. IR-DRGs also use a severity adjustment. IR-DRGs were designed to help compare one country with another.

Long-Term Care DRG (LTC-DRG) DRGs established by CMS for long-term care patients.

Medicare DRG (MDRG) Inpatient DRGs established by CMS. The list is revised every October 1st.

Pediatric-Modified DRG (PM-DRG) DRGs for the classification of pediatric medical conditions. These include, for example, additional DRGs for neonates that take into account birth weight, duration of mechanical ventilation, multiple major problems, and surgical procedures. PM-DRGs were developed by the National Association of Children's Hospitals and

Related Institutions, Inc. (NACHRI) in a research project funded by HCFA (now CMS).

Refined DRG (RDRG) Modified DRGs that revised the use of complications and comorbidities (CC) in the original Medicare DRGs. A secondary diagnosis is considered a CC if it causes a significant increase in hospital resource use. Refined DRGs were the result of a Yale University project (mid-1980s) funded by HCFA (now CMS).

Severity DRG (SDRG) A 1993 modification of Medicare DRGs by HCFA (now CMS) resulting from the re-evaluation of the use of complications and comorbidities to adjust for severity of illness. Sometimes also referred to as Severity Refined DRGs or SR-DRGs.

transfer DRG A DRG on the CMS list of DRGs for which acute-care hospitals receive payment under the *post-acute care transfer (PACT) policy*.

DRG coordinator A hospital employee with duties regarding the prospective payment system (PPS). The duties typically are to determine at an early date (the first hospital day, if possible) the DRG of the patient, inform the attending physician of the normal length of stay (LOS) for that DRG and its price, assist in discharge planning, and provide feedback from the case mix management information system.

DRG cost weight A number, or weight, assigned to each DRG by the federal government. It reflects the DRG's use of resources in relation to the cost of the average Medicare patient as determined by the federal government. The average Medicare patient's cost, when multiplied by the DRG cost weight, gives the price for the DRG in question.

DRG creep A change in the distribution of patients among DRGs without a real change in the distribution of patients treated in the hospital. It was feared that hospitals and physicians would change their record-keeping and reporting so that more patients would appear in higher-priced DRGs, and thus hospital income would be increased without a corresponding increase in cost—the creep would be "upward," and would represent exploitation of the payment system. This term is sometimes inappropriately used when the apparent creep simply represents a systematic improvement in record-keeping and coding. When this is the case, of course, there should be a one-time adjustment, which the PPS system should recognize as laudable. Sometimes called "code creep."

DRG enhancer A computer program that arranges the medical data for billing to Medicare so as to achieve the best DRG classification (i.e., the one with the biggest price tag).

DRG payment system Originally, slang for the prospective payment system (PPS) of Medicare. However, this term may now be appropriate usage when payment by other than the Medicare program (insurance plans, for example) is also based on DRGs.

DRG-specific price blending See *price blending*.

DRG system See *prospective payment system*.

drip A medical device used for the administration of a drug or other substance by means of *infusion*.

DRS See *designated record set*.

drug Any substance, other than food, used medicinally, that is, in the prevention, diagnosis, or treatment of disease. In health care, the term "medication" ("med" for short) is used to cover both prescription drugs and nonprescription drugs.

analog drug A drug that is similar in chemical structure to another drug but is slightly different in physiological effect. Drugs that are already in use, and thus have known effectiveness and safety, are a fruitful starting point for developing other drugs with more or less potency and hopefully fewer side effects. Researchers start with an analog of the original drug. These analog drugs may have similar, different, or even opposite effects. Also spelled analogue.

The same analog process that is used to develop legitimate drugs can be used to create illicit drugs; see *designer drug*, below.

brand name drug See *generic equivalent*.

breakthrough drug The first innovator drug to use a new therapeutic mechanism. See also *me-too drug*, below.

designer drug A term usually applied to an *analog drug* (see above) that produces the same or similar effects as a narcotic or other illicit drug. Designer drugs, because they are not identical to the controlled substances they copy, are more difficult to control, although there are laws to curb the production, sale, and use of these designer drugs. Sometimes called "controlled substance analog."

The term is also sometimes—confusingly—applied to legitimate drugs created (or prescribed) in response to an individual's genetic makeup; see *pharmacogenomics*.

follow-on drug See *me-too drug*, below.

generic drug See *generic equivalent*.

innovator drug See *generic equivalent*.

investigational new drug (IND) A drug not yet approved by the Food and Drug Administration (FDA) and so not yet available to the general public. Before the drug can be used on humans, the FDA must approve an IND application, which gives reports of animal toxicity tests with the drug, a description of proposed clinical trials, and a list of names and qualifications of the investigators conducting the studies. Once the IND application is approved, the drug may be used only experimentally, to determine its safety and effectiveness, and only authorized persons may prescribe it.

legend drug See *prescription drug*, below.

me-too drug A brand-name drug that is structurally similar to an existing drug and uses the same therapeutic mechanism. For example, Tagamet was a *breakthrough drug*—the first drug to relieve ulcers by blocking the histamine 2 (H2) receptors in the lining of the stomach from stimulating acid production by the parietal cells. A few years later, a second H2 antagonist, Zantac, was approved. It did not violate the patent on Tagamet because it was not exactly the same structure, but it competed directly with Tagamet because it did the same thing. Synonym: follow-on drug.

multiple-source drug A drug for which the patent has expired, so it is available not only from the original brand-name manufacturer, but also from generic companies.

nonprescription drug A drug that may be purchased without a drug prescription from a physician, dentist, or other authorized provider. Synonyms: over-the-counter (OTC) drug, patent drug, patent medicine.

over-the-counter (OTC) drug See *nonprescription drug*, above.

patent drug See *nonprescription drug*, above.

prescription drug A drug that can only be provided to a patient on the prescription of a physician, dentist, or other authorized provider. Synonym: legend drug. See also *generic equivalent*.

single-source drug A drug that is still under patent, and thus available (usually) only from the original manufacturer.

drug abuse See *substance abuse*.

drug administration See *medication administration*.

drug category See *PDP formulary* under *formulary (health plan)*.

drug class See *PDP formulary* under *formulary (health plan)*.

drug dependence See *substance dependence*.

drug dispensing A portion of the process of providing prescription drugs to patients. It involves the preparation (if not a preprepared product), packaging, labeling, recording, and delivery of the drug (one or more doses) to the patient, the patient's representative, or an agent of the hospital, such as a nurse.

Drug Enforcement Administration (DEA) The federal agency that has to do with licensing the physician, hospital, and others to handle controlled substances, such as narcotics, and with enforcing the drug laws generally. The predecessor agency was the Bureau of Narcotics and Dangerous Drugs (BNDD). **www.dea.gov**

drug error See *medication error*.

drug formulary See *formulary* (health plan, hospital, pharmaceutical).

drug incompatibilities The interference by certain drugs or foods with the actions of certain other drugs. See also *drug interaction*.

drug information service The service of providing readily accessible information about drugs, such as their properties, effects, dosage, contraindications, and drug interactions.

drug interaction The effects (actions) of one or more drugs when two or more drugs are given simultaneously. If each drug acts as though no other drug were being administered, there is no interaction. However, if the action on the body of one or more of the drugs is different than if given by itself, there is a drug interaction. Such interactions are increasingly known, and watched for by physicians and pharmacists; computer systems are being introduced to check for interactions among the list of medications for a given patient. A known drug interaction may or may not be a reason to not use a drug on a given patient, depending on whether the altered effect would be harmful. See also *adverse drug event*, *contraindication*, and *drug incompatibilities*.

drug prescription A written order, by a licensed physician, dentist, or other authorized individual, for a prescription drug to be dispensed by a pharmacy or given in a hospital to a specific patient. When such an order is given in a hospital for a drug to be given to an inpatient, it is called a *medication order*. (Medication orders are required for any drug to be given an inpatient, even if the drug is a nonprescription drug.)

drug reaction See *adverse drug event*.

drug utilization A term that usually refers to the patterns of use of drugs by individual physicians and in hospitals and other facilities.

drug utilization review (DUR) Review of the use of drugs. This may involve looking at a single prescription (either before or after it has been filled), a single patient (reviewing all medications being taken by that patient), patterns of prescribing behavior of individual physicians, or patterns of drug use in a hospital or other facility. The term usually refers to the federal Omnibus Budget Reconciliation Act of 1990 (OBRA 90) requirement that pharmacies participating in Medicaid must perform DUR on both a prospective and retrospective basis.

Prospective DUR (Pro-DUR) seeks to avoid potential problems with a medication order (for an inpatient) or drug prescription (for an outpatient) *before* the order is dispensed or prescription filled. Such problems might include incorrect dosage, premature refill, undesired drug interactions or allergies, and age or gender conflicts with the prescribed drug. Prospective DUR often involves the use of computers that have been programmed to compare the proposed prescription against the patient's age, sex, and prior prescription drug history. This type of DUR can also help prevent medication errors.

In contrast to prospective DUR, retrospective DUR occurs after the prescription is filled to determine whether a drug prescription is appropriate, medically necessary, and not likely to result in an adverse event. This type of review can warn if a problem has occurred, detect patterns, and provide for corrective actions. The purpose of DUR programs of either type is to decrease costs and improve outcomes. Sometimes called drug use review.

DSCC See *Disease-Specific Care Certification*.

DSH See *disproportionate share hospital* under *hospital*.

DSM Disease state management. See *disease management*.

DSM-IV *Diagnostic and Statistical Manual of Mental Disorders, Fourth Edition*. The definitive authority in the United States on psychiatric terminology, published by the American Psychiatric Association. The first edition appeared in 1952, the fourth in 1994. The fifth edition is planned for publication in 2011.

DSMO See *Designated Standard Maintenance Organization*.

DSRF See *debt service reserve fund* under *fund*.

DSS See *decision-support software*.

DT See *dietetic technician* and *drama therapy*.

DTC See *direct-to-consumer*.

DTR See *Dance Therapists Registered* under *dance therapist*, and *Dietetic Technician, Registered* under *dietetic technician*.

dual-benefit calculation A benefit payment practice used by some health insurers, and for some Medicare benefits, in which the beneficiary is billed for the contractual copayment percentage of the *retail* price of a given service, while the insurance company or Medicare pays only on a *discounted* price for the service. This practice passes a higher percentage of the real, out-of-pocket cost on to the beneficiary than the amount stated in the contract.

For example, in the case of a service that has a retail price of $1,000, the insurance contract may require the beneficiary to pay 20%, $200. The insurance company may, in fact, be obtaining the service at a discounted price of $600, so the beneficiary is actually paying 33% of the $600. In some cases the percentage paid by the beneficiary has actually been as high as 60% to 70%.

The practice has been overturned in a number of lawsuits and refunds issued to policyholders. In Minnesota, Blue Cross Blue Shield (BC/BS) was sued over this issue and ended up settling the case for $3.9 million in the summer of 1995. BC/BS also agreed to change the way it computes coinsurance payments levied against subscribers who have that cost-sharing mechanism. Suits have been filed in other states as well.

Reportedly requiring Medicare to charge beneficiaries only the *true percentage* rather than the inflated percentage could increase Medicare costs by over $134 billion over the next ten years.

dual capacity doctrine A legal doctrine used to permit an employee to sue his or her employer despite workers' compensation, which ordinarily employs the **exclusive remedy** doctrine (see under **remedy**). It is used in circumstances where the employer has provided medical treatment for an employee's work-related injury, and has caused additional injury through negligent treatment. The employer may not be sued as an employer because of the exclusive remedy provision; however, some states allow the employer to be sued for malpractice in its second capacity, that of healthcare provider.

dual eligibles People who qualify for both Medicare and Medicaid—those who have low incomes and are also over age sixty-five or otherwise qualify (see **Medicare Part A** under **Medicare**).

dual injury doctrine A legal doctrine used to permit an employee to sue his or her employer despite workers' compensation, which ordinarily employs the **exclusive remedy** doctrine (see under **remedy**). The dual injury doctrine is used in circumstances where the employer concealed the injury or illness from the employee, such as where the company physician detects asbestos poisoning but fails to tell the employee. The first injury is the poisoning, which falls under the exclusive remedy doctrine; the second injury is the aggravation of the first due to the concealment, which does not fall under the exclusive remedy doctrine.

due process A fair, just method to determine a person's rights or duties. The law defines two kinds of due process: "procedural" due process concerns fairness in the process by which rights are decided; "substantive" due process requires that laws not be arbitrary or unfairly discriminate among classes of persons. In common usage, "due process" usually means procedural due process.

The Fourteenth Amendment to the U.S. Constitution states that no one shall be deprived of life, liberty, or property without "due process" of law. The kind and amount of process that is "due" depends on the nature of the rights and duties to be determined, and upon who is doing the determination. The Constitution applies to actions of the federal or state government; however, the courts have, for various reasons, extended the principle to require fairness in a variety of previously private arenas. In addition, some federal and state laws prescribe due process requirements for specific actions.

Basic principles of procedural due process require that a person facing an allegation or adverse action be given reasonable notice of and an opportunity to challenge the allegation, and to present evidence on her or his own behalf. The law requires hospitals to provide a certain amount of due process to physicians who may have their medical staff privileges denied, reduced, or revoked. The Health Care Quality Improvement Act of 1986 (HCQIA) in particular describes minimum due process requirements that a hospital must meet in order to obtain the protection of the act.

DUHP Duke-UNC Health Profile. See *Duke Health Profile* under *quality of life scale*.

DUKE See *Duke Health Profile* under *quality of life scale*.

Duke Endowment A private foundation established in 1924 by industrialist and philanthropist James B. Duke (who also funded Duke University). Its mission is to serve the people of North Carolina and South Carolina by supporting selected programs of higher education, health care, children's welfare, and spiritual life. **www.dukeendowment.org**

Duke Health Profile (DUKE) See under *quality of life scale*.

Duke's system A method of staging tumors. See *staging (tumors)*.

dumping The denial or limitation of the provision of medical care to, or the transfer elsewhere of, patients who are not able to pay or for which the payment method (for example, the prospective payment system (PPS)) does not pay the hospital enough to cover its costs. Laws intended to prevent dumping typically prohibit the transfer of patients if the transfer cannot be justified by medical necessity. See also *Emergency Medical Treatment and Labor Act*. Synonyms: patient dumping, case shifting.

    granny dumping The practice of abandoning an ill, elderly, indigent person at a hospital or other healthcare facility.

DUR See *drug utilization review*.

durable medical equipment (DME) Medical equipment, such as a wheelchair, breathing equipment, home dialysis equipment, or other equipment, that is prescribed by the physician. The term is most often applied when DME is used in the home.

durable medical equipment regional carrier (DMERC) An insurance company contracted by CMS to process durable medical equipment, prosthetics, orthotics, and supplies (DME-POS) claims for the Medicare program. Replaced in 2006 with DME *Medicare Administrative Contractor* (DME MAC).

durable power of attorney See under *power of attorney*.

duty (legal) A "legal" duty is distinctly different from other, general duties, in that failing to perform a legal duty may land you in jail, or have other dire consequences. Having a legal duty also means having a corresponding legal liability for failing in that duty. Like the well-known action/reaction rule in physics, a "legal duty" owed by one gives rise to an enforceable "**legal right**" in another. Rights are often classified by type, such as "property" rights or "civil" rights.

    Legal rights and duties typically arise from either a statute (legislative law), a court's decision in a particular case (case law), an administrative agency's rule (based on authority derived from a statute), or a contract (agreement) between parties. See also *accountability (governance)* and *liability (legal)*.

Dx See *diagnosis*.

E

e- Electronic. A jargon shorthand prefix used to denote that something exists in *cyberspace* (on the Internet, via email, etc.) rather than in hard, physical form. Common examples are "email" and "e-business."

E&M See *evaluation and management services*.

EAP See *employee assistance program*.

Early and Periodic Screening Diagnosis and Treatment Program (EPSDT) A program required of states by Medicaid for children under age nineteen in families receiving Aid to Families with Dependent Children (AFDC). EPSDT is designed to detect physical and mental defects and arrange treatment.

early offer A system for compensating patients who suffer harm as a result of some aspect of health care, proposed as an alternative to malpractice litigation.

The name "early offer" comes from the way the system works: A statute would provide that when a patient suffers harm, the health provider has an option to make an offer of defined compensation within a limited time (for example, 120 days). The compensation would cover (1) economic damages, including costs of the added care required as a result of the harm, loss of income, and/or added expense resulting from the harm (for example, homemaker services); and (2) attorney's fees. The offer would not cover noneconomic losses, such as pain and suffering or punitive damages. If the patient accepts the offer, payment is made within six months (or in periodic payments), and litigation is precluded. If the patient rejects the offer, he or she may pursue a lawsuit, but must show *gross negligence* (see under *negligence*) on the part of the healthcare provider, with the standard of proof raised significantly. Under today's malpractice standards, the patient need only prove that it was more likely than not that the caregiver was negligent (see *professional negligence* under negligence). A patient going to trial after rejecting an early offer, however, must prove *gross* negligence by "clear and convincing evidence" or even "beyond a reasonable doubt," depending on which criterion the statute provides. This proposal is based on a variant of the well-established *business judgment rule*.

Proponents of the system cite as advantages that (1) many more patients harmed are compensated (in a fashion similar to workers' compensation), (2) the compensation is provided when it is needed (unlike litigation, in which compensation must wait, usually for years, for settlement or trial of the suit), (3) the costs of litigation are greatly lessened, and (4) malpractice premiums may be reduced. Critics contend, among other things, that the absence of common law punishment of offenders lessens the "quality control" aspect of litigation.

Early offer, first proposed by Jeffrey O'Connell in the 1980s, is attracting new attention in view of the escalation in liability insurance costs, coupled with a 2001 Joint Commission on Accreditation of Healthcare Organizations (JCAHO) "Patient Rights" standard calling for informing patients "about the outcomes of care, including unanticipated outcomes" (RI 1.2.2). Early offer is discussed thoroughly in an article by O'Connell and Boutros, "Treating Medical Malpractice Claims Under a Variant of the Business Judgment Rule" (*Notre Dame Law Review,* 2002;77:373). Sometimes called "neo-no fault" or "patients' compensation."

Eastern medicine See *Oriental medicine* under *medicine (system)*.

EBHC See *evidence-based health care*.

EBM See *evidence-based medicine*.

Ebola disease African hemorrhagic fever. A disease, first recognized in 1967, caused by the Ebola virus, a virus somewhat resembling physically the rabies virus, but of a different family of viruses. The case-fatality rate is high. Epidemics have occurred in Zaire and the Sudan in recent years. The spread of infection has been controlled by isolation and protective clothing, but there is no known treatment for infected individuals. A closely related virus, the Marburg virus, causes what appears to be the same clinical disease (but called Marburg disease).

EBT See *electronic beam tomography* and *eye bank technician*.

EC Sometimes used to abbreviate "e-commerce" (electronic commerce).

ECF Extended care facility. See *skilled nursing facility*.

ECFMG See *Educational Commission for Foreign Medical Graduates*.

ECG See *electrocardiogram*.

ECGT See *electronic clinical guidance tools*.

echocardiography The use of *sonography* to visualize the heart and its structures.

echoencephalography The use of *sonography* to visualize the brain.

E-CMO A *chief medical officer (CMO)* whose job is focused on the use of information technology (such as the Internet) to link providers with health plan members.

ecological fallacy A statistical term for a logical fallacy in trying to take information from group studies and apply it to individuals.

economic index See under *index (numerical)*.

economic system The way in which goods and services are produced, distributed, and consumed. In health care, the traditional provider-driven system is moving toward a market-driven system.

> **market-driven system** An economic system that responds to the demands of the market, that is, those of the purchaser. The term is currently being applied in health care with the emergence of competitive healthcare delivery plans that seek to attract "customers" by offering (1) more of what the customers want (amenities as well as services) or (2) attractive prices (that is, price competition). Note that the customer is the person paying for the service, and is not necessarily the consumer (the patient).

> **provider-driven system** An economic system in which providers (in health care—physicians, other professionals, and institutions) "prescribe" and furnish those services that they consider to be the best care for the patients. Such a system is intended to meet the needs of the patients as determined by the providers rather than to meet the demands of the purchasers of care.

ECRI In the 1960s the acronym "ECRI" stood for Emergency Care Research Institute, an organization that focused on the development and evaluation of new emergency medical devices. Now this nonprofit organization prefers to be known as ECRI only, because emergency medicine is only a small part of its worldwide role. In 1968, ECRI conducted a study of manually operated resuscitators and found half of them to be dangerous and eliminated them from the marketplace. That study started ECRI down its current path of being an independent evaluator and information provider in the areas of healthcare technology assessment and management. ECRI projects include the *Universal Medical Device Nomenclature System (UMDNS)* and the *Medical Device Safety Reports (MDSR)*. ECRI's mission is to promote the highest standards of safety, quality, and cost-effectiveness in health care through research, publishing, education, and consulting. ECRI is (in 2007) an *Evidence- based Practice Center (EPC)*. **www.ecri.org**

ECS See *Clinical Electrophysiologic Certified Specialist* under *physical therapist*.

ECU Extended care unit. See *skilled nursing unit*.

ED See *Department of Education* and *emergency department*.

Eden Alternative A movement to improve the quality of life for residents of long-term care facilities. The core concept is to see care environments as habitats for human beings rather than facilities for the frail and elderly, and to create vibrant, vigorous habitats. The first principle is that loneliness, helplessness, and boredom account for the bulk of human suffering. These can be alleviated by making human and animal companionship readily available, including access to children and plants in the environment (for example, having child daycare on-site), and using quality improvement techniques to enhance quality of life, not just quality of care. Research has shown that Eden facilities have lower medication use, fewer infections, and lower employee turnover.

Eden Alternative is trademarked by Summer Hill Company, Inc., of Sherburne, New York, which provides training, software, and other tools for implementing the philosophy locally. The process of change is called "Edenizing." Facilities dedicated to the philosophy are called "Eden Homes" and may apply to be listed in the "Eden Registry" maintained by Summer Hill. **www.edenalt.com**

e-detailing The process by which pharmaceutical companies use telecommunications to sell drugs to physicians. E-detailing supplements and supports the activities of the pharmaceutical sales representative ("detailer"). Methods include telephone support, a web site with information, video conferencing, and online drug sample ordering. Synonym: eDetailing. See also *detailing*.

EDI See *electronic data interchange*.

EDIFACT International standards for Electronic Data Interchange for Administration, Commerce and Transport. They are developed and maintained under the auspices of the United Nations Economic Commission for Europe. These standards facilitate information flow among trading partners in many industries. The scope and format of these standards is similar, but not identical, to those developed by the United States (see *ANSI ASC X12N*). **www.unece.org/trade**

education The acquisition of knowledge and skills; see also *continuing education* and *training*.

health education Education directed at increasing the information of individuals and populations, especially communities, about health and its maintenance and the prevention of disease and injury; bringing about modifications in the behavior of individuals so as to achieve better health; and changing social policy in the direction of a more healthful environment and practices.

in-service education Education for healthcare employees, which is part of their employment and usually takes place on-site, without serious interruption of their duties.

medical education The formal education of physicians. See also *continuing medical education* under *continuing education*.

direct graduate medical education (DGME) Refers to a subsidy paid by Medicare to a teaching hospital to compensate the hospital for some of the costs directly related to the graduate training of physicians. The amount is determined by the number of residents at the hospital, the cost of their training, and the hospital's "Medicare patient load," which is the fraction of total inpatient days that Medicare beneficiaries represent. See also *indirect medical education*, below. Synonym: direct medical education (DME).

direct medical education (DME) See *direct graduate medical education* (above).

graduate medical education (GME) Formal education in residency programs. Graduate medical education is only available to *physicians*.

indirect medical education (IME) Refers to a subsidy (the IME adjustment) paid by Medicare to a teaching hospital, as an add-on payment for each case paid by the inpatient prospective payment system (IPPS). The amount is determined by a formula based on the ratio of residents to beds. See also *direct medical education*, above.

undergraduate medical education (UGME) Education in medicine prior to the granting of the Doctor of Medicine (MD) or Doctor of Osteopathic Medicine (DO) degree.

patient education Teaching patients what they need to know about their illness or condition, especially how to care for themselves.

Educational Commission for Foreign Medical Graduates (ECFMG) A nonprofit organization responsible for examining credentials, testing medical knowledge and English-language competency, and granting certification to all foreign-educated (except Canadian) physicians who seek to enter clinical training programs in U.S. medical centers. ECFMG is sponsored by the American Medical Association (AMA), American Board of Medical Specialties (ABMS),

National Medical Association (NMA), Federation of State Medical Boards (FSMB), Association of American Medical Colleges (AAMC), and Association for Hospital Medical Education (AHME). **www.ecfmg.org**

education department The department of an institution responsible for arranging and coordinating education and training programs (both in-service and continuing education) for employees, employee orientation, and, in some circumstances, community health education programs and patient education programs.

EEG See *electroencephalogram*.

EEGT See *electroencephalographic technologist*.

effectiveness The degree to which the effort expended, or the action taken, achieves the desired effect (result or objective). For example, one drug is more effective than another if it relieves certain symptoms to a greater extent, or in a higher proportion of patients. This is also called "clinical effectiveness." The cost or other amount of resources required to obtain the desired effect is not part of the measure of effectiveness, as it would be for the measure of *efficiency*, which is often confused with effectiveness.

  If the effort or intervention is carried out under carefully controlled conditions, as in a laboratory test, the word **efficacy** is more commonly used to describe the degree of success. When the Food and Drug Administration (FDA) tests a new drug, for instance, it will report its findings in terms of safety and efficacy. Whether the drug will be clinically effective, or efficient, are questions not answered by FDA testing.

efficacy See *effectiveness*.

efficiency The relationship of the amount of work accomplished to the amount of effort required. A given hospital's food service is more efficient than another hospital's in one measure if, for example, it can furnish meals to patients for a lower average cost per meal (assuming that the meals are of equal quality). Although efficiency is usually thought of in terms of cost, it can equally well be measured in other ways, such as time; for example, the automobile racing crew that can change a set of tires in the shortest time is the most efficient. See also *effectiveness*, which is often confused with efficiency.

EFM See *electronic fetal monitoring*.

eGov Electronic government. An initiative in the Office of Management and Budget (OMB) to coordinate efforts within the federal government to utilize technology to improve functioning and services. eGov includes several "Line of Business" initiatives: Case Management (CM), Financial Management (FM), Grants Management (GM), Human Resources Management (HR), Federal Health Architecture (FHA), IT Security (ITS), Budget Formulation and Evaluation (BFE), Geospatial LoB (Line of Business), and IT Infrastructure Optimization Initiative (IOI). **www.whitehouse.gov/omb/egov**

eHealth See *telehealth*.

eHealth Initiative (eHI) The eHealth Initiative and the **Foundation for eHealth Initiative** are independent, nonprofit affiliated organizations whose missions are the same: to drive improvement in the quality, safety, and efficiency of health care through information and information technology. Members include hospitals and other healthcare organizations, clinician groups, consumer and patient groups, employers and purchasers, health plans, healthcare information technology organizations, manufacturers, public health agencies, academic and research institutions, and public sector stakeholders. One sponsored program is *Connecting Communities for Better Health*. **www.ehealthinitiative.org**

eHI See *eHealth Initiative*.

EHIBCC See *Health Industry Business Communications Council*.

e-HIM See under *health information management*.

EHL Electrohydraulic lithotripsy. See *lithotripsy*.

EHNAC See *Electronic Healthcare Network Accreditation Commission*.

EHR See *electronic health record* and *evidence-based hospital referral*.

EHRS See *electronic health record system*.

EIN See *Employer Identification Number*.

Eisenberg Patient Safety Awards Awards created in 2002 by the Joint Commission on Accreditation of Healthcare Organizations (JCAHO) and the National Quality Forum (NQF) to recognize individuals and healthcare organizations that have made significant contributions to improving patient safety. The awards are named for John M. Eisenberg, former leader of the Agency for Healthcare Research and Quality (AHRQ).

EIT Electronic and information technology. Federal regulations require EIT to be equally accessible to those with and without disabilities.

EKG See *electrocardiogram*.

eldercare Services provided to the *elderly* so that they may remain independent and in their homes. Sometimes used specifically to refer to services provided by friends and relatives. Some use eldercare to refer to the full spectrum of health care and other support services available for seniors. Synonym: elder care. The U.S. government has an "Eldercare Locater" connecting individuals with community services: **www.eldercare.gov**.

elderly Somewhat old; past middle age. The term refers to a person's chronological age, not their physical or mental condition. Elder simply means older. Generally, statutes define elderly as being sixty-five years of age or older. The *area agencies on aging*, however, use age sixty as their measurement. AARP members need only be fifty.

e-learning A loosely defined concept that involves the presentation of instructional content using electronic devices. When presented over telecommunication channels, such as the Internet, it is also known as distance learning (or an online course). E-learning can be focused on general educational subjects, so as to supplement or even replace high school or college courses, or on specific training needs. One use for e-learning in the healthcare arena is training people to use software tools to assist in coding diagnoses and procedures. Although developing the content for use in e-learning programs can be substantial, it is often less expensive to deploy to many recipients, especially if they are in remote locations. E-learning can be synchronous (in real time, often with a "live" instructor), asynchronous (participants learn on their own schedules), or even blended (a mix of various methods, even "face-to-face" learning). Although it doesn't need to be, much e-learning content is interactive, either allowing or requiring responses from the participant.

elective Treatment that is medically advisable, but not critical. Elective care (such as hospitalization, treatment, or surgery) can be scheduled in advance, in contrast to emergency care, which must be rendered immediately to avoid death or serious disability. See *elective surgery* under *surgery (treatment)*.

electrocardiogram (ECG, EKG) The recording made in the diagnostic procedure called electrocardiography. EKG is used interchangeably with ECG as an abbreviation.

electrocardiography A diagnostic procedure that records, or shows on a screen, the electrical activity of the heart muscle as it contracts and relaxes with the heartbeat. The recording is called an electrocardiogram (ECG, EKG). Although ECGs may be taken directly from the heart during surgery, they are routinely taken for diagnostic purposes as well. ECG involves placing perhaps a dozen electrodes (small plates that conduct electricity) on the skin at various locations (leads), and connecting (leading) the plates with the recording instrument (electrocardiograph). This provides a variety of views, which appear as "tracings" on the screen or recording paper. A large body of experience has been developed that permits the translation of the patient's particular array of views into diagnostic information for the physician.

electroconvulsive therapy (ECT) The process of administering brief, carefully measured electrical current, through electrodes attached to the head, to alter the brain's electrical activity. The patient is first given an anesthetic and a muscle relaxant. ECT is used to treat certain mental disorders, including depression. Numerous sessions are usually required. Today's

ECT is far safer than early applications of the technology. Sometimes called "shock therapy" or "electroshock therapy."

electroencephalogram (EEG) The record of the electrical activity of the brain obtained by electroencephalography.

electroencephalographic technologist (EEGT) An electroneurodiagnostic technologist who specializes in electroencephalography.

> **Registered Electroencephalographic Technologist (R. EEG T.)** An electroneurodiagnostic technologist who is registered in electroencephalography by the American Board of Registration of Electroencephalographic and Evoked Potential Technologists (ABRET). **www.abret.org**

electroencephalography An electroneurodiagnostic procedure for determining the electrical activity of the brain by the use of equipment that makes recordings (or video displays) from electrodes (electrical contacts), which pick up the electrical impulses. The electrodes are ordinarily placed on the scalp but may, during surgery, be placed on the surface of the brain or in its interior.

electrohydraulic lithotripsy (EHL) See *lithotripsy*.

electromagnetic therapy See *bioelectromagnetic therapy*.

electromyogram (EMG) The record of the electrical activity of the muscles obtained by electromyography.

electromyography The use of electroneurodiagnostic procedures to record and evaluate electrical activity of the muscles.

electroneurodiagnostics (END) The science of recording and studying the electrical activity of the brain and nervous system. Includes *electroencephalography*, *electromyography*, *electronystagmography*, *evoked potentials*, *intraoperative monitoring*, *nerve conduction studies*, and *polysomnography* (sleep studies).

electroneurodiagnostic technologist (ENDT) A health professional qualified to perform certain electroneurodiagnostic procedures. ENDTs may specialize in several areas (see individual listings):

> *electroencephalographic technologist*
> *evoked potential technologist*
> *intraoperative monitoring technologist*
> *nerve conduction technologist*
> *polysomnographic technologist*

electronic beam tomography (EBT) A noninvasive imaging technique that can detect early calcification (hardening) of the coronary arteries. It is being studied as a factor to motivate patients to follow prescribed programs for the prevention of heart disease.

Electronic Benefits Transfer (EBT) The use of information technology (IT) ("debit card technology") to deliver federal and state government benefits (for example, AFDC, Social Security, Veterans Compensation Pension) electronically. The beneficiary uses a **Benefit Security Card** to obtain cash benefits at automated teller machines (ATMs) and point of sale (POS) devices.

electronic clinical guidance tools (ECGT) Computer and Internet-based software and systems that (1) correlate patient-specific data with the best biomedical evidence, (2) tailor the result to specific decisions and decision makers in real-time, (3) provide intelligent alerts and reminders, and (4) facilitate and record communications among all participants in the care process. The gold standard for an information system for patient care is one that provides guidance for handling the actual problems of the individual patient. A computer program that checks a drug being prescribed for compatibility with the other treatments that patient is receiving is an example of such guidance. A much more elegant example is found in *Problem-Knowledge Couplers*.

electronic data interchange (EDI) The exchange of routine business transactions via computer. EDI enforces a level of standardization in the way the electronically transmitted data are formatted, making it possible for a variety of different computer systems to exchange data. The term is used in health care primarily in connection with claims and other financial transactions.

electronic fetal monitoring (EFM) The process of listening to the heart rate of the fetus, sometimes during the course of labor and delivery.

Certificate of Added Qualification in Electronic Fetal Monitoring A certificate of added qualification available to registered nurses, physicians, and physicians' assistants who pass an examination in electronic fetal monitoring given by the National Certification Corporation (NCC). **www.nccnet.org**

electronic government *See eGov.*

Electronic Healthcare Network Accreditation Commission (EHNAC) An independent, nonprofit organization that establishes criteria for and accredits healthcare networks and information security systems. It grew out of the 1993 Workgroup for Electronic Data Interchange (WEDI). **www.ehnac.org**

electronic health record (EHR) A term used to refer to a variety of forms of electronic health and healthcare information. Often, it is used as a generic, "umbrella" term to describe the full range of record systems. Sometimes it is used synonymously with electronic medical record (EMR), computer-based patient record (CPR), or one of the other terms defined below. The Healthcare Information and Management Systems Society (HIMSS) provides the following definition:

> The Electronic Health Record (EHR) is a secure, real-time, point-of-care, patient-centric information resource for clinicians. The EHR aids clinicians' decisionmaking by providing access to patient health record information where and when they need it and by incorporating evidence-based decision support. The EHR automates and streamlines the clinician's workflow, closing loops in communication and response that result in delays or gaps in care. The EHR also supports the collection of data for uses other than direct clinical care, such as billing, quality management, outcomes reporting, resource planning, and public health disease surveillance and reporting. (Definitional Model 1.0, November 6, 2003)

The two leading EHR concepts are the CPR and the EMR (defined below). One distinction between them is interoperability: The CPR must be interoperable among all providers, insurers, and systems, whereas the EMR need only be interoperable within a physician's office or institution. Another is content: The CPR is longitudinal and contains continuing chronological data, whereas an EMR may contain only the patient's record within one clinic or for one hospital stay. Each of the terms below reflects a specific vision of what an EHR should be and do. None of these actually exists in a complete stage, because standards, capabilities, and visions are evolving. See also *Continuity of Care Record* (under *data set*), *electronic health record system*, *medical record*, *Patient Medical Record Information*, *translucent medical record*, and *VistA*.

computer-based patient record (CPR) An electronic health record that is longitudinal and includes all of a person's health data, from prenatal to current (and eventually postmortem), including all providers (it "goes beyond the walls" of a single hospital or practice), diagnoses, treatments, surgeries, medications, and so forth. The Computer-based Patient Record Institute (CPRI; see *CPRI-HOST*) was formed in 1991 to pursue and coordinate efforts to develop the CPR. CPRI defined it as follows:

> A CPR is electronically maintained information about an individual's lifetime health status and health care. The computer-based patient record replaces the paper medical record as the primary source of information for health care meeting all clinical, legal and administrative requirements. It is seen as a virtual compilation of non-redundant health data about a person across a lifetime, including facts, observations, interpretations, plans, actions and outcomes. The CPR is supported by a system that captures, stores, processes,

communicates, secures and presents information from multiple disparate locations as required. ("Definition of Electronic Medical Record." American Medical Association, November 10, 2000. http://www.ama-assn.org/ama/pub/category/2900.html)

In 1991 the Institute of Medicine (IOM) published a report, *The Computer-Based Patient Record: An Essential Technology for Health Care*, advocating the development of the CPR and identifying twelve critical attributes for a CPR system, called the "Gold Standard": (1) provides problem lists, (2) measures health status and functional levels, (3) documents clinical reasoning/rationale, (4) provides longitudinal and timely CPR linkages with other patient records, (5) guarantees confidentiality and audit trails, (6) provides continuous authorized-user access, (7) supports simultaneous user views in the CPR, (8) provides access to local or remote information resources, (9) facilitates clinical problem solving, (10) supports direct physician entry, (11) supports practitioners in measuring and managing costs and in improving quality, and (12) provides flexibility to support existing and evolving needs of each specialty. A key feature of the CPR is interoperability, with freedom to exchange information among providers and between various systems. This distinguishes it from the *electronic medical record* (EMR; see below), which need not necessarily be interoperable outside the enterprise. Synonyms: computerized patient record (this is the term used by the Veterans Administration in its VistA system), electronic patient record.

computerized medical record (CMR) A medical record that is electronic only because paper documents have been digitized. This means that traditionally recorded paper documents have been scanned into a computer system.

computerized patient record (CPR) See *computer-based patient record*, above.

digital health record (DHR) See *electronic medical record*, below.

digital medical record (DMR) An electronic health record that is kept on the Internet, and providers can access it using an Internet browser. Patient information is posted on the web site and accessed ("pulled") as needed, rather than sent to providers as email messages ("pushed"). The technology is based on an XML-based generic standard that allows communication as well as data management. There is no specific content; the DMR might have the functionality of the electronic medical record (EMR) or computer-based patient record (CPR), for example. In this usage, digital medical record is not as broad a term as *online medical record* (see below) in that the patient doesn't necessarily have access. However, some may use the terms synonymously.

electronic medical record (EMR) An electronic health record covering the care provided to a patient within a single enterprise (for example, clinic, hospital, physician's office, or health plan; sometimes called the "care delivery organization" (CDO)). The EMR ideally has interoperability within the enterprise, among all departments and systems. Some say that an essential feature of the EMR is that the physician must enter data into the computer while examining the patient (the computer is in the examination room).

The EMR can contain all information contained in the traditional medical record: diagnoses, surgeries, nursing notes, laboratory reports, physicians' orders, drugs administered and known interactions, images of such record elements as electrocardiographic tracings, and other data. In addition, the EMR promises many advantages over the paper record. For example, it can present information at the touch of a finger, with legibility and helpful display techniques. Time series of laboratory values can be shown graphically and abnormal values can be color-coded. The computer can automatically check for potential drug interactions. Patient education can be both triggered and provided within the sophisticated systems. Patient and physician reminder notices—health checkpoints—can be generated automatically. Medical care can be made much more efficient and less error-prone.

Another advantage of the EMR is that, unlike a paper record, it can be accessible simultaneously to several users in several places (e.g., to consultants, billing clerks, attending physician, in the office and at the hospital).

Despite its many advantages, adoption of the EMR has been slow, largely because it has required changes in the habits of physicians and other caregivers, and because the input methods have slowed down the care process (at least initially). Physicians have been loath to devote learning time. Time saved later in care—the promise of "delayed gratification"—has not always been enough to overcome these problems. Synonyms: paperless medical record, digital health record (DHR).

electronic patient record (EPR) Some use this as a synonym for *computer-based patient record (CPR)*; others use it more generally, similar to electronic health record. The *Medical Records Institute (MRI)* sees it as similar to the CPR but focusing on relevant information and not necessarily covering the patient's lifetime, and not including dental, behavioral, or alternative care.

Government Computer-based Patient Record (G-CPR) A collaborative project of the Department of Veterans Affairs (VA), the Department of Defense (DoD), Indian Health Service (IHS) (and originally Louisiana State University Medical Center (LSUMC)) to develop an *infrastructure* (see *information infrastructure*) and *standards* (see *standard (norm)*) for a *computer-based patient record (CPR)* system. The effort was initiated in 1998. It led to the *Federal Health Information Exchange (FHIE)*. See also *VistA*.

online medical record (OMR) An electronic medical record (EMR) kept online. Access is via any type of computer terminal, which in the early 21st century includes devices such as cell phones. Caution must be used when using this term, because *any* EMR is "online" to some extent; otherwise, data couldn't be entered or retrieved by anyone. Most people today use "online" synonymously with "on the Internet." Use of this term implies an EMR that is accessible to a wider audience than just the provider, including the patient. See also *digital medical record*, above.

patient-carried record (PCR) A concept introduced (and explored) in the 1980s. The patient was envisioned as being the connecting entity for all his or her health information. The patient (consumer) would have a device, such as a smart card, that contained the patient's essential health information. Providers could swipe the card to receive and update information. The vision failed by the late 1980s (after a cost of about $500 million to the healthcare industry) due to technical card problems, difficulties with interoperability concerning content and terminology, and lack of an infrastructure that would permit every provider to record and read cards. In the 2000s, however, the patient-centric concept is being revisited; see *personal health record*, below. Synonym: patient-carried medical record.

personal health record (PHR) An electronic health record that is patient-centric, rather than focused on provider needs. The concept is that the patient (consumer) can carry his or her own health information (perhaps in a cell phone; see *Consumer Health Manager*) and update it as needed. Ideally, this would be in a system interoperable with providers' systems, so the patient could simply upload and download information to and from the provider (like loading music into an iPod). The content of the personal health record has not been defined. Some see the PHR as being kept online and accessed via the Internet.

personal information carrier (PIC) A portable, electronic device the size of a "dog tag" that carries a soldier's personal medical history. It is a rugged, low power consumption, flash memory device that is hardware and operating system independent, with a storage capacity of 8 to 128 megabytes. The PIC works with a computer-based patient record (CPR) and can store x-rays, MRIs, EKGs, and other information. Data are stored on the PIC, in the CPR database, and when there is connectivity (wireless LAN, radio, etc.) the data are also stored in a central database server. The PIC is designed to be readily accessed and updated by first responder medical personnel via laptop or hand-held computers when real-time connectivity to a database is unavailable. Synonym: digital dog tag.

electronic health record system (EHRS) A collection of software applications, including the *electronic health record (EHR)*, that supports a variety of functions related to health care.

The system may automate the provider's workflow, support billing, provide decision support, generate reports, relay medication and other orders, and so forth. A committee of the Institute of Medicine (IOM) has identified eight core functions that EHR systems should be capable of performing in order to promote greater safety, quality, and efficiency in healthcare delivery. HL7 is using this list to devise a common industry standard for EHR functionality. The core functions are:

- Health information and data
- Result management
- Order management
- Decision support
- Electronic communication and connectivity
- Patient support
- Administrative processes and reporting
- Reporting and population health

Some include the necessary hardware in the term "electronic health record system."

electronic medical record (EMR) See under *electronic health record*.

electronic neural network See *neural network*.

electronic patient record (EPR) See under *electronic health record*.

electronic prescribing See *e-prescribing*.

electronic signature A method using encryption technology (see *cryptography*) whereby an individual can securely attach a special kind of electronic data to some other digitized information, for the purpose of proving that the data came from that individual. An electronic signature, if approved by applicable statutes, carries the same legal force as a traditional written signature, including that of *nonrepudiation*. This term should not be confused with the graphic picture that is the result of optically scanning an individual's written signature, and storing it on a computer in digital form. Synonym: digital signature. See also *authentication* and *public key infrastructure*.

electronic transaction See *Transactions and Code Sets*.

electronic transactions standards (ETS) Technological standards for the electronic transmission of health information, issued by the Department of Health and Human Services under the administrative simplification provisions of HIPAA. See *Transactions and Code Sets*.

electronystagmogram (ENG) The record of the electrical activity of the eyes obtained by electronystagmography.

electronystagmography An electroneurodiagnostic procedure that records electrical activity of the eyes to study involuntary movement of the eyeballs. Also used to evaluate dizziness because it can distinguish between inner ear and central nervous system involvement.

electrophoresis A laboratory technique that takes advantage of the fact that various substances (molecules) move at different speeds when exposed to an electric field. This fact is used to separate the substances in various analyses and in working with genetic materials.

electrophysiology The study of the relationship of the body to electricity, including the production of electric currents by, and the effect of electrical stimulation on, organs and tissues.

electrotransport A process, also known as "iontophoresis," that uses small amounts of electricity to make drugs or other compounds pass through the surface of the skin. This process is usually implemented via a transdermal ("through-the-skin") device known as a "patch," which is fastened to the skin, or even implanted. A small battery powers the electrical circuit, which allows a positively charged drug molecule to move from the positive pole of the patch through the skin to the negatively charged pole of the patch. The bloodstream absorbs the drug molecules on the way. It is hoped this system can replace shots and vaccinations because it allows for greater control over the timing and amount of drugs dispensed, as well as the fact that it doesn't hurt. This process can be used to administer almost any biotech compound, even large complex molecules such as insulin, for example.

element (chemical) A substance that cannot be decomposed by the ordinary types of chemical change, or made by chemical union. An *atom* is the smallest particle of an element.

element (data) An "item of information." When used in connection with computers, a data element may be one part of a data record (a logically connected group of data elements); see *database*.

Element of Performance (EOP) A specific expectation within a standard of the Joint Commission on Accreditation of Healthcare Organizations (JCAHO). Each standard has one or more Elements of Performance. JCAHO defines EOPs as "specific performance expectations that must be in place for an organization to provide safe, high quality care, treatment and services." During an accreditation survey, each EOP is scored on a three-point scale: 0 = insufficient compliance, 1 = partial compliance, 2 = satisfactory compliance.

ELF radiation See *extremely low frequency (electromagnetic) radiation* under *radiation*.

eligibility A term usually used in health care with reference to whether an individual may be enrolled in a given insurance plan, governmental program, or other health plan. Also may refer to the qualification of a health plan to contract with CMS to provide services to Medicare beneficiaries.

eligibility period The period of time a new employee has to sign up for life or health insurance without having to take a physical examination or otherwise show insurability. After the eligibility period has expired, the employee may be denied insurance because of a preexisting condition, or have to pay higher premiums.

email Electronic mail. This is used to describe a variety of messages that are not only transmitted electronically, but also intended to be read and replied to electronically as well. Consequently, email does not include faxes, telegrams, or other such messages, which are transmitted electronically but routinely presented to the receiver as "hard copy" (paper).

embargo Refers to a situation in which information concerning a forthcoming (print) article is furnished by a publisher to the media (TV, radio, etc.), with the understanding that the media not make public (broadcast) any of the disclosed information until the specific time and/or date set by the publisher (or other source). Very occasionally the source may decide that the public interest would be best served by the immediate release of the information, prior to the source's normal publication date. The media generally abides by the embargo rules, but occasionally a member of the media will ignore the embargo date. In this case, the source may retaliate by not furnishing advance copies of journal articles, statements, and the like in the future. This type of embargo is strictly an informal arrangement voluntarily accepted by all parties.

embryo An organism in the very early stages of development. From fertilization of the ovum until the eighth week of growth, a human is usually considered an embryo; thereafter it is called a fetus. See also *stem cell*.

EMBS See *Engineering in Medicine and Biology Society*.

EMCRO See *experimental medical care review organization*.

emergency A situation requiring immediate attention in order to prevent death or severe disability. A situation less critical is "urgent." The least critical level is "elective."

emergency center, free-standing (FEC) A free-standing facility, separate from the hospital, that provides services to patients needing immediate care. Such a facility has x-ray and laboratory services, and has arrangements for transportation and hospitalization of patients who require it.

emergency department (ED) A hospital department that gives care for patients who need prompt attention. By definition, patients may not become continuing patients of an emergency department; the entire episode of emergency care is one visit. Ordinarily, an emergency department is available twenty-four hours a day. Synonym: emergency room (ER).

emergency medical facility A physical structure, excluding mobile vehicles, that has been approved by the appropriate regulatory authority to receive emergency patients and that is equipped and staffed to evaluate and treat patients with life-threatening conditions.

emergency medical services (EMS) A broad term covering all services required to care for patients in emergencies, at the sites of the emergencies, in transit, and at emergency facilities. It includes emergency medical treatment; transportation arrangements; communication among vehicles, personnel, and facilities; triage of patients prior to and following transportation; and mobilization of personnel and resources as necessary.

emergency medical services board (EMS board) A term sometimes used for the state agency with responsibility for, among other things, licensing emergency medical technicians, approving ambulances and emergency medical facilities, and similar functions. See also *board (credentialing)*.

emergency medical services region (EMS region) A defined geographic area used for emergency medical services planning, development, and coordination.

emergency medical services system (EMS or EMSS) A coordinated system for providing emergency medical services within a designated geographic area organized to respond to medical emergencies, regardless of the cause. It includes personnel, transportation, communication, equipment, and sometimes facilities. Such systems are subject to regulation by federal, state, and local agencies with respect to personnel qualifications, equipment and its maintenance, and the like. See also *National Disaster Medical System*.

emergency medical technician (EMT) A health professional with special training in on-site and in-transit care of injured and emergency medical patients (victims). All states require certification of EMTs, although specific requirements vary from state to state. The National Highway Traffic Safety Administration of the U.S. Department of Transportation has established a standard curriculum for EMT training. The National Registry of Emergency Medical Technicians (NREMT) (**www.nremt.org**) offers five levels of registry examinations:

First Responder A person trained in basic emergency medical care. Many fire fighters and police officers have this level of training, which is aimed at the first people to arrive at the scene of an accident.

Emergency Medical Technician—Basic (EMT-Basic) An EMT who has been trained to assess a patient's condition and manage respiratory, cardiac, and trauma emergencies, both at the scene of an accident and during transport to the hospital, under medical direction.

Emergency Medical Technician—Intermediate/85 (EMT-Intermediate/85) An EMT with more advanced training who is able to administer intravenous fluids, use a manual defibrillator, and use advanced airway techniques and equipment in a respiratory emergency. "85" denotes that the EMT has completed an approved course of study that equals or exceeds the education objectives of the 1985 EMT-Intermediate National Standard curriculum as promulgated by the U.S. Department of Transportation.

Emergency Medical Technician—Intermediate/99 (EMT-Intermediate/99) An intermediate-level EMT who has completed an approved course of study that equals or exceeds the education objectives of the 1999 EMT-Intermediate National Standard curriculum as promulgated by the U.S. Department of Transportation. This is a higher level of training than the *Emergency Medical Technician—Intermediate/85* (see above).

Emergency Medical Technician—Paramedic (EMT-Paramedic) The highest level of EMT, this person is trained to administer drugs orally and intravenously, interpret electrocardiograms (EKGs), perform endotracheal intubations, use monitors and other complex equipment, and perform other advanced skills.

Emergency Medical Treatment and Labor Act (EMTALA) This federal law requires hospitals that participate in the federal Medicare program to provide an "appropriate" medical screening exam to *any* patient who comes to their emergency room. If the condition is an emergency, the hospital must stabilize the patient unless the patient requests a transfer in writing and the physician considers the transfer to be more beneficial than risky. The equipment used to transfer must be adequate.

Although the word "appropriate" is not defined by the statute, CMS states that an appropriate medical screening exam will take into account the current condition and past history of the patient, as well as the capabilities of the hospital's emergency department. However, treatment should not be delayed while the hospital verifies patient-provided information, economic or otherwise.

Hospitals and doctors who violate the EMTALA provisions can be fined for each violation and can be excluded from Medicare. In addition, the patient can sue the hospital. (However, the federal courts have basically held that this statute cannot be used as a basis for malpractice claims, which must be brought under state law.) Although the law was passed to prevent hospitals from withholding emergency medical care for uninsured or economically disadvantaged patients, courts have generally not required suing patients to prove that the hospital was motivated by economic factors.

This act, also known as the "Anti-Dumping Act," was passed as a part of the Consolidated Omnibus Budget Reconciliation Act of 1985 (COBRA 1985). A report issued in 2001 found that 527 hospitals, or roughly 10% of U.S. hospitals, were found to have violated the act's screening, treatment, and transfer provisions in the preceding several years.

New rules effective in 2003 reduced some of the burden on hospitals by, among other things, making it clear that not all hospitals have to have physicians on call twenty-four hours a day, seven days a week, and that EMTALA no longer applies to an individual who is admitted as an inpatient. The Medicare Modernization Act required that determinations of medical necessity be made based on information available to the provider at the time an item or service was ordered or furnished, rather than on the patient's principal diagnosis. 42 U.S.C. § 1395dd (2004).

emergency medicine The area of medicine dealing with sudden illness or injury requiring immediate attention, from onset until the patient is released from the emergency treatment facility.

emergency nursing The area of nursing focused on the needs of patients with sudden illness or injury that requires immediate attention.

Certified Emergency Nurse (CEN) A specialist in emergency nursing who has passed an examination of the Board of Certification for Emergency Nursing (BCEN). **www.ena.org/bcen**

emergency physician (EP) A physician who specializes in emergency medicine. Often works in the emergency department (ED) of a hospital (where the physician is often called an "emergency department physician") or in a free-standing emergency center (FEC). The emergency physician, by definition, sees the patient only once; continuing care is provided elsewhere, such as in a private physician's office, the outpatient department, or in the hospital, as appropriate.

emergency room (ER) See *emergency department*.

Emergency System for Advance Registration of Volunteer Health Professionals (ESAR-VHP) A national program to "preregister" volunteer health professionals so that they may respond immediately in a crisis situation. In mass disasters, such as 9/11, many medical personnel make themselves available to help, but must be turned away because there is not time nor a mechanism to verify their identities and credentials. The ESAR-VHP, administered by the Health Resources and Services Administration (HRSA), assists states in establishing standardized preregistration systems that provide readily available, verifiable, up-to-date information regarding each volunteer's identity, licensure, credentials, and privileges in hospitals or other medical facilities. **www.hrsa.gov/esarvhp**

Emergency Use Authorization (EUA) Permission by the Food and Drug Administration (FDA) to use an unapproved drug, or an approved drug for an unapproved use, in the event of an emergency. The Secretary of Health and Human Services must first issue a "declaration of emergency," based on a determination by the Secretary of Homeland Security, Secretary of Defense, or Secretary of Health and Human Services that there is a domestic emergency, military emergency, or threat to national security involving a specified biologic, chemical, radiological, or nuclear agent or agents. The FDA may then approve the drug for emergency use if it determines that the potential benefits outweigh the risks under the circumstances. Drug companies may submit drugs to the FDA for consideration for potential EUAs prior to an emergency, to save time in the event of an emergency. This is called a pre-EUA. See also *compassionate use.*

emeritus staff See *honorary medical staff* under *medical staff member.*

EMG See *electromyogram.*

emotional distress A legal term referring to a nonphysical injury caused by malpractice or other wrongdoing. "Emotional distress" is used in the context of deciding what kinds of injury are compensable; that is, the kinds of injury for which a plaintiff can recover money from the wrongdoer. Normally, money damages are awarded for actual economic loss, such as medical expenses and lost earnings, and for noneconomic loss such as the pain and suffering that accompany physical injury. Although emotional distress is acknowledged by the courts to be very real, money damages for emotional distress alone are usually not allowed unless the wrongdoing that caused it was intentional or grossly reckless. Most medical malpractice cases do not involve the type of malice or recklessness required for the allowance of damages for emotional distress.

Emotional distress is most often claimed by a third party, that is, someone who was not physically injured by the malpractice, but was nevertheless terribly disturbed. An example of such a third party would be a mother who witnesses her newborn baby being dropped by a hospital attendant; although the baby is seriously injured, the mother herself is not put in danger by the act. Therefore, the mother cannot recover for her own emotional distress. Denying the mother damages for emotional distress is an example of the "line-drawing" that courts do to limit liability, especially for unintentional behavior. Synonym: mental distress.

intentional infliction of emotional distress A *tort* where the wrongdoing consists of intentional outrageous conduct that causes extreme mental suffering—for example, falsely telling a parent that her child has just been killed. This tort is also called outrage.

negligent infliction of emotional distress A *tort* where the wrongdoing consists of negligence that causes extreme mental suffering. For example, a physician was liable for the breakup of a patient's marriage after misdiagnosing a sexually transmitted disease. Not all states recognize this cause of action.

emotional support animal See *service animal.*

employee A person who works for and is paid by another (the employer), and who is under the control of the employer. An employee is to be distinguished from an *independent contractor*, who works for him- or herself. The line between the two is often fuzzy, but the legal consequences are important. Different tests to determine whether someone is an employee or independent contractor are used for different purposes—taxes, workers' compensation, liability, unemployment insurance, and so forth. The same person can easily be both an employee and an independent contractor, at the same time, for different purposes.

employee assistance program (EAP) An occupational health service program that helps employees with substance abuse or physical or behavioral problems deal with these problems when they affect job performance. The assistance may be provided within the organization or by referral to outside resources.

employee health benefit plan An organization's plan for health benefits for its employees and their dependents. The term generally refers to the "package" of benefits that are provided. Such plans are among the "fringe benefits" of the employees, and thus are not part of the employee's salary. The employees may or may not contribute to paying the cost by deductions from their salaries.

employee health service A service provided by an organization to examine persons prior to employment and to give certain health care (and, often, counseling) to employees.

Employee Retirement Income Security Act (ERISA) The federal law adopted in 1974 in response to fraud and mismanagement of employee pension funds and benefit plans. ERISA, among other things, preempts state regulation of health benefit plans offered by self-insured employers. It does not preempt state laws that regulate insurance—a highly litigated distinction. ERISA offers remedies for improper denial of health benefits, but regulates in a way not as pervasive as state regulation. Employers who directly contract with providers assert that these relationships are not subject to state regulation because they fall within the broad ERISA preemption. Insurance regulators argue that employers who contract with providers on a capitated basis are essentially providing insurance and should be regulated at the state level. 29 U.S.C. § § 1001–1461 (2005).

employee stock ownership plan (ESOP) A qualified stock bonus or combination money purchase and stock bonus plan designed to invest primarily in employer securities. Specific Internal Revenue Service (IRS) requirements must be met for setting up such a plan.

employee welfare benefit plan (EWBP) A plan, fund, or program established by an employer or employee organization for the purpose of providing employees, through insurance or otherwise, medical, surgical, or hospital care or benefits, or benefits in the event of sickness, accident, disability, or death. The term is fully defined in the Employee Retirement Income Security Act (ERISA).

Employer Identification Number (EIN) A unique number for an employer, issued by the Internal Revenue Service (IRS), similar to a Social Security number for an individual. The EIN has been adopted by CMS as the standard unique *identifier* (mandated by HIPAA) for employers in the filing and processing of healthcare claims and other transactions.

employer mandate See under *mandate*.

employer shared responsibility (ESR) See *Healthy Americans Act*.

employer-sponsored health care An approach used by mid- to large-sized employers to augment conventional managed care or pharmacy benefits management (PBM) plans by contracting for primary care and pharmacy services in a way that is both cost-effective and convenient for employees (possibly including dependents and retirees). The motivation for this approach comes from reported industry data that suggest that persons who must leave the workplace to get health care use twelve to sixteen times as much time as those who get it on the job. Employee participation is voluntary. Employer-sponsored healthcare programs are tailored to meet the employer's and employees' needs, and each will be unique in its configuration. Ironically, this is in many ways a return to the earlier part of the twentieth century, when large factories and work sites had on-site health clinics.

Another major motivating factor is that pharmaceuticals are the fastest growing cost element in health care at the beginning of the 21st century. An employer-sponsored pharmacy that offers prescription services exclusively to its covered population ("closed-door pharmacy") can get these pharmaceuticals at a significantly deeper discount than it could by other means. Also, employer-sponsored health care can help an employer achieve Voluntary Protection Program (VPP) status with the Occupational Safety and Health Administration (OSHA).

employment at will Employment of an individual without a personal or union contract. The employee may be let go at any time for any reason, except for cases of *wrongful discharge*.

emporiatrics The study of the prevention, diagnosis, and treatment of diseases encountered in travel. Synonym: travel medicine.

empowerment See *patient empowerment*.

EMR See *electronic medical record* under *electronic health record*.

EMS See *emergency medical services* and *emergency medical services system*.

EMS board See *emergency medical services board*.

EMS region See *emergency medical services region*.

EMSS See *emergency medical services system*.

EMS system See *emergency medical services system*.

EMT See *emergency medical technician*.

EMTALA See *Emergency Medical Treatment and Labor Act*.

EMT-Basic See *Emergency Medical Technician—Basic* under *emergency medical technician*.

EMT-Intermediate/85 See *Emergency Medical Technician—Intermediate/85* under *emergency medical technician*.

EMT-Intermediate/99 See *Emergency Medical Technician—Intermediate/99* under *emergency medical technician*.

EMT-Paramedic See *Emergency Medical Technician—Paramedic* under *emergency medical technician*.

encoder Computer software (program) for assisting in the assignment of a code to a word or phrase expressed in natural language (human language, such as English). See *computer-assisted coding*.

encoding (genetics) The information within a strand of DNA that provides instructions for the body's production of proteins, polypeptides, and RNA molecules, and of their constituent groups.

encoding (information management) Converting information into code.

encounter The personal contact between the patient and a professional healthcare giver. This term is typically used only with respect to personnel involved in assessment or treatment, or providing social services, not with obtaining a prescription drug from a pharmacy, for example.

> **standardized patient encounter (SPE)** An encounter between a physician or other healthcare worker and a "standardized patient" (SP) (a nonphysician trained to simulate a patient encounter accurately and consistently) for teaching and for evaluating the performance of the physician or worker. The SP may be a patient or simply be acting out the part.

encryption See *cryptography*.

END See *electroneurodiagnostics*.

endemic Constantly present in a specific population or geographic area. The adjective may be applied, for example, to a disease or an infectious agent. A **holoendemic** disease is one that has a high prevalence in children, and that is less common in the adult population. Malaria is often a holoendemic disease. A **hyperendemic** disease is one that affects all age groups equally, and that has a high prevalence in an area.

endocrine A kind of organ that produces and secretes into the body itself, generally into the blood, chemical substances called hormones that have effects on one or more other organs. The pancreas, which secretes insulin (a hormone involved in the body's use of sugar, and in diabetes), is an endocrine organ.

endocrinology The study of the organs of internal secretion, that is, organs that produce chemicals essential to specific body functions. Such chemicals (and organs) include, for example, insulin (from the pancreas) and adrenalin (from the adrenal glands).

end of life care Healthcare and other services provided to a person who is dying. The focus is to make the quality of life as high as possible during this time. A study found that from the patient's perspective, five areas were important for quality end of life care: (1) receiving adequate pain and symptom management, (2) avoiding inappropriate prolongation of dying, (3) achieving a sense of control, (4) relieving the burden, and (5) strengthening relationships with loved ones. (Singer, P., Martin, D., & Kelner, M. "Quality End-of-Life Care: Patients' Perspectives." *Journal of the American Medical Association, 1999*;281(2):163–168.)

end stage renal disease (ESRD) Renal (kidney) disease in which the kidneys no longer function enough to sustain life, a condition known as renal insufficiency. Life may be sustained by kidney transplant in some instances, or by *hemodialysis* (see under *dialysis*). Specific benefits are available for patients with ESRD under Medicare, which may be the primary source for paying for long-term hemodialysis, either in the hospital or in the home.

ENDT See *electroneurodiagnostic technologist*.

energy agent See under *agent (facilitator)*.

ENG See *electronystagmogram*.

Engineering in Medicine and Biology Society (EMBS) An international society of biomedical engineers. Affiliated with the *Institute of Electrical and Electronics Engineers (IEEE)*. One of EMBS's projects is *MEDIX*. **www.embs.org**

enrollee As used in health insurance and with prepayment plans, a person who is covered (receives benefits) under a contract for care. Sometimes called "member" or "covered person." See also *subscriber*.

ENT See *otorhinolaryngology*.

enteral Given via the alimentary tract or lungs, as taken by mouth or injection into the rectum (enteron = intestine). See also *nutrition support* and *parenteral*.

enteric Having to do with the intestines (enteron = intestine).

enteric disease A disease caused by microorganisms, parasites, viruses, or other pathogens in the intestines, often characterized by diarrhea and/or vomiting. An infectious disease, it is often transmitted via food, fecal matter, or water, or carelessness about hand washing and sanitation of objects handled.

enterostomal therapy nursing (ETN) See *wound, ostomy, and incontinence nursing*.

entity One of the items making up a universe.

entity coding See under *coding*.

entrepreneur A person who organizes a new venture and assumes the risk. See also *intrapreneur*.

entropy prevention The set of management activities directed at maintaining quality and enthusiasm in the performance of established activities and duties that are not in need of change. Entropy is a term taken from physics for the tendency of any system (process) to lose energy, to "run down," if no additional energy is provided. An appreciable amount of management energy is applied to change that, although resisted, is seen as "where the action is." However, an equal or even greater amount of management energy must be applied to keep ongoing activities (systems) interesting and exciting, and to prevent quality from declining and change from occurring.

entry See *medical record entry*.

enumerated See *National Provider Identifier*.

Enumerator See *National Provider Identifier*.

environmental assessment A planning technique in which influences and events external to the organization that are felt likely to present either problems or opportunities are listed. An attempt is then made to predict the effects of these factors on the organization, and to suggest the appropriate responses. It can be contrasted with "environmental impact," in which the effects of the organization's actions on its environment are assessed.

Environmental Protection Agency (EPA) The agency of the federal government charged with protecting human health and the natural environment. **www.epa.gov**

environmental services Services in a hospital or other facility involved in providing for the patients, employees, and visitors a "clean" environment. It may include housekeeping, laundry, and solid and liquid waste control; however, maintenance, radiation protection, and air conditioning, for example, are unlikely to be included in this term.

enzyme A specific type of chemical (a protein) that can speed up a specific chemical reaction, but that is not changed or used up in the reaction; a biological catalyst.

EOP See *Element of Performance*.

EP See *emergency physician* and *evoked potentials*.

EPA See *Environmental Protection Agency*.

EPC See *Evidence-based Practice Center*.

EPI See *Estes Park Institute*.

Epidemic and Pandemic Alert and Response (EPR) A program of the World Health Organization (WHO) to support world-wide efforts to prevent, detect, and respond rapidly to public health emergencies of international concern. EPR supports member states in implementing laboratory capacities, early warning alert and response systems, and other capabilities; supports training programs; coordinates pandemic and seasonal influenza preparedness and response; develops standardized approaches for readiness and response to major epidemic-prone diseases (e.g., meningitis, yellow fever, plague); strengthens biosafety, biosecurity, and readiness for outbreaks of dangerous and emerging pathogens (e.g., SARS, viral hemorrhagic fevers); and maintains and develops a global operational platform to support outbreak response and support regional offices. **www.who.int/csr/don/en**

epidemiologic autopsy See under *autopsy*.

epidemiologist A physician or other health professional specializing in epidemiology.

hospital epidemiologist The person who has charge of a hospital's infection control program. The hospital epidemiologist may be a qualified epidemiologist or a physician or other individual assigned to the task.

medical epidemiologist An epidemiologist who is a physician.

nurse epidemiologist An epidemiologist who is a nurse.

epidemiology The study of diseases or causes of disease in relationship to a population, such as a hospital or a community. Epidemiology deals primarily with the analysis of existing data rather than data collected prospectively in an experimental design.

black box epidemiology A method of epidemiology that permits drawing inferences without examining, knowing, or understanding all of the factors responsible—the group or groups of unknowns are the *black box*. For example, smoking has been implicated in the causation of lung cancer without an understanding of all of the biological mechanisms by which the effect is caused. These biological mechanisms are the black boxes. Some criticize the approach as being unscientific, whereas others point out that it permits action to prevent disease even before understanding of the disease mechanism is complete. The competing style of epidemiology is *mechanistic epidemiology* (see below), in which the processes in the black box are the focus—in the preceding example, the biological mechanisms triggered in the lung by smoking. A movement is afoot to see the two approaches as complementary.

genetic epidemiology The study of diseases in groups of relatives, and of inherited diseases within populations.

mechanistic epidemiology A method of epidemiology that tries to understand the mechanisms by which a factor (or factors) causes a biological effect. For example, in the epidemiological relationship between smoking and lung cancer, mechanistic epidemiology studies the biological mechanisms by which the smoke triggers the cancer. See also *black box epidemiology* (above).

molecular epidemiology The study of the specific strains of pathogenic organisms that are responsible for the production of disease and epidemics. Toxicity alone is apparently not enough; the organism must also be able to colonize and invade.

epigenetics The study of all factors that influence expression of a gene. DNA sequence alone does not determine the final characteristics of an organism; information stored "above and beyond the gene" affects, among other things, whether a gene is activated, and to what extent.

episode A series of events that is distinct in itself. For example, a period of fever that disappears may be an episode of fever within a continuous process, such as a chronic illness.

episode of care A continuous course of care by a hospital or physician for a specific medical problem or condition. Often the term has a specific definition under a federal or state statute.

EPO See *exclusive provider organization*.

EPR See *electronic patient record* (under *electronic health record*) and *Epidemic and Pandemic Alert and Response*.

EPRA Ethics in Patient Referrals Act; see *Stark I*.

e-prescribing The use of an electronic data entry system (handheld, PC, or other) to generate a prescription, rather than writing it on paper. The prescription may be printed out and given to an outpatient or faxed or electronically transmitted to the nurses' station or pharmacy. Synonyms: eRx, electronic prescribing. See also *computerized physician order entry*.

EPSDT See *Early and Periodic Screening Diagnosis and Treatment Program*.

EPT See *evoked potential technologist*.

equity (access) Fairness. This is one great impetus to healthcare reform; inequities among regions of the country, between rural and urban settings, among ethnic groups, and among socioeconomic groups, in access to and quality of both preventive and curative services, are widely reported.

equity (finance) Assets minus liabilities; also called "net worth." See *asset* and *liability (financial)*.

ER Emergency room. See *emergency department*.

E-Rate Support A program to provide discounts in telecommunications rates to assist schools and libraries in having access to the Internet. See *Universal Service Fund*.

ergonomics Commonly describes the study of ways to make a more comfortable and productive fit between humans and their machines and work environments. The International Ergonomics Association (IEA) (**www.iea.cc**) gives the following definition: "Ergonomics (or human factors) is the scientific discipline concerned with the understanding of interactions among humans and other elements of a system, and the profession that applies theory, principles, data and methods to design in order to optimize human well-being and overall system performance."

Unlike the very obvious safety concerns represented by regulatory efforts such as the Occupational Safety and Health Administration (OSHA), ergonomics still has very few standards of any kind, and even less regulation, at least in the United States. Sweden's regulation of cathode ray tube (CRT) or video display terminal (VDT) emissions is one of the better known governmental efforts to create and enforce an ergonomic standard.

Apparently ergonomics got its first boost as a discipline during World War II when it became increasingly obvious that the human being was the weak link in sophisticated military weaponry. Today, much of the interest in ergonomics comes from office workers having problems related to spending many hours working in front of computers. One category of such problems is repetitive stress injuries (RSIs), whose best known example is carpal tunnel syndrome. Synonym: human factors.

ergonomist A specialist in *ergonomics*. According to the International Ergonomics Association (IEA), "ergonomists contribute to the design and evaluation of tasks, jobs, products, environments and systems in order to make them compatible with the needs, abilities and limitations of people." **www.iea.cc**

   Certified Ergonomics Associate (CEA) A person with a bachelor's degree plus training and experience in ergonomics who has been certified by the Board of Certification in Professional Ergonomics (BCPE). **bcpe.org**

   Certified Human Factors Professional (CHFP) A specialist in ergonomics with a master's degree in human factors (or equivalent) who has been certified by the Board of Certification in Professional Ergonomics (BCPE). **bcpe.org**

   Certified Professional Ergonomist (CPE) A specialist in ergonomics with a master's degree in ergonomics (or equivalent) who has been certified by the Board of Certification in Professional Ergonomics (BCPE). **bcpe.org**

ERISA See *Employee Retirement Income Security Act*.

eRx See *e-prescribing*.

ESAR-VHP See *Emergency System for Advance Registration of Volunteer Health Professionals*.

e-signature See *electronic signature*.

ESOP See *employee stock ownership plan*.

ESR Employer shared responsibility; see *Healthy Americans Act*.

ESRD See *end stage renal disease*.

ESRD Network A federally mandated organization that contracts with CMS to provide certain services relating to Medicare patients with end stage renal disease (ESRD) within a state or region. In 2002, eighteen networks encompassed 299,591 patients and 4,443 providers. Each network operates on a three-year Statement of Work cycle, and is responsible for conducting activities in the following areas: quality improvement, community information and resources, administration, information management, and special studies. **www.esrdnetworks.org**

Estes Park Institute (EPI) An independent nonprofit corporation providing education and other services for the healthcare community. EPI believes that "health care must have a moral center and that health care professionals, trustees and managers of hospitals and health systems have the highest duty and responsibility in our society." EPI's mission is "to educate teams of physicians, board members and health care managers so that they can better serve their patients and all people in their local communities and can exercise leadership in the field." Its main programs are national conferences for hospital medical staff officers, hospital and other healthcare administrators and trustees, and community members. **www.estespark.org**

ethics (moral) The study and theory of *moral* principles. In health care, the field is often called "bioethics." Important bioethical principles include *autonomy*, *beneficence*, and *distributive justice*.

ethics (professional) The set of standards and rules promulgated by the various professions and enforced against their members. For example, lawyers are governed by the *Model Rules of Professional Conduct* and the *Model Code of Professional Responsibility*. Physicians must follow the *Code of Ethics* of the American Medical Association (AMA), and psychiatrists must follow the American Psychiatric Association (APA) *Code of Ethics*.

Members of professions may and do find themselves at odds with the standards they must follow. One can arguably be an ethical person (see *ethics (moral)*), but also be an unethical lawyer or doctor at the same time, due to behaving, or not behaving, in a particular way. The codes of ethics and standards are merely the accepted behavior for the professionals in light of the responsibility they have by being members of their profession. It should be remembered that professional ethics are the result of consensus, and as such they are subject to change over time and circumstances.

ethics committee A hospital committee, typically with a broad representation from the medical staff, hospital administration, nursing, the clergy, social services, and others, that is concerned with education of hospital personnel on biomedical ethical issues (see *ethics (moral)*) and decision-making processes, formulation of institutional policies on medical-ethical issues (for example, "do not resuscitate" policies), and review of and consultation on cases presenting ethical problems. Such committees do not make decisions on the care of individual patients, but rather act, if consulted, in an advisory and educational capacity. The role of the ethics committee varies from hospital to hospital (or other healthcare institution).

Ethics in Patient Referrals Act See *Stark I*.

E31 Committee on Health Informatics See *ASTM E31 Committee on Health Informatics*.

etiology In common usage, the cause of a disease or disorder. Technically, however, the term "etiology" means the study of causes.

ETN Enterostomal therapy nursing. See *wound, ostomy, and incontinence nursing*.

ETS See *electronic transactions standards*.

E2B A standard for the definition of an electronic *adverse drug event* case, developed by *ICH*.

EUA See *Emergency Use Authorization*.

eugenics Efforts to control reproduction as a means of improving a race, either by eliminating traits that are thought undesirable (negative eugenics) or by enhancing the frequency of traits thought desirable (positive eugenics).

Europäisches Komitee für Normung German for "Comité Européen de Normalisation." See *CEN*.

European Committee for Standardization English for "Comité Européen de Normalisation." See *CEN*.

European Health Industry Business Communications Council (EHIBCC) See *Health Industry Business Communications Council*.

euthanasia Permitting the death of a hopelessly ill or injured person (passive euthanasia), or causing the death of that individual in a reasonably painless manner (active euthanasia) as an act of mercy. The term "euthanasia" (which means literally "good death") may be applied to the policy as well as to the act. The line between active and passive euthanasia is not always clear, and some believe that asserting the right to die (refusing or withdrawing life-sustaining treatment) on behalf of an incompetent individual is a form of euthanasia. Synonym: mercy killing. See also *physician-assisted suicide* under *suicide*.

evaluation and management (E&M) documentation guidelines CMS requirements for what must be in the patient's medical record to support the "level of care" in the health insurance claim form or billing statement as coded in CPT and ICD-9-CM. Three to five levels of care are defined by the codes. The purpose of the E&M guidelines is to ensure that the level billed for is merited—higher level, higher fee.

The guidelines include basic requirements for the medical record (e.g., completeness and legibility, documentation for each encounter, rationale for diagnostic and other services, availability of past information, identification of risk factors, course of the patient's progress). Different levels of service requirements apply to new and to established patients. Specific, detailed guidelines are given for documentation of the patient's history; chief complaint and/or reason for encounter; history of present illness; review of systems; past, family, and/or social history; examination of the patient; medical decision making; and counseling and/or coordination of care.

evaluation and management (E&M) services Relates to a policy of Medicare that is explained in the "Evaluation and Management Services Guide," a thirty-two-page document published by CMS and available at its web site with the proviso that "Medicare policy changes frequently. . . ." The policy states:

The more work performed by the physician, the higher the level of code [higher levels command higher reimbursement] he or she may bill within the appropriate category. The billing specialist or alternate source reviews the physician's documented services and assists with selecting codes that best reflect the extent of the physician's personal work necessary to furnish the services.

Thus, the fee claimed is indicated by the "level" of care shown by the code submitted on the bill and documented in the medical record. Factors involved in determining the level include whether the patient is a new or established patient, the complexity or seriousness of the patient's problem, and the amount of face-to-face time required of the physician—a predicted ten minutes for Level 1, with a problem focus and "straightforward medical decision making," twenty minutes for Level 2, thirty minutes for Level 3, forty-five minutes for Level 4, and sixty minutes for Level 5, which requires comprehensive study and "medical decision making of high complexity."

evaluation of care Assessment of the degree to which care measures up to accepted standards.

evidence-based health care (EBHC) An evolutionary broadening of *evidence-based medicine (EBM)*, which includes disciplines other than medicine in recognition of the many factors affecting a person's health.

evidence-based hospital referral (EHR) A method to increase patient safety by making sure that patients with high-risk conditions are treated at hospitals with characteristics shown to be associated with better outcomes for those conditions. An initiative of the *Leapfrog Group*.

evidence-based medicine (EBM) Using the current best information in making decisions about the care of individual patients. EBM means combining the healthcare provider's clinical expertise and experience with the best available external clinical evidence from a variety of sources, preferably from systematic research.

Evidence-based Practice Center (EPC) An institution that has a contract with the Agency for Healthcare Research and Quality (AHRQ) to study topics relevant to clinical, social science/behavioral, economic, and other healthcare organization and delivery issues—specifically those that are common, expensive, and/or significant for the Medicare and Medicaid populations. The EPCs review all relevant scientific literature on selected topics to produce evidence reports and technology assessments. These reports are used for informing and developing coverage decisions, quality measures, educational materials and tools, guidelines, and research agendas. The EPCs also conduct research on methodology of systematic reviews. Topics are nominated by nonfederal partners such as professional societies, health plans, insurers, employers, and patient groups. The goal of the program is "to improve the quality, effectiveness, and appropriateness of health care by synthesizing the evidence and facilitating the translation of evidence-based research findings." The following institutions had five-year EPC contracts beginning in 2002:

> Blue Cross and Blue Shield Association, Technology Evaluation Center
> Duke University
> ECRI
> Johns Hopkins University
> McMaster University
> Oregon Evidence-based Practice Center RTI International—University of North Carolina
> Southern California Evidence-based Practice Center—RAND
> Stanford University—University of California, San Francisco Evidence-based Practice Center
> Tufts University—New England Medical Center
> University of Alberta
> University of Minnesota
> University of Ottawa

e-visit A doctor's "visit" that consists of email communication between patient and physician. This can be especially useful for care of ongoing conditions such as diabetes, high blood pressure, or asthma. Health plans have traditionally only covered face-to-face visits, but some are now paying for e-visits as well. See also *telehealth*.

evoked potentials (EP) An electroneurodiagnostic procedure that records electrical activity of the brain, spinal nerves, and sensory receptors that occurs in direct response to external stimuli. These "evoked potentials" are a series of waves that can help evaluate the functional state of sensory pathways.

evoked potential technologist (EPT) An electroneurodiagnostic technologist who specializes in evoked potentials.

Registered Evoked Potential Technologist (R. EP T.) An electroneurodiagnostic technologist who is registered in evoked potentials by the American Board of Registration of Electroencephalographic and Evoked Potential Technologists (ABRET). **www.abret.org**

EWBP See *employee welfare benefit plan*.

excess benefit transaction rule A provision in the federal Taxpayer Bill of Rights that exposes trustees and managers of tax-exempt organizations (such as nonprofit hospitals) to individual (personal) financial liability for certain contracts the organization enters into with an "insider" of that organization. In essence, the law is designed to assure that no individuals wrongly benefit from the nonprofit status of the organization (see *inurement*). If an organization, such as a typical hospital, enters into a contract with someone the IRS deems to be an insider and pays that insider more than fair market value for something, each trustee or board member who knowingly participated in the contract formation may be liable. The nature of the liability is such that the trustee may be required to personally pay up to $10,000 as an "excise tax" on the amount of the contract considered to be above fair market value.

The law and the IRS regulations refer to insiders as "disqualified persons," defining them as persons who are in a position to exercise substantial influence over the affairs of the organization—such as board members and trustees. Whether physicians appointed to the medical staff would be included in this definition apparently depends on the particular facts of each case. Also known as the "intermediate sanctions rule."

excess coverage See under *insurance coverage*.

Exclusions List See *List of Excluded Individuals/Entities*.

exclusive contract See under *contract*.

exclusive dealing An agreement between a seller and buyer, for the seller to sell only to the buyer (or the buyer to buy only from the seller). When such an arrangement unfavorably affects competition, it may violate the federal antitrust laws.

exclusive provider organization (EPO) A health plan that is basically a *preferred provider organization (PPO)*, but that restricts beneficiaries to use of the facilities and providers that form the panel of the EPO. Some EPOs allow beneficiaries to obtain care outside the plan but with reduced benefits (same as a *preferred provider option*).

exclusive remedy See under *remedy*.

exculpatory Excusing, clearing from guilt. In some states, clinical practice guidelines can be used as an affirmative defense in a medical malpractice claim if the physician can prove that she or he followed them. The defense is exculpatory in that it can excuse a physician if evidence of compliance is offered and proven. See *clinical practice guidelines* (under *guidelines*), *malpractice crisis*, and *rebuttable presumption*.

exculpatory clause A clause in a contract that releases a party from liability for its acts. Such clauses are not always enforceable.

executive An individual who is a high-level manager, and who has authority to make significant decisions. Similar authority is implied by use of the terms employed for corporate officers, such as "president" and "vice president." The trend is to use these terms in healthcare organizations where formerly such persons might have been called "administrators," implying that the decisions came from elsewhere and the person simply carried them out. See also *healthcare executive*.

executive director See *chief executive officer*.

ex officio Membership by virtue of holding a position or office. An ex officio member of a body (such as a board of directors or a committee) may or may not have authority to vote, depending on the bylaws of the body.

expenditure target A goal for attempting to hold down the rate of growth in expenditures. Such a target may be mandated by law and limit the payments that may be made, for example, to a physician in a given year. One such target was the Medicare Volume Performance Standards (MVPS).

expense The using up of an asset (as in depreciation), or the cost of providing services or making a product, during an accounting period. The subtraction of expenses from revenue gives the net income.

experience rating See under *rating*.

experimental medical care review organization (EMCRO) Prior to the establishment of the professional standards review organization (PSRO) as part of the Medicare administration, several organizations were set up under federal grants to experiment with the concept of having a body composed of physicians, external to the hospital, review the medical necessity, appropriateness, and quality of services provided to beneficiaries of the Medicare program. After experience was gained with their operation, the EMCROs were disbanded, and legislation was enacted that established the PSRO program on a nationwide basis. Later, in 1982, PSROs were replaced by peer review organizations (PROs).

Experiment in Patient Injury Compensation (EPIC) A 1995 research project in Utah that combined features of no-fault and enterprise liability systems for compensation for injuries sustained by patients in the healthcare system. The sponsor of EPIC was the Utah Alliance for Health Care, a coalition of medical, hospital, business, labor, and other community organizations.

expert system A group of rules that outlines a reasoning process. The rules are statements made by experts in a given field of expertise. The system is applied to a database and results in deductions being made. Expert systems often revolve around a computer program that elicits answers from a nonexpert operator (acquisition of data), and then applies the previously stored rules (embedded in the software) to this new data to come up with a conclusion. An expert system might be used in a bank, for example, to ask a clerk to enter certain relevant information from a loan applicant into its database, and then have the expert system decide whether the applicant qualifies for a loan given the bank's rules. In health care, an expert system could accept a patient's medical history and symptoms, and then apply these data to stored rules to suggest possible diagnoses. See also *Problem Knowledge Couplers*.

explicit Specifically stated. For example, if there are conditions tied to one's income that state nothing can be spent on travel, that is an *explicit* limitation. If there are no conditions, but the income will not permit both a vacation trip and painting the house, the necessity for choice (or establishing priorities) is *implicit*; it goes "naturally" with the idea of limited funds. In financing medical and hospital care, limited funds require choices as to how to spend them. In the past, the rationing of funds has been implicit, but some states are beginning to use explicit methods; see *Oregon Health Plan*.

exposure prone procedure A procedure where a healthcare worker's fingers and a needle or other sharp object are both in a "poorly visualized or highly confined anatomic site," or any other procedure where there is a significant risk of contact between the worker's blood or body fluids and those of the patient. The term occurs in regulations concerning the prevention of transmitting hepatitis B, AIDS, and similar diseases.

express A term used in genetics meaning to manifest a characteristic that is specified by a gene. With hereditary diseases, for example, a person can carry the gene for such a disease but not actually have the disease. In this case the gene is not "expressed."

extended care See *skilled nursing care* under *nursing care*.

extended care facility (ECF) See *skilled nursing facility*.

extended care unit (ECU) See *skilled nursing unit*.

extern A person, usually in medicine or dentistry, who provides medical or dental care, under professional supervision, while still a student.

external cardiac massage See *closed-chest cardiac massage*.

extracorporeal shock wave lithotripsy (ESWL) See *lithotripsy*.

extracorporeal technologist See *perfusionist*.

extraordinary treatment See under *treatment*.

eye bank technician (EBT) A health professional trained in the procurement and processing of corneas and other eye tissue.

Certified Eye Bank Technician (CEBT) An eye bank technician who has at least a high school diploma or GED and six months of technical experience and has passed an examination of the Eye Bank Association of America (EBAA). **www.restoresight.org**

F

FA See *functional administration* under *administration*.

FAAHC Fellow of the American Association of Healthcare Consultants. See *Certified Healthcare Consultant* under *healthcare consultant*.

FAAN Fellow of the *American Academy of Nursing*.

FACCT See *Foundation for Accountability*.

face time Time spent by two or more people together physically, face-to-face; used to distinguish from nonphysical encounters: phone calls, emails, text messages, and so on. In health care, face time is time spent by a physician or other caregiver together with the patient. In 2006, Medicare issued a new rule to reward physicians for spending more time with patients, discussing their health and ways to maintain or improve it. The rule did this by increasing financial reimbursement for *evaluation and management (E&M)* services.

FACHA Fellow of the *American College of Hospital Administrators*.

FACHE Fellow of the American College of Healthcare Executives. See *Certified Healthcare Executive* under *healthcare executive*.

facility Formerly used to refer to an institution organized to provide ambulatory, inpatient, residential, or other health care. However "facilities and services" now are commonly used together, with a listing of a varied mixture of things: physical facilities (for example, long-term care facility, urgent care center), activities (support groups, health fairs), types of care (such as assisted living), equipment (CT scanner), and other hospital attributes or healthcare services.

  The *AHA Guide to the Health Care Field* in 1989 listed fifty-four categories of facilities. The 2007 *AHA Guide* listed 126 facilities and services.

FACMPE Fellow of the American College of Medical Practice Executives. See *Certified Medical Practice Executive* under *medical practice management*.

FACPE Fellow of the *American College of Physician Executives*.

factor A term used in the *International Classification of Diseases* (ICD) referring to reasons (other than disease or injury) why people come into contact with the healthcare system. See *problem*.

faculty practice plan See *medical practice plan*.

FADA Fellow of the *American Dietetic Association*; see *Registered Dietitian* under *dietitian*.

FAH See *Federation of American Hospitals*.

fail first See *step therapy*.

failure to diagnose A type of medical malpractice claim that became a leading cause of litigation in the 1990s. Some explain this trend because of the prevalence of managed care and its financial disincentives to perform as many tests and evaluations as previously.

faith-based organization (FBO) A generic term covering all religious organizations, including nonprofit groups affiliated with a church or religion. Such organizations, which exist in all communities, often address social issues and provide food, clothing, and health care to the needy. The federal government is "partnering" with faith-based ("religiously affiliated") and community organizations to provide social services by offering grants to the organizations so that they can "help those in need." Synonyms: faith community, faith organization.

false claim A claim filed for services or an item that was not actually provided. The filing of false claims is a way some providers defraud the Medicare and Medicaid programs in order to make money. It is a felony to file a false claim under Medicare, Medicaid, or a state health program that is funded by a federal block grant. See also *fraud and abuse*.

False Claims Act (FCA) A federal statute that provides that private citizens who know of anyone defrauding the government (not just in healthcare payment claims) may sue on the government's behalf and be eligible for a share of the suit's proceeds. Citizens who bring these law suits are called qui tam relators or, more commonly, "whistleblowers."

The first False Claims Act was passed in 1863 at the behest of President Abraham Lincoln, who was attempting to keep the federal government from paying for lame horses and broken rifles being sold to the Union Army during the Civil War. Amendments to the act in 1943 severely restricted its use, and the number of cases brought declined sharply. In 1986, Congress again amended the act, this time making it much easier to bring (and win) a claim, as well as providing for treble damages. According to the Department of Justice (DOJ), these incentives have resulted in a dramatic increase in the number of actions successfully brought under the act, many of them related to fraudulent healthcare claims. By the year 2000, the largest payment to a single whistleblower was $52 million, in a case against SmithKline Beecham Clinical Laboratories, Inc. Also known as the Civil False Claims Act. 31 U.S.C. § 3129 et seq. (2005).

false imprisonment A *tort* in which the wrongdoing consists of depriving a person of his freedom against his will, and without legal right.

false negative A diagnostic test result indicating that the patient does *not* have the condition being tested for, when in fact the patient *does* have it. A false negative leads to failure to treat a patient who has the condition in question, and a false sense of security on the part of the patient.

false positive A diagnostic test result indicating that the patient *has* the condition being tested for, when in fact the patient does *not*. A false positive could lead to unnecessary treatment and psychological trauma.

family Traditionally, this has been used in the healthcare setting to mean "blood" (or adopted) relatives (i.e., legal relatives). For example, a hospital patient may be permitted as visitors only the patient's "immediate family," defined as spouse, parents, and sometimes children of the patient. Also, this group is consulted during the care of the patient, kept informed, and involved in the decision-making process. This arbitrary definition obviously excludes unmarried persons, including homosexuals, and other friends, regardless of the nature and strength of the ties. In recent years, society has begun to recognize the fact that the people who play the role of family in a person's life—those closest to the person—are often not related by blood or law, and in fact the legal relatives may be completely out of the picture.

The Joint Commission on Accreditation of Healthcare Organizations (JCAHO) has defined a patient's family as "the person(s) who plays a significant role in the patient's life." This would include an individual not legally related to the patient. This person(s) is often referred to as a surrogate decision maker if authorized to make care decisions for a patient should the patient lose decision-making capacity.

Family and Medical Leave Act (FMLA) A 1993 federal law requiring employers with fifty or more employees to provide employees twelve weeks of unpaid leave per year for birth or adoption of a child, to care for a sick family member, or for an employee with a serious health condition. The act defines a health condition as an "illness, injury, or impairment or physical or mental condition." The condition must involve either continuing treatment by a provider or inpatient care. Pub. L. No. 103-3, 107 Stat. 6 (1993).

family birth center A family-centered unit in the hospital where mothers with normal pregnancies may, if they wish, deliver their babies in a hospital, but in a homelike environment.

family care home (FCH) A family residence that provides *rest home care* (see under nursing care) to a limited number of persons. Usually the number of persons who can be cared for is stipulated by law or regulations as, for example, six or fewer. (A greater number of persons turns the facility into a "rest home" and places it under rest home licensure and supervision requirements.) May also be called "adult foster home."

family-centered maternity/newborn care An approach to maternity and newborn care that emphasizes the physical and social needs of the entire family—mother, baby, and others.

family medicine The medical specialty that is "concerned with the total health care of the individual and the family. It is the specialty in breadth which integrates the biological, clinical, and behavioral sciences. The scope of family medicine is not limited by age, sex, organ system, or disease entity." (Definition adopted by the American Board of Family Medicine.) The care provided is *primary care*.

family nursing The area of nursing focusing on *primary care* for individuals and families.

    Family Nurse Practitioner A registered nurse with a master's degree or higher who is qualified in family nursing and has passed an examination of the American Nurses Credentialing Center (ANCC) (**nursingworld.org/ancc**). The credential is APRN,BC (Advanced Practice Registered Nurse, Board Certified).

Family Opportunity Act (FOA) See *Deficit Reduction Act of 2005*.

family planning Efforts to determine the number of children and their spacing in a family by the use of birth control methods.

family practice (FP) The former term for *family medicine*.

FAO See *Food and Agriculture Organization*.

FAQs Frequently asked questions, and answers to them. This is a page that is found on many web sites, and is self-explanatory. The term "FAQ" originated as the data file, usually in simple text format and no more than several pages long, that resides on host computer systems. FAQs evolved from the README.TXT file as a practical solution to giving new users the information they are most likely to need, when and where they need it. This also eases the burden of technical support staff from having to answer the same questions over and over again.

FAS See *fetal alcohol syndrome*.

FASB See *Financial Accounting Standards Board*.

FBO See *faith-based organization*.

FCA See *False Claims Act*.

FCC See *Federal Coordinating Center* under *National Disaster Medical System*.

FCE See *functional capacity evaluation*.

FCH See *family care home*.

FDA See *Food and Drug Administration*.

FDA defense A legal defense that limits liability in medical products liability cases if the medical product has been approved by the Food and Drug Administration (FDA). Michigan enacted such a law in 1996; it provides drug manufacturers and sellers with an absolute defense in products liability actions if the drug was approved by the FDA, and the approval was not obtained by fraud or bribery.

FEC See *free-standing emergency center*.

Federal Coordinating Center (FCC) See under *National Disaster Medical System*.

Federal Emergency Management Agency (FEMA) An agency of the federal government, within the Department of Homeland Security (DHS), responsible for national preparedness for all kinds of emergencies, natural or otherwise. FEMA's emergency plans are detailed in the **National Response Plan**. See also *National Disaster Medical System*. **www.fema.gov**

Federal Employee Health Benefits Program (FEHBP, FEP) A voluntary group health insurance program covering federal employees, retirees, and dependents. The program is administered by the Office of Personnel Management (OPM). See also *TRICARE*. **www.opm.gov/insure/health**

Federal Food and Drugs Act of 1906 (the "Wiley Act") A federal law, signed by Teddy Roosevelt in 1906, whose purpose was "preventing the manufacture, sale, or transportation of adulterated or misbranded or poisonous or deleterious foods, drugs, medicines, and liquors, and for regulating traffic therein, and for other purposes." The law was reportedly passed at least in part as a reaction to Upton Sinclair's novel *The Jungle*, which dealt with the unsanitary conditions prevalent in meat packing plants at the time. The law acquired its common name from Dr. Harvey W. Wiley, a chemist who promoted food adulteration studies and campaigned for a federal law. Dr. Wiley was called the "Crusading Chemist" and "Father of the Pure Food and Drugs Act."

In spite of the apparent seriousness of manufacturing and selling poisonous food, violating the law was only a misdemeanor. Furthermore, food adulteration continued because there was no specific authority in the law for the standards of purity and content that the Food and Drug Administration (FDA) had set up. A significant amendment to the law was passed in 1913. Known as the Gould Amendment, it required that food package contents be "plainly and conspicuously marked on the outside of the package in terms of weight, measure, or numerical count."

By 1933, so many changes had occurred in the food and drug industry that the FDA recommended a complete revision of the 1906 law and its amendments, which the FDA now considered to be obsolete. The first bill containing sweeping changes, introduced into the Senate that year, launched a five-year legislative battle. In what unfortunately was to become a pattern in the passage of consumer protection legislation, a tragedy in 1937 provided the impetus to get the new law passed. A drug known as Elixir Sulfanilamide, containing the poisonous solvent diethylene glycol, killed 107 persons, many of whom were children. The following year the *Federal Food, Drug, and Cosmetic Act of 1938* was passed by Congress, and the original 1906 law was repealed. Pub. L. No. 59-384, 34 Stat. 768 (1906).

Federal Food, Drug, and Cosmetic Act of 1938 A 1938 federal law, signed by President Franklin D. Roosevelt, that essentially replaced the *Federal Food and Drugs Act of 1906 (the "Wiley Act")*. The act contained the following key provisions:

- Extended control to cosmetics and therapeutic devices.
- Required new drugs to be shown safe before marketing (which started a new system of drug regulation).
- Eliminated the Sherley Amendment to the prior 1906 law, which required proof of intent to defraud in drug misbranding cases.
- Provided that safe tolerances be set for unavoidable poisonous substances.
- Authorized standards of identity, quality, and fill-of-container for foods.
- Authorized factory inspections.
- Added the remedy of court injunctions to the penalties of seizures and prosecutions that existed under the 1906 law.

This law was further modified by the *Safe Medical Devices Act of 1990 (SMDA)*. 21 U.S.C. § 301 et seq. (2005).

Federal Health Architecture (FHA) An initiative managed by the Office of the National Coordinator for Health Information Technology (ONC) that seeks to establish a federal health information technology environment that is interoperable with the private sector and supports the Strategic Framework. The "managing partner" of the effort is the Department of Health and Human Services (HHS), with the Department of Defense (DoD) and Department of Veterans Affairs (VA) as "lead partners." Also participating are more than twenty federal agencies involved in health care. **www.hhs.gov/fedhealtharch**

Federal Health Information Exchange (FHIE) A system to exchange health information between the Department of Defense (DoD) and the Department of Veterans Affairs (VA) to ensure that the VA has accurate medical records for military personnel who come into the VA system. After the FHIE system was up and running, a **Bi-directional Health Information Exchange (BHIE)** system was created so that the DoD has timely health information on those coming from the VA system to the DoD. The BHIE connects the VA's Computerized Patient Record System (see *VistA*) with the DoD's Composite Health Care System.

Federal Information Processing Standard (FIPS) A standard approved for use within federal government agencies to process or exchange information. Many such standards already exist, and new ones are approved by the federal government as technology changes. A FIPS is not created, owned, or controlled by the government, so it is not a standard in the sense of one created by a standards development organization (SDO). However, the government may require that information or documents submitted to it comply with one or more FIPS. Examples of FIPSs include the database language SQL and the document processing language SGML. Various cryptography methods have also been approved as FIPS, and will likely be of interest for anyone concerned with exchanging protected health information (PHI) under HIPAA. See also *Consolidated Health Informatics*.

Federal Information Security Management Act (FISMA) A federal law enacted in 2002 that requires every government agency to secure the information and information systems that support its operations and assets, including those provided or managed by another agency, contractor, or other source. 44 U.S.C. § 3541 et seq. (2004). FISMA is Title III of the E-Government Act of 2002 (Pub. L. No. 107-347, 116 Stat. 2899).

federalism A form of association between organizations that are independent but that delegate certain common functions to a central body. The United States is a federation. There is increasing interest in forming local federations among healthcare providers and agencies in order to allow organizations and institutions to retain their identities and yet to avoid duplication and thus to meet the unique healthcare needs of the individual community in the most appropriate and economical fashion.

Federally Funded Research and Development Center (FFRDC) A private, nonprofit organization that assists the U.S. government with scientific research and analysis, development and acquisition, and/or systems engineering and integration, usually in a long-term "partnership" arrangement. FFRDCs are typically sponsored by a federal agency and receive most of their funding from the government, but may receive up to 30% from private sources. Many are administered by universities or other nonprofits. FFRDCs are independent entities but have limitations and restrictions on their activities; for example, they are not permitted to compete with commercial enterprises. In fact, FFRDCs commonly transfer the practical results of their work to the public through such methods as cooperative research and development, technology licensing, open source participation, and contributions to industry standards. In 2007, the Departments of Energy, Defense, Health and Human Services, Homeland Security, Transportation, and Treasury; the National Aeronautics and Space Administration; the Nuclear Regulatory Commission; and the National Science Foundation were sponsoring a total of thirty-six FFRDCs.

Federally Qualified Health Center (FQHC) A local, community-based organization that provides preventive, primary care, and other services to those who might not otherwise have access to health care; sometimes called a community health center (CHC). To be "federally qualified," the health center must have the following features:

- Is tax-exempt nonprofit or public.
- Is located in or serves a high-need community (low-income, lack of access, or otherwise underserved).
- Provides comprehensive primary healthcare services, referrals, and other services needed to facilitate access to care, such as case management, translation, and transportation.
- Serves everyone in the community regardless of ability to pay.
- Is governed by a community board with the majority of members patients of the health center.

These "safety net" providers are part of the Health Center Program administered by the Health Resources and Services Administration (HRSA), Bureau of Primary Health Care (BPHC). FQHCs receive enhanced Medicare and Medicaid reimbursement, lower prices on drugs through the 340B Drug Pricing Program, medical malpractice coverage through the Federal Tort Claims Act (FTCA), access to the National Health Service Corps (NHSC) through designation as a Health Professional Shortage Area (HPSA), access to the Vaccine for Children program, and eligibility for various other federal programs and grants. There are three types of FQHCs: *Section 330 Health Centers*, *FQHC Look-Alikes*, and *Indian Health Service FQHCs* (see below).

The first health centers were for migrant workers, established by the Migrant Health Act of 1962. In the next ten years or so, approximately 100 neighborhood health centers were established under the Economic Opportunity Act of 1964, which was central to the Johnson Administration's "War on Poverty." With the phase-out of the Office of Economic Opportunity in the early 1970s, the coordinating responsibility was transferred to the Public Health Service. In 1975, the Community Health Center program was authorized under Section 330 of the Public Health Service Act (Public Law 94-63). The Health Care for the Homeless program was established by the Stewart B. McKinney Homeless Assistance Act of 1987. The Public Housing Primary Care program was a result of the Minority Health Improvement Act of 1990. Finally, in 1996, the Health Centers Consolidation Act brought together the community, migrant, homeless, and public housing primary healthcare programs under one grant structure, Section 330. The centers were reauthorized by the Health Care Safety Net Amendments of 2002. Section 330 grants provide approximately 25% of the funds needed to operate the centers; the rest come from state and local grants, Medicaid, Medicare, SCHIP, and other funding.

In 2007, over 1,000 health centers served urban and rural communities in every state and territory, covering 15 million people. About half of the patients live in rural areas and half in urban areas. Further information can be obtained from the National Association of Community Health Centers, **www.nachc.com**, and from the Indian Health Service, **www.ihs.gov**. See also *Rural Health Clinic*.

FQHC Look-Alike A Federally Qualified Health Center (FQHC) that meets the requirements for Section 330 funding, but does not receive Section 330 grants. An FQHC Look-Alike is, however, eligible for enhanced Medicaid and Medicare reimbursement, participates in the 340B Drug Pricing program, and receives an automatic Health Professional Shortage Area designation.

Indian Health Service FQHC An outpatient health program or facility operated by a tribe or tribal organization under the Indian Self-Determination Act or by an Urban Indian Health Program receiving funds under Title V of the Indian Health Care Improvement Act (see *Indian Health Service*). These programs may receive Section 330 funding and are exempt from the member governing board requirement.

Section 330 Health Center A Federally Qualified Health Center (FQHC) that receives grants under Section 330 (now Section 254b) of the Public Health Service Act. Organizations that may qualify for Section 330 grants include Community Health Centers (CHCs), Migrant Health Centers (MHCs), Health Care for the Homeless (HCH) Health Centers, and Public Housing Primary Care (PHPC) Health Centers.

Federally Qualified Health Center Look-Alike (FQHC Look-Alike) See under *Federally Qualified Health Center*.

federally qualified HMO (FQHMO) A health maintenance organization (HMO) that has applied for and received a designation by CMS that makes the HMO eligible to apply for a Medicare contract. The HMO must meet a number of requirements, which are stricter than those required for a *competitive medical plan (CMP)*. A federally qualified HMO may offer more diverse products than a CMP. It is also eligible for loans and loan guarantees not available to nonqualified plans.

Federal Register (FR) The daily (Monday through Friday, excluding holidays) publication of the U.S. government in which federal administrative agencies officially publish their rules and regulations (including proposed rules subject to public comment). The *Federal Register* also serves as the vehicle for the publication of legal notices, such as presidential proclamations and Executive Orders. A federal law provides that the contents of the *Federal Register* amount to judicial notice. Rules that are approved are then codified (officially entered and numbered) in the *Code of Federal Regulations (CFR)*.

A citation of the *Federal Register* consists of a volume number, plus *FR*, plus the page number. For example, a citation of 59 FR 63410 refers to volume 59 of the *Federal Register*, page number 63410. In this case, it is the 235th daily edition of this volume, published on December 8, 1994. Page numbering continuing across daily issues of the *Federal Register* accounts for the relatively high page number (the first page in this daily volume (59) being number 63241!).

Federal Tort Claims Act (FTCA) Generally, under the theory of "sovereign immunity" the United States may not be sued. However, in 1946, the federal government passed the Federal Tort Claims Act, which granted consent for the federal government to be sued for the negligent acts of its *employees*. For example, an Army doctor is an employee of the federal government. The FTCA provides relief to those injured by federal employees who were acting within the "scope of their employment," so a patient injured by the doctor's malpractice could sue the government. The FTCA was amended in 1988 by the Federal Employees Liability Reform & Tort Compensation Act (FELRTCA) (28 U.S.C. § 2679 (2005)), which provides that suit against the government pursuant to the FTCA is the exclusive remedy for those claims. In other words, the patient cannot also sue the negligent doctor. FTCA is codified at 28 U.S.C. § 1346(b) and 28 U.S.C. §§ 2671–2680 (2005). See also *tort*.

Federal Trade Commission (FTC) The federal agency that has jurisdiction over unfair and deceptive trade practices, including those that violate the federal antitrust laws. The agency includes the Bureaus of Consumer Protection, Competition, and Economics. **www.ftc.gov**

Federation Licensing Examination (FLEX) See *United States Medical Licensing Examination*.

Federation of American Hospitals (FAH) A national organization representing investor-owned or managed community hospitals and health systems throughout the United States. FAH provides representation and advocacy on behalf of its members to the federal government, the judiciary, media, academia, accrediting organizations, and the public. **www.fahs.com**

Federation of State Medical Boards (FSMB) An organization formed in 1912 committed to improving methods to determine fitness for licensure and the practice of medicine. Its members include the boards (see *state medical board* under *board (credentialing)*) of all fifty states, the District of Columbia, Puerto Rico, Guam, the Virgin Islands, the Commonwealth of the Northern Mariana Islands, and fourteen state boards of osteopathic medicine. See also *International Association of Medical Regulatory Authorities*. **www.fsmb.org**

fee A charge for a service rendered.

fee-for-service (FFS) A method of paying physicians and other healthcare providers in which each service (for example, a doctor's office visit or procedure) carries a fee. See also *capitation* and *prospective payment system*.

private fee-for-service (PFFS) A health plan with coverage very similar to Medicare, offered by private insurers as an alternative to Medicare. The federal government pays a subsidy to the private insurer for each patient. The amount of the subsidy was increased by the Medicare Modernization Act of 2003.

fee schedule A list of charges (or allowances) for specific procedures and services. See *antitrust* and *HCPCS*.

negotiated fee schedule A fee schedule for paying physicians or other healthcare providers, determined through negotiations (and contract) between payer and provider(s) ahead of time. Synonym: negotiated payment schedule.

FEHBP See *Federal Employee Health Benefits Program*.

fellow A person who has been granted status (fellowship) higher than that of membership by an association, for example, the American College of Healthcare Executives (ACHE) or the American College of Physicians (ACP). The status is usually given after the candidate has met strict requirements for education and performance.

The term is also used for certain individuals whose positions are supported by special stipends for advanced study and research, such as a "fellow in cardiology."

FEMA See *Federal Emergency Management Agency*.

fen-phen A contraction formed from the combination of fenfluramine (fen) (or a closely related drug, dexfenfluramine) and phentermine (phen), two commonly prescribed appetite suppressants, used as weight-loss medications. In 1996, in the United States, 18 million prescriptions for fen-phen were written each month. Both drugs had been separately approved by the Food and Drug Administration (FDA). The drugs had been frequently prescribed in combination due to greater effectiveness at lower dosages, and fewer perceived side effects.

In 1997, the Mayo Clinic reported clinical findings (not a formal study) of unusual valvular heart disease linked to the use of fen-phen. The findings were triggered by the observations of Pam Ruff, an echocardiogram sonographer at a North Dakota clinic, who first noticed a possible link between damaged heart valves and the use of fen-phen in 1994. (Cardiologists did not at first respond to her suspicion, so she gathered data over the next two years on twenty patients who had taken fen-phen and had valvular heart disease. At this point, in 1996, her observations were taken seriously.) As a result of the Mayo and similar reports, the FDA asked the manufacturers to voluntarily remove fenfluramine and dexfenfluramine from the market (phentermine was not withdrawn).

FEP See *Federal Employee Health Benefits Program*.

fertile Capable of reproducing. Distinguished from *infertile* or *sterile (nonreproductive)*.

fertility drug A drug that enhances the ability of an individual to reproduce.

fertilization The process of uniting the components necessary for reproduction, for example, a sperm and an egg, and thus starting the development of a new individual.

fetal alcohol syndrome (FAS) A pattern of birth defects found in babies as a result of the consumption of alcohol by their mothers.

fetus An unborn baby from the eighth week after conception until the moment of birth. Prior to the eighth week, it is called an *embryo*. See also *stem cells*.

FFRDC See *Federally Funded Research and Development Center*.

FFS See *fee-for-service*.

FHA See *Federal Health Architecture*.

FHFMA Fellow of the Healthcare Financial Management Association. See *Certified Healthcare Finance Professional* under *healthcare finance professional*.

FHIE See *Federal Health Information Exchange*.

FI See *fiscal intermediary*.

FIC See *John E. Fogarty International Center* under *National Institutes of Health*.

FICSIT Trials See *Frailty and Injuries: Cooperative Studies of Intervention Techniques*.

fiduciary A person who has a legal duty, created by his or her undertaking, to act primarily for the benefit of another or others in matters connected with the undertaking. The fiduciary owes a higher duty of care than a person acting only for his or her own benefit. Guardians, trustees, directors, and executors are traditional fiduciaries. Also, as managed care takes hold, and an intermediary (managed care plan or insurance company, for instance) makes decisions concerning an individual's access to medical care, it is becoming clear that the intermediary is a fiduciary and must act in the best interests of the patient. It must be noted that courts have traditionally been very protective of those to whom a fiduciary duty is owed, so a "breach" of that duty can have very serious consequences.

"Fiduciary" is also used as an adjective, to describe the duty of a fiduciary: a trustee has a fiduciary duty to protect the assets of the hospital.

FIM See *Functional Independence Measure*.

Final Rule See *rule*.

Financial Accounting Standards Board (FASB) A professional group that establishes standards for record-keeping, performance, reporting, and ethics (see *ethics (professional)*) for the accounting profession. **www.fasb.org**

financial director See *chief financial officer*.

financial statement A "picture" of the financial condition of an institution, which consists of a *balance sheet* and an *income and expense statement*.

financial structure The portion of an organization's balance sheet that shows how its assets are financed.

financing (finance) A method of obtaining money. Types available to hospitals include debt financing (borrowing money), equity financing (selling ownership—shares of stock—in the institution), tax-exempt bond financing (if available), and obtaining donations.

debt financing Obtaining money by borrowing.

equity financing Obtaining money by selling ownership in the organization (usually shares of stock).

tax-exempt bond financing The sale of *tax-exempt bonds* (see under *bond*) in order to raise money. In some instances, nonprofit hospitals are permitted to issue tax-exempt bonds (a privilege ordinarily held only by government entities) and thus may use this form of financing.

financing (health care) A method of paying for health care ("healthcare financing").

finding See *diagnosis*.

FIPS See *Federal Information Processing Standard*.

firewall A defensive security system consisting of either, or both, hardware and software designed to protect computers from unwanted outside electronic intrusion, rather than direct physical tampering or theft. The term has gained significance as more and more computers are connected to each other via electronic networks, such as the Internet, where such unwanted electronic intrusion is now not only possible, but likely. A computer that is never physically connected to an outside network would not typically need a firewall of this type. It is likely that this term will also be applied to other situations in which, for instance, part of a patient's electronic medical record (EMR) needs a high level of privacy protection as opposed to another part that doesn't need such protection.

firmware Computer software that is embedded in hardware, typically in one or more integrated circuits ("IC chips"). The use of firmware allows the manufacture of "smart" devices whose brains can be updated, without having to replace the device itself. The firmware, sometimes referred to as "non-volatile random access memory" (NVRAM), can be upgraded over time, as new technology becomes available, or as "bugs" are discovered and fixed. Common devices containing firmware include pacemakers and cell phones.

first aid Initial treatment of an injured or ill person, prior to the arrival of a physician or transportation to a treatment facility. See also *emergency medical technician*.

first assistant A health professional who is specially qualified to serve as a *surgical assistant*.

Certified First Assistant (CST,CFA) A *Certified Surgical Technologist (CST)* (see under *surgical technologist*) who has met additional requirements and is certified to serve as a surgical assistant by the Liaison Council on Certification for the Surgical Technologist (LCC-ST). **www.lcc-st.org**

Certified Registered Nurse First Assistant (CRNFA) A registered nurse, specially trained as a first assistant, who has passed an examination of the Competency and Credentialing Institute (CCI) (formerly Certification Board Perioperative Nursing). A retired CRNFA may use the credential CRNFA(E) (emeritus). **www.cc-institute.org**

first-dollar coverage See under *insurance coverage*.

First Responder See under *emergency medical technician*.

first year resident physician See under *physician*.

fiscal Having to do with finance.

fiscal function The sum of the activities, wherever performed, through which the hospital (or other organization) achieves fiscal (financial) soundness.

fiscal intermediary (FI) Previously, a private company that had contracted with CMS to pay Medicare Part B claims. Sometimes referred to simply as an "intermediary." See *Medicare Administrative Contractor*.

fiscal period An accounting period. A fiscal period is usually a year, and is therefore called a fiscal year (FY).

fiscal year (FY) An accounting period that covers exactly one year, at the end of which books are closed, and the year's financial situation summarized. The fiscal year may or may not be the calendar year.

FISMA See *Federal Information Security Management Act*.

fitness program A program intended to achieve and maintain a state of physical well-being that permits optimal performance.

5 Million Lives Campaign A continuation of the *100,000 Lives Campaign*. The new campaign, launched on December 12, 2006, by the Institute for Healthcare Improvement (IHI), asks hospitals to improve safety more rapidly than before in order to protect patients from 5 million incidents of *medical harm* over a twenty-four-month period, ending December 9, 2008. It is being sponsored principally by the U.S. Blue Cross and Blue Shield health plans. Six interventions from the 100,000 Lives Campaign are continued, plus six new ones were added:

- Prevent methicillin-resistant *Staphylococcus aureus* (MRSA) infection by reliably implementing scientifically proven infection control practices throughout the hospital.
- Reduce harm from high-alert medications starting with a focus on anticoagulants, sedatives, narcotics, and insulin.
- Reduce surgical complications by reliably implementing the changes in care recommended by the *Surgical Care Improvement Project (SCIP)*.
- Prevent pressure ulcers by reliably using science-based guidelines for prevention of this serious and common complication.
- Deliver reliable, evidence-based care for congestive heart failure to reduce readmissions.
- Get boards on board by defining and spreading new and leveraged processes for hospital Boards of Directors, so that they can become far more effective in accelerating the improvement of care.

501(c)(*) Section 501(section)(numbered paragraph) of the U.S. Internal Revenue Code of 1954 (as subsequently amended). Section 501(c) is the section dealing with *nonprofit* organizations exempt from federal income taxes. Any organization, to qualify for tax-exempt status under the Internal Revenue Code, must be incorporated in a given state as a nonprofit organization. Such incorporation, of itself, is not sufficient to grant exemption from federal income taxes. This exemption is granted only if the IRS, following application by the organization, makes a "determination" that the organization is properly qualified under a specific paragraph. Each numbered paragraph deals with a "class" of such qualified nonprofit organizations. For example, 501(c)(1) organizations are those exempt from income taxes because they have been organized under Acts of Congress; 501(c)(16) organizations are those organized to finance crop operations.

Three classes of organizations in health care find the 501(c)(*) classification useful for two primary reasons: (1) relief from income taxes gives all of them a substantial savings, and (2) for those qualifying for 501(c)(3) classification, the ability to obtain tax-deductible contributions from foundations and individuals may provide significant income. The three classifications are:

501(c)(3) The classification reserved for nonprofit organizations that are primarily charitable, scientific, religious, or educational. Nonprofit hospitals fall into this category, as do churches and educational institutions. **501(c)(3) organizations** are able to obtain tax-deductible donations from individuals and grants from foundations. (Foundations ordinarily are not able to make grants to organizations, even though the organizations are nonprofit, unless the grantee has obtained this designation from the IRS.) Foundations routinely request evidence that the applicant has obtained the 501(c)(3) determination from the IRS.

If a 501(c)(3) organization is a healthcare provider, the Internal Revenue Code requires that it must provide care to the indigent (*charity care*).

501(c)(4) The classification for nonprofit organizations that, although they may be similar to hospitals in many respects, do not satisfy the IRS that they are charitable. HMOs and PHOs typically are given this classification. They are then exempt from paying federal income taxes (this results in a substantial reduction in their operating costs), but contributions to them are not tax-deductible to the donor. Thus they are ineligible for grants from foundations and tax-deductible gifts from individuals.

501(c)(6) The classification typically described as that for nonprofit "trade associations." State and national professional associations, such as those of physicians, and associations of organizations, such as hospitals, usually qualify for this classification.

FLEX Federation Licensing Examination. See *United States Medical Licensing Examination*.

flexible benefit plan See *cafeteria plan*.

flexible spending account (FSA) An account managed by an employer that allows employees to set aside pretax funds for medical, dental, legal, and day-care services. An FSA may be a component of a cafeteria plan for providing health care, which allows employees to choose among various levels of benefits. Sometimes called flexible spending arrangement.

Flexner Report (The) A 1910 report, authored by Adam Flexner, commissioned by the Carnegie Foundation, and produced with help from the AMA, which proposed that medical education follow the "university-hospital" model used by Johns Hopkins University. This report revolutionized medical education in the United States. It suggested that the then-used "guild-apprenticeship" model be abolished.

flight nursing A subspecialty of *transport nursing*, which focuses on the needs of patients being transported by air.

Certified Flight Registered Nurse (CFRN) A specialist in flight nursing who has passed an examination of the Board of Certification for Emergency Nursing (BCEN). **www.ena.org/bcen**

float pool A pool (group) of nurses without regular assignment to a patient care unit who are kept in readiness to serve as float nurses, that is, to be assigned wherever needed to fill in for absences or to meet extraordinary workloads.

flowchart A type of diagram depicting the steps in a process and their sequence. Flowcharts are used, for example, in quality management to better view a process and find ways to simplify or otherwise improve it.

fluoroscope A device by which x-ray images may be viewed directly as the x-rays pass through the patient. The x-rays are projected on a screen, which responds to being hit by the rays in the same manner as a film does. The viewer can see in the fluoroscope the movement of the body organs and the passage of radiopaque substances. The physician carrying out a barium enema, for example, can manipulate the abdomen and get a variety of views of the bowel. (She also takes films for detailed study and permanent records.)

FMC See *foundation for medical care*.

FMG See *foreign medical graduate*.

FMLA See *Family and Medical Leave Act*.

FNIC See *Food and Nutrition Information Center*.

FNP Family Nurse Practitioner; see *family nursing*.

FNS See *Food and Nutrition Service*.

FOA Family Opportunity Act. See *Deficit Reduction Act of 2005*.

focus charting A charting system based on "focus statements." A focus may be a nursing diagnosis, a patient concern or behavior, a significant change in the patient, or a significant event in therapy. After the nursing assessment is conducted, a column is created with a list of focus statements instead of nursing diagnoses/problems, and a care plan is written. Nursing notes use focus statements, with the organization DAR: D = data about the patient, A = action (actual or planned nursing interventions), and R = response (patient's). The system was developed at Eitel Hospital in Minneapolis in 1980.

focused factory A manufacturing plant that limits production to one or just a few products and processes. The term is also being applied to a specialty hospital where physicians perform a high volume of a narrow range of procedures. See also *limited-service hospital* under *hospital*.

focus group A group of individuals convened to give their thoughts on a given subject. Focus groups are used in market research, for example.

FOIA See *Freedom of Information Act*.

Food and Agriculture Organization (FAO) The largest autonomous agency within the United Nations system, with the mandate of raising levels of nutrition and standards of living, to improve agricultural productivity, and to better the condition of rural populations. Areas of focus include land and water development, plant and animal production, forestry, fisheries, economic and social policy, investment, nutrition, food standards, commodities and trade, and food and agricultural emergencies. A major priority is encouraging sustainable agriculture and rural development, a long-term strategy for the conservation and management of natural resources. **www.fao.org**

Food and Drug Administration (FDA) An agency within the U.S. Department of Health and Human Services (HHS) responsible for protecting the health of the nation against impure and unsafe foods, drugs, cosmetics, biological substances, and other potential hazards. A major part of the FDA's activity is controlling the sale, distribution, and use of drugs and medical devices, including the licensing of new drugs for use by humans. The FDA's law enforcement functions have been in existence (under different agency names) since 1907, when the *Federal Food and Drugs Act of 1906 (the "Wiley Act")* became effective. The FDA got its current name from the Agriculture Appropriation Act of 1931. Previously it was known as the Food, Drug, and Insecticide Administration.

The FDA includes the *Center for Biologics Evaluation and Research (CBER)*, *Center for Drug Evaluation and Research (CDER)*, *Center for Food Safety and Applied Nutrition (CFSAN)*, *Center for Devices and Radiological Health (CDRH)*, *Center for Veterinary Medicine (CVM)*, *National Center for Toxicological Research (NCTR)*, Office of the Commissioner (OC), Office of Regulatory Affairs (ORA), and regional field offices. **www.fda.gov**

Food and Nutrition Information Center (FNIC) A service of the U.S. Department of Agriculture (USDA) that provides food and human nutrition information to nutrition and health professionals, educators, government personnel, and consumers. **fnic.nal.usda.gov**

Food and Nutrition Service (FNS) The agency of the federal government, within the U.S. Department of Agriculture (USDA), responsible for administering the variety of food assistance programs created by federal legislation. FNS programs include the school lunch and breakfast programs; Food Stamps; Women, Infants, and Children (WIC); and others. The primary emphasis of these programs is to improve the nutrition of children and low-income adults. **www.fns.usda.gov**

Foodborne Diseases Active Surveillance Network (FoodNet) A collaboration among state health departments, the U.S. Department of Agriculture (USDA), and the Food and Drug Administration (FDA) that closely monitors the human health burden of foodborne diseases in the United States. FoodNet consists of active surveillance at over 650 clinical laboratories, from which is collected information on all of the laboratory-confirmed cases of diarrheal illness. **www.cdc.gov/foodnet**

FoodNet See *Foodborne Diseases Active Surveillance Network*.

Food Safety and Inspection Service (FSIS) An agency of the U.S. Department of Agriculture (USDA) charged with assuring that the nation's meat, poultry, and egg supply is safe, wholesome, unadulterated, and properly labeled and packaged. The FSIS frequently cooperates with the Food and Drug Administration (FDA) in combating foodborne illnesses, such as salmonella infections caused by improperly handled eggs. **www.fsis.usda.gov**

food service Provision of meals and other nourishment to patients and personnel, and special nutritional services for patients, such as diet modification. Synonym: dietary service.

foot doctor A pejorative term for *podiatrist*.

FORE See *Foundation of Research and Education in Health Information Management*.

foreign medical graduate (FMG) A graduate from a medical school outside the United States and Canada. In order to practice in the United States, an FMG must be certified by the Educational Commission for Foreign Medical Graduates (ECFMG), have one or more years of accredited residency training, and meet other requirements of the state medical board.

alien foreign medical graduate (alien FMG) A foreign medical graduate who was not a U.S. citizen at the time of obtaining his or her medical education.

U.S. foreign medical graduate (USFMG) A foreign medical graduate (FMG) who was a U.S. citizen when he or she obtained medical education in a foreign country.

forensic Pertaining to the law.

forensic medicine The branch of medicine that deals with legal questions, such as poisonings, causes of death and injury, and the like.

forensic nursing The area of nursing focusing on the needs of law enforcement, including investigation and treatment of victims of assault or abuse, criminals, mass casualty, and unexplained or accidental death. Examples of forensic nurses are nurse coroner, nurse investigator, and correctional nurse. See also *sexual assault examiner*.

formulary (health plan) A list of all drugs that are covered by a health plan (or other payer). These drugs are usually chosen for their efficacy, safety, and cost-effectiveness. The formulary is sometimes "tiered" into several levels (tiers), with lower tiers (such as generic drugs) being fully covered by the plan (or having lower copayments), and higher tiers (such as brand name drugs) having higher copayments. Drugs not included in the formulary may not be covered by the plan at all unless under an exception.

PDP formulary Medicare prescription drug plans (PDPs) must follow guidelines, developed by the United States Pharmacopeia (USP) pursuant to the Medicare Modernization Act (MMA), in developing their formularies. The USP first divided drugs into **therapeutic categories** according to either their therapeutic use or an organ system, based on ICD-9-CM classifications. For example, a drug may be categorized as "analgesic," "antiparkinson," or "cardiovascular." Within the categories, drugs are subdivided into **pharmacologic classes** based either on the chemical structure of the drug or on its mechanism of action (how it works to achieve its results). The category analgesic, for example, includes the classes of "opioids" (such as codeine or morphine) and "non-opioids" (such as ibuprofen or aspirin). Some classes are further subdivided.

PDP formularies following the guidelines must include at least two drugs from each class in a category. If a class has subdivisions, the PDP must include one drug from each subdivision. If a category has no classes, the formulary must include at least two drugs from the category. Medicare Part D requires that there be an exceptions process for a beneficiary to challenge the placement or exclusion of a drug.

formulary (hospital) A list of drugs that are routinely stocked by the hospital (or other institution) pharmacy and that are available for immediate dispensing; drugs not in the formulary will have to be obtained by special order from other sources.

formulary (pharmaceutical) A document containing recipes for the preparation (compounding) of medicinal drugs but, unlike a pharmacopeia, not containing standards as to their strength and purity. See also *United States Pharmacopeia—National Formulary*.

for-profit An entity organized under any of various business forms (corporation, partnership, sole proprietorship, etc.) whose profits (excess of income over expenses) are returned to its members (shareholders, investors, owners) as dividends. See *for-profit corporation* under *corporation*, and *for-profit hospital* under *hospital*. Distinguish from *nonprofit*.

F/OSS Free and/or *Open Source* software.

foster care home A facility that provides *rest home care* (see under *nursing care*).

Foundation for Accountability (FACCT) A nonprofit organization dedicated to helping Americans make better healthcare decisions. It was formed by large healthcare purchasers in 1995 as a result of a series of meetings sponsored by the Jackson Hole Group. After the failure of national health reform measures in 1994, the participants sought ways to hold providers accountable and improve the quality of health care. FACCT worked on methods of evaluating quality of care, educating the public, requiring disclosure of information about healthcare providers and health plans, and supporting consumers in making complex decisions concerning their health care. FACCT has ceased operations, but its key healthcare policy and research documents remain accessible to the public at the Markle Foundation web site. **www.markle.org/resources/facct**

Foundation for eHealth Initiative See *eHealth Initiative*.

Foundation for Informed Medical Decision Making (FIMDM) A nonprofit corporation organized in 1989 in Hanover, New Hampshire, to obtain and make available the information needed to enable informed medical decision making. Its goals are to provide accurate and understandable information, to study and improve methods of communication to patients, and to develop, produce, evaluate, and disseminate programs that provide patients with information they can share in the decision-making process with their physicians (see *Shared Decision Making Programs*). Co-founders were John E. Wennberg, MD, and Albert J. Mulley, MD. **www.fimdm.org**

foundation for medical care (FMC) A nonprofit organization, usually of physicians, that provides *medical services review* (see under *review*) or *utilization review* of a specific population under a prepayment plan for health care.

Foundation of Research and Education in Health Information Management (FORE) A charitable foundation of the American Health Information Management Association (AHIMA) that promotes education and research in the health information management field. **www.ahima.org/fore**

fourth party payer See under *payer*.

FP Family practice or family practitioner. See *family medicine*.

FQHC See *Federally Qualified Health Center*.

FQHC Look-Alike See *Federally Qualified Health Center*.

FQHMO See *federally qualified HMO*.

Frailty and Injuries: Cooperative Studies of Intervention Techniques (FICSIT) A multicentered study sponsored by the National Institute on Aging and the National Institute of Nursing Research and carried out by eight independent clinical trials that assessed the efficacy and feasibility of a variety of intervention strategies, including exercise, in reducing falls and/or frailty in the elderly. Synonym: FICSIT Trials.

Framework for Strategic Action (FSA) See *Strategic Framework*.

Framingham Heart Study An ongoing study instituted in Framingham, Massachusetts, in 1948 by the National Heart, Lung and Blood Institute (NHLBI). Framingham is a community thought to have a reasonably stable population that could be studied over a long time. Its design was to enroll a large number of persons; give them thorough physical, laboratory, and x-ray examinations every two years; and record their medical histories throughout their lives. Originally, 5,209 men and women between the ages of thirty and sixty-two years were enrolled. In 1971, the study enrolled a second-generation group—5,124 of the original participants' adult children and their spouses.

Numerous scientific papers have been written from the study, and a substantial amount of important information has been added to the field of medicine, including the identification of the major cardiovascular disease (CVD) "risk factors" (a term coined by the study)—high blood pressure, high blood cholesterol, smoking, obesity, diabetes, and physical inactivity. In addition, significant studies have been performed regarding peripheral arterial disease, stroke, cardiac arrhythmia, dementia, cancer, arthritis, and other conditions. The study has now amassed a DNA library from two generations of participants—over 5,000 blood samples—as a basis for further investigations. Sometimes called simply the "Framingham Study." The study is now conducted in collaboration with Boston University. **www.nhlbi.nih.gov/about/framingham**

Franklin Award of Distinction An award created in 2002 by the American Case Management Association (ACMA) and the Joint Commission on Accreditation of Healthcare Organizations (JCAHO) to recognize exceptional hospital and health system case management. The award is named for Benjamin Franklin, co-founder of the first organized hospital in the United States. "His personal character, integrity and credibility as well as his notoriety as an entrepreneur and inventor represents the type of leadership and forward thinking required by the Hospital/Health System that wins this award."

fraud Obtaining products, services, or reimbursement by intentional false statements. Fraud includes such acts as misrepresenting eligibility or need for services, and claiming reimbursement for services not rendered or for nonexistent patients. Fraud is illegal and may carry civil and criminal penalties. See also *fraud and abuse*.

fraud and abuse The federal body of law applying to Medicare and Medicaid providers that prohibits three things: (1) the filing of false claims, (2) paying or receiving bribes or kickbacks for referrals, and (3) self-referral schemes. The practical effect of this legislation is greater concentration in the healthcare delivery system because it encourages physicians to form groups or become employees of a healthcare system. Violations of these laws can result in both civil penalties and criminal punishment. The Office of Inspector General (OIG) of the Department of Health and Human Services (HHS) enforces the civil penalties. The Department of Justice (DOJ) enforces the criminal penalties. Also known as the "Medicare and Medicaid fraud and abuse law." See also *Medicare Integrity Program*, *Stark I*, *Stark II*, *safe harbor regulations*, *Antikickback Statute*, and *false claim*.

freedom of choice A policy that permits patients to choose their own physicians. Such choice is at least restricted for persons who are members of an HMO or other managed care plan (MCP), because they must go to physicians within the plan (or themselves pay or pay more for care obtained elsewhere). In some HMOs patients must be satisfied with the physician on call.

freedom-of-choice waiver A waiver that excuses the purchaser of care from permitting freedom of choice to the beneficiaries. Freedom of choice is a normal requirement for Medicaid; a state, for example, wishing to carry out its Medicaid plan via managed care would need such a waiver from CMS.

Freedom of Information Act (FOIA) A federal law enacted in 1966 to establish an effective legal right of access to government information. The FOIA provides access to all "agency records," except those that are specifically exempted. Requests under the FOIA may be made by "any person," which is rather broadly defined. Although the FOIA applies only to federal agencies, each state has laws guaranteeing its citizens access to the records of its agencies. If the information you are seeking from the agency is about yourself, you can also make the request under the federal **Privacy Act of 1974**. Indeed, you should probably make requests for personal records under both the FOIA and the Privacy Act, since the Privacy Act also gives you the right to amend or delete information about you that is inaccurate or outdated. This is similar to the rights that individuals have regarding their protected health information under the HIPAA *Privacy Rule*.

FOIA was amended in 1974, and again in 1996 via the Electronic Freedom of Information Act Amendments of 1996 to include the many electronic media types that have come into widespread usage. The later amendment also extended the legal response period to twenty days from the ten days formerly required. Because many FOIA requests are so broad and complex that they cannot be completed even within this longer period, the amendment established procedures for a government agency to negotiate with the requester for an extension of time to respond. 5 U.S.C. § 552 (2005).

free-standing emergency center (FEC) See *emergency center, free-standing*.

free-standing facility A facility that is not a physical part of a hospital or other healthcare facility. A free-standing facility may be a facility for carrying out ambulatory surgery, urgent care, emergency care, or other care. "Free-standing" does not necessarily indicate separate ownership; a hospital may operate a free-standing facility or the facility may be owned by a separate organization.

FRG See *Function Related Group*.

FSA See *flexible spending account*. Also Framework for Strategic Action; see *Strategic Framework*.

FSIS See *Food Safety and Inspection Service*.

FSMB See *Federation of State Medical Boards*.

FTC See *Federal Trade Commission*.

FTCA See *Federal Tort Claims Act*.

FTE See *full-time equivalent*.

full-risk capitation See *capitation*.

full-time equivalent (FTE) A concept used in developing statistics on the size of a work force. The idea is to express a work force made up of both full- and part-time employees as the number of workers that would be employed if all were full time. It is computed by dividing the total hours worked by all employees in a given time period by the number of work hours in the time period. Thus an FTE would be, for example, one person working a normal work week, two people working half time, and so on.

fully integrated systems See *integrated health delivery network* and *network (health care)*.

functional administration (FA) See under *administration*.

functional capacity evaluation (FCE) A systematic process for assessing a person's physical capacities and functional abilities, particularly in relation to the demands of a specific work activity or occupation. It is used in connection with determining occupational disability status. It may be performed by a *disability examiner*.

functional food See *nutraceutical*.

Functional Independence Measure (FIM) A tool to document the functioning of a rehabilitation patient. It measures functioning in eighteen activities of daily living: thirteen motor items covering self-care, sphincter control, transfers, and locomotion, and five cognition items covering communication and social cognition. In each activity, the patient is observed or interviewed by a clinician and rated on the level of independence, from 1 meaning total assistance needed (by a person or device) to 7 meaning total independence. "0" means that the activity did not occur during the assessment period. The FIM is the core of the Inpatient Rehabilitation Facility Patient Assessment Instrument (IRF-PAI).

Function Related Group (FRG) A classification system for rehabilitation patients, based on the Functional Independence Measure (FIM). The "FIM-FRG" system is used to classify patients at the time of admission to rehabilitation to facilitate prediction of the length of stay and the level of function that can be achieved during rehabilitation, and to make comparisons between patients. Patients are classified by type of impairment and by severity of disability—there are fourteen severity groups for stroke, for example.

fund (noun) An asset set aside for a given purpose (e.g., a building fund), which is to be used only for that purpose.

bond sinking fund A fund in which assets are accumulated in order to liquidate bonds at or before their maturity dates.

debt service fund See *debt service reserve fund*, below.

debt service reserve fund (DSRF) A fund to account for accumulating and paying out the funds necessary to retire long-term debt that is not to be paid from specific sources. The term is used especially in government accounting. Synonym: debt service fund.

endowment fund A fund whose principal must be kept intact; only the interest income from the fund may be used. Sometimes called a permanent fund.

general fund Money that can be used; that is, money that has not been set aside ("funded") for a specific purpose. In governmental usage, the "general fund" has the same meaning, that is, it has not been set aside for Social Security, for example. Synonym: unrestricted fund.

permanent fund See *endowment fund*, above.

sinking fund Usually refers to a fund in which money is set aside to pay off financial obligations, for example, to retire bonds.

specific-purpose fund A fund whose principal and interest can only be used for the purpose specified. The restriction may be imposed by the terms of a gift or by governing body action.

unrestricted fund See *general fund*, above.

fund (verb) To set aside an asset for a specific purpose; for example, to "fund depreciation" means to set aside money at a rate determined by estimating the time before a given piece of equipment will have to be replaced so that, at the end of that time, there will be enough money to replace it.

fund balance A term often used by nonprofit organizations in their financial statements to indicate the difference between assets and liabilities. A positive fund balance is sometimes called a gain; in the profit sector, it would be called a profit. A negative fund balance is a loss in either sector. Nonprofit organizations may also refer to the fund balance as "revenues over (under) expenses."

fund-raising Planned and coordinated activities by which the organization seeks gifts. Fund-raising often goes under the term "development," and the fund-raising director is called "the director of development."

funds Available money resources. Several kinds are discussed in connection with hospital finance:

board-designated funds Funds that were unrestricted funds but were later set aside by action of the governing body for specific purposes or projects.

restricted funds Funds that can be expended only for the specific purpose for which they were obtained.

unrestricted funds Funds that the governing body can use at its discretion.

furry prozac An emotional-needs animal; see *service animal*.

futile care Useless; vain. Treatment, other than comfort care, that will not result in improvement or cure and that could not, in the opinion of the physician (and, usually, consultants), reasonably be expected to result in a quality of life that would be acceptable to the patient. For example, if a ventilator cannot extend the life of a patient, the doctor does not have to offer or provide it, even upon request of the family. Synonym: futile treatment.

futility policy A hospital policy dealing with the issues presented by *futile care*.

FY See *fiscal year*.

FYI For your information.

G

Gabrieli Medical Nomenclature (GMN) A medical nomenclature developed by Dr. Elemér Gabrieli, a pioneer in the use of computers in clinical medicine, to support automated medical text processing. It is hierarchical and includes 189,000 primary terms and 300,000 synonyms. It was originally developed as a lexicon designed to represent every medical word, phrase, or expression that may occur in a patient record, whether in canonical ("academically proper") form, layperson's terms ("head cold"), or vernacular metaphor ("my marriage ran out of gas"). Terms are classified into six categories: anatomy, physiology, diagnostic modality, clinical terminology, etiology of illness, and therapy. The codes include the source of the information—for example, if 4 represents clinical terminology, the code would be subdivided as follows:

4-1 = stated by the patient: symptom

4-2 = observed by the examiner: sign

4-3 = summary conclusion: diagnosis

and so on

The subsequent code units list the steps of subdivision leading to that particular term, for example, 4-3-9-1-1 for anemia, where 4 = clinical terminology, 3 = diagnosis, 9 = hematology, 1 = red cell disorder, and the final 1 = anemia. Thus the code chain describes the partitioning process until the term in focus is reached. Code chains may be long—eight or ten digits or more—but because they function as "medical machine language," the length is unimportant. A second, "local" code, which is totally random (not hierarchical), is also assigned to each term, so the term receives a "stable" code that does not change even if the term is moved within the hierarchy. Other codes include grammatical codes (part of speech), ambiguity codes, cross reference to ICD, CPT, and so on; these are all attached to the local code.

GAF Geographic Adjustment Factor. See *Geographic Practice Cost Indices*.

gagging A practice of some health plans of forbidding physicians from telling patients about alternative, more expensive forms of treatment than those authorized by the plan.

gainsharing A term without a fixed definition, it is commonly used to describe a variety of compensation arrangements that are designed to align the economic interests of hospitals and physicians. The typical intent is to provide cost-effective health care and to share in the resultant cost savings. This is accomplished through some combination of a fixed (or hourly) fee, or percentage payment. It may also refer to sharing with employees any increase in revenue that is the result of gains in productivity. Gainsharing is a form of incentive program or profit-sharing. (The term "profit" is not used in the nonprofit environment.)

Under a prospective payment system (PPS), where Medicare dollars are fixed, a hospital using gainsharing would typically share a portion of its Medicare Part A cost savings with the participating physicians. In 1999, the Office of Inspector General (OIG) of the Department of Health and Human Services (HHS) issued a Special Advisory Bulletin (SAB) that essentially outlawed traditional gainsharing programs. However, in later advisory opinions, the OIG approved arrangements between hospitals and physician groups to share the savings gained from reducing operating expenses as long as appropriate safeguards were adopted to protect against fraud and abuse. In 2002, the Internal Revenue Service (IRS) issued an information letter outlining ten factors that should be considered in any physician incentive compensation plan.

GALEN Generalised Architecture for Languages, Encyclopaedias and Nomenclatures in medicine. Formerly a project at the University of Manchester, U.K., GALEN was established to develop a model of clinical terminology "represented in a formal language, and associated with sophisticated support for different natural languages and conversion between different coding schemes." It was designed to provide a computer-based multilingual coding system for medicine for terminology covering "(1) elementary clinical concepts such as 'fracture', 'bone', 'left', and 'humerus'; (2) relationships such as 'fractures can occur in bones', that control how these may be combined; and (3) complex concepts such as 'fracture of the left humerus' composed from simpler ones."

GALEN is now being operated by **OpenGALEN**, a nonprofit organization formed to "enable the widest possible exploitation of some of the results of the GALEN Programme, in a more commercially-oriented framework." OpenGALEN's slogan is "making the impossible very difficult." It aims to persuade the GALEN community to contribute material as an Open Source effort to help complete a shared, central, application-independent part of the Common Reference Model, i.e., of the GALEN model of medical concepts (or "clinical terminology") that captures "'medical concepts'—the ideas we use to talk about medicine." Output in XML format is planned. OpenGALEN expects to fund maintenance and distribution of the resource. **www.opengalen.org**

Galen Institute A nonprofit organization founded in 1995 dedicated to research and education on health and tax policy. Its mission is to promote a more informed public debate about ideas that advance individual freedom, consumer choice, and competition in the health sector. **www.galen.org**

gambling counselor A counselor specially trained in the needs of individuals with gambling problems.

National Certified Gambling Counselor (NCGC) A gambling counselor with education in behavioral health who has met the certification requirements of the National Gambling Counselor Certification Board (NGCCB). **www.ncpgambling.org**

gaming Attempting to manipulate "the system" in an illegal or unethical manner. The terms "gaming" and "to game the system" are used, for example, in connection with efforts to bill under the prospective payment system (PPS) in such a way as to maximize income by giving as the principal diagnosis that which places the patient in the highest-priced DRG, even though a lower-priced one more correctly reflects the patient's problem and the services rendered. See also *coding (billing)*.

GAO See *Government Accountability Office*.

gaps Health services that are not covered by insurance. In particular, the costs or services that are not covered under the *Original Medicare Plan* (see under *Medicare*). See also *doughnut hole* and *Medigap*.

gastroenterology (GI) The medical discipline pertaining to the digestive (gastrointestinal (GI)) system.

gastroenterology associate A health professional who assists in caring for patients with digestive and other intestinal disorders, but who is not a nurse.

gastroenterology nursing The area of nursing focused on the needs of patients with digestive and other intestinal disorders.

Certified Gastroenterology Nurse (CGN) A licensed vocational/practical nurse who has passed an examination of the Certifying Board of Gastroenterology Nurses and Associates (CBGNA). **www.cbgna.org**

Certified Gastroenterology Registered Nurse (CGRN) A registered nurse who has passed an examination of the Certifying Board of Gastroenterology Nurses and Associates (CBGNA). **www.cbgna.org**

gastroenterology technician A health professional with special training in using technical instruments to measure pressure and acidity in the gastrointestinal system.

gatekeeper (health care) The person responsible for determining the services to be provided to a patient and coordinating the provision of the appropriate care. The purposes of the gatekeeper's function are: (1) to improve the quality of care by considering the whole patient, that is, all the patient's problems and other relevant factors; (2) to ensure that all necessary care is obtained; and (3) to reduce unnecessary care (and cost). When, as is often the case, the gatekeeper is a physician, she or he is a primary care physician and usually must, except in an emergency, give the first level of care to the patient before the patient is permitted to be seen by a secondary care physician. Synonyms: primary care manager (PCM), patient care manager. See also **case management**.

gatekeeper (judicial) A trial judge's role in ruling on the admissibility of expert testimony. The rules the judge must follow in doing this depend on the relevant state or federal statutory rules and case law. See **Daubert test**.

gatekeeping history A record of judicial challenges to the testimony of an expert witness. In a lawsuit, the trial judge must act as "gatekeeper" and decide whether an expert witness's testimony is both relevant and reliable before it will be allowed in evidence. The gatekeeping history would show how often a given expert witness was challenged, whether the testimony was ruled admissible or not, and, if possible, on what grounds. See **Daubert test**.

gateway (computer) In computer networking terms, any method by which a user can access the resources of one online network while being connected to another. Gateways can simplify life for the user because there is only a single entry point that needs to be learned and maintained, yet access to resources is limited only by the number of gateways the service provider makes available. See, e.g., **NLM Gateway**.

gateway (organization) An organization or system that provides a single point of access to a given universe of products or services. Unlike "directory assistance," which simply gives a referral "address," a gateway organization (1) provides service directly or, if it does not offer the desired service, (2) makes sure that the customer "makes contact" or reaches the proper destination.

health gateway A gateway organization that offers "one-stop health shopping" to a community. It not only provides one access point for the traditional healthcare services (for example, physicians, hospital care, and home care), but also offers a single, integrated link to the entire array of facilities and services that contribute to a **healthy community** and healthy individuals. The aim of the health gateway is to simplify the individual's access to the greatest degree possible, often by making appointments on the spot.

An information system (typically computer-based) is essential to the gateway's successful operation. It maintains a current inventory of all resources and contacts and assists in finding the requested resource. The individual may access the gateway via a variety of portals, for example, telephone (e.g., "Call 4HEALTH"), walkup "gateway information" stations (automated or human-staffed), a web site, and so on.

A health gateway should not be confused with a health **gatekeeper (health care)**. Whereas a gatekeeper sometimes makes the determination as to whether the individual should receive care (and, if so, what the care should be), the health gateway does not make judgments, but simply facilitates the individual's access to the requested service or resource. The table below illustrates some services that may usefully be accessed via a health gateway.

Type of Services	Examples	
Health Care	Physicians Other health professionals Mental health services Hospice services Home nursing services Immunization Prenatal care	Indigent health care Managed care plans Migrant health services Adult dental services Children's dental services Alternative health services

Type of Services	Examples	
Health Facilities	Hospital inpatient services Outpatient services Nursing home care	Hospice Assisted living
Home Services	Home nursing Therapeutic services Physical therapy Homemaker services	Fitness Companionship for shut-ins Elder day care
Appointments and Coordination	Physicians' appointments: "Who is on call?" Laboratory appointments	Hospital Consultations Education classes Time dollars for volunteers
Prevention Programs	Immunization Teenage pregnancy Screening Alcohol abuse prevention	Drug abuse prevention Child abuse prevention Domestic violence prevention
Health Education Programs	Firearm safety Fitness programs Water safety	First aid instruction Injury prevention
Health Information Resources	Health library services Video libraries	Internet
Links to Agencies and Organizations	Public health Public safety Social welfare School health	Parish nursing Environmental control Loan closets Health insurance
Human Services	Housing for the homeless "Sharing house" Transportation	Emergency shelters Employment services
Employer Services	Health risk appraisal Environmental consultation	Safety instruction Industrial health
Counseling	Substance abuse Domestic violence	Marital Family
Support Groups	AA Cancer	Bereavement

GB See *governing body*.

GCN See *Genetic Clinical Nurse* under *genetic nursing*.

GCP See *Good Clinical Practice*.

G-CPR See *Government Computer-based Patient Record* under *electronic health record*.

GCS See *Geriatric Certified Specialist* under *physical therapist*.

GDP See *gross domestic product*.

GDSA See *Governor Designated Shortage Area*.

GE See *genetically engineered*.

GEHR See *Good Electronic Health Record*.

gender identity disorder (GID) A DSM-IV psychiatric diagnosis sometimes given to *transgender* individuals. Highly controversial, the diagnosis is needed in many instances for reimbursement of clinical services (for example, sexual reassignment surgery (SRS)). It has many social and legal implications, as well, and there is a movement to change or remove it.

gene The basic unit of heredity, carried on a chromosome. It consists of a specific sequence of *DNA* nucleotides that carry the information required for constructing proteins, which make up the structural components of cells, tissues, and enzymes for essential biochemical reactions. See also *allele*.

gene-altered See *transgenic*, *genetic engineering*, and *biotechnology*.

General Accounting Office (GAO) Former name (until 2004) of the *Government Accountability Office*.

general nursing The area of nursing concerned with the health needs of a diverse population, throughout the life span, and that includes wellness and prevention as well as acute and chronic care.

general nursing practice A specialist in general nursing who has met the requirements of the American Nurses Credentialing Center (ANCC). **www.nursingworld.org/ancc**

general practitioner (GP) A physician who does not hold specialty qualifications, and who does not restrict his or her practice to any particular field of medicine. Most physicians who would formerly have been general practitioners are now specialists in family medicine or internal medicine.

generic Relating to or characteristic of a whole group. The term is often used in connection with drugs, where the meaning is slightly different; see *generic equivalent*.

"Generic" is also used in this book to describe a term that applies to a class of things, of which there are several types, each of which would be a specific rather than a generic type. For example, the term "steering committee" is described as "generic," whereas the term "building program steering committee" would be "specific."

branded generic See *generic equivalent*.

generic equivalent A drug that is identical in chemical composition to a brand name drug but sold under its chemical (generic) name. The first company that produces a drug, and holds the patent, is called the originator (or innovator) and the drug is called the **innovator drug** (or brand name drug). For example, Xanax is the innovator drug for alprazolam (its generic name). When the patent expires, other companies may produce the drug. If they sell the drug under its generic name, it is called a **generic drug**. If the generic equivalent is sold under a trade name other than the product's approved generic name, it is called a **branded generic**. Sometimes the originator competes with the generic manufacturers by producing its own generic of its innovator drug, for example, by allowing another company to produce it as an "authorized" generic or by using the company's own subsidiary corporation. It is often then sold for less than the generic companies' products, thus maintaining market share for the originator.

Generic equivalents are generally less costly than innovator drugs. In many states, substitution of a generic equivalent by a pharmacist is permitted (or required) unless the physician specifically orders that the brand name product be dispensed. In this case, the drug prescription or medication order would include the notation "dispense as written" (DAW). The physician who specifically prescribes a brand name product may feel that the generic drug has some differences not detectable by simple chemical analysis; for example, he may believe that its ability to dissolve may not be as good as the brand name product, or that it is not produced with as good quality control as that of a major drug firm that he trusts. The physician's reasons for choosing a brand name product over a generic one are often well founded.

To help control healthcare costs, some payers or providers impose a **maximum allowable cost (MAC)** provision. Under a MAC program, the payer pays only the price of a commonly available generic equivalent, whether or not it or a more expensive brand name drug was actually prescribed or filled.

A generic equivalent may or may not also be a *therapeutic equivalent* (TE) drug. See also *drug*. Synonyms: generic drug, nonproprietary drug.

generic product identifier (GPI) A coding system with a fourteen-digit number grouping drugs according to pharmaceutical equivalence. Products having the same GPI are identical with respect to active ingredient(s), dosage form, route of administration, and strength or concentration. The GPI does not consider the presence of inactive ingredients. See also *generic equivalent* and *identifier*.

generic screening See under *screening (quality)*.

gene testing Direct examination of an individual's DNA to detect mutations or matches. Such testing is done to screen for genetic diseases that may be passed to offspring, prenatal diagnostic testing, prediction of adult-onset inherited disorders or risk of other disease, and forensic identification. Earlier genetic testing methods used biochemical tests or examination of chromosomes, but not the DNA molecule itself. Synonym: DNA-based test.

gene therapy The treatment or prevention of disease by changing an individual's genetic material.

germline gene therapy Changing the germ cells (egg and sperm cells of the parent) to affect the offspring. Currently, no federal funds are being used for research into human germline gene therapy, due to ethical concerns. Although genetic information is sometimes used to make reproductive decisions, no cells are actually being changed.

somatic gene therapy Changing body (somatic) cells to help an individual. The change is not passed to the next generation.

genetic Pertaining to *genes*.

genetically engineered (GE) A product of *genetic engineering*. Often refers to food.

Genetically Engineered Food Right to Know Act A proposed federal law that would require any genetically engineered (GE) food to be labeled as follows:

Genetically Engineered: This product contains genetically engineered material, or was produced with a genetically engineered material.

genetically modified organism (GMO) A plant, animal, or microorganism whose basic genetic material (DNA) has been manipulated to achieve a specific result, such as resistance to an organism or a chemical, increase of life span, or to contain more nutrients. This is an application of the same bioengineering methods used to produce such drugs as interferon, insulin, and growth hormone. See also *genetic engineering*.

genetic code The instructions in a gene for making a specific protein. A single code contains three of the letters A, T, G, and C, which represent the bases in DNA. The term "genetic code" may also refer to a table showing all of the combinations.

genetic counseling Providing information and support to families who are at risk for, or already have, birth defects or genetic disorders or diseases.

genetic counselor A health professional with at least a master's degree in genetic counseling. Genetic counselors come from a variety of backgrounds, such as biology/biosciences, psychology, genetics, and nursing.

Certified Genetic Counselor (CGC) A genetic counselor who has passed certification examinations of the American Board of Genetic Counseling (ABGC). **www.abgc.net**

genetic disease A disease caused by an individual's genetic material. The disease may be one that continues from generation to generation due to a continuing genetic fault, or one due to a noninherited mutation.

genetic drift Random changes in genes and chromosomes; unpredictable changes without a known cause.

genetic engineering The purposeful manipulation of an organism's genetic material. Genetic engineering may be done at the molecular level by advanced technologies. It has also been done for centuries by farmers and biologists using selective breeding and other means of artificial selection, such as destruction of unwanted individuals so that they would not reproduce. However, until recent technological advances, these "natural" efforts have been confined to the same species. New techniques now permit transferring genes among species, creating transgenic organisms that are entirely new. For example, an "antifreeze" gene from a fish was used to create a tomato that could withstand ordinary frost. See also *genetically modified organism*.

genetic epidemiology See under *epidemiology*.

geneticist A scientist who studies genetics. Usually holds a PhD or MD and may work in research, laboratory, or teaching.

geneticization A term coined by Abby Lippman referring to the social process of making distinctions between individuals based on their DNA, defining diseases, disorders, behaviors, and other social differences as being genetically determined.

genetic linkage Two genes on the same chromosome that are not passed on independently, but are transmitted together.

genetic map A linear map of the relative position of genes along a chromosome.

genetic mapping Determining the physical location of a gene or genetic marker on a chromosome.

genetic material See *genome*.

genetic nursing The area of nursing that provides care to individuals and families who have a known genetic condition, are at risk to develop a genetic condition, or have children with genetic conditions.

    Advanced Practice Nurse in Genetics (APNG) An advanced practice nurse with at least a master's degree and experience in genetic nursing who has met the certification requirements of the Genetic Nursing Credentialing Commission (GNCC). **www.geneticnurse.org**

    Genetic Clinical Nurse (GCN) A registered nurse with a bachelor's degree and experience in genetic nursing who has met the certification requirements of the Genetic Nursing Credentialing Commission (GNCC). **www.geneticnurse.org**

genetics The study of genes and heredity. See also *genetic counseling*, *genetic epidemiology* (under *epidemiology*), *genomics*, and *pharmacogenomics*.

    behavioral genetics The study of how genetics and the environment contribute to individual variations in human behavior.

    biochemical genetics The study of the biochemistry of genes.

    clinical genetics The application of the science of genetics in a clinical setting, including counseling, diagnosis, treatment, and research.

    cytogenetics The study of genetics at the cellular level.

    human genetics The science of genetics in humans.

    medical genetics The application of genetics to human health.

    molecular genetics The science of genetics at the molecular level.

    population genetics The study of genetics at the level of populations.

    public health genetics The study of genetics in relation to public health and the prevention of disease.

genetic test Testing to find out if an individual has an inherited disorder, has a predisposition for any such disorders, or is a carrier.

Genew See *Human Gene Nomenclature*.

genius grant See *MacArthur Foundation*.

genome The complete set of genetic material that is passed from one generation of an organism to the next. The genome contains the instructions for all cellular structures and activities for the lifetime of the cell or organism. The human genome consists of tightly coiled threads of deoxyribonucleic acid (see **DNA**) and associated protein molecules, organized into structures called chromosomes. Every nucleus of a person's many trillions of cells contains the genome. The term was coined from *gene* and chromos*ome*. See also **Human Genome Project**.

genome sequencing strategies In the human genome sequencing effort, two "competing" strategies have been employed. One is called the "whole shotgun" approach, in which the human genome is broken into many fragments, which are then analyzed as to their DNA sequences, and later reassembled by the use of computer algorithms that determine where they overlap. The **Human Genome Project** used a different technique, the "nested shotgun" approach, in which the human genome is "chopped" into segments of decreasing size that are placed in rough order, analyzed as to their DNA sequences, and then reassembled into their known relative order.

Genomes to Life (GTL) See *Genomics:GTL*.

genomic library A repository of fragments of *DNA*.

genomic medicine See *medical genetics* under *genetics*.

genomics The study of genomes on a large scale. The term was created by the Human Genome Project to cover the expanded range of investigation and discovery about genetics and their application to human health. See also **proteomics**.

structural genomics The three-dimensional study of the proteins forming and associated with the human genome.

Genomics:GTL Subtitled "Systems Biology for Energy and Environment," Genomics:GTL is a research project of the Department of Energy (DOE) to use new genomic data and high technologies to study microbes and plants at the molecular, cellular, and community levels. The goal is to learn about fundamental biological processes and then translate the knowledge into new technologies—"biobased solutions"—for energy and environmental problems. For example, the DOE has already sponsored the genome sequencing of key plants and some 200 microbes relevant to generating clean energy, cleaning up toxic waste from nuclear weapons development, and cycling carbon from the atmosphere. "GTL" comes from an earlier DOE proposal for the next stage of the Human Genome Project, and stands for "Genomes to Life." genomicsgtl.energy.gov

genotype The genetic makeup of an organism, as contrasted with its physical appearance, which is called its phenotype.

genuine progress indicator (GPI) A measure of the national economy that takes into account such factors as depletion of natural resources, the costs of crime, the household and volunteer economy, defensive expenditures (other than against crime), the distribution of income, and the loss of leisure. The GPI is a start toward an economic indicator to replace the gross domestic product (GDP), which is based entirely on money and industrial and service production data and thus does not allow for other factors that bear on the satisfaction of people with the condition of the nation. It is suggested by its authors that such an indicator would be a better guide to public policy than the GDP. The GPI is the product of Redefining Progress, a nonprofit public-policy organization in San Francisco.

Geographic Adjustment Factor (GAF) See *Geographic Practice Cost Indices*.

Geographic Practice Cost Indices (GPCIs) A method used to adjust payments made to Medicare providers based on their geographical location. Pronounced "gypsies." Sometimes referred to as the Geographic Adjustment Factor (GAF). See **Omnibus Budget Reconciliation Act of 1989**.

geriatric Pertaining to *elderly* people.

geriatric consultation team An in-hospital team, typically consisting of a physician, a registered nurse, and a social worker, all of whom are specialists in geriatric medicine and the problems of the elderly. Such a team evaluates the needs of a geriatric patient on admission to the hospital and provides recommendations on the patient's care to the direct care providers.

geriatrician A physician specializing in the care of patients with multiple chronic diseases who may not be able to be cured but whose care can be managed. Care for such patients involves collaboration of a team of physicians, nurses, therapists, and other caregivers appropriate to the needs of the individual patient. Special efforts are made to educate and empower the patients, other caregivers, and other providers in the care process. Because the chronic diseases usually accumulate through aging, most of the patients are older, but because the disability may arise from any cause, such as cerebral palsy, Down's syndrome, trauma (e.g., veterans), lifestyle choices, or the environment, the geriatrician is not restricted to the care of the elderly.

geriatrics The branch of medicine concerned with the medical problems and care of the elderly. This is the traditional definition, but the field is broadening; see *geriatrician*. See also *gerontology*.

German-style system A regulated multipayer system of health care. In Germany, approximately 1,200 nonprofit insurance plans, called *Krankenkasse* or "sickness funds," are organized by employers, labor unions, and professional groups. The plans are funded by equal payroll taxes on both employers and employees. Self-employed and wealthier employees may purchase private insurance. Funds are turned over to regional networks of physicians, who reimburse doctors in private practice, and to hospitals, who pay their staff physicians. Physician networks oversee their members' utilization. The government oversees fee negotiations, which set global budgets, and also covers the poor and the unemployed.

germline gene therapy See under *gene therapy*.

gerodentistry Dentistry of geriatric patients.

gerontological nursing The area of nursing concerned with the health needs of older adults.

    Board Certified Gerontological Nurse A registered nurse with a Bachelor of Science in Nursing (BSN) degree who is qualified in gerontological nursing and has passed an examination of the American Nurses Credentialing Center (ANCC) (**www.nursingworld.org/ancc**). The credential is RN,BC (Registered Nurse, Board Certified).

    Certified Gerontological Nurse A registered nurse with an associate degree or diploma who is qualified in gerontological nursing and has passed an examination of the American Nurses Credentialing Center (ANCC) (**www.nursingworld.org/ancc**). The credential is RN,C (Registered Nurse, Certified).

    Clinical Specialist in Gerontological Nursing A clinical nurse specialist with a graduate degree who is qualified in gerontological nursing and has passed an examination of the American Nurses Credentialing Center (ANCC) (**www.nursingworld.org/ancc**). The credential is APRN,BC (Advanced Practice Registered Nurse, Board Certified).

    Gerontological Nurse Practitioner (GNP) A nurse practitioner with a master's degree from a gerontological nursing practitioner program. A GNP who has passed the GNP examination of the American Nurses Credentialing Center (ANCC) (**www.nursingworld.org/ancc**) may use the credential APRN,BC (Advanced Practice Registered Nurse, Board Certified).

gerontology The multidisciplinary study of the biological, psychological, and social processes of aging and the elderly. See also *geriatrics*.

    preventive gerontology Preventive services for the elderly in order to avoid illness and disability.

GHAA Group Health Association of America. See *American Association of Health Plans*.

ghost PPO See *silent PPO*.

GI See *gastroenterology*.

GID See *gender identity disorder*.

global budget A limit on total healthcare spending for a given unit of population, taking into account all sources of funds. In healthcare reform discussions and proposals, it usually means that caps will be placed on (1) employers' expenditures, based on payroll; (2) individuals' expenditures for insurance, based on income; (3) institutional budgets' "core spending";

and (4) personal out-of-pocket expenditures. Problem areas include how the information on total spending data is obtained and how the "cap" is enforced.

global capitation See *capitation*.

global fee A single fee charged for certain medical services that would otherwise be broken down into a number of separate fees. Managed care plans frequently use this method to achieve greater predictability of costs, because there otherwise could be significant variations in what separate services the provider actually bills for. For any complex surgery, for instance, there are office visits before and after the actual surgery, and a global fee encompasses all of these services in one single fee. See also *unbundling*.

Global Utilization of Streptokinase and Tissue Plasminogen Activator for Occluded Coronary Arteries (GUSTO) An international randomized clinical trial that compared four strategies for using thrombolytic agents for acute myocardial infarction. The study was organized in 1989, begun in 1990, and completed in 1993. A total of 1,081 hospitals in North America, Europe, Israel, New Zealand, and Australia participated in the study, which included 41,021 patients.

GME See *graduate medical education* under *medical education*, under *education*.

GMENAC See *Graduate Medical Education National Advisory Committee*.

GMN See *Gabrieli Medical Nomenclature*.

GMO See *genetically modified organism*.

GNP See *Gerontological Nurse Practitioner* (under *gerontological nursing*) and *gross national product*.

going bare Slang for practicing without professional liability insurance coverage.

Gold Seal of Approval A symbol, proprietary to the Joint Commission on Accreditation of Healthcare Organizations (JCAHO), that may be displayed by healthcare organizations that have been accredited or certified by JCAHO.

Good Clinical Practice (GCP) A standard established by the Food and Drug Administration (FDA) for the design, conduct, performance, monitoring, auditing, recording, analysis, and reporting of FDA-regulated clinical trials.

Good Electronic Health Record (GEHR) A three-year project (1991–1995) within the European Health Telematics research program (Advanced Informatics in Medicine) that developed a comprehensive multimedia data architecture for using and sharing electronic health records. The GEHR project consortium involved twenty-one participating organizations in seven European countries, and included clinicians from different professions and disciplines, computer scientists in commercial and academic institutions, and major multinational companies. The architecture object model, exchange format, term sets, and specifications of access and integration tools were placed in the public domain.

good faith A legal term that means "honest in fact," and describes the state of mind of someone acting without intent to defraud or injure, but with the intent of carrying out his or her legal and professional duties honestly and fairly, without ulterior or dishonest motive. See also *duty (legal)* and *liability (legal)*.

Good Samaritan statute A state law that protects a volunteer who stops at the scene of an accident and assists the victims, making that volunteer immune from suit as long as she or he did not act maliciously or recklessly. Most states have such a law.

governing body The body that is legally responsible for a hospital's policies, organization, management, and quality of care. The governing body is accountable to the owner of the hospital, which may, for example, be a corporation, a unit of government, or the community (see *accountability (governance)*). The governing body is often called the "hospital board," "board of trustees," "governing board," or "board of directors." Individual members of the body are "trustees" or "directors," depending on the name of the body. There is a growing tendency to call the governing body the "board of directors" in order to emphasize its role in establishing policy and directing the hospital toward goals. The term "board of trustees" is losing some favor because trusteeship may be equated with safeguarding rather than achieving. Synonyms: hospital board, board of trustees, governing board, board of directors.

Government Accountability Office (GAO) The agency of the federal government that is the auditing arm of the legislative branch and its financial consultant. Independent and nonpartisan, the GAO is sometimes called the "congressional watchdog." Formerly (until 2004) called the General Accounting Office. **www.gao.gov**

Government Computer-based Patient Record (G-CPR) See under *electronic health record*.

Governor-Designated Shortage Area (GDSA) An area in a state that has been designated by the state's governor as medically underserved. It may or may not also be federally designated as a Medically Underserved Area (MUA).

GP See *general practitioner*.

GPCIs Pronounced "gypsies." See *Geographic Practice Cost Indices*.

GPI See *genuine progress indicator*.

GPO Group purchasing organization. An alliance formed to take advantage of *group purchasing* (see under *purchasing*).

GPWW Group practice without walls; see *clinic without walls*.

graduate An individual who has attained a given academic degree or has been certified as completing an education program not leading to a degree.

graduate medical education (GME) See under *medical education*, under *education*.

Graduate Medical Education National Advisory Committee (GMENAC) A task force established in 1976 by the Department of Health, Education and Welfare (now HHS) to study the need for physicians in the United States. There had been a general consensus that there was a physician shortage. The GMENAC issued a report in 1980 that predicted the United States would have a surplus of 70,000 physicians by 1990, and that this would grow to 145,000 by 2000. It also estimated that there would be shortages in psychiatry, preventive medicine, and emergency medicine, but that the needs for family medicine, general internal medicine, and general pediatrics would be nearly balanced.

graduate year one (GY-1) The term applied to the residency position for a physician who has already had formal training in medicine, and who is now obtaining his or her first year of supervised practical training. This position may also be called a "first year residency," and the person may be called a "first year resident physician."

The term "internship" was formerly given to this position, but "intern" is no longer restricted to physicians; the term is applied in many disciplines.

graft See *transplant*.

granny dumping See under *dumping*.

grant A sum of money given by the government, a foundation, or another organization to support a program, project, organization, or individual.

    block grant A type of health grant from the federal government in which a "block" of money is provided, and the recipient is given relatively broad discretion in its use.

    categorical grant Federal funds that have been provided for specific purposes; for example, the treatment of cancer or the establishment of a burn center.

GRASP A workload management system used in hospitals, nursing homes, and home health on a system-wide basis and within units, including nursing, ancillary, and support departments. Work is divided into four components: process, teaching and emotional support (in clinical settings), direct care, and indirect care. Data, collected manually or through the institution's automated systems, are analyzed and presented using GRASP software. The result provides both information and essential documentation, and is used for budgeting, meeting regulatory requirements, process improvement, quality improvement, scheduling, skill-mix analysis, staffing, and work redesign.

GRASP is an initialism for "Grace Reynolds Application and Study of PETO," extended research completed in 1973 at Grace Hospital in Morgantown, North Carolina, funded by the

Kate B. Reynolds Trust to study and extend the applications of the *PETO* system. GRASP is now a product of GRASP Systems International, Inc. **www.graspinc.com**

GRATEFUL MED Software offered by the National Library of Medicine (NLM) for both PC and Macintosh computers to facilitate searching NLM's Medical Literature Analysis and Retrieval System (MEDLARS). **Internet Grateful Med (IGM)** was developed for access via the Internet, but has been replaced by the *NLM Gateway*.

green cleaning Using healthy, safe, and environmentally friendly cleaning products and technologies. The American Society for Healthcare Environmental Services has adopted a position encouraging healthcare facilities to use green practices for cleaning and disinfection, but to make sure that the procedures are clinically proven to be effective.

gross domestic product (GDP) The market value of all goods and services produced by labor and property *within* the United States during a particular period of time. Income from overseas operations of a domestic corporation would not be included in the GDP, but activities carried on within U.S. borders by a foreign company would be. The GDP measures how the U.S. *economy* is doing.

In 1991, the GDP replaced the *gross national product (GNP)* to bring the United States into greater conformity with international measures of national income. See also *national health expenditures* and *Genuine Progress Indicator*.

gross national product (GNP) The market value of all goods and services produced by labor and property supplied by residents of the United States during a particular period of time. Income from overseas operations of a domestic corporation would be included in the GNP, which measures how U.S. *residents* are doing economically. See *gross domestic product*.

Grouper A software program (logic) by which patient bills under Medicare are classified to their DRGs, using the *Uniform Hospital Discharge Data Set (UHDDS)* (see under *data set*), which contains *diagnoses* and *procedures* coded to ICD-9-CM along with other standardized information about the patient. This program is also used for other classification; see *HIPPS code*. Grouper is distributed by the *National Technical Information Service (NTIS)*.

Group Health Association of America (GHAA) See *American Association of Health Plans*.

group practice See under *practice (business)*.

group practice without walls (GPWW) See *clinic without walls*.

group purchasing See under *purchasing*.

GTL See *Genomics:GTL*.

guanine (G) See *DNA*.

guaranty fund A pool of money, funded by assessing insurers, that is designed to protect healthcare providers and consumers if an insurer becomes insolvent.

guardian A person who has the legal responsibility, and the authority to make decisions, for an incompetent person or a minor. A guardian is appointed by a court. Sometimes the guardian will only make decisions about money and property management (in this case the guardian is usually called a "conservator"), and the protected person may still make personal decisions. In other cases, a guardian of the person is appointed to make personal decisions, such as those regarding health care. Some guardians have the authority to make both personal and property-management decisions. The written guardianship order specifically states the authority of the guardian. Synonym: committee of the incompetent.

guardian ad litem A guardian appointed by a court to represent the interests of a minor or incompetent person during a lawsuit or other court proceeding. A guardian ad litem normally has no authority over the person or property of the ward.

guardian of the person A guardian who has the authority to make personal decisions concerning the incompetent (mental) person, such as those regarding health care. Usually, the guardian of the person does not control the finances of the incompetent person.

guest bed program See *hotel-hospital*.

guidance counselor See *school counselor*.

guidelines Directing principles that lay out a suggested policy or procedure.

administrative guidelines Suggestions promulgated by an administrative agency as to procedure or interpretations of law. Guidelines are not binding as are regulations, which have the force of law. However, they are strongly influential.

clinical practice guidelines Statements by authoritative bodies as to the procedures appropriate for a physician to employ for certain diagnoses, conditions, or situations. They are intended to change providers' practice styles, reduce inappropriate and unnecessary care, and cut costs (see also *utilization control*). The first guidelines were for the management of a given diagnosis or of the treatment planned. More recently, other topics pertaining to health have appeared, for example, "Driving Following a Single Seizure."

The Agency for Health Care Policy and Research (AHCPR) has been charged with responsibility for producing "Clinical Practice Guidelines (CPGs)," and has issued a number of them. Several medical associations and specialty societies, as well as hospitals, have also published guidelines for various kinds of patients. Thousands of such guidelines have been published, some of which are subsequently rewritten or withdrawn entirely, so the number of and titles of those *in force* are constantly changing.

Guidelines are not the answer to controlling or improving quality, or controlling cost. Guidelines must necessarily be so broad that they will only identify extreme *under-* and *over-*utilization for a given diagnosis or procedure, or disclose conspicuously egregious practice. There is no way they can be tailored to the individual patient. They also raise serious questions with regard to malpractice, just a few of which are: (1) Is it OK to do *everything* in a guideline? (2) *Must* one do everything within a guideline? (3) If one stays within a guideline does this grant immunity from malpractice? (Yes; in some jurisdictions this is an affirmative defense.) (4) What if a guideline is withdrawn (or rewritten) and a physician still follows it? For potentially better solutions, see *clinical path* and *Problem Knowledge Couplers*.

Synonyms: practice guidelines, practice parameters, physician practice guidelines, guidelines for medical care. See also *protocol* and *performance measure*.

Guide to the Health Care Field See *AHA Guide to the Health Care Field*.

GUSTO See *Global Utilization of Streptokinase and Tissue Plasminogen Activator for Occluded Coronary Arteries*.

GY-1 See *graduate year one*.

gynecologic/reproductive health care nursing The area of nursing focusing on women's health needs, specifically concerning the reproductive system.

gynecology The branch of medicine dealing with disorders of the female reproductive system.

gypsies Common pronunciation for *Geographic Practice Cost Indices (GPCIs)*.

H

H See *Hematology Technologist* under *clinical laboratory technologist*.
HA See *health alliance*.
HAA See *Healthy Americans Act*.
HAB See *HIV/AIDS Bureau*.
HAD See *healthcare alternatives development*.
halfway house A facility, which includes living quarters, for persons who require continuing treatment for mental illness or substance abuse (including alcoholism), but who no longer need hospitalization. The rehabilitation services provided include guidance. Synonym: community living facility.
HAN See *Health Alert Network*.
HAPI Healthy Americans Private Insurance. See *Healthy Americans Act*.
hardware The physical components of the computer (keyboard, monitor, disk drives, and so on), as contrasted with the computer programs, which are called "software." Synonym: computer hardware. See also *firmware*.
harm See *medical harm*.
harmonization The coordination process used by standards development organizations (SDOs) to make standards work together.
Hastings Center A nonprofit organization dedicated to public service and education in the field of biomedical ethics (see *ethics (moral)*). Its staff conducts research in the field, and provides assistance to educators, students, ethics committee members, physicians, attorneys, researchers, and journalists. It publishes, bimonthly, the *Hastings Center Report* and *IRB: Ethics & Human Research*. Topics on which it has published include surrogate parenting, AIDS issues, allocation of health care, physician-assisted suicide, embryo research, genetic technologies, reproductive technologies, environmental ethics, chronic illness and long-term care, doctor-patient relationships, organ transplantation, and methodology in bioethics. **www.thehastingscenter.org**
HAV Hepatitis A virus. See *hepatitis A*.
Hawaii plan The healthcare reform plan instituted in Hawaii in 1974 with passage of a law (the Prepaid Health Care Act) that required all employers to provide health insurance for all employees working twenty hours a week or more. This is called *employer mandate* (see under *mandate*).
hazardous area A term used in healthcare facilities usually to mean an area with a fire hazard greater than usual. Specific definition in this usage can be found in the *Life Safety Code*.
hazardous materials (HAZMAT) Substances, such as radioactive or chemical materials, that are dangerous to humans and other living things. Many hospitals have "hazardous materials plans," which are similar to (and sometimes incorporated within) their disaster preparedness plans and that deal specifically with handling emergencies involving hazardous materials. In the event of a nuclear or toxic chemical accident, the plan would go into effect.

For example, a special entrance to the hospital is required to permit control over incoming patients, so that they and their clothing may be decontaminated; hospital staff must be specially garmented; air flow must be controlled to prevent contamination of other areas of the hospital; and so on.
hazardous waste Waste materials that are dangerous to living things, and so require special precautions for disposal. Hazardous waste includes radioactive materials, toxic chemicals, and biological waste (blood, tissue, etc.) that can transmit disease (also called "medical waste" or "infectious waste"). In health care, items disposed of regularly include used hypodermic needles, surgical sponges, and other products containing blood and body fluids. A

special concern is contaminated needles; a needlestick is one way in which AIDS and hepatitis B can be transmitted. Hospitals are taking great care to ensure proper disposal of hazardous waste; precautions include special, stick-proof containers for needles; colored bags to signal biological waste (red, for example); and other special handling.

Hazelden Foundation A nonprofit organization located in Minnesota dedicated to helping people recover from alcoholism and other drug addiction. It provides residential and outpatient treatment for adults and young people, programs for families affected by chemical dependency, and training for a variety of professionals. It also publishes information on this subject and related areas. **www.hazelden.org**

HAZMAT See *hazardous materials*.

HBO, HBOT See *hyperbaric oxygen therapy*.

HBV Hepatitis B virus. See *hepatitis B*.

HCAHPS See *Hospital Consumer Assessment of Healthcare Providers and Systems*.

HCBSP See *Hospital Community Benefits Standards Program*.

HCCA Health Centers Consolidation Act; see *Federally Qualified Health Center*.

HCEC See *Health Care eBusiness Collaborative*.

HCFA Health Care Financing Administration. The former name (until 2001) of the Centers for Medicare and Medicaid Services (see *CMS*).

HCFAC See *Health Care Fraud and Abuse Control Program*.

HCFA-1450 See *UB-92*.

HCFA-1500 A standardized or "universal" form for physicians to submit claims to payers for health services, developed by HCFA (now CMS) and the American Medical Association.

HCH See *Health Care for the Homeless*.

HCI See *Health Commons Institute*.

HCIdea A national database containing unique identifying information for individuals authorized to write drug prescriptions. Created by the National Council for Prescription Drug Programs (NCPDP), it contains over 1 million records, each with at least one additional industry-recognized identifier. Once *National Provider Identifiers (NPIs)* are available, HCIdea will provide a crosswalk to those identifiers. (However, not all prescribers will have an NPI.)

HCIT Health care information technology. See *information technology*.

HCO See *healthcare organization*.

HCP See *Human Cognome Project*.

HCPCS CMS (formerly Health Care Financing Administration) Common Procedure Coding System. A federal coding system used to identify medical services and supplies provided to Medicare patients. Pronounced "hick-picks." There are three levels of the system:

1. The CPT codes copyrighted by the American Medical Association form Level 1 of HCPCS. These codes are entirely numeric.
2. Level 2 are called the "national codes." They cover primarily durable items, but also injections, chemotherapy drugs, medical and surgical supplies, and so on. Level 2 codes are five characters long, with the first a restricted alphabetic character. Certain alphabetic characters are reserved for CMS; others are controlled by a panel.
3. Level 3 are "local codes" available individually to Medicare carriers. W, X, Y, and Z are reserved for this level. Alphanumeric modifiers may be used with both Level 2 and Level 3 codes.

Examples of alphanumeric codes: A0010 for an ambulance ride, A4927 for gloves, A9300 for exercise equipment, D7130 for a tooth root removal, G0008 for a flu shot ("Admin influenza virus vac"), P9610 for collecting a urine specimen, and V2020 for a pair of glasses (no kidding!).

HCPOTP Health care professionals other than physicians.

HCPR Health Care Policy and Research. See *Agency for Health Care Policy and Research*.

HCQIA See *Health Care Quality Improvement Act*.

HCQII See *Health Care Quality Improvement Initiative*.

HCQIP See *Health Care Quality Improvement Program*.

HCQM See *Health Care Quality Management and Patient Safety Certification* under *quality management professional*.

HCSL See *HealthCare Standards Landscape*.

HCSNA See *Health Care Safety Net Amendments of 2002*.

HCUP See *Healthcare Cost and Utilization Project*.

HCV Hepatitis C virus. See *hepatitis C*.

HCW See *healthcare worker*.

HDHP See *high-deductible health plan*.

health As defined by the World Health Organization (WHO), "health is a state of complete physical, mental and social well-being and not merely the absence of disease or infirmity."

health advocacy An allied health field that originated as "patient advocacy," efforts to help resolve patients' complaints in relation to medical care and hospital and other healthcare services and with the protection of their rights. Thus health advocacy was originally the field of the patient advocate or patient representative, also known as an "ombudsperson."

Today, however, the person who serves as the advocate of an individual patient's interests is but one variety of "health advocate." Health advocacy is also practiced by advocates for groups of people in health programs, by program specialists in health foundations, by advocates for special populations or interest groups, and by legislative specialists in health. The current trend is for this broader advocacy to be a joint effort of consumers and professionals.

Health Alert Network (HAN) A nationwide, integrated information and communications system serving as a platform for distribution of health alerts, dissemination of prevention guidelines and other information, distance learning, national disease surveillance, and electronic laboratory reporting, as well as for the Centers for Disease Control and Prevention's (CDC's) bioterrorism and related initiatives, to strengthen preparedness at the local and state levels. Funding for HAN supports connections to the Internet, training of the public health workforce via distance learning systems (satellite, Internet, or both), and the capacity to send urgent health alerts to local agencies via information broadcast technologies (e.g., broadcast fax services, autodialing).

health alliance (HA) An organization proposed in legislation in the early 1990s as a feature of the "managed competition" approach to healthcare reform. The HA was to serve as a "sponsor" for populations that would otherwise have no intermediary between their beneficiaries and organizations that provided care. Its basic functions were to bargain with and purchase health insurance from accountable health plans (AHPs) or other sources of health care on behalf of consumers, and to furnish information to consumers on the services provided by the competing AHPs, an evaluation of their quality of care, participant satisfaction, and price.

Health alliances would not be needed for groups such as corporations with many employees, state governments, and similar institutions that were large enough effectively to carry out the purchasing function themselves.

Initially, the organization was called a "health insurance purchasing corporation" (HIPC). This was then changed to "health insurance purchasing cooperative" (HIPC) and, later, "health plan purchasing cooperative" (HPPC). All were referred to as "hippick," an acronym no one could look up in a glossary. Another synonym was "insurance purchasing pool." The terminology seemed to settle on "health alliance."

health care or healthcare Services provided for (1) health promotion, (2) prevention of illness and injury, (3) monitoring of health, (4) maintenance of health, and (5) treatment of diseases, disorders, and injuries in order to obtain cure or, failing that, optimum comfort and function (quality of life).

During the 1990s the term "health care" increasingly began to appear as the single word "healthcare." A web search on Alta Vista in late 1998 yielded 966,901 hits for the two-word term, but 1,585,551 hits for the single word version. In July 2001, the same search turned up slightly more hits for "healthcare" (2,177,466) and even less (555,997) for "health care." Similarly, Google found 3,510,000 hits for "healthcare" and less for "health care" (2,820,000). However, in 2007, Google found 208,000,000 hits for "healthcare" but 357,000,000 for "health care."

At this point, usage is still mixed. We now have the Joint Commission on Accreditation of Healthcare Organizations and the American College of Healthcare Executives, but we also have the American College of Health Care Administrators. This book uses *healthcare* when the term is used as an adjective ("healthcare financing"), and *health care* when the main term is "care" ("higher quality health care"). The exception is a proper name or title, such as *Slee's Health Care Terms*.

healthcare administration See under *administration*.

healthcare alternatives development (HAD) A term that refers to the development of alternative delivery systems and alternative financing systems. One must seek the context of this term to understand just what is meant.

healthcare clearinghouse In the context of HIPAA, a public or private entity that processes or facilitates the processing of nonstandard data elements of health information into standard data elements. As such, it is deemed to be a *covered entity* under the act.

healthcare coalition An organization working on broad healthcare concerns, ordinarily including hospital and healthcare costs, and typically with provider, business, and consumer participation. Often there is government participation as well.

    business healthcare coalition A healthcare coalition composed of or organized by business firms concerned with healthcare problems, primarily those problems affecting employees of the member companies. Such a coalition is also likely to have providers and consumers as members.

healthcare consultant A person who holds herself or himself out as an independent contractor to provide professional advice and services to hospitals, often concerning management matters and planning. The American Association of Healthcare Consultants (AAHC) recognizes consultants in several specialties: strategic planning and marketing, organization and management, human resource management, facilities programming and planning, finance, operations and information systems, and health specialist. Synonym: hospital consultant.

    Certified Healthcare Consultant (CHC) A credential awarded by the American Association of Healthcare Consultants (AAHC) (**www.aahc.net**) to members who meet certain requirements, but who are not yet ready for Fellowship in the Association. This credential may be used after the individual's name until qualified as a **Fellow of AAHC**, after which **FAAHC** replaces it.

healthcare consumerism A system in which the buyer of healthcare services is the patient (the consumer), rather than the employer, insurer, or other third party. This puts control over health and health care in the hands of the consumer, which in turn requires that the consumer have access to complete, credible information with which to make important decisions about quality, cost, and effectiveness of healthcare services. This includes data about specific providers and their services, prices, and results so that comparisons can be made. It also includes information about health, wellness, and disease management so that the consumer can maintain and improve health, and can make informed decisions about treatment.

    Several trends are evidence of this emerging system. One is the movement toward *patient empowerment*. Another is the *consumer-driven health plan* (CDHP). A third is the direct marketing and advertising of healthcare products, such as pharmaceuticals, to consumers rather than to healthcare providers. Synonyms: consumer-driven health care (CDHC), consumer-directed health care, patient-driven health care.

Healthcare Cost and Utilization Project (HCUP) A project of the Agency for Healthcare Research and Quality (AHRQ) to develop clinical quality indicators. These became the *AHRQ Quality Indicators*; see under *quality indicator*, under *indicator*.

healthcare delivery A term sometimes used as a synonym for "comprehensive healthcare delivery system." However, the term "healthcare delivery" applies to providing any of the wide array of healthcare services as well as to the totality.

healthcare delivery system A term without specific definition, referring to all the facilities and services, along with methods for financing them, through which health care is provided.

Health Care eBusiness Collaborative (HCEC) A national nonprofit membership association working for improvement of electronic business (eBusiness) efficiencies in the healthcare industry. Membership is open to all healthcare providers and their trading partners. Formerly Healthcare Electronic Data Infrastructure Coalition (HEDIC). **www.hcec.org**

Healthcare Electronic Data Infrastructure Coalition (HEDIC) Former name of the *Health Care eBusiness Collaborative*.

healthcare executive An individual who works in administration and/or management within the healthcare field. Positions range from department head to chief executive officer (CEO), and may be within a hospital or other facility, healthcare association, home health agency, managed care organization—anywhere throughout the industry.

Certified Healthcare Executive (CHE) A credential awarded by the American College of Healthcare Executives (ACHE) (**www.ache.org**) to members who meet certain requirements, but are not yet ready for Fellowship in the College. This credential may be used after the individual's name until he or she is qualified to be a **Fellow of the American College of Healthcare Executives**, after which **FACHE** replaces it.

Certified Home/Hospice Care Executive (CHCE) A healthcare executive specializing in home and/or hospice care, certified by the National Association for Home Care & Hospice (NAHC). **www.nahc.org**

healthcare finance professional (HFP) A financial management professional working in health care. These include chief financial officers (CFOs), controllers, patient accounts managers, accountants, and others, employed in hospitals, integrated delivery systems, managed care organizations, medical group practices, public accounting and consulting firms, insurance companies, government agencies, other healthcare organizations, or as consultants.

Certified Healthcare Finance Professional (CHFP) A healthcare finance professional who has passed an examination of the Healthcare Financial Management Association (HFMA) (**www.hfma.org**). HFMA also offers certification in four subspecialty areas: accounting and finance, financial management of physician practices, managed care, and patient financial services. With further qualification, a CHFP may convert status to **Fellow of HFMA (FHFMA)**.

Healthcare Financial Management Association (HFMA) A national membership organization for healthcare finance professionals. **www.hfma.org**

Health Care Financing Administration (HCFA) The former name (until 2001) of the Centers for Medicare and Medicaid Services (see *CMS*).

Health Care Financing Administration Common Procedure Coding System (HCPCS) See *HCPCS*.

Health Care for the Homeless (HCH) A federal program to provide preventive and primary health services to homeless people. The program was established under the Stewart B. McKinney Homeless Assistance Act of 1987, and reauthorized under Section 330(h) of the Health Centers Consolidation Act. See also *Federally Qualified Health Center*.

Health Care Fraud and Abuse Control Program (HCFAC) A program established under HIPAA to combat fraud committed against all health plans, both public and private, and designed to coordinate federal, state, and local law enforcement activities with respect to healthcare fraud and abuse. HCFAC is operated under the joint direction of the U.S. Attorney

General and the Secretary of the Department of Health and Human Services (HHS), acting through the HHS Office of Inspector General (OIG). HIPAA requires that the program issue an annual report of the amounts deposited and appropriated to the Medicare Trust Fund, and the source of those deposits.

healthcare informatics See *medical informatics* under *informatics*.

Healthcare Informatics Standards Board (HISB) A multi-stakeholder ANSI group that supported the development of a common data model that could be shared by developers of healthcare informatics standards. HISB coordinated standards for:

Healthcare models and electronic healthcare records.

Interchange of healthcare data, images, sounds, and signals within and between organizations and practices. See *MEDIX*.

Healthcare codes and terminology.

Communication with diagnostic instruments and healthcare devices.

Representation and communication of healthcare protocols, knowledge, and statistical databases.

Privacy, confidentiality, and security of healthcare information.

Identifiers for healthcare providers, patients, entities, and so on.

HISB discontinued activities in 2005, and was superceded by the *Healthcare Information Technology Standards Panel (HITSP)*.

Healthcare Information and Management Systems Society (HIMSS) A nonprofit organization focused on providing leadership for the optimal use of healthcare information technology and management systems for the betterment of health care. It has over 20,000 individual members and over 300 corporate members. HIMSS united with CPRI-HOST in 2002. Activities in which HIMSS collaborates include the Alliance for Nursing Informatics (ANI), Certification Commission for Health Information Technology (CCHIT), Continuity of Care Record (CCR), IHE, and others. **HIMSS EMEA** has initiatives in Europe, the Middle East, and Africa (hence "EMEA"). **www.himss.org**

Healthcare Information Standards Planning Panel (HISPP) The precursor to the ANSI *Healthcare Informatics Standards Board (HISB)*. In the late 1980s, CEN, a European standards development organization (SDO), was actively working to establish healthcare informatics standards, and asked ANSI to coordinate U.S. efforts with those already underway in Europe. The formation of a planning panel is a mechanism that ANSI uses to foster collaboration in a field when there are several groups developing overlapping standards. HISPP was the result, formed in 1992.

Healthcare Information Technology Standards Panel (HITSP) An ANSI panel established in 2005 to facilitate the harmonization of consensus-based standards necessary to enable the widespread interoperability of healthcare information in the United States. Over 100 member organizations include standards development organizations, healthcare providers, public health agencies, consumers, and government agencies. The panel is assisting in the development of the Nationwide Health Information Network (NHIN) by addressing issues such as interoperability, privacy, and security. ANSI HITSP has recommended, for example, interoperability specifications in the areas of electronic health records, biosurveillance, and consumer empowerment. The Healthcare Information and Management Systems Society (HIMSS), the Advanced Technology Institute (ATI), and Booz Allen Hamilton (a consulting firm) serve as strategic partners with ANSI in this initiative, which has the oversight and backing of the Office of the National Coordinator for Health Information Technology (ONCHIT). See also *ONCHIT1*.

healthcare institution As commonly used, any institution dealing with health. Some definitions state that an institution, to qualify for this term, must have an organized professional staff. However, there are no regulations, such as standards for the licensure or registry of institutions, that currently restrict the use of this term.

Healthcare Integrity and Protection Data Bank (HIPDB) A national data collection program to help protect against healthcare *fraud and abuse*. HIPDB has procedures for reporting and disclosing specified "final adverse actions" taken against healthcare providers and suppliers. It was created under HIPAA. **www.npdb-hipdb.com**

Health Care Market Analysis System (HCMAS) A software program used by the Hospital Council of Western Pennsylvania, developed by Weston Medical Data Systems in Massachusetts. It provided reports comparing the council's hospitals with groups of hospitals and with individual hospitals in Pennsylvania. The data source was the data set the state required each hospital to report on every hospital discharge.

Health Care Network Accreditation Program An accreditation program provided by *URAC* for healthcare networks. The Joint Commission on Accreditation of Healthcare Organizations (JCAHO) also had a program, but it was discontinued effective January 1, 2006.

Healthcare Open Systems and Trials (HOST) See *CPRI-HOST*.

healthcare organization (HCO) An organizational form for healthcare delivery, such as a hospital or health plan. The Joint Commission on Accreditation of Healthcare Organizations (JCAHO) defines it for the purposes of performance measurement: "The business entity which is participating in a performance measurement system (e.g., health care organization level data describes information about the business entity)."

healthcare plan See *health plan*.

Health Care Policy and Research Agency for Health Care Policy and Research. Former name of the *Agency for Healthcare Research and Quality*.

Health Care Prepayment Plan (HCPP) A prepaid plan serving Medicare beneficiaries based on reimbursement, not risk. CMS will provide reimbursement for services actually provided. Distinguished from HMOs and similar plans in that HCPPs do not need to provide all Medicare covered services, do not have to offer open enrollment, and can avoid member appeal rights. HCPPs are frequently used by labor organizations to provide services for their members only.

healthcare professional See *health professional*.

healthcare provider See under *provider*.

healthcare proxy See *advance directive*.

Health Care Quality Improvement Act (HCQIA) A federal act of 1986 that (1) gave certain protection from lawsuits to physicians and hospitals for peer review activities and (2) set up a national clearinghouse of information on disciplinary and malpractice actions against physicians.

The title of the section concerning peer review is "Encouraging Good Faith Professional Review Activities." Participants in peer review activities who comply with the law are protected from liability, except for violation of civil rights or government enforcement of antitrust or other laws. The peer review must be done in good faith (without malice or ulterior motive, such as driving a competitor out of business), and anyone providing information to a review committee must also provide it in good faith.

Hospitals under the act also receive certain protection from liability for peer review activities and physician sanctions. To obtain the protection, the hospital must provide specified minimum due process procedures (basically, a fair hearing) to physicians prior to taking adverse action on privileges. The second portion of the act created the *National Practitioner Data Bank*. 42 U.S.C. §§ 11101–11152 (2004).

Health Care Quality Improvement Initiative (HCQII) A program launched in 1992 by HCFA (now CMS) to change the focus of peer review organizations (PROs) (now called quality improvement organizations) from individual clinical cases to patterns of care and outcomes so that healthcare quality could be improved. This was partly in response to reports from the Institute of Medicine (IOM), which stated that individual instances of poor quality care were usually due to problems in the larger system of care. The aim of the HCQII was to establish a collaborative relationship between providers and PROs. The HCQII evolved into the Health Care Quality Improvement Program (HCQIP). See also *Quality Initiative*.

Health Care Quality Improvement Program (HCQIP) A program of CMS that utilizes quality improvement organizations (QIOs) to improve healthcare quality and safety in the United States. QIO contracts are revised every three years and include a **Statement of Work (SOW)** that sets out the tasks to be completed by the QIO during the next three-year period. These SOWs have been numbered since their inception in 1982; the 8th Statement of Work, or "SOW8," covers 2005–2008. SOW8 requires, in addition to its ongoing tasks (review, etc.), that the QIO undertake quality improvement programs in the following areas:

1. Nursing homes
2. Home health agencies
3. Hospitals (including rural and critical access hospitals)
4. Physicians' offices

The programs for physicians' offices, for example, are to focus on more widespread adoption and use of health information technology; improving the quality, safety, and effectiveness of pharmacotherapy; and reducing disparities in care received by underserved populations. SOW8 will also focus on Medicare Advantage and prescription drug plans, electronic health records, and e-prescribing.

An extension of the Health Care Quality Improvement Initiative (HCQII), the HCQIP established quality-improvement projects as the primary function of the QIO (then called peer review organization (PRO)) in the mid-1990s. See also *Quality Initiative*.

healthcare reform A term without a clear definition, which is applied to the efforts on the federal, state, and local levels to make changes in the healthcare delivery "system" so that (1) costs are reduced or "contained," (2) everyone has health insurance coverage, (3) all citizens have access to health care, (4) financing is assured, and (5) quality of care is controlled or, preferably, improved. The options as to "management" of the healthcare system range from highly centralized, federal controls, through the setting of certain requirements at the federal or state level but allowing local innovation as to implementation, through local solutions even if nothing is done at the state or national level.

Health Care Safety Net Amendments of 2002 (HCSNA) Federal legislation that reauthorized the "community health centers program" (see *Federally Qualified Health Center*) and the *National Health Service Corps*, and made other provisions to strengthen health care for rural and underserved areas. The law provided automatic facility status as Health Professional Shortage Areas (HPSAs) to all FQHCs, and to those Rural Health Clinics (RHCs) that provide access to health care to all without regard to ability to pay. Beginning in 2008, however, the FQHCs and RHCs will have to demonstrate that they actually qualify for the designation. Pub. L. No. 107-251, 116 Stat. 1621 (2002).

HealthCare Standards Landscape (HCSL) A public web site containing information about healthcare technology standards; the organizations that develop, promote, or use these standards; related healthcare standards information; and links to external resources. Sponsored by the National Institute of Standards and Technology (NIST) and supported by a number of contributing organizations (for example, the Agency for Healthcare Research and Quality (AHRQ), Healthcare Information and Management Systems Society (HIMSS), Healthcare Information Technology Standards Panel (HITSP), and HL7). **hcsl.sdct.nist.gov:8080/hcsl**

healthcare system A system designed to take responsibility only for the *care* of those who seek it out. It responds to the needs of individual patients who present themselves with illness or injury. See also *health system*.

healthcare worker (HCW) The definition depends upon the context, but will generally include physicians, residents, interns, supervising nurses, nurses, nursing assistants, emergency medical technicians (EMTs)—anyone who comes into direct contact with patients. The term is used most often in regards to HIV/AIDS. For example, Texas passed a statute requiring that all "healthcare workers" follow universal precautions. Tex. Bus. & Com. Code § 85.203(a).

health center See *Federally Qualified Health Center*.

Health Centers Consolidation Act (HCCA) See *Federally Qualified Health Center*.

Health Commons Institute (HCI) A nonprofit corporation established in 1992 based on the belief that the potential exists for a quantum improvement in the quality and safety of health care. Factors supporting this belief include the (1) growth of biomedical knowledge, (2) advance of evidence-based medicine, (3) accessibility of information, (4) trend toward *patient-caregiver collaboration (PCC)*, and (5) availability of tools to adapt knowledge to the individual patient. However, even with patient and physician approaching parity in "raw" biomedical information, and even when information tools are used that reduce the burden of collecting and correlating data for both physician and patient, patients still need the help of the health professional in the analysis of their problems, in interpretation of the biomedical information, and in making wise choices among their options as to health maintenance, disease prevention, health problem solving, and therapy. HCI's mission is to study and facilitate this paradigm shift with respect to its implications for physician (and other professional) education, patient education, public education, healthcare practice design, information system design and technology, medical record system design, computer hardware and software development and application, and other relevant factors.

health court A proposed alternative justice system for people injured by medical errors. This method of *tort reform* would establish an administrative process to compensate injured patients, similar to the workers' compensation system. The health court (which is outside of the regular court system) would be presided over by a specially trained judge, who would make the decision (there would be no jury). The court, rather than plaintiff and defendant, would hire neutral, independent expert witnesses to assist it. The judge would issue a written, public opinion to provide guidance to prevent future injuries. Notably, the standard for liability would be broadened: If an injury would have been avoidable had best practices been followed, it would be compensated, unlike the present standard, which requires that negligence be proved.

A trial would be avoided when possible. An injured patient would first file a claim. The court would do a preliminary investigation and determine whether the injury was avoidable according to a predetermined list of avoidable classes of events called **accelerated compensation events (ACEs)**. For example, a sponge left in after surgery might be on the list. If the event was an ACE, the patient would be awarded compensation. This, too, would be guided by a predetermined schedule and would include both economic and noneconomic compensation. If the event was obviously not avoidable, the claim would be dismissed (an appeals process would be available). Only if there was an issue as to avoidability would the case go to trial.

Health courts would also be available to adjudicate claims of improper denial of coverage by insurance companies and health plans. The court would resolve the issue of medical necessity, and award compensation if appropriate.

The concept of health courts was developed by the national advocacy organization Common Good (**www.cgood.org**) working with a research team from the Harvard School of Public Health, supported by the Robert Wood Johnson Foundation. Federal and state legislation was introduced in 2006 to create health court pilot projects.

health department See *local health department*.

health economics The branch of economics (a social science) that deals with the provision of healthcare services, their delivery, and their use, with special attention to quantifying the demands for such services, the costs of such services and of their delivery, and the benefits obtained. More emphasis is given to the costs and benefits of health care to a population than to the individual.

health education See under *education*.

HealtheVet An "ideal" health information system under development by the Department of Veterans Affairs (VA) during the mid-2000s, to improve upon and expand *VistA* (also called HealtheVet-VistA). HealtheVet will integrate a number of additional capabilities:

- The Health Data Repository (HDR) will create a longitudinal health record, including information from both VA and non-VA sources.
- Provider systems include the Computerized Patient Record System (CPRS), VistA Imaging, Blood Bank, Pharmacy, Laboratory, Federal Health Information Exchange (FHIE), and Scheduling.
- Management and financial systems include the Financial Management System, Billing and Accounts Receivable (AR), and Fee Basis (paying providers).
- Information and education systems include prescription refills, appointments, fillable forms online, and "My HealtheVet" (where a patient can access his or her health record, online health assessment tools, and high quality health information).
- Registration, enrollment, and eligibility systems.

health facility licensing agency A state agency that sets standards and issues permits for the operation of health facilities.

health fair A type of community health education activity in which exhibits are the main method used and in which free diagnostic services such as chest x-rays and multiphasic screening are sometimes offered.

healthfinder An Internet web site sponsored by the Office of Disease Prevention and Health Promotion (ODPHP) that provides consumer health information to the public. Healthfinder offers online access to 400 other government web sites, as well as approximately 5,000 links to other resources such as publications, libraries, referral services, research and clinical information, and discussion and self-help groups. See also *National Health Information Center*.
www.healthfinder.gov

health hazard appraisal (HHA) See *health risk appraisal*.

Health Help Agency (HHA) See *Healthy Americans Act*.

health home See *Healthy Americans Act*.

Health Industry Bar Code (HIBC) A two-part standard developed in the early 1980s by a task force consisting of healthcare industry stakeholders, and hosted by the American Hospital Association (AHA). The first standard is the "HIBC Supplier Labeling Standard," which is the basis for the *Universal Product Number (UPN)*. This standard covers the labeling formats used by *suppliers* of healthcare products. The second part is the "HIBC Provider Applications Standard," which covers the formats used internally by healthcare providers themselves. ANSI has approved both standards. After developing the HIBC standard, the task force then formed the *Health Industry Business Communications Council (HIBCC)* to administer HIBC and perform related tasks. (Note the unfortunately confusing similarity of the HIBC and HIBCC initialisms.) See also *bar code* and *identifier*.

Health Industry Business Communications Council (HIBCC) A consortium of healthcare stakeholders formed in the early 1980s to administer and develop standards for use in the healthcare industry, especially the *Health Industry Bar Code (HIBC)*. In 1988, the European Health Industry Business Communications Council (EHIBCC) was formed to serve as a partner to HIBCC and administer the HIBC standard in Europe.

A major HIBCC effort is the **Health Industry Number (HIN)**, an identifier for healthcare facilities, providers, and retail pharmacies to use in electronic communications. A randomly assigned, nine-character, alpha-numeric identifier, the HIN can identify not only specific healthcare facilities, but also specific locations and/or departments within them. Another HIBCC project is the **Labeler Identification Code (LIC)**, which identifies manufacturers and distributors, and is used (with and without bar codes) for products and supplies distributed in the healthcare industry. The LIC, assigned by HIBCC, consists of a letter followed by three numbers. There is also support for the *Universal Product Number (UPN)*. See also *bar code* and *identifier*. **www.hibcc.org**

Health Industry Number (HIN) See *Health Industry Business Communications Council*.

health information Information such as that contained in the medical record, which includes demographic information, dates, diagnoses, medications, treatments, and much more about each patient. The term is often used in a broader sense to include patient information from the billing department, pharmacy, lab, and generally any data involved in health and the delivery of health care, including information about wellness, disease prevention, and health promotion for an individual.

HIPAA defines health information as "any information, whether oral or recorded in any form or medium, that (1) is created or received by a health care provider, health plan, public health authority, employer, life insurer, school or university, or health care clearinghouse; and (2) relates to the past, present, or future physical or mental health or condition of an individual; the provision of health care to an individual; or the past, present, or future payment for the provision of health care to an individual" (45 C.F.R. § 160.103 (October 1, 2006)). See also *de-identification*, *Patient Medical Record Information*, and *protected health information*.

health information administrator (HIA) A health professional with advanced education and training in health information science, including management of the medical record department. Formerly called medical record administrator (MRA) or medical record librarian.

Registered Health Information Administrator (RHIA) An HIA who has met the requirements (including at least a bachelor's degree) of the American Health Information Management Association (AHIMA) (**www.ahima.org**). The credential formerly was RRA, for registered record administrator.

health information community initiative (HICI) See *American Health Information Community*.

health information exchange (HIE) Describes the concept of interoperable electronic exchange of secure health data. The term is used variously in different contexts; it may mean the ability to share information, the infrastructure that permits sharing of information, or an organization that shares information. Sometimes used interchangeably with regional health information organization (RHIO). See also *Federal Health Information Exchange*.

health information management (HIM) The field of *informatics* as applied to healthcare.

e-HIM Electronic health information management. e-HIM is a registered trademark of the American Health Information Management Association (AHIMA), which uses it in conjunction with its focus on promoting the use of electronic health record systems (EHR-S) to improve information management.

health information management professional A specialist in health information management (HIM). See also *privacy and security professionals*.

Certified Professional in Healthcare Information and Management Systems (CPHIMS) A health information management professional who has met the requirements of the Healthcare Information and Management Systems Society (HIMSS). **www.himss.org**

health information technician (HIT) A health professional trained in organizing medical records, checking them for completeness and accuracy, assigning codes to patient information, and other tasks within the medical record department. Formerly called medical record technician (MRT).

Registered Health Information Technician (RHIT) An HIT who has met the requirements of the American Health Information Management Association (AHIMA) (**www.ahima.org**). The credential formerly was ART, for Accredited Record Technician.

health information technology (HIT) See *information technology*.

Health Insurance Association of America (HIAA) A trade association made up of companies writing health insurance for the private healthcare system. HIAA has merged into *America's Health Insurance Plans (AHIP)*.

Health Insurance for the Aged See *Medicare*.

Health Insurance Portability and Accountability Act of 1996 (HIPAA) See *HIPAA*.

health insurance prospective payment system (HIPPS) See *prospective payment system*.

Health Insurance Reform Act of 1996 An early, alternate name for the *Health Insurance Portability and Accountability Act of 1996 (HIPAA)*.

health insuring organization (HIO) An organization that contracts with a state Medicaid agency to serve as a fiscal intermediary.

health IRA See *Health Savings Account*.

Health Level Seven See *HL7*.

health literacy The extent to which a person is able to find, understand, and act on health information—to make informed choices. This information includes prescription instructions, test results, insurance forms, advice from a physician or nurse, disease information, and so forth. Two tests are widely used to assess an individual's health literacy; see *Rapid Estimate of Adult Literacy in Medicine* and *Test of Functional Health Literacy in Adults*.

health maintenance All efforts carried out in order to preserve health. As used in the term "health maintenance organization (HMO)," however, the term is not so inclusive, but rather simply includes those healthcare services that are included in the particular benefit package of the enrollee.

Health Maintenance Act of 1990 The model act developed by the National Association of Insurance Commissioners (NAIC), which has been used by most states as a pattern for their health maintenance organization (HMO) legislation. The model act requires the HMO to have a certificate of authority to do business in the state and requires detailed information to be provided to the state, including the HMO's financial status and quality assurance programs.

health maintenance organization (HMO) A healthcare-providing organization that ordinarily has a closed group ("panel") of physicians (and sometimes other health professionals), along with either its own hospital or allocated beds in one or more hospitals. Individuals (usually families) "join" an HMO, which agrees to provide all the medical and hospital care they need for a fixed, predetermined fee. Actually, each subscriber is under a contract stipulating the limits of the service (not necessarily "all" the care needed is provided). Such a contract is called a risk contract, and the HMO is therefore called a "risk contractor."

    group model HMO A health maintenance organization that contracts with a single multispecialty group practice to provide care to members. The HMO pays the group a negotiated, per capita rate for each member.

    network model HMO A health maintenance organization that contracts with multiple physician groups to provide services to HMO members. The physician groups may have both HMO and non-HMO patients. See also *independent practice association*.

    open-ended HMO See *point-of-service*.

    social HMO (S/HMO) A type of long-term care (LTC) "alternative" organization under experimentation since 1984 in which a provider, under a capitation payment (a fixed fee for each individual covered), furnishes social, long-term, and healthcare services for (currently) low income individuals. The demonstration sites are financed by a combination of capitation payments from Medicare and member premiums and copayments.

    staff model HMO A type of closed-panel health maintenance organization in which the physicians are employees of the HMO, and see patients in the HMO's facilities. Patients are limited to services provided by HMO staff physicians.

Health Maintenance Organization Act of 1973 A federal act that helped create the environment that encouraged the growth of HMOs on a large scale in the United States. Preempting restrictive state laws that had previously hindered HMO development, this act also created a federal grant and loan program, established standards for federal qualification of HMOs, and required employers to offer an HMO option under certain circumstances. The stage was set for this legislation in President Nixon's 1971 Health Message to Congress, which endorsed HMOs as cost-efficient providers of quality health care. Pub. L. No. 93-222, 87 Stat. 914 (1973).

Health Opportunity Account (HOA) See *Deficit Reduction Act of 2005*.

health outcomes assessment See *quality of life scale*.

health outcomes research See *outcomes research*.

health physicist See under *physicist*.

health plan An organized service to provide stipulated medical, hospital, and related services (benefits) to individuals under a prepayment contract. It may be offered by a Blue Cross Blue Shield plan, an insurance company, a health maintenance organization (HMO), a healthcare organization (HCO), or other organization. Synonym: healthcare plan. See also *managed care plan*.

Health Plan Employer Data and Information Set See under *data set*.

Health Plan ID See *National Payer ID*.

health planning See under *planning*.

health plan purchasing cooperative (HPPC) See *health alliance*.

health plan sponsor See *plan sponsor*.

Health Policy Agenda for the American People (HPA) A program spearheaded by the American Medical Association (AMA) in the mid-1980s to develop a set of proposals for improving health and health care in the United States. Among organizations represented in the policy-making process were the American Association of Retired Persons, American Nurses Association, Blue Cross and Blue Shield Association, Business Roundtable, Health Insurance Association of America, U.S. Chamber of Commerce, and various state and national medical and specialty associations. Completion of the agenda development was accomplished in 1986, and a summary giving the 195 recommendations was published. (Balfe, B.E., et al. "A Health Policy Agenda for the American People. The Issues and Their Development." *Journal of the American Medical Association*, 1986;256(8):1021–6.)

health professional A comprehensive term covering people working in the field of health care who have some special training and/or education. The degree of education, training, and other qualifications varies greatly with the nature of the profession, and with the state regulating its practice. There are three relevant aspects to the qualifications of any health professional:

Education and training: This may vary from a short course of several weeks or on-the-job training, to programs of a year or more, those requiring associate or bachelor's degrees, and those requiring work at the master's or doctoral level. Practical experience is usually part of the training program. A certificate or diploma is issued to those who successfully complete the program.

Professional credentials: Most professions offer additional credentials to those meeting certain requirements, which often include passing an examination. These credentials are offered by professional associations or boards that specify criteria and standards for various levels of accomplishment. The individual meeting the requirements becomes certified or board certified. Increasingly, such credentials have a limited "life," and recertification is required at specified intervals (every three years, for example).

State regulation: States regulate the practice of the health professions in varying degrees, from a great deal to very little or not at all. The most restrictive regulation is licensure, less restrictive is certification, and (usually) least restrictive is registration. Note, however, that licensure in one area may actually have less stringent requirements than registration in another. A registered nurse, for example, must complete an associate or bachelor's degree, and pass a state examination.

Some individuals may call themselves "professional" with little or no training or credentials. When state licensure is required, practicing without it is illegal. But if the requirement is certification or registration, a person often may legally practice without either. To assess the qualifications of any healthcare practitioner—regardless of what they call themselves—the consumer must find out about that particular specialty area and what education and credentials are required or desirable. A good health professional should be happy to assist in that quest. For more about the health professions, see *health science discipline*, *medical specialty*, and *nursing specialty*.

Health Professional Shortage Area (HPSA) An urban or rural area, population, or public or private nonprofit medical facility that the Secretary of the Department of Health and Human Services (HHS) determines has a shortage of primary medical care, dental care, or mental health care providers. Physicians practicing within an HPSA receive bonuses for services provided to Medicare beneficiaries. These areas can also apply for the assignment of National Health Service Corps personnel. See also *Medically Underserved Area*, *Medically Underserved Population*, and *Physician Scarcity Area*.

health promotion Efforts to change peoples' behavior in order to promote healthy lives and, to the extent possible, prevent illnesses and accidents and to minimize their effects, rather than having people use the healthcare system for "repairs." A health promotion program may include health risk appraisal of the individuals, and may give attention to fitness, stress management, smoking, cholesterol reduction, weight control, nutrition, cancer screening, and other matters on the basis of the risks detected. Synonym: wellness program. See also *demand management*.

health record A record of a person's health information; there is no single definition. Sometimes used as a synonym for *medical record*. See also *electronic health record*.

health record analyst (HRA) A person who analyzes data from medical records and other sources for hospital management and medical staff. An HRA may abstract data from the records for computer input; however, analysis and abstracting are distinctly different functions, ordinarily carried out by different people. Analysis requires interpretation, whereas abstracting is basically a clerical function. An HRA is the same as a medical record analyst (MRA).

health record bank (HRB) A repository for electronic health records (EHRs). See *independent health record bank*.

health reimbursement account (HRA) An arrangement in which the employer reimburses an employee for qualified health expenses not covered by the group health insurance plan—deductibles or co-insurance amounts, for example. Sometimes called personal care account, health reimbursement arrangement, or Section 105 HRA plan.

health-related care institution A facility providing some kind of health care to inpatients who do not require full nursing services.

health-related quality of life (HRQOL) See under *quality of life*.

health-related services A term apparently used to include everything in the healthcare field except medical care (physician services).

health resources Personnel (both professional and supportive), facilities, funds, and technology that are available or could be made available for health services.

Health Resources and Services Administration (HRSA) The federal agency within the Department of Health and Human Services (HHS) that deals with issues relating to access, equity, quality, and cost of care. HRSA supports states and local communities in their efforts to organize and deliver health care, especially to underserved populations and other groups with special health needs, such as mothers and children. HRSA is also the focal point for programs that currently have a high national priority, such as organ donation and transplantation, bioterrorism, rural health care, and health information technology. HRSA calls itself the "Access Agency," and defines its mission as assuring equal access to comprehensive, culturally competent, quality health care for all. **www.hrsa.gov**

health risk appraisal (HRA) A technique for determining for a given individual the factors most likely to result in illness, injury, or premature death. The determination is based on comparing a set of data about the individual (her or his database) with statistics on the likelihood of specific illnesses, injuries, and causes of death among large groups of persons for whom the same database has been collected and analyzed. Included in the database are the individual's age, sex, physical condition, genetic background, behavior, environment, and other factors, obtained by examination of the individual, laboratory tests, and information obtained from the person by interview or questionnaire.

The purpose of the appraisal is preventive, that is, to be able to prescribe measures and programs to counter the risks detected. For example, elevated blood pressure would be a risk whenever it occurs, inability to swim would be an especially great risk factor in a child exposed to water sports, and driving a motor vehicle would be a risk factor when a patient requires certain drugs that interfere with the ability to drive. Synonyms: health hazard appraisal, health risk assessment.

Health Savings Account (HSA) A replacement for the medical savings account (MSA), created by the Medicare Modernization Act of 2003 to help individuals pay for healthcare services. Unlike the MSA, which had restricted eligibility, the HSA is available to anyone under the age of 65 who has a qualified high-deductible health plan (HDHP) and is not covered by other health insurance. The HSA is structured much like an independent retirement account (IRA). Contributions to the HSA up to the amount of the deductible or a specified dollar limit (whichever is less) are tax-deductible. The cash in the account is available to pay for deductibles, copayments, and other "qualified medical expenses" not paid by the holder's insurance; withdrawals for other purposes will be penalized and taxed. After age 65, the money may be withdrawn for any purpose without penalty (although it will be taxed). Sometimes called a health IRA or medical IRA.

health science discipline A very broad term that includes a range of scientific and other fields related to health care, including medicine and nursing. Recently it is being used most to describe those professions other than physician, nurse, dentist, or pharmacist, because the terms previously used—"allied health professions" or "paramedical personnel"—were too narrow or nondescriptive of many of the disciplines. The term "applied health sciences" is also being used. See also ***allied health professional***, ***health professional***, ***medical specialty***, and ***nursing specialty***. Following are some current occupations (see individual listings for more details):

acupuncturist
alcoholism counselor
anesthesiologist assistant
art therapist
athletic trainer
audiologist
biomedical instrumentation technologist
bone densitometrist
cardiovascular technologist
care manager
case manager
chaplain
childbirth educator
clinical engineer
clinical laboratory specialist
clinical laboratory technician
clinical laboratory technologist
clinical medical librarian
coding specialist
community counselor

computed tomography technologist
contact lens technician
Cytotechnologist (see under *clinical laboratory technologist*)
dental assistant
dental hygienist
dental laboratory technician
diabetes educator
diagnostic medical sonographer
dietetic technician
dietitian
dispensing optician
diving medical technician
doula
electroencephalographic technologist
electroneurodiagnostic technologist
emergency medical technician
evoked potential technologist
eye bank technician
first assistant
gambling counselor
gastroenterology associate
gastroenterology technician
genetic counselor
health information administrator
health information technician
health physicist (see under physicist)
health science librarian
hemodialysis technician
histologic technician (see under *clinical laboratory technician*)
histotechnologist (see under *clinical laboratory technologist*)
horticultural therapist
hyperbaric technologist
informationist
intraoperative monitoring technologist
kinesiotherapist
lactation consultant
low vision therapist
magnetic resonance imaging technologist
mammographer
manual arts therapist
marriage and family counselor
marriage and family therapist
massage therapist
mastectomy fitter
medical administrative specialist
medical assistant
medical dosimetrist
medical illustrator
medical physicist (see under *physicist*)
Medical Technologist (see under *clinical laboratory technologist*)
medical transcriptionist

mental health counselor
music therapist
myofascial trigger point therapist
nerve conduction technologist
nuclear medicine scientist
nuclear medicine technologist
occupational therapist
occupational therapy assistant
ocularist
ophthalmic laboratory technician
ophthalmic medical assistant
ophthalmic medical technologist
ophthalmic technician
ophthalmic ultrasound biometrist
orientation and mobility specialist
orthopedic technologist
orthoptist
orthotist
pathologist's assistant
pedorthist
perfusionist
personal trainer
physical therapist
physical therapist assistant
physician assistant
polysomnographic technologist
privacy and security professionals
prosthetist
quality management technologist
radiation therapist
radiographer
radiologic technologist
rehabilitation counselor
respiratory therapist
respiratory therapy technician
school counselor
speech-language pathologist
student affairs practitioner
substance abuse counselor
surgical technologist
therapeutic recreation specialist
tobacco addiction counselor
vision rehabilitation therapist

health science librarian A health professional, usually with a master's degree in library science (MLS), who specializes in helping physicians, other providers, patients, and students access information on health, medicine, and health care. See also ***clinical medical librarian***.

health security Protection against threats to public health, such as infectious disease; potential pandemics; chemical, biological, and radionuclear threats; the effects of the globalization of travel and trade; global warming; and the increasing frequency and severity of natural disasters. The World Health Organization (WHO) defines health security as the "provision and maintenance of measures aimed at preserving and protecting the health of the population" and also as "the policy areas in which national security and public health concerns overlap."

Health Security Act (HSA) President Clinton's proposal for healthcare reform, which was defeated in 1993.

health service area A specific geographic area considered in the governmental health planning process. The boundaries of health service areas were established in compliance with 1974 federal legislation on the basis of population, political subdivisions, geography, and other factors. The term "health service area" may also be used more loosely to mean service area, the area from which a facility or program actually draws its patients or clients, that is, its "catchment area."

health services A term without specific definition that pertains to any services that are health related. See also *health care* or *healthcare*.

health services research Research pertaining to the efficiency and effectiveness of various organizational forms for healthcare delivery, administrative approaches, relationship to needs, and like matters.

health status The state of health of an individual or population. A description of health status is usually given either in vague lay terms, for example, "good," or as a *health status index*, which may appear more objective and meaningful than it really is.

health status assessment See *quality of life scale*.

health status index A statistic that attempts to quantify the *health status* of an individual or a population. Such indices are developed using *health status indicators*. Statements of health status have not been developed to the point that they have standard definitions; each publication using such indices should give full details on the indicators used, their aggregation into the indices themselves, and any other pertinent methodological detail, such as the sampling techniques used (in the case of health status indices for populations).

health status indicator A measurement of some attribute of individual or community health that is considered to reflect *health status*. Each attribute is given a numerical value, and a score (a health status index) is calculated for the individual or community from the aggregate of these values.

To the extent possible, the indicators are objective; that is, they are facts for which various observers or investigators would each find the same value. In the case of a community, such statistics as mortality and morbidity rates are sometimes used. For the health status of individuals (and thus of the group), data may be obtained by sampling (obtaining data on only a properly selected portion of the population). Such facts may be obtained by examination of individuals or by questionnaires inquiring as to physical function, quality of life, activities of daily living (ADL), emotional well-being, episodes of medical care, and the like.

An example of health status indicators are those defined in 1991 by the Centers for Disease Control and Prevention (CDC) as part of *Healthy People 2000*. The eighteen indicators included measures of health status and/or factors that put individuals at increased risk of disease or premature mortality; for example:

Race/ethnicity-specific infant mortality as measured by the rate (per 1,000)
Motor vehicle crash deaths per 100,000 population
Suicides per 100,000 population
Lung cancer deaths per 100,000 population
Reported incidence (per 100,000 population) of tuberculosis

health survey An investigation of individuals, an area, or a population in order to obtain information about some aspect of the health of those surveyed (health problems, health resources, or anything else pertaining to health). Such a survey typically employs sampling, and may obtain information from direct observations, questionnaires, published data, or other sources. Examples of surveys in health care include *BASIS-32*, *Current Population Survey (CPS)*, *Hospital Consumer Assessment of Healthcare Providers and Systems (HCAHPS)*,

Medical Expenditure Panel Survey (MEPS), *National Health and Nutrition Examination Survey (NHANES)*, *National Health Interview Survey (NHIS)*, *National Hospital Discharge Survey (NHDS)*, and *SF-36 Health Survey* (see under *quality of life scale*).

health system A system designed to take responsibility for the *health* of its defined community; it involves "outreach" rather than "response" or "reaction." This is in contrast with a health*care* system (see *healthcare system*).

health technology The drugs, biologicals, devices, and medical and surgical procedures used in health care, as well as measures for prevention and rehabilitation of disease, and the organizational and support systems in which health care is provided.

health technology assessment (HTA) A process of using scientific evidence to evaluate the medical, social, economic, and ethical implications of *health technology*. The purpose of HTA is to inform and/or advise technology-related policy and decision making.

Health Technology Assessment International (HTAi) An international organization whose mission is to support the development, communication, understanding, and use of *health technology assessment* around the world as a means of promoting effective innovations and effective use of resources in health care. HTAi was launched at the nineteenth Annual Meeting of the *International Society of Technology Assessment in Health Care (ISTAHC)* in June 2003 in Canada. See also *vortal*. www.htai.org

Health Technology Assessment Reports (HTAR) See *Office of Health Technology Assessment*.

Health Web Site Accreditation See *URAC*.

Healthy Americans Act (HAA) Federal legislation proposed in 2006 by Oregon Senator Ron Wyden to provide health insurance coverage for all Americans through "individual mandate"—everyone, except Medicare beneficiaries and those receiving health care through the military (and certain others), would be required to purchase private health insurance. Insurers would offer **Healthy Americans Private Insurance (HAPI)** plans that meet the requirements of the act. These plans must provide benefits at least equivalent to the Blue Cross Blue Shield Standard Plan provided under the Federal Employees Health Benefit Program as of January 1, 2007. HAPIs could offer additional benefits. The plans must encourage wellness and include catastrophic coverage, and must provide for **personal responsibility contributions (PRCs)** (payments made by the insured other than for premiums; presumably coinsurance, copayments, or deductibles) except for preventive care or services for early detection. The HAPI would designate a healthcare provider, such as a primary care physician, nurse practitioner, or other qualified healthcare provider, to monitor the health and health care of the covered individual; this provider would be called the **health home** of the individual.

Employers would no longer provide health benefits for employees, but would phase out their health plans and instead pay the amount saved to employees so that they can purchase their own insurance. Eventually all employers would pay an **employer shared responsibility (ESR)** contribution to help subsidize the system. Federal funds would also be provided.

The system would be coordinated in each state by a state **Health Help Agency (HHA)**, which would provide consumers with information on available HAPIs and the quality of healthcare providers. The HHA must make sure that at least two HAPI plans are offered. To help individuals pay for their health insurance, the HHA would provide subsidies to qualified low income individuals for premiums and/or personal responsibility contributions. A penalty would be imposed on individuals who did not purchase insurance. Enforcement would be left to the states.

Healthy Americans Private Insurance (HAPI) See *Healthy Americans Act*.

healthy communities movement A movement that contends that the goal of the healthcare system should be the health of the community, and that every community is responsible for its own health, that is, for having its own "health system"—of which traditional health care is only a part. To that end, there must be wide involvement of all agencies, organizations, and citizens, and the hospital must fit into the total scheme for achievement of optimum health of all, even though this alters its traditional role of simply providing care to those who present themselves to it. See also *healthy community*.

healthy community An unofficial label that a community often gives itself when it has established and continues an organized effort to achieve optimum health for all its residents and visitors, using the resources available, and in response to its own perceived needs. Such a community is part of the *healthy communities movement*.

A healthy community finds that it has human resources that can be tapped and mobilized in new and novel ways and financial resources that can be pooled. Organizations and agencies that often have provided duplicate services and competed with one another become collaborators. Services are taken to where the needs are. Physicians, other health professionals, and hospitals increase their outreach programs.

Among the projects reported in healthy communities are:
Child abuse prevention
Community health information networks
Community-knowledge-based managed care
Companionship for shut-ins
Consumer health education
Consumer health informatics
Dental services to children
Domestic violence prevention
Elder day care
Environmental monitoring
Firearm safety
Fitness
Housing for the homeless
Immunization
Indigent care
Injury prevention
Migrant worker health care
Parish nursing
Prenatal care
Preventive medicine
Safety education
School health
Teenage pregnancy programs
Time banking for volunteer services
Voice mail guidance to prenatal care
Voice mail triage into health care
Water safety instruction
Women's health
"One-stop shopping" for community services
"One-stop shopping" for health care
See also *health gateway* under *gateway (organization)*.

Healthy People Consortium An alliance of over 350 national health organizations, state and federal agencies, and others concerned about the nation's health. It was first convened in 1988 by the Institute of Medicine of the National Academy of Sciences, at the request of the U.S. Public Health Service. It produced the *Healthy People 2000* report, and has released an update, the Healthy People 2010 initiative. Now managed by the Office of Disease Prevention and Health Promotion within the *Office of Public Health and Science (OPHS)*. **www.healthypeople.gov**

Healthy People 2000 A report published by the U.S. Public Health Service in 1990 outlining health promotion and disease prevention goals for Americans for the year 2000. The report states that meeting the goals requires acceptance of shared responsibilities by citizens, health professionals, government at all levels, the media, and communities. The goals included such specifics as an increased life span accompanied by a high quality of life (QOL) factor, improving the health of populations deemed to be particularly disadvantaged, and providing all Americans with preventive health services. It has since been updated in *Healthy People 2010*; see *Healthy People Consortium*. See also *health status indicator*.

Healthy People 2010 A national initiative setting forth goals of promoting health and preventing disease; an update of *Healthy People 2000*. See also *Healthy People Consortium* and *Leading Health Indicators*.

hearsay A statement made out of the courtroom, which is offered into evidence during a trial to prove the substance of what was said. The "hearsay rule" makes hearsay not admissible as evidence; however, there are many exceptions. A notable exception for hospitals is the *business record* exception, which makes admissible written statements made in the ordinary course of business. The medical record is usually accepted as a business record; thus its contents are admissible in court unless excluded for other reasons (such as privilege or irrelevancy). See *legal medical record*, under *medical record*, and *privileged communication*.

heart attack See *myocardial infarction* under *infarction*.

heart-lung machine A machine through which a patient's blood is circulated, bypassing the patient's heart, during surgery on the heart. The machine supplies the heart's pumping function during the operation, and also acts as a lung, supplying oxygen to the blood.

HEDIC Healthcare Electronic Data Infrastructure Coalition. See *Health Care eBusiness Collaborative*.

HEDIS See *Health Plan Employer Data and Information Set* under *data set*.

HELP See *Committee on Health, Education, Labor, and Pensions*.

hemapheresis See *apheresis*.

hematology The study of blood and blood-forming tissues: chemistry, structure, physiology, biology, and diseases.

Hematology Technologist (H) See under *clinical laboratory technologist*.

Hemlock Society See *Compassion & Choices*.

hemodialysis See under *dialysis*.

hemodialysis nurse See *Certified Hemodialysis Nurse* under *dialysis nursing*.

hemodialysis technician A health professional trained to perform hemodialysis services, often in outpatient dialysis units. See also *dialysis nursing*.

Certified Clinical Hemodialysis Technician (CCHT) A hemodialysis technician who has passed an examination of the Nephrology Nursing Certification Commission (NNCC). **www.nncc-exam.org**

Certified Hemodialysis Technologist/Technician (CHT) A hemodialysis technician who has passed an examination of the Board of Nephrology Examiners, Inc. Nursing and Technology (BONENT). **www.bonent.org**

hemodialysis unit A unit of the hospital set up to treat patients with certain renal (kidney) disorders by the use of *hemodialysis* (see under *dialysis*). Synonyms: renal dialysis unit, dialysis unit.

heparin Heparin sodium. A drug that acts as an anticoagulant (keeps blood from clotting). Often used to reduce the incidence of heart attacks by helping to keep the arteries unclogged. See also *hirudin*.

hepatitis A An infection of the liver caused by the hepatitis A virus (HAV). The disease is communicable by ingestion (i.e., by eating or drinking contaminated food or beverage). Vaccines are now available for long-term prevention for those two years old and over. Immune globulin is available for short-term prevention for all ages.

hepatitis B Hepatitis (inflammation of the liver) caused by hepatitis B virus (HBV). The disease can cause lifelong infection, cirrhosis (scarring) of the liver, liver cancer, liver failure, and death. The virus is most commonly transmitted by contaminated needles (see **needlestick**), blood, or blood products. However, hepatitis B may also be transmitted when bodily secretions such as saliva or semen are in contact with mucous membranes, particularly during sexual contacts; thus, hepatitis B is classified as a sexually transmitted disease (STD). Vaccination against hepatitis B is available and is recommended for healthcare workers and for other groups, such as school teachers and employees. HBV is more readily transmitted than HIV, and its prevalence provides a strong argument for the insistence on **universal precautions** (see under **precautions**) in healthcare facilities. Synonyms: serum hepatitis, transfusion hepatitis.

hepatitis C An infection of the liver caused by the hepatitis C virus (HCV). A disease similar in symptoms, pathology, and transmission to hepatitis B, but caused by a different virus. A study conducted in 2000 found that each year, 1,000 new cases of HCV infection are identified among healthcare workers and result in treatment costs of $15 billion annually.

herbalist A person who practices herbal medicine.

herbal medicine The therapeutic use of herbs. An herb is a plant containing chemical substances that have an effect on the body. Synonym: herbology.

Chinese herbal medicine The body of knowledge in traditional Chinese medicine concerning the therapeutic use of herbs.

herbologist One who practices herbal medicine.

Diplomate of Chinese Herbology (Dipl. C.H.) An herbologist specializing in Chinese herbal medicine who has met the requirements for eligibility and passed an examination of the National Certification Commission for Acupuncture and Oriental Medicine (NCCAOM). **www.nccaom.org**

hereditary Having to do with the transmission or characteristics, through the cellular structure of the individual, from parent to offspring.

heredity The transmission of characteristics from parent to offspring.

hermaphrodite See *intersexed*.

heroic treatment See *extraordinary treatment* under *treatment*.

heterogeneous Composed of a mixture of things. For example, a DRG that is heterogeneous is one that is composed of patients with a variety of diagnoses, as contrasted with a "homogeneous" or "single-diagnosis" group, in which all the patients have the same diagnosis.

heterograft See *xenograft*.

HEW A short abbreviation for the former federal *Department of Health, Education, and Welfare (DHEW)*.

HFMA See *Healthcare Financial Management Association*.

HFP See *healthcare finance professional*.

HGP See *Human Genome Project*.

HHA Health hazard appraisal; see *health risk appraisal*. Also Health Help Agency; see *Healthy Americans Act*. See also *home health agency*.

HHCC See *Home Health Care Classification*.

HH MAC Home health/hospice *Medicare Administrative Contractor*.

HH-PPS See *home health prospective payment system* under *prospective payment system*.

HHQI Home Health Quality Initiative. See *Quality Initiative*.

HHRG See *Home Health Resource Group*.

HHS See *Department of Health and Human Services*.

HI Hospital Insurance; see *Medicare Part A* under *Medicare*. Also *health information*.

HIA See *health information administrator*.

HIAA See *Health Insurance Association of America*.

HIBC See *Health Industry Bar Code*.

HIBCC See *Health Industry Business Communications Council.*

HICI Health information community initiative. See *American Health Information Community.*

hickfa or hickva Common pronunciations of the initialism HCFA (the former name of CMS).

hick-picks Common pronunciation of *HCPCS.*

hicky Common pronunciation of HCQI, for "health care quality improvement" (HCQI). See *quality improvement.*

HIE See *health information exchange.*

hierarchy A system in which persons or things are in graded ranks. Authority in an organization is usually hierarchical; perhaps the best example is the military. In a hospital, "line authority" illustrates the principle: a floor nurse reports to a head nurse, who in turn reports to the chief of nursing, who in turn reports to the chief executive officer of the hospital who, finally, reports to the governing body. Only a person higher in this series is authorized to "give orders" to a person lower in the series.

high-deductible health plan (HDHP) Health insurance or a health plan with an exceptionally high deductible. To qualify for a Health Savings Account (HSA), the deductible must be at least $1,050 for an individual or $2,100 for a family (in 2006).

hikva A common pronunciation for the acronym HCFA (the former name of CMS).

Hill-Burton Act Federal legislation resulting in a post-World War II federal program of financial assistance for the construction and renovation of hospitals and other healthcare facilities. The intent was to increase the number of hospital beds in poor or underserved communities of the United States. The Hill-Burton Act also required that community hospitals receiving support under this program provide reasonable medical services to all people living in the hospital's service area, regardless of their ability to pay. The Department of Health and Human Service (HHS) issued regulations that established standards for uncompensated care and specified that the care provided to Medicare and Medicaid patients was not considered uncompensated care. Technically known as the Hospital Survey and Construction Act, it was signed by President Truman in August 1946. By 1978, when the law expired, 500,000 hospital beds had been built, at a cost of about $13.5 billion. Pub. L. No. 79-725, 60 Stat. 1040 (1946), codified at 42 U.S.C. § 291 (2004).

HIM See *health information management.*

HIMSS See *Healthcare Information and Management Systems Society.*

HIMSS EMEA See *Healthcare Information and Management Systems Society.*

HIN Health Industry Number. See *Health Industry Business Communications Council.*

HINN See *hospital-issued notice of non-coverage.*

HIO See *health insuring organization.*

HIP Hospital Insurance Program (Medicare Part A); see *Medicare.*

HIPAA Health Insurance Portability and Accountability Act of 1996. Federal legislation whose primary purpose is to provide continuity of healthcare coverage. It does this partly by providing limitations on preexisting condition exclusions, as well as prohibiting discrimination against individuals based on health status. The law also guarantees that insured workers will be eligible to keep their insurance if they leave their jobs. HIPAA created the medical savings account (MSA) to help individuals pay for their health care. It also made amendments to other legislation, including the Employee Retirement Income Security Act (ERISA), the Internal Revenue Code (IRC), and the Public Health Service Act.

For healthcare providers, however, HIPAA imposed sweeping requirements for the electronic transmission of health information (see *administrative simplification provisions*) and protection of patient privacy (see *Privacy Rule*). The passage of this legislation created a new interest in healthcare standards (see *standard (norm)*), because this law focuses on standards for data interchange in the areas of healthcare plans, claims, and reimbursement (see *data standards* and *electronic transactions standards*). Failure to comply with some of the act's provisions can result in severe criminal penalties (up to ten years in prison).

HIPAA was originally known as the "Kennedy-Kassebaum bill (K2)" for its two leading sponsors in the U.S. Senate. It was the House version, however, known as the "Health Insurance Reform Act of 1996" that was actually passed by the Senate in lieu of the Kassebaum/Kennedy bill. Pub. L. No. 104-191, 110 Stat. 1936 (1996).

HIPC Health insurance purchasing cooperative. See *health alliance*.

HIPDB See *Healthcare Integrity and Protection Data Bank*.

HIPPA A fairly common misrepresentation of the acronym *HIPAA*.

hippick Common pronunciation of HIPC or HPPC, for "health insurance purchasing cooperative" (HIPC) or "health plan purchasing cooperative" (HPPC). See *health alliance*.

hippotherapy Treatment with the help of a horse. Support and accreditation in this area are available from the North American Riding for the Handicapped Association (NARHA). **www.narha.org**

HIPPS Health insurance prospective payment system. See *prospective payment system*.

HIPPS code Health insurance prospective payment system code. A payment code representing a case-mix group that has been assigned by Grouper software, which interprets a standard patient assessment instrument using an algorithm. Institutional providers use HIPPS codes on claims in association with special revenue codes. One revenue code is defined for each *prospective payment system* that requires HIPPS codes. These include the skilled nursing facility prospective payment system (SNF-PPS), the home health prospective payment system (HH-PPS), and the inpatient rehabilitation facility prospective payment system (IRF-PPS).

hirudin A protein found in the saliva of leeches that acts as an anticoagulant (keeps blood from clotting). Researchers have found a way to genetically engineer the hirudin compound for medicinal use. At least one study has shown hirudin to be more effective in reducing blood-clot formation in humans than the generally used anticoagulant heparin. These medicines are used to reduce the incidence of heart attacks by helping to keep the arteries unclogged.

HIS See *healthcare information system* or *hospital information system* under *information system*.

HISB See *Healthcare Informatics Standards Board*.

HISPP See *Healthcare Information Standards Planning Panel*.

histology See under *anatomy*.

history Information about a patient obtained by questioning the patient and the patient's family, in contrast to information obtained through testing and physical examination.

medical history The portion of the patient's medical record containing the essential medical (and social) information about the patient and his or her family (ancestors, blood relatives, and siblings), spouse and household, past personal injuries and illnesses, and development of the present problems. The history may be recorded using the traditional method of "systems review," under headings such as "respiratory," "past illnesses," "cardiac," and the like, or it may be recorded in the newer method, the problem oriented medical record (POMR), in which each of the patient's problems is traced separately. A medical history is often referred to simply as a "history."

natural history The ordinary course of a disease. For example, the common cold has an incubation period before symptoms and signs appear, a period when the patient is noticeably ill, and then a recovery phase; this is the natural history of the common cold. Treatment is intended to modify the natural history of the disease.

values history See under *advance directive*.

Histotechnician (HT) See under *clinical laboratory technician*.

Histotechnologist (HTL) See under *clinical laboratory technologist*.

HIT Health information technology; see *information technology*. Also *health information technician*.

HITSP See *Healthcare Information Technology Standards Panel*.

HIV (human immunodeficiency virus) The virus that causes *AIDS*. HIV is usually passed from one person to another through blood-to-blood or sexual contact. However, an infected pregnant woman can pass HIV to her baby during pregnancy or delivery, or through breast-feeding. Additional body fluids that may transmit the virus to healthcare workers include cerebrospinal fluid surrounding the brain and the spinal cord, synovial fluid surrounding bone joints, and the amniotic fluid surrounding a fetus. People with HIV are called **HIV positive** and have **HIV infection**; most will develop *AIDS*.

HIV/AIDS Bureau (HAB) One of the key program areas of the Health Resources and Services Administration (HRSA). HAB was formed in August 1997 to consolidate all programs funded under the Ryan White CARE (Comprehensive AIDS Resources Emergency Care) Act. It is the largest single source, next to the Medicaid and Medicare programs, of federal funding for HIV/AIDS care for low-income, un- and underinsured individuals in the United States. **hab.hrsa.gov**

HIV/AIDS nursing The nursing specialty focused on the needs of *HIV* and *AIDS* patients.

Advanced AIDS Certified Registered Nurse (AACRN) A registered nurse with at least a master's degree and experience in HIV/AIDS nursing, who has passed an advanced examination of the HIV/AIDS Nursing Certification Board (HANCB). **www.hancb.org**

AIDS Certified Registered Nurse (ACRN) A registered nurse practicing in HIV/AIDS nursing who has passed an examination of the HIV/AIDS Nursing Certification Board (HANCB). **www.hancb.org**

HL7 Health Level Seven. A nonprofit *standards development organization (SDO)* developing standards for the electronic interchange of clinical, financial, and administrative information among differing computer systems and applications in the healthcare industry. "Level Seven" is a reference to the "application level," the highest of the seven levels of OSI (the Open Systems Interconnection reference model).

Founded in 1987 and based in Ann Arbor, Michigan, HL7 has gained wide acceptance both in the United States and abroad. Members include users, hospitals, vendors, consultants, and others. *ANSI* accredited HL7 as an SDO in 1994. In 1995, ANSI approved the fourth version of the HL7 standard (version 2.2), thereby making it the first American National Standard for the exchange of clinical data.

Although other healthcare standards development efforts are underway that deal with particular departments, HL7 was formed to focus on the interface requirements of the entire healthcare organization.

"HL7" is also used to refer to the standard itself. HL7 is a messaging standard in which certain "trigger" events in the healthcare arena cause the transmission of a specific message relating to the trigger event. HL7 defines the format of the messages according to the standard, allowing healthcare data to be interchanged among a variety of information systems in which the data themselves may be in a proprietary format internally. **www.hl7.org**

HMO See *health maintenance organization*.

HN-BC See *Holistic Nurse—Board Certified* under *holistic nursing*.

HOA Health Opportunity Account. See *Deficit Reduction Act of 2005*.

holding company A corporation organized for the purpose of owning the stock of another corporation or corporations; or any company that owns such a large portion of the stock of a corporation that it controls that corporation.

holistic health A view of health as consisting of the health of the "whole" person—body, mind, and spirit. That view requires coordinated attention to all three components by the several disciplines involved, and places major responsibility for health on the individual. Synonym: wholistic health. See also *noetic*.

holistic medicine A term originally applied to the principle that the whole person should be treated, rather than just the person's disease, disturbance of function, or injury. This principle has always guided the provision of health care of good quality, which stresses the importance of personal responsibility, prevention, exercise, nutrition, rest, moderation, personal habits, and so on. Holistic medicine became the focus of a movement in the 1960s with the formation of the International Association of Holistic Health Practitioners (IAHHP) in 1970.

The term has come under criticism by the medical profession and others in recent years because it has come to include a variety of treatment methods, some of which are incompatible with others, and some of which have scientific proof whereas others do not. For example, such a mixed bag of concepts as astrology, nutrition, faith healing, graphology, macrobiotics, naturopathy, numerology, acupuncture, psychocalisthenics, self-massage, psychotherapy, and touch encounter have at various times been listed as being among the tools of holistic medicine. Synonym: wholistic medicine. See also *complementary and alternative medicine*, *mind-body medicine*, and *noetic*.

holistic nursing The area of nursing that focuses on the *holistic health* of a person from birth to death. The holistic nurse is a facilitator, working in partnership with the individual.

Advanced Holistic Nurse—Board Certified (AHN-BC) A registered nurse with a master's or doctorate degree in nursing who has passed an examination in holistic nursing given by the American Holistic Nurses' Certification Corporation (AHNCC). **www.ahncc.org**

Holistic Nurse—Board Certified (HN-BC) A registered nurse with a bachelor's degree who has passed an examination in holistic nursing given by the American Holistic Nurses' Certification Corporation (AHNCC). **www.ahncc.org**

holoendemic See *endemic*.

home Health home; see *Healthy Americans Act*.

homebound A term used by Medicare for a patient who is unable to leave the home without "considerable and taxing effort," and who leaves home infrequently and for "short duration" or to receive medical treatment. An individual must be "homebound" to qualify for Medicare home healthcare benefits. The Medicare Modernization Act (MMA) required a demonstration project to test an expanded definition to allow more freedom for the homebound person. Sometimes called "confined to the home."

home care See *home health care*.

home care program See *home healthcare program*.

home health agency (HHA) Essentially the same as a home healthcare program in that it provides medical and other health services in the patient's home. Unlike the home healthcare program, which provides services itself, the home health agency has the option of arranging the services by contracting with others. The term "home health agency" is applied to both nonprofit and proprietary bodies.

home health aide See under *aide*.

home health care Care at the levels of skilled nursing care and intermediate care (see *nursing care*) provided in the patient's home through an agency or program that has the resources necessary to provide that care. The care is given under the prescription of a physician by nurses and other health professionals (social workers, physical therapists, and so forth), as appropriate. Services may also include homemaking and personal care services.

Home health care is a growing alternative to skilled nursing facilities and units (SNFs and SNUs) and to intermediate care facilities (ICFs) and units. Also called "in-home care" and "home care." See also *home life care*.

Often home health care is divided into three categories, depending on the intensity:

intensive home health care Home care for persons who are seriously ill and require intensive medical and nursing attention.

intermediate home health care Home care for persons with an active but reasonably stable disease, that is, whose condition is not expected to change rapidly, and for whom less medical and nursing care is required than in the case of intensive home health care.

maintenance home health care Home care for persons needing mostly personal care and support.

Home Health Care Classification (HHCC) The former name of the *Clinical Care Classification (CCC)*.

home healthcare program An organization that provides medical and other health services in the patient's home. Synonym: home care program.

home health nursing The area of nursing focusing on the needs of patients who require nursing care in their own home.

Certified Home Health Nurse A specialist in home health nursing who has met the requirements of the American Nurses Credentialing Center (ANCC). The certification examination was eliminated in 2005. **www.nursingworld.org/ancc**

Clinical Specialist in Home Health Nursing A specialist in home health nursing with advanced training and experience, who has passed an examination of the American Nurses Credentialing Center (ANCC). The certification examination was eliminated in 2005. **www.nursingworld.org/ancc**

home health prospective payment system (HH-PPS) See under *prospective payment system*.

Home Health Resource Group (HHRG) A patient classification (similar to DRGs) used by CMS to pay for home health care for Medicare patients. See *home health prospective payment system* under *prospective payment system*.

home health services See *home health care*.

home life care Supportive services provided by an agency in order to permit an individual who is able to carry out the activities of daily living (ADL) to remain at home rather than being placed in an institution. The services are given by homemakers and home aides rather than by nurses. One benefit of having such trained assistance in the home is that the worker going into the home is in a position to detect the need for and to obtain nursing services as required. Home life care is distinguished from home health care in that home health care includes nursing services under the direction of a physician rather than simply homemaking care. See also *home health care*.

homeopathy See under *medicine*.

homogeneous Composed of things that are the same, in contrast to "heterogeneous," which refers to a mixture. For example, in a homogeneous or "single-diagnosis" DRG, all the patients have the same diagnosis; on the other hand, a heterogeneous DRG is composed of patients with a variety of diagnoses.

homograft See *allograft*.

homology Similarity between structures or functions that are thought to indicate a common evolutionary origin.

homunculus A small model of a man, used to show anatomy.

horizontal transmission Transmission of a disease from one individual to another in the same generation. In contrast, vertical transmission is from one generation to another, such as transmission of HIV infection from a mother to her offspring.

hormone A chemical substance, produced in the body and secreted internally, usually into the blood, which has effects on organs other than those in which it is produced. Most hormones are produced by endocrine organs.

horse therapy See *hippotherapy*.

horticultural therapist A health professional specially trained in horticultural therapy. Many colleges and universities offer courses or programs in HT.

Horticultural Therapist Assistant (HTA) A basic credential for horticultural therapists, offered by the American Horticultural Therapist Association (AHTA) for those transitioning into the field. HT volunteer work, employment in HT and related fields, and various educational and professional experiences are credited toward attaining this credential. **www.ahta.org**

Horticultural Therapist Registered (HTR) The primary level of registration for a horticultural therapist. A minimum of 2,000 hours of HT employment experience is required. The credential is offered by the American Horticultural Therapist Association (AHTA). **www.ahta.org**

Master Horticultural Therapist (HTM) A certified horticultural therapist with extensive educational and professional backgrounds and at least 8,000 hours of HT experience. The credential is offered by the American Horticultural Therapist Association (AHTA). **www.ahta.org**

horticultural therapy (HT) The use of gardening and plants to improve a person's social, psychological, educational, and physical adjustment.

Horty, Springer & Mattern, PC The nation's first law firm to devote its practice entirely to healthcare law, as well as being the first to combine training and publishing with the practice of law. This firm publishes the well-known *Action Kit* series of newsletters for hospital trustees and others involved in health care. **www.hortyspringer.com**

Hoshin planning A Total Quality Management (TQM) system to work toward breakthrough improvement. Used by industry for a number of years, Hoshin planning is now being tried by some hospitals as part of their TQM programs. The system was developed in Japan after World War II to plan new processes. It uses seven tools, which are used individually or in combination: affinity diagrams, arrow diagrams, interrelationship digraphs, matrix diagrams, prioritization matrices, process decision program charts, and systematic diagrams. Other terms for the approach include policy deployment, structured breakthrough planning, and management by planning. See also *quality management*.

hospice A program that assists with the physical, emotional, spiritual, psychological, social, financial, and legal needs of the dying patient and her or his family. The service may be provided in the patient's home or in an institution (or division of an institution) set up for the purpose. Volunteers are usually integral parts of the staff. Bereavement care for the family is also included.

hospice and palliative medicine (HPM) An interdisciplinary approach to studying and caring for patients with a limited prognosis, where the main focus is on quality of life.

hospice and palliative nursing The area of nursing focusing on the needs of those dying, and/or for whom no therapy is appropriate other than that required to alleviate pain and suffering (see also *hospice* and *palliative care*).

Advanced Practice Certified Hospice and Palliative Nurse (ACHPN) An advanced practice nurse with at least a master's degree who has been certified by the National Board for Certification of Hospice and Palliative Nurses (NBCHPN). **www.nbchpn.org**

Certified Hospice and Palliative Licensed Nurse (CHPLN) A licensed practical or vocational nurse who has been certified by the National Board for Certification of Hospice and Palliative Nurses (NBCHPN). **www.nbchpn.org**

Certified Hospice and Palliative Nurse (CHPN) A registered nurse who has been certified in hospice and palliative nursing by the National Board for Certification of Hospice and Palliative Nurses (NBCHPN). **www.nbchpn.org**

Certified Hospice and Palliative Nursing Assistant (CHPNA) A nursing assistant with at least 2,000 hours of hospice and palliative nursing assistant practice under the supervision of a registered nurse, who has been certified by the National Board for Certification of Hospice and Palliative Nurses (NBCHPN). **www.nbchpn.org**

hospital The traditional definition of "hospital" is that it is a healthcare institution that has an organized professional staff and *medical staff*, and inpatient facilities, and which provides medical, nursing, and related services. States have specific definitions for what may be called a "hospital," including, for example, a minimum number of beds, and the services that must be available.

However, in an increasing number of communities, the term "hospital" is being applied to a geographic region occupied by a virtual healthcare organization with multiple programs operating in multiple locations. This emerging hospital is a deinstitutionalized, decentralized, electronically integrated community healthcare network, which includes churches, schools, neighborhoods, and workplaces. Services are being provided where the people reside and spend their time rather than expecting the people to go to the hospital, except for a narrow range of procedural or other services requiring its extraordinary resources.

A given hospital may fit one or more of the following definitions:

accredited hospital A hospital meeting the standards of the Joint Commission on Accreditation of Healthcare Organizations (JCAHO) and so certified by JCAHO (or, in Canada, by the Canadian Council on Health Facilities Accreditation (CCHFA)).

acute care hospital A hospital that cares primarily for patients with acute diseases and injuries (that is, those with an average length of stay (ALOS) of thirty days or less), or in which more than half the patients are admitted to units with an ALOS of thirty days or less. Synonyms: acute hospital, short-term hospital.

affiliated hospital A hospital that has some connection with another hospital, a training program, a multihospital system, a medical center, or some other organization.

AHA-registered hospital A hospital recognized by the American Hospital Association (AHA) as meeting its definition of a hospital and approved by its Board of Trustees for registration. Sometimes called simply "registered hospital."

certified hospital A hospital recognized by CMS as meeting the standards necessary to be a provider for Medicare.

chronic disease hospital See *long-term acute care hospital*, below.

city hospital A hospital controlled by a city government. Although a hospital operated by a city is often referred to as a "municipal hospital" (and properly can be called that), the term municipal hospital refers to a hospital operated by any local unit of government.

closed-staff hospital A hospital that has a *closed medical staff* (see under *medical staff*).

community hospital A hospital established primarily to provide services to the residents of the community in which it is located. Most community hospitals are nonprofit, nonfederal, and for short-term patients.

community-owned hospital See *nonprofit hospital*, below.

county hospital A hospital controlled by county government.

Critical Access Hospital (CAH) See *Critical Access Hospital Program*.

day care hospital A hospital that treats, during the day, patients who are able to return to their homes at night.

delegated hospital A hospital to which the former local professional standards review organization (PSRO) delegated authority to carry out review functions—admissions review and continued stay review (see under *review*), and *medical care evaluation*—for Medicare, Medicaid, and maternal and child health (MCH) patients. The delegated hospital's own determinations on these matters had to be accepted by the paying agency.

disproportionate share hospital (DSH) A hospital serving a higher than average proportion of low-income patients who are also Medicaid beneficiaries. Medicaid providers classified as a DSH are paid a higher rate under the prospective payment system (PPS) for inpatient services to help cover the higher cost of caring for these patients; the higher payment rate is intended to help ensure the continued viability of these *safety net hospitals* (see below). Large inner-city hospitals and many rural hospitals typically qualify as DSHs.

district hospital A hospital controlled by a special political subdivision (a "hospital district") created solely to operate the hospital and other healthcare institutions.

federal government hospital A hospital controlled and operated by the federal government.

for-profit hospital A hospital operated by a for-profit corporation, in which the profits are paid in the form of dividends to shareholders who own the corporation. A for-profit hospital is the same as an investor-owned hospital and a proprietary hospital; see also *publicly owned hospital*, below.

full-service hospital A hospital that provides a complete range of services needed by a community, including 24/7 emergency services, and serves all community members, regardless of ability to pay, insurance status, or medical condition. See also *limited-service hospital*, below.

general hospital A hospital offering care for a variety of conditions and age groups. It is contrasted with a specialty hospital (for example, a children's hospital, or an "eye and ear" or psychiatric hospital).

government hospital A hospital operated by a unit of government, usually the federal government. Hospitals operated by states are usually called state hospitals, and those operated by cities are usually called municipal hospitals.

investor-owned hospital See *for-profit hospital*, above.

licensed hospital A hospital licensed by the state licensing agency.

limited-service hospital A specialty hospital that focuses on a narrow range of procedures and/or services, in contrast to a *full-service hospital* (see above). These hospitals (often owned by physicians, who refer their patients to them) tend to limit services to those that are financially rewarding, such as orthopaedics or cardiac care, and their patients to those that can pay. This takes some of the lucrative business away from traditional community full-service hospitals (which fulfill essential needs, such as providing emergency services and care to the uninsured)—this in turn puts a strain on the community hospital's budget and threatens the availability of essential services.

In addition, Medicare antikickback regulations prohibit a physician from referring Medicare and Medicaid patients to a medical facility in which the physician has a financial interest, with an exception for "whole hospitals"—thus a loophole was found. In response to the growing number of physician-owned limited-service hospitals, the Medicare Modernization Act (MMA) mandated an eighteen-month moratorium prohibiting billing Medicare for self-referrals to new physician-owned specialty hospitals. This was extended by the Deficit Reduction Act of 2005 so that the issue could be studied by the Department of Health and Human Services (HHS). Synonym: limited-access facility.

long-term acute care hospital (LTACH) A hospital providing *long-term acute care*. Synonym: chronic disease hospital.

Medicare Dependent Hospital (MDH) A hospital that qualifies for certain advantages under the *Medicare Dependent Hospital (MDH) Program*.

municipal hospital A hospital operated by a municipal government, usually a city.

night hospital A hospital that treats, only at night, patients who are able to be out during the day.

nondelegated hospital A hospital not qualified under its professional standards review organization (PSRO) to perform review functions (see *delegated hospital*, above).

nonprofit hospital A hospital owned and operated by a corporation whose "profits" (excess of income over expense) are used for hospital purposes rather than returned to shareholders or investors as dividends. "Nonprofit" does not necessarily mean "tax-exempt." To be tax-exempt, an organization must not only be nonprofit, but also qualify under paragraph 501(c)(3) of the Internal Revenue Code as "scientific, religious, educational, or charitable" and have a determination to this effect from the IRS. The organization must also meet state requirements to be exempt from state taxes. Synonyms: community-owned hospital, not-for-profit hospital.

open-staff hospital A hospital that has an *open medical staff* (see under *medical staff*).

private hospital A hospital not operated by a government agency. A private hospital may be either for-profit or nonprofit.

proprietary hospital See *for-profit hospital*, above.

psychiatric hospital A hospital specializing in the care of patients with mental illness.

publicly owned hospital A hospital operated by a corporation that offers ownership of shares to the general public. The term is currently being applied to for-profit, investor-owned (proprietary) hospitals.

registered hospital Short for *AHA-registered hospital* (see above).

rehabilitation hospital A hospital specializing in rehabilitation care.

rural hospital A hospital serving a *rural area*. For Medicare purposes, most rural hospitals are qualified as either Critical Access Hospital (CAHs) (56%) (see *Critical Access Hospital Program*), *Sole Community Hospitals* (SCHs; see below) (18%), or Medicare Dependent Hospitals (MDHs) (6%) (see *Medicare Dependent Hospital Program*) (2007 figures).

safety net hospital A hospital, whether public or nonprofit, that by public mandate or its own commitment provides access to care for people with limited or no access to care because of their health condition or insurance status. Safety net hospitals, in addition, provide more than their proportionate share of public health and specialty services, including trauma, emergency psychiatric, pediatric and neonatal intensive care, alcoholism inpatient care, HIV/AIDS services, crisis prevention, and burn care. In the context of Medicaid, a hospital of this type is referred to as a *disproportionate share hospital* (DSH; see above). See also *Emergency Medical Treatment and Labor Act* and *safety net provider*.

satellite hospital A hospital operated by another, "parent," hospital, at a location different than that of the parent hospital.

self-insured hospital A hospital carrying *self-insurance* (see under *insurance*).

short-term hospital See *acute care hospital*, above.

Sole Community Hospital (SCH) A hospital that is the only reasonably available inpatient facility in a given geographic area, due to the absence of other hospitals, travel time or difficulty, or other reasons. Being classified as an SCH typically carries with it certain advantages under federal legislation, such as higher reimbursement rates under the Medicare program.

specialty hospital See *limited-service hospital*, above.

state hospital A hospital operated by a state. Such hospitals are usually specialized, particularly for the care of contagious disease and psychiatric patients.

teaching hospital A hospital with one or more accredited education programs in medicine, nursing, or other health science disciplines.

university hospital A hospital that is owned by or affiliated with a medical school and that is used in the education of physicians.

virtual hospital See *Virtual Hospital* (separate listing).

voluntary hospital A hospital that is private (nongovernmental), autonomous, and self-supported.

whole hospital An entire hospital, in contrast to a department or facility, such as an ambulatory surgical center (ASC). See *limited-service hospital*, above.

hospital auxiliary See under *auxiliary*.

hospital board See *governing body*.

hospital chain See *multihospital system*.

Hospital Community Benefits Standards Program (HCBSP) A voluntary demonstration certification program for hospitals launched in 1990, created at New York University by Robert Sigmond and Anthony Kovner, under grant support from the W.K. Kellogg Foundation. The purpose of the program was to stimulate hospitals to provide community benefits, and to reward them with special certification when they did.

The hospital had to meet four standards to be certified: (1) the hospital's governing board must define the boundaries of the community and approve the goals and operations plan of the community benefit program, (2) the hospital must sponsor projects that improve the overall health standards in the community, (3) the hospital must identify community health problems and ways to solve them (this effort can be conducted in conjunction with other community organizations and projects), and (4) the hospital must encourage the involvement of a wide range of hospital employees, medical staff members, and volunteers.

Hospital Compare A consumer-oriented web site sponsored by CMS that presents data on the performance of hospitals in relation to *National Hospital Quality Measures (NHQMs)*.

It is similar to the Joint Commission on Accreditation of Healthcare Organizations' **Quality Check**, but includes both accredited and nonaccredited hospitals. Performance at Quality Check will be compared with all JCAHO-accredited hospitals; at Hospital Compare, it will be compared with all reporting hospitals.

The performance measures used at both sites are identical (called NHQMs at Hospital Compare and National Quality Improvement Goals (NQIGs) at Quality Check), although not all measures will be found for all hospitals, nor all at both sites. For example, Quality Check reports mortality for AMI, but Hospital Compare does not. In addition, the interpretation and/or presentation of the data at each site may vary. See also **transparency initiative**. **www.hospitalcompare.hhs.gov**

hospital consultant See **healthcare consultant**.

Hospital Consumer Assessment of Healthcare Providers and Systems (HCAHPS) A standardized survey instrument for measuring patient satisfaction with hospital care, designed to permit comparisons among hospitals. It has a core set of questions, which may be combined with customized, hospital-specific questions. It was developed by CMS and the Agency for Healthcare Research and Quality (AHRQ). HCAHPS is one of the **National Hospital Quality Measures**. Synonym: CAHPS Hospital Survey. See **Consumer Assessment of Healthcare Providers and Systems**.

hospital discharge abstract system A system in which a number of hospitals submit coded, computer-ready summaries (discharge abstracts) of clinical records to a central shared computer service. The summaries may be submitted on paper or via computer media. In return, the hospitals receive reports and analyses of their own data, which they need for their internal operations. In addition, by using standardized information, hospitals may obtain interhospital comparisons, and may establish a database that may be used, under the confidentiality rules of the system, for research. The prototype of such systems was the **Professional Activity Study (PAS)**.

hospital district A special political subdivision created solely to operate the hospital and other healthcare institutions.

hospital engineer A term sometimes used to designate the person responsible for the operation and maintenance of the hospital's equipment and physical plant.

Hospital Health Plan (HHP) A specific model of a physician-hospital organization (PHO) whose managed care plan (MCP) is an alternative to the typical health maintenance organization (HMO). To the extent that groups and members of the community work with the hospital and physicians in a collaborative effort to create the plan, it is better called a "community health plan." The model was developed by Richard Ya Deau, MD, in 1984. A Hospital Health Plan has specific attributes:

1. An HHP is designed to provide the services needed for its own defined population; it is "community rated" in benefits as well as in premium structure (see **community rating** under **rating**). Its health services are those required for prevention of disease, injury, and disability and for provision of optimal care, with the goal of achieving optimal health for the community rather than simply health care for those who present themselves. It is designed to manage care rather than manage dollars.

2. An HHP can only be established after a thorough feasibility study and actuarial analysis, which provides evidence that the proposed plan will (1) have an adequate enrollment, (2) have adequate participation by providers and others, (3) be able to offer its locally defined benefit package for a saleable premium, (4) have a sound business and capitalization plan, and (5) be able to meet the state's requirements for licensure as an insurance company (reinsurance protects against unexpected loss). As a result of this careful preparation, several HHPs are in successful operation (including repaying their start-up financing) with as few as 12,000–15,000 enrollees.

3. An HHP is nonprofit, and because none of the premium income is committed to shareholders or equity investors, it is able to function with a **medical loss ratio** (portion of

the premium spent on benefits) reported to be about 91%. In a nonprofit operation, the higher this ratio is, the better, because the plan exists to provide care. (In a for-profit insurance company, the incentive is to keep this number low (often lower than 75%) in order to reward the investors.) Thus the nonprofit plan can provide more care with a lower premium.

4. Governance of an HHP is by a local board of directors representing physicians, health-care facilities, and enrollees.
5. The physicians in the HHP develop the medical policies and oversee their implementation, rather than being overseen by an "outside" HMO.
6. The hospital's financial survival is insured by including in the financing of the HHP a capitation amount for the predicted hospitalizations for the enrolled population.
7. Physicians may be paid by either fee-for-service from a capitated pool or directly capitated, depending on the policies of the plan and individual preference.

An HHP has available to it a management information system (MIS) that provides all necessary online transactional processing (OLTP) resources for a managed care plan and an on-demand knowledge-based analytic processing system. See discussion of these processing types under *Online Analytical Processing* and *knowledge-based management*.

hospital information system (HIS) See under *information system*.

Hospital Insurance Program (HI) See *Medicare Part A* under *Medicare*.

hospital-issued notice of noncoverage (HINN) A notice given to a Medicare beneficiary by a hospital when, in the hospital's opinion, Medicare will not cover the patient's admission or continued stay because (1) the services are not reasonable and necessary for the diagnosis or treatment of illness or injury, (2) the services are not being delivered in the appropriate setting, or (3) the services constitute custodial care. May be issued prior to admission, during the stay, or upon discharge. The notice is not an official Medicare coverage decision, but Medicare generally will not pay for inpatient care where the hospital has issued an HINN. Sometimes called a discharge notice or continued stay denial notice (CSDN). See also *notice of discharge and Medicare appeal rights* and *notice of Medicare non-coverage*.

hospitalist A physician who specializes in inpatient medicine. A hospitalist manages the care of inpatients (hospitalized patients) in the same way that a primary care physician (PCP) manages the care of outpatients. The *Society of Hospital Medicine* defines hospitalists as "physicians whose primary professional focus is the general medical care of hospitalized patients. Their activities include patient care, teaching research, and leadership related to Hospital Medicine." Hospitalists have long been common in urban hospitals in Canada and Great Britain, but had been scarce in the United States until the late 1990s. The rapid rise of managed care is believed to have led to increased numbers of hospitalists.

The term was coined by Drs. Robert Wachter and Lee Goldman in a 1996 article (Wachter, R.M., & Goldman, L. "The Emerging Role of 'Hospitalists' in the American Health Care System." *New England Journal of Medicine*, 1996;335:514–517).

hospitalization A period of stay in the hospital, where the patient stays in the hospital overnight. Also, the placing of a patient in the hospital.

partial hospitalization A structured program of treatment where a patient spends a certain number of hours at a hospital (or other facility) during each day, but returns to his or her home at night. Often used to provide psychiatric or drug treatment services where hospitalization is not necessary or desirable.

hospitalize To admit a patient to a hospital in which that patient will be lodged. The patient, once admitted, becomes an "inpatient." See *admission (hospital)*.

hospital medicine The medical specialty practiced by *hospitalists*.

hospital nursing care See under *nursing care*.

Hospital Payment Monitoring Program (HPMP) A program carried out by quality improvement organizations (QIOs) to prevent payment errors by prospective payment system hospitals. It was established by CMS to protect the Medicare Trust Fund by ensuring that Medicare pays only for services that are reasonable and medically necessary. QIOs monitor the incidence of improper fee-for-service payments for acute care inpatient hospital stays by analyzing data, conducting focused audits, and helping hospitals to implement system changes to prevent payment errors.

The program was originally called the Payment Error Prevention Program (PEPP) and carried out by peer review organizations (PROs, now QIOs) to reduce the **payment error rate**. Audits by the Office of Inspector General (OIG) of Medicare payments made in 1996 and 1997 estimated that billions of dollars per year were actually "incorrect payments." It was also estimated that 20% of these incorrect payments were related to inpatient services; hence the HPMP. The following types of payment errors were believed to be most common:

1. Incorrectly coded services (see **coding (billing)**).
2. Billing for services that are not medically necessary (see **medical necessity**).
3. Billing for non-covered services.
4. Billing for insufficiently documented services (see **evaluation and management documentation guidelines** and **physician query form**).

Payments for claims other than inpatient hospitals stays are reviewed by the **Comprehensive Error Rate Testing** (CERT) program.

Hospital Quality Alliance (HQA) A public-private collaboration to improve the quality of care provided by the nation's hospitals by measuring and publicly reporting on that care. Hospitals voluntarily report their performance on a number of **National Hospital Quality Measures**, and the results can be seen by consumers via the **Hospital Compare** web site.

HQA includes the CMS, American Hospital Association (AHA), Federation of American Hospitals (FAH), and Association of American Medical Colleges (AAMC), and is supported by other organizations such as the Agency for Healthcare Research and Quality (AHRQ), National Quality Forum (NQF), Joint Commission on Accreditation of Healthcare Organizations (JCAHO), American Medical Association (AMA), American Nurses Association (ANA), National Association of Children's Hospitals and Related Institutions, Consumer-Purchaser Disclosure Project, AFL-CIO, AARP, and U.S. Chamber of Commerce.

The full name of the alliance is The Hospital Quality Alliance: Improving Care Through Information. Originally called the National Voluntary Hospital Reporting Initiative (NVHRI). See also **AQA** and **Quality Alliance Steering Committee**. **www.aha.org/aha_app/ issues/HQA**

Hospital Quality Initiative (HQI) See **Quality Initiative**.

Hospital Quality Measures (HQMs) See **National Hospital Quality Measures**.

Hospital Research and Educational Trust (HRET) A nonprofit research arm of the American Hospital Association (AHA), which supports activities to improve hospitals and health services. **www.hret.org**

Hospitals & Health Networks The official monthly publication of the American Hospital Association (AHA).

hospital service A term used interchangeably with "department" when referring to elements of the hospital organization, and which may refer to the hospital or its medical staff. The nursing department may be called the nursing service, the pharmacy the pharmacy service, the housekeeping department the housekeeping service, and so on. When used in the plural, "hospital services" more commonly refers to the clinical services or clinical departments of the medical staff than to the hospital's administrative units.

hospital-specific relative value (HSRV) A method for adjusting the relative weights given to certain DRGs in order to take into account the severity of illnesses encountered and the cost of providing their care in a given hospital, so that hospital payment under Medicare better reflects the relative volume and types of diagnostic, therapeutic, and bed services required for the unique mix of patients treated at each hospital.

Hospital Statistics The annual publication of the American Hospital Association (AHA) covering hospitals in the United States, and giving descriptions of each as well as tabulated data on hospitals. Subtitled *The AHA Profile of U.S. Hospitals*. See also **AHA Guide to the Health Care Field**.

HOST Healthcare Open Systems and Trials. See **CPRI-HOST**.

hotel-hospital A hotel facility operated by a hospital, at hotel rates, for use by patients and their families before and after hospitalization. Such facilities are sometimes used for temporary care for elderly patients in order to give their family caregivers a rest. If separated from the hospital, the hotel-hospital often provides shuttle bus service. Synonym: guest bed program.

hotel, medical care See **medical care hotel**.

house staff See under **staff (group)**.

HP See **Hemapheresis Practitioner** under **clinical laboratory specialist**.

HPA See **Health Policy Agenda for the American People**.

HPMP See **Hospital Payment Monitoring Program**.

HPPC Health plan purchasing cooperative. See **health alliance**.

HPSA See **Health Professional Shortage Area**.

HQA See **Hospital Quality Alliance**.

HQI Hospital Quality Initiative. See **Quality Initiative**.

HQM Hospital Quality Measures. See **National Hospital Quality Measures**.

HRA See **health record analyst**, **health reimbursement account**, and **health risk appraisal**.

HRB See **health record bank**.

HRET See **Hospital Research and Educational Trust**.

HRQOL See **health-related quality of life** under **quality of life**.

HRSA See **Health Resources and Services Administration**.

HSA See **Health Savings Account**.

HSRV See **hospital-specific relative value**.

HT See **Histotechnician** under **clinical laboratory technician**, and **horticultural therapy**.

HTA See **health technology assessment**, and **Horticultural Therapist Assistant** (under **horticultural therapist**).

HTAi See **Health Technology Assessment International**.

HTAR Health Technology Assessment Reports. See **Office of Health Technology Assessment**.

HTL See **Histotechnologist** under **clinical laboratory technologist**.

HTM See **Master Horticultural Therapist** under **horticultural therapist**.

HTR See **Horticultural Therapist Registered** under **horticultural therapist**.

HTT Horticultural Therapist Technician; see **Horticultural Therapist Assistant** under **horticultural therapist**.

hub site See **distant site**.

HUGN See **Human Gene Nomenclature**.

HUGO See **Human Genome Organisation**.

Hui OpenVistA See under **VistA**.

Human Cognome Project (HCP) A proposed multidisciplinary project, comparable to the Human Genome Project, to chart the structure and functions of the human mind. It was suggested by Robert E. Horn, Stanford University, and was subsequently recommended in a 2002 report of the National Science Foundation, *Converging Technologies for Improving Human Performance: Nanotechnology, Biotechnology, Information Technology, and Cognitive Science*. (Horn coined the term "**cognome**" to parallel "genome.")

human factors engineering See **ergonomics**.

Human Gene Nomenclature (HUGN) A database containing the approved names and unique symbols (short-form abbreviations) of all known human genes. For example, the gene named "steroidogenic acute regulator" has the symbol "STAR"; "arginine-fifty homeobox pseudogene 1" has the symbol "ARGFXP1." HUGN is developed and maintained by the HUGO Gene Nomenclature Committee (HGNC) (see *Human Genome Organisation*), which approves the names and symbols. All approved symbols are stored in **Genew**, the Human Gene Nomenclature Database. In 2007, HGNC had approved names and symbols for over 20,000 genes (for each of which there could be at least one disorder with a unique diagnosis). The Consolidated Health Informatics (CHI) initiative has adopted HUGN as a standard. **www.gene.ucl.ac.uk/nomenclature**

human genetics See under *genetics*.

Human Genome Organisation (HUGO) An international organization of scientists involved in human genetics, established in 1989 by a group of the world's leading human geneticists. HUGO's primary mission is to promote and sustain international collaboration in the field of human genetics. The HUGO Gene Nomenclature Committee (HGNC) is responsible for maintaining the *Human Gene Nomenclature*. **www.hugo-international.org**

Human Genome Project (HGP) A thirteen-year effort, begun in 1990, to discover all the estimated 20,000–25,000 human genes and make them accessible for further biological study. Another project goal was to determine the complete sequence of the 3 billion DNA subunits (bases in the human genome). As part of the HGP, parallel studies were carried out on selected model organisms such as the bacterium *E. coli* and the mouse to help develop the technology and interpret human gene function. The HGP also studied the societal implications (ethical, legal, and social issues (ELSI)) of doing genetic research in the first place. The project was coordinated by the National Institutes of Health (NIH) and the U.S. Department of Energy (DOE). International partners included the United Kingdom, France, Germany, Japan, and China. The HGP was originally planned to last fifteen years, but rapid technological advances accelerated the completion date to 2003. See also *Genomics:GTL*, *Human Gene Nomenclature*, *National Human Genome Research Institute* (under *National Institutes of Health*), and *United Nations Educational, Scientific and Cultural Organization*. **genomics.energy.gov**

human immunodeficiency virus (HIV) See *HIV (human immunodeficiency virus)*.

human leukocyte antigen (HLA) Chemicals found in blood that are often responsible for rejection of bone marrow and other organ transplants. The body's reaction to these antigens may also interfere with transfusion of blood platelets. See also *leukoreduction*.

hybrid The offspring of parents with dissimilar genes.

hybridization The process of producing offspring, hybrids, from parents with dissimilar genes. The process can produce hybrid plants or animals, or hybrid cells, called hybridomas, which are used in producing monoclonal antibodies.

hybridoma A hybrid cell formed by fusing two cells of different origins. In monoclonal antibody (MAB) technology in cancer therapy the hybridoma is formed by fusing a cancer cell and an antibody-producing cell.

Hyde Amendment An amendment to the Departments of Labor and Health, Education, and Welfare Appropriation Act of 1976, revised in 1980, which forbids federal funds to reimburse the cost of non-therapeutic abortions under the Medicaid program. The 1980 revisions allowed federal funds to be used if a woman was raped or abused by incest and she promptly reported the incident to the police or a public health service. This funding restriction was named after Representative Hyde, the Congressional sponsor of the amendment. The Hyde Amendment withstood serious Constitutional attack in *Harris v. McRae*, 448 U.S. 297 (1980).

hyperbaric Pertaining to gas pressure greater than one atmosphere absolute (ATA), which is the pressure of air at sea level.

hyperbaric medicine Study of the effect of increased gas pressures on the human body, and use of such pressure for medical treatment. See *hyperbaric oxygen therapy* and *hyperbaric therapy*. See also *undersea medicine*.

hyperbaric nursing See *baromedical nursing*.

hyperbaric oxygen therapy (HBO, HBOT) The use of increased oxygen pressure to treat illness or injury. The entire body is enclosed in a *hyperbaric* chamber, where the patient breathes 100% oxygen intermittently while pressure is increased to greater than one atmosphere absolute (ATA). HBO is being used for an increasing number of conditions, such as air or gas embolism, carbon monoxide poisoning, crush injuries, certain wounds, radiation injury, and burns.

hyperbaric technologist A health professional with special training in hyperbaric therapy and hyperbaric oxygen therapy (HBO).

Certified Hyperbaric Technologist (CHT) A hyperbaric technologist who has met the certification requirements of the National Board of Diving and Hyperbaric Medical Technology (NBDHMT) (**www.nbdhmt.com**). To qualify, the candidate must be one of the following (in addition to meeting training and competency standards): respiratory therapist, diving medical technician, physician assistant, corpsman, medical services specialist, emergency medical technician, paramedic, registered nurse, licensed practical nurse, nurse practitioner, physician, life support technician, certified nurse aide, medical assistant, chamber technician, physiologist, or medical researcher.

hyperbaric therapy The therapeutic use of hyperbaric gas pressures by enclosing an extremity of the body or the entire body in a chamber where the pressure can be increased. Sometimes ordinary atmosphere (21% oxygen) and sometimes pure (100%) oxygen is used (see *hyperbaric oxygen therapy*). Hyperbaric treatment is best known for treatment of the bends (the accumulation of nitrogen bubbles in the blood stream when divers ascend too rapidly from submersion).

hyperendemic See *endemic*.

hyperthermia Treatment by raising the body's temperature.

hypoallergenic A term without clinical or scientific meaning, used by cosmetic and other manufacturers to imply that their product is less likely to cause an allergic reaction. There are no standards, definitions, or Food and Drug Administration (FDA) regulations governing the use of this term.

I

IA See *intra-arterial*.

IACUC See *institutional animal care and use committee*.

IAD See *instructional advance directive* under *advance directive*.

IADL See *Instrumental Activities of Daily Living scale*.

IAMRA See *International Association of Medical Regulatory Authorities*.

iatrogenic An illness or injury resulting from a diagnostic procedure, therapy, or other element of health care. A significant category of iatrogenic injury results from the **adverse drug event (ADE)**, as pointed out by the 1999 Institute of Medicine (IOM) report, *To Err Is Human* (see **patient safety**). An iatrogenic illness is often confused with a "nosocomial" illness, which simply means an illness "occurring in a hospital."

IBB See *interest-based bargaining*.

IBCLC See *International Board Certified Lactation Consultant* under *lactation consultant*.

IBNR See *incurred but not reported*.

IC See *Infection Control*.

ICCS See *International Classification of Clinical Services*.

ICD (classification) *International Classification of Diseases*. A publication of the World Health Organization (WHO), revised periodically and now in its Tenth Revision, dated 1994. The full title is *International Statistical Classification of Diseases and Related Health Problems*. This classification, which originated for use in deaths, is used worldwide for that purpose. In addition, it has been used widely in the United States for hospital diagnosis classification since about 1955 through adaptations and modifications made in the United States of the Seventh, Eighth, and Ninth Revisions. Modification was required for hospital use because, as discussed under **classification (scheme)**, the purpose of the classification determines the pigeonholes; for example, "death pigeonholes" are quite different, in many instances, from those for illnesses and injuries. The current modification, *International Classification of Diseases, Ninth Revision, Clinical Modification (ICD-9-CM) (1978)*, has been in official use in the United States since 1979.

ICD (device) See *implantable cardioverter-defibrillator* under *defibrillator*.

ICD-9 The Ninth Revision of the *International Classification of Diseases* (see **ICD**). The 1975 revision of the World Health Organization (WHO) series of statistical classifications, which was expanded for North American use into the *International Classification of Diseases, Ninth Revision, Clinical Modification (ICD-9-CM)*. One often finds reference to use of ICD-9 as the disease classification system being employed in clinical settings, research, and reimbursement systems in the United States. This is incorrect; the system being used is ICD-9-CM, except in references to the international exchange of statistical information at the national level.

ICD-9-CM *International Classification of Diseases, Ninth Revision, Clinical Modification*. The classification in current use for coding of diagnoses and procedures for indexing medical records by diagnoses and operations, for compiling hospital statistics, and for submitting bills in the prospective payment system (PPS).

ICD-O See *International Classification of Diseases for Oncology*.

ICD-10 *International Statistical Classification of Diseases and Related Health Problems*, the Tenth Revision of the *International Classification of Diseases*, published by the World Health Organization (WHO) in 1992. The original volume, published in 1900, was called *The International List of Causes of Death*. Subsequent revisions, about every ten years, have broadened the scope of the volume to include causes of injury and illness, their external causes, and "other factors influencing health status and contact with health services." The name was changed with the Seventh Revision (1955) to *The International Classification of Diseases, Injuries, and Causes of Death*. This title was used for the Eighth and Ninth Revisions as well. With the Tenth Revision, the title shown above has been adopted. In view of the widespread use of ICD-9 in the United States, the Tenth Revision is referred to as "ICD-10," despite the fact that this short title no longer reflects the actual title of the classification.

Major changes from the Ninth Revision include the adoption of alphanumeric codes (previously most of the codes were numeric), the provision of categories for additional "other factors" (see **problem**), changes in the details of categories throughout the classification, changes in the chapters and chapter headings, and the inclusion of the previous "supplementary classifications" as chapters within the classification itself. A comparison between ICD-9 and ICD-10 is shown in the table below.

Table 1: ICD-9 vs. ICD-10: Comparison of Chapters, Codes, and Titles

Ch.	ICD-9	ICD-10	ICD-9 Chapter Title	ICD-10 Chapter Title
I	001–139	A00–B99	Infectious and Parasitic Diseases	Certain Infectious and Parasitic Diseases
II	140–239	C00–D48	Neoplasms	Neoplasms
III	240–279		Endocrine, Nutritional and Metabolic Diseases and Immunity Disorders	
		D50–D89		Diseases of Blood and Blood-Forming Organs and Certain Disorders Involving the Immune Mechanism
IV	280–289		Diseases of Blood and Blood-Forming Organs	
		E00–E90		Endocrine, Nutritional, and Metabolic Diseases
V	290–319	F00–F99	Mental Disorders	Mental and Behavioral Disorders
VI	320–389	G00–G99	Diseases of the Nervous System and Sense Organs	Diseases of the Nervous System
VII	390–459		Diseases of the Circulatory System	
		H00–H59		Diseases of the Eye and Adnexa
VIII	460–519		Diseases of the Respiratory System	

Ch.	ICD-9	ICD-10	ICD-9 Chapter Title	ICD-10 Chapter Title
		H60–H95		Diseases of the Ear and Mastoid Process
IX	520–579		Diseases of the Digestive System	
		I00–I99		Diseases of the Circulatory System
X	580–629		Diseases of the Genitourinary System	
		J00–J99		Diseases of the Respiratory System
XI	630–676		Complications of Pregnancy, Childbirth, and the Puerperium	
		K00–K93		Diseases of the Digestive System
XII	680–709	L00–L99	Diseases of the Skin and Subcutaneous Tissue	Diseases of the Skin and Subcutaneous Tissue
XIII	710–739	M00–M99	Diseases of the Musculoskeletal System and Connective Tissue	Diseases of the Musculoskeletal System and Connective Tissue
XIV	740–759		Congenital Anomalies	
		N00–N99		Diseases of the Genitourinary System
XV	760–779		Certain Conditions Originating in the Perinatal Period	
		O00–O99		Pregnancy, Childbirth, and Puerperium
XVI	780–799		Symptoms, Signs, and Ill-Defined Conditions	
		P00–P96		Certain Conditions Originating in the Perinatal Period
XVII	800–999		Injury and Poisoning	

Ch.	ICD-9	ICD-10	ICD-9 Chapter Title	ICD-10 Chapter Title
		Q00–Q99		Congenital Malformations, Deformations, and Chromosomal Abnormalities
XVIII		R00–R99		Symptoms, Signs, and Abnormal Clinical and Laboratory Findings Not Elsewhere Classified
XIX		S00–T98		Injury, Poisoning, and Certain Other Consequences of External Causes
XX		V01–Y98		External Causes of Morbidity and Mortality
XXI		Z00–Z99		Factors Influencing Health Status and Contact with Health Services
	E800–E999		Supplementary Classification of External Causes of Injury and Poisoning	
	V01–V82		Supplementary Classification of Factors Influencing Health Status and Contact with Health Services	

ICD-10-CM *International Classification of Diseases, Tenth Revision, Clinical Modification.* The version of **ICD-10** that has been modified by the National Center for Health Statistics (NCHS) for use in the United States as the sequel to **ICD-9-CM**. The work was essentially completed in 1997, but implementation has been delayed at least until 2011. The volumes are similar to **ICD-9-CM** in that diagnoses are classified according to the basic categories of **ICD-10** (see table above). **ICD-10-CM** differs in at least two major respects from **ICD-9-CM**: (1) no procedure classification is supplied because ICD-10 has no procedure classification (but see **ICD-10-PCS**); (2) there is a great proliferation in the numbers of categories, but the added categories increase the complexity of the system rather than its specificity because they are primarily **combination categories** (see under **category**).

ICD-10-PCS *ICD-10 Procedure Coding System.* The coding system for procedures being built under contract for CMS as a companion to **ICD-10-CM** (although in spite of its title, **ICD-10 PCS** has no relationship to **ICD-10**). Essentially ready for use in 2001, it was not yet implemented in 2007.

    ICD-10-PCS is an extremely complete but complex system that, like **SNOMED**, requires the coupling of elements from several modules to form the code (with its nomenclature) for cedure. There are seven lists (modules), each with a potential of thirty-four alphanumeric entries (unlike in ICD-10, the letters "I" and "O" have been omitted to avoid confusion). Not all of the 52 billion possible combinations have been used, but some 200,640 codes are available for the male reproductive system, and 482,000 for the female. No diagnostic information is included.

ICD-10-PCS is a **coding** system, not a **classification (scheme)**. It cannot be considered a replacement for the procedure classification in ICD-9-CM because ICD-10-PCS does not group procedures at levels suitable for describing clinical practice or resource use in statistics or for billing.

ICD-10 Procedure Coding System See *ICD-10-PCS*.

ICF See *intermediate care facility* and *International Classification of Functioning, Disability, and Health*.

ICF/MR See *intermediate care facility for the mentally retarded*.

ICH International Conference on Harmonisation of Technical Requirements for Registration of Pharmaceuticals for Human Use. An international effort to standardize the pharmaceutical regulatory environment worldwide. **www.ich.org**

ICHI See *International Classification of Health Interventions*.

ICIDH International Classification of Impairments, Disabilities, and Handicaps. See *International Classification of Functioning, Disability, and Health*.

ICN See *International Council of Nurses*.

ICNP See *International Classification for Nursing Practice*.

ICP See *infection control professional*. Also means interdisciplinary care plan; see *interdisciplinary patient care plan*.

ICRC See *infant care review committee*.

ICT See *information and communication technology*.

ICU See *intensive care unit*.

ICU physician staffing (IPS) A method to improve patient safety by making sure that hospital intensive care units (ICUs) are staffed by qualified physicians specializing in intensive care (called intensivists). An initiative of the *Leapfrog Group*.

identifier Any of a variety of codes used to identify people, products, or services. When used in the context of products and services, these identifiers are typically used to improve efficiencies in what is called "supply chain management." Identifiers are typically numeric (digits) or alphanumeric (letters and digits), but may include special characters or symbols.

"Uniform" (or "universal") identifiers typically have a sponsoring organization that defines and maintains necessary information about that identifier, such as its structure and rules for its use. Examples include the Social Security number used to identify people, the ISBN number that identifies books, and the Universal Product Code (UPC) that identifies items in retail stores (including groceries). Identifiers (the message) should not be confused with the method used to represent them (the medium). One of the most popular mediums used to represent identifiers is the *bar code*.

Identifiers are important in any system that must keep track of many unique entities, and they are critical if that system is to be automated or take advantage of new information system technologies. The healthcare industry has been moving toward usage of identifiers in many areas; see *Health Industry Bar Code*, *National Drug Code*, *National Health Plan Identifier*, *National Patient Identifier*, *National Payer ID*, *National Provider Identifier*, *unique device identifier*, *unique identifier number*, and *Universal Product Number*.

IDN Integrated delivery network. See *integrated health delivery network*.

IDS Integrated delivery system. See *integrated health delivery network*.

IEC See *Independent Ethics Committee*.

IEEE Institute of Electrical and Electronics Engineers, a national organization. Recognized and accredited by ANSI, IEEE has a group working on computer standards, some of which apply to medical systems. See *MEDIX*.

IEEE EMBS A task group working on an effort to develop standards for the exchange of data between hospital computer systems. See *MEDIX*.

IEEE 1073 A task group developing standards for medical device communications.

IFIC See *International Food Information Council*.

IG Inspector General. See *Office of Inspector General*.

IGNet See *Office of Inspector General*.

IHC See *interactive health communication*.

IHCA Individual health care account. See *Medical Savings Account*.

IHCIA Indian Health Care Improvement Act. See *Indian Health Service*.

IHE An initiative by healthcare professionals and industry to improve the way computer systems in health care share information. IHE promotes the coordinated use of established standards, such as DICOM and HL7, to address specific clinical needs in support of optimal patient care. Sponsored in North America by the American College of Cardiology (ACC), Healthcare Information and Management Systems Society (HIMSS), and Radiological Society of North America (RSNA). There are also an IHE Europe and IHE Japan. IHE stands for Integrating the Healthcare Enterprise. **www.ihe.net**

IHI See *Institute for Healthcare Improvement*.

IHR See *International Health Regulations*.

IHRB See *independent health record bank*.

IHS See *Indian Health Service*. Also integrated healthcare system; see *integrated health delivery network*.

IHTSDO See *International Health Terminology Standards Development Organisation*.

IIHI See *individually identifiable health information*.

IISP See *Information Infrastructure Standards Panel*.

ILS See *intermediate life support* under *life support*.

IM See *internal medicine*, *intramuscular*, and *intraoperative monitoring*. See also *information management department*.

imaging (archival) The process of storing analog and digital images of documents (including text, x-rays, electrocardiograph tracings, etc.), especially in medical records, on CD-ROM or some other electronic medium. This electronic storage is a replacement, in the main, for microfilming.

imaging (diagnostic) A term that covers the variety of technologies that result in pictures (images) of body structures or functioning. The first imaging technology was, perhaps, medical illustration. Then came conventional radiology (x-ray). The next technology to gain prominence was computed tomography (CT) scanning. To these have been added magnetic resonance imaging (MRI), functional MRI, diagnostic ultrasound, single photon emission computer tomography (SPECT), and positron emission tomography (PET). Many former Departments of Radiology in hospitals are now called Departments of Imaging.

IMC See *indigent medical care*.

IMD exclusion A rule in the Medicaid program that prohibits coverage of medical assistance for services provided to any individual over age twenty-one and under age sixty-five who resides in an **institution for mental disease (IMD)**, even for treatment unrelated to mental illness, and even for treatment provided outside the facility itself. The Department of Health and Human Services (HHS) defines an IMD as "an institution that is primarily engaged in providing diagnosis, treatment or care of persons with mental diseases." A hospital, skilled nursing facility (SNF), or intermediate care facility (ICF), for example, can also be an IMD for Medicaid purposes; the "overall character" of the institution governs. The IMD exclusion conflicts with the *Emergency Medical Treatment and Labor Act (EMTALA)* because EMTALA requires both general and psychiatric hospitals to provide emergency treatment regardless of the patient's ability to pay, but under the IMD exclusion, Medicaid would not pay the psychiatric hospital for that treatment. Legislation (the **Medicaid Psychiatric Hospital Fairness Act**) has been introduced to remedy this conflict.

IME See *indirect medical education* under *medical education*, under *education*.

IMHO In my humble opinion.

IMIA See *International Medical Informatics Association*.

IMIS Integrated management information system. See *management information system* under *information system*.

IMM See *Important Message from Medicare*.

immobilization A method of disposing of plutonium in which the plutonium is embedded within the structure of a durable, solid material, such as molten glass or ceramic.

immortalized cell In genetics, refers to a cell taken from a culture of cells reproduced outside the body. See also *primary cell*.

immune system The organs, cells, and other components that work together to fight against disease and other foreign agents to protect the body.

immunity The condition of being immune or insusceptible to an agent. The term is most often used in regard to resistance to infectious disease—immunity to smallpox, diphtheria, colds, AIDS, and the like. However, one may also speak, for example, of **stress immunity**, the ability to resist stress, or **cold immunity**, the ability to withstand cold. Immunity is relative, in that almost any immunity may be overwhelmed by either (1) a massive attack (such as contamination of a wound by barnyard dirt loaded with tetanus) or (2) a general lack of resistance, often referred to as **immunodeficiency** (an emaciated, starving person is unlikely to resist pneumonia); the combination of a massive attack and lack of resistance makes infection even more likely.

acquired immunity Immunity to infection that is the result of (1) infection, or (2) the administration of an agent, such as a vaccine, either of which may stimulate the body to develop active immunity.

active immunity A type of acquired immunity in which the body is stimulated to produce its own antibodies. This occurs either: (1) in response to an infection (which may or may not produce symptoms); or (2) in response to the inoculation of a vaccine, either a strain of killed bacteria or other infectious agent, or an attenuated (weakened) strain of the infectious agent (a strain that is able to stimulate the body to produce antibodies but not symptoms).

herd immunity The relative immunity of a group of persons or animals as a result of the immunity of an adequate number (proportion) of the individuals in the group. The immunity may be active immunity or passive immunity. Herd immunity is actually an immunity against an epidemic, rather than the immunity of individuals against infection. For an epidemic to succeed, it must be possible for the disease to travel from one individual to another. When enough individuals are immune (perhaps 70% to 80%), the epidemic simply dies out. Herd immunity is fortunate for the public health control of contagious diseases, because the chance of being able to get everyone immunized is practically zero.

passive immunity A type of acquired immunity that is conferred by giving to the person (or animal) immune substances developed in another animal or human. One example is tetanus antitoxin, an immune substance developed in a laboratory animal and transferred to the human patient by inoculation (injection). Such an antibody is prefabricated and immediately ready to repel the invasion of the infection (in this case, tetanus). Its protection is temporary, because the body eliminates the antitoxin as fast as it can (it is also a foreign substance), and thereafter the body is susceptible to tetanus again.

immunodeficiency See *immunity*.

immunology The study of the *immune system* and its disorders.

impaired A descriptive term that, when applied to a professional such as a physician, usually encompasses problems such as alcoholism, drug dependence, senility, physical or mental illness, or behavior problems, which may interfere with the physician's competency to practice.

The protection of the **impaired physician**'s patients should be the first priority, while getting help for the physician him- or herself should immediately follow. Sometimes the impaired physician will admit to the impairment or agree to seek help only if the impairment is not reported to the state medical board. Within a hospital, an impaired physician will generally first get the attention of his or her **peer review committee**. See also **state medical board** under **board (credentialing)**.

implant To place a substitute organ, tissue, or device in a living body. The difference between implanting and transplanting is that implanting may involve a device (for example, a cardiac pacemaker, an artificial hip joint, or a capsule of radioactive material) or an organ or tissue, whereas transplanting involves only organs or tissues. The term "implant" may also be used as a noun to indicate the organ or tissue implanted.

implicit "Naturally" a part of, although not specifically stated. See **explicit** for further discussion.

Important Message from Medicare (IMM) A document that must be given to a Medicare beneficiary upon that person's admission to a hospital. The IMM explains the beneficiary's rights under Medicare, including the right to remain in the hospital as long as it is medically necessary.

Improper Payments Information Act of 2002 (IPIA) Federal legislation designed to save money by reducing the amount of "improper payments" (defined as payments that should not have been made or were made in an incorrect amount) made by federal agencies. Annually, the head of each agency must submit estimates of the amount of improper payments made by its programs and activities to Congress, along with an action plan to reduce improper payments for any program for which those payments exceeded $10 million. CMS derives its improper payment estimate for Medicare through the Comprehensive Error Rate Testing (CERT) program and the Hospital Payment Monitoring Program (HPMP). Pub. L. No. 107-300, 116 Stat. 2350 (2002), codified at 31 U.S.C. § 3321 (2005).

IMSystem Indicator Measurement System. A program developed by the Joint Commission on Accreditation of Healthcare Organizations (JCAHO) in 1988 to "gauge and compare the actual performance of health care organizations, stimulate improved patient care, and to generate reports on performance to meet the needs of patients, purchasers and regulators of health care." It included seven indicator sets for perioperative care, obstetrics, cardiovascular care, oncology, trauma, medication use, and infection control. The system, set to begin in 1995 with accredited hospitals collecting and transmitting data, was never put into place. However, it did set the stage for the **ORYX** initiative and the development of **performance measures**.

IMT See **intraoperative monitoring technologist**.

IN Informatics nurse; see **informatics nursing**.

incentive A reward for desired behavior. In health care, this term is used in regard to rewards to institutions and individuals for decreasing hospital and physician costs, and for encouraging patients to be frugal in demands for health care. See also **disincentive**.

incentive benefit plan A health benefits plan that provides a built-in incentive for its beneficiaries to reduce their use of the plan's services. The incentive may consist of monetary or other rewards.

incentive pay plan A plan for rewarding the performance of individuals in an institution with added compensation. The incentives typically are in the form of annual bonuses or percentage increments above the base salary if specified financial, productivity, or quality performance goals are met, although some institutions use long-term incentives. Although these incentives typically apply to top executive personnel, many employers offer group incentives (i.e., incentives to the personnel in various organizational units of the institution).

incidence See **prevalence**.

incident An event in the hospital that does not comport with the standards of the hospital, or that is unexpected and undesirable. For example, a patient leaving against medical advice (AMA) or a patient's adverse reaction to administration of a drug might be classified by a hospital as "incidents." Sometimes "incident" is used more narrowly to mean an accident (such as a fall) in which a patient is injured (or might have been injured) and for which the hospital may be liable. An incident report is completed for each incident, to assist in quality management and risk management. See also *adverse patient occurrence*.

incidental Happening by chance or as a minor consequence; not intentional. See *incidental surgery* under *surgery (treatment)*.

income Money earned during an accounting period, in contrast with revenue, which is the increase in assets or the decrease in liabilities during the accounting period.

income and expense statement A standard part of a financial statement that shows the revenues, costs, and expenses of the organization for the accounting period. The other part of the financial statement is the *balance sheet*. Synonyms: profit and loss statement (P & L), operating statement, income statement.

incompetent (ability) An individual who is considered unable to perform a task in an acceptable manner.

incompetent (legal capacity) Lacking the ability to make decisions. Competency is relative, and standards of legal competency will vary according to the type of decision to be made. For example, competency to make decisions about one's own healthcare treatment requires the ability to understand one's condition, the options available, and the potential consequences of the various alternatives.

A person who is involuntarily committed to a psychiatric institution is not, just because of the commitment, legally incompetent. For example, that person would ordinarily still be able to make his or her own treatment decisions, and could legally enter into a contract. On the other hand, a comatose person is clearly incompetent to make decisions. Some classes of persons, for example minors (children), may be incompetent by law. See *minor*.

If a person is declared incompetent by a court, a legal guardian is appointed for that person. The person may be judged only unable to handle her or his financial affairs, and so the guardian will only make decisions about money and property management (in that case the guardian is usually called a conservator), and the incompetent person may still make personal decisions, such as those regarding health care. In other cases, a "guardian of the person" is appointed to make personal decisions. Some guardians have the power to make both personal and property-related decisions. In any case, the court document appointing the guardian will state the authority of the guardian.

A legally incompetent person may still be sufficiently competent to make a valid will, because the requirements for competency in this area are less stringent. The testator (the person making a will) need only understand what property he owns, and be able to recognize the "natural objects of his bounty" (for example, his wife and children).

incremental An adjective that describes a process that proceeds step by step, and each step adds an increment (increase in quantity or value) to the step preceding. The term is being used with a different meaning in healthcare reform discussions to mean a process of change that happens bit by bit rather than all at once; action in contrast with an approach in which substantial healthcare reform steps would occur simultaneously. A better word might be "additive."

Various actions of reform, such as cost controls and tort reform, for example, taken incrementally would be taken separately. Changes made one at a time might be less traumatic, but would extend the whole reform process over a considerable time, all essential changes might never occur, and generally the end result is not likely to be as complete a change as might be desirable. Furthermore, the pieces, when finally in place, may not fit together well. However, it appears that there is consensus that the incremental approach to improving the healthcare system is the only feasible one; see *Leapfrog Group*.

incubator A special bed for an infant who needs control of his or her environment: temperature, humidity, and breathing (such as supplementary oxygen). An incubator also provides isolation for the infant. Incubators are used for premature infants and other infants with special problems, whether born in the hospital or elsewhere.

inculpatory Anything that will aid in establishing guilt, or an admission of guilt. For example, if a defendant in a medical malpractice trial testified that she forgot to scrub before surgery, that statement would be inculpatory. Distinguish from *exculpatory*.

incurred but not reported (IBNR) An obligation of a managed care plan under its benefit structure that the patient has received, but that has not been reported to the plan. Distinguish from *reported but not incurred*.

IND See *investigational new drug* under *drug*.

indemnity benefits See under *benefits*.

indemnity contract See under *contract*.

independent contractor A person who works for him- or herself and is not controlled by another, as distinguished from an employee. See *employee* for further discussion.

independent ethics committee (IEC) A body analogous to an *institutional review board (IRB)* in countries outside the United States. Its responsibility is to protect the rights, safety, and welfare of human subjects in research.

independent health record bank (IHRB) A proposed independent, nonprofit, member-owned institution that would serve as a repository for lifetime electronic health records (EHRs). Consumers would be free to choose an IHRB to maintain their health records, and would be able to access that information (perhaps with a health card) and give permission for others to access it. Providers could access the account at the point of care to gain medical and health plan (payment) information. In an emergency, providers would have immediate access, anywhere in the country, to a pre-authorized, limited data set. The IHRBs collectively would create a nationwide network of health information, similar to the nationwide financial network created by MasterCard and Visa associations.

According to proposed legislation (2006), IHRBs would be registered and regulated through the Federal Trade Commission (FTC) and the U.S. Attorney General. The IHRB could make money by selling consumer-approved, blinded (the patient's identity would not be revealed) data for research or other authorized means. (Note that the research value of these medical records would be severely limited by the nature of the "sample" of patients electing to use the IHRB as well as their willingness to give consent to release of information.) The revenue would be considered tax-free income and split between the IHRB and the consumer. Providers and payers could also receive payment for data they deposit into the IHRB. See also *Nationwide Health Information Network*.

independent/integrated physician association (IPA) Former synonym for *independent practice association*.

independent medical examination (IME) A physical examination of an individual performed by a physician other than the primary doctor treating the patient, done for the purpose of clarifying or documenting medical and work-related issues. The term is used in the context of workers' compensation, where the insurance carrier or employer (if self-insured) has a legal right to have an IME of an employee submitting a claim. It may also be requested by the employee or by an agency.

independent practice association (IPA) A type of healthcare provider organization composed of physicians, in which the physicians maintain their own practices but agree to furnish services to patients of a managed care organization (MCO) in which the physician services are supplied by the IPA. An IPA is a provider network, but is not a health maintenance organization (HMO), a health care organization (HCO), or a preferred provider organization (PPO). Formerly called individual practice association and independent physician association. See also *physician-hospital organization*, especially regarding antitrust implications for an IPA.

independent practitioner A health professional, usually a person who gives patient care, who practices without supervision. See also *licensed independent practitioner*, under *allied health professional*, and *midlevel practitioner*.

Independent Study Program in Coding (ISP/Coding) A program administered by the American Health Information Management Association (AHIMA) to prepare students to become *coding specialists*.

index (list) A list, alphabetical or numerical, of items, created for the purpose of helping one find the items. Indexes (or indices) are common in books.

medical record index A system of indexing medical records so that they can be located according to several factors, such as by patient name, diagnoses, procedures, physicians, and surgeons.

index (numerical) A number expressing the relative size of a given statistic (number calculated from data) when compared with a reference value for that statistic. It is the result of dividing the given value of the statistic by the reference value.

Consumer Price Index (CPI) A statistic produced by the U.S. Department of Labor's Bureau of Labor Statistics (BLS) to measure inflation. The CPI compares the price of a "market basket" of goods and services in specified cities during a certain month against the average price of the same market basket during a base period.

Changes in hospital and medical costs are compared with changes in a specific portion of the CPI called the **Consumer Price Index—Medical Care Services (CPI-MSC)**. It should be understood that such comparisons may be faulty in that the CPI uses in its computation the cost of hospital services to private patients paying *list* prices. Recent evidence suggests that actual price inflation for hospitals (net rather than list) may be about one half the figure used in the CPI. This is because of the fact that *very few patients pay list prices*. A growing number of organizations paying for care negotiate discounts, and such discounts are said to be increasing in size. Thus hospital price inflation is far less divergent from the overall CPI than usually stated.

The CPI also has a pharmaceutical component, CPI-Rx, which uses retail prices of various types of drugs.

Related to the CPI is the **Producer Price Index—Hospital (PPI-H)**, introduced by the BLS in 1993, which measures net changes in hospital prices (as opposed to costs) for a standardized patient against a baseline using the same computation for December 1992. Thus the CPI-MSC and the PPI-H are measuring different aspects of healthcare costs or prices.

economic index A statistical measure of the economy. One such index is the consumer price index.

wage index A component used by CMS in adjusting payments (prices) under the Medicare prospective payment system (PPS). The wage index is derived by CMS starting with data supplied by hospitals in response to a questionnaire; it takes into account normal work hours, as well as part-time and overtime work hours.

rural area wage index A wage index computed by Medicare for hospitals it classifies as rural hospitals.

Index Medicus A bibliographic listing (in print) of references to articles from biomedical journals worldwide, published by the National Library of Medicine (NLM). Index Medicus ceased publication with the December 2004 edition (Volume 45). It has been superceded by its electronic equivalent, *MEDLINE*.

Indian Health Care Improvement Act (IHCIA) See *Indian Health Service*.

Indian Health Service (IHS) An agency within the Department of Health and Human Services (HHS) whose goal is "to assure that comprehensive, culturally acceptable personal and public health services are available and accessible to American Indian and Alaska Native people." The IHS manages a comprehensive healthcare delivery system for more than 561 federally recognized Indian tribes in 35 states. The population served includes approximately 1.8 million members living on or near reservations, and 600,000 living in urban areas. The system includes IHS direct health services, tribally operated health services, Urban Indian Health Program (UIHP) centers, and non-IHS service providers under contract with IHS. It should be noted that, as U.S. citizens, American Indians and Alaska Native (AI/AN) people are not limited to IHS services, but are entitled to participate in Medicaid, Medicare, and all other public, private, federal, and state health programs available to the general population.

Significant legislation providing funding for AI/AN health services includes the Snyder Act of 1921 (25 U.S.C. § 13 (2005)), which is the basic and first legislative authority for Congress to appropriate funds specifically for health care provided by the Indian Health Service; the Indian Self-Determination and Education Assistance Act of 1975 (25 U.S.C. § 450 et seq.), which gives tribes the option of operating IHS programs in their own communities; and the Indian Health Care Improvement Act of 1976 (IHCIA) (25 U.S.C. § 1601 et seq.), considered to be the "cornerstone" legal authority for the provision of health care to American Indians and Alaska Natives. The IHCIA was passed after findings that the health status of American Indians ranked far below that of the general U.S. population. The act expired at the end of 2001, and had not yet been reauthorized as of 2007. See also *Federally Qualified Health Center*. www.ihs.gov

indicated A term used by physicians meaning that, taking into account the patient's problems and condition, carrying out a given diagnostic procedure or treatment would be the wise course of action. For example, appendectomy (surgical removal of the appendix) is indicated in suspected acute appendicitis, unless there are factors in the patient's condition that outweigh the medical necessity for the operation. Such a factor might be, for instance, a concomitant illness that would add an intolerable risk to that of the surgery or anesthesia. See also *contraindication*.

indication A finding or piece of information that suggests or points to the proper next step in diagnosis or treatment of the patient. A certain set of symptoms and physical findings, for example, is an "indication" for diagnostic x-rays in a suspected fracture. See also *contraindication*.

indicator Something that shows how things are; it measures performance or results. In health care, indicators are used to measure many aspects of management as well as the processes and outcomes of the care itself. Indicators are becoming prominent tools in hospitals with the increasing attention to quality of care (including patient safety) and effective management. An indicator has four attributes:

1. A *parameter*: The thing to be *evaluated*. Each parameter must be explicitly defined.
2. A *measurement*: An objective way to look at the parameter.
3. A *reference point*: A value against which to compare the measurement. In health care, this is often called a benchmark.
4. A *target*: Criteria for the relationship to the reference point. Is the desired result above, below, or at the reference point?

Examples:

- One indicator for performance of an automobile concerns (1) engine temperature. The gauge measures (2) the degrees of the engine. A red area shows where (3) dangerous temperatures begin. To avoid a destroyed engine, the needle must (4) stay out of the red zone.
- A business office keeps track of (1) "days in accounts receivable" (DAR). The measurement is the (2) average number of days between the submission of bills and receipt of their payment. The reference point is typically (3) 60 days (standard business practice). Management will investigate if the DAR (4) exceeds 60 days.
- One important aspect of a patient's condition is (1) body temperature. Measurement is (2) degrees Fahrenheit/Celsius. The reference point is (3) 98.6°F (average normal temperature). Fever is present if the temperature (4) exceeds 98.6°F.

See also *benchmark*, *dashboard*, and *performance measure*.

quality indicator (QI) In health care, a quality indicator is a tool used to monitor performance or outcome to achieve or maintain a desired level. Some pertain to management activities (see **dashboard**). Increasingly, the context is clinical, with "quality indicator" being shorthand for "clinical quality indicator" (CQI).

The use of beta blockers in post–acute myocardial infarction (AMI) patients provides a good example for a clinical quality indicator. Experts agree that "all AMI patients (all things being equal) should be placed on a treatment using beta blocking drugs." "All things being equal" is shorthand for acknowledging that an individual patient may have a contraindication to using a beta blocker. For those patients, the medical record must document the contraindication.

To measure the hospital's performance in this area, the indicator will need:

1. A *parameter*: In this case, the use of beta blockers for post-AMI patients.
2. A *measurement*: The percentage of post-AMI patients who receive beta blockers.
3. A *reference point*: The *Journal of the American Medical Association* (December 2000) reported that only about 8% of individuals have contraindications for using beta blockers.
4. A *target*: The hospital expects beta blocker usage in at least 90% of post-AMI cases. If actual usage falls below 90%, this will trigger close watching and perhaps investigation to find out why.

Most groups now call these **performance measures**. See also **quality management**.

AHRQ Quality Indicators (QIs) Quality indicators published by the Agency for Healthcare Research and Quality (AHRQ) that make use of readily available hospital inpatient administrative data. There are four modules:

1. *Prevention QIs*, to identify hospital admissions that evidence suggests could have been avoided, at least in part, through high-quality outpatient care. Examples: Diabetes Short-term Complications Admission Rate (PQI 1), Perforated Appendix Admission Rate (PQI 2).
2. *Inpatient QIs*, to reflect the quality of care inside the hospital, including inpatient mortality for medical conditions and surgical procedures. Examples: Acute Myocardial Infarction (AMI) Mortality Rate (IQI 15), Cesarean Delivery Rate (IQI 21).
3. *Patient Safety QIs*, which also reflect quality of care inside the hospital, but focus on potentially avoidable complications and iatrogenic events. Examples: Complications of Anesthesia (PSI 1), Postoperative Hip Fracture (PSI 8).
4. *Pediatric QIs*, which both reflect quality of care inside the hospital and identify potentially avoidable hospitalizations among children. Examples: Pediatric Heart Surgery Mortality (PDI 6), Asthma Admission Rate (PDI 14).

The complete list of indicators and specifications can be downloaded at **www.qualityindicators.ahrq.gov**.

HCUP Quality Indicators The precursers to **AHRQ Quality Indicators** (above).

Indicator Measurement System See **IMSystem**.

indigence The condition of being **indigent**.

indigent Lacking the necessities of life; not having sufficient resources. "Indigent" will have different definitions for different purposes; for example, to qualify for a public assistance program.

medically indigent The condition, as defined by the federal, state, or local government, of lacking the financial ability to pay for one's medical care. Any individual whose income and other resources fall below the defined level is declared to be medically indigent and may qualify for public assistance.

indigent medical care (IMC) Care for patients whose income falls below a level usually set by statute or regulation as defining indigence. Such care is provided without charge or for reduced charges, but the institution must find the resources by "overcharges" to other patients (or their payers), supplementary appropriations, public subscription, or elsewhere. See also **charity care**.

Indigo Institute A nonprofit organization founded by attorney John Horty, LLB, that conducts and disseminates research on the organization, function, and financing of health care. Its position on healthcare reform is that a single national solution to all the problems is not possible, and that the movement already under way, in which healthcare reform is emerging in local communities from the bottom up in response to those communities' specific needs and resources, should be facilitated.

Legislative changes that would encourage local innovation in healthcare organization and payment are encouraged, as are changes in favor of tort reform and provision for portable benefits. Use of local solutions, perhaps with federal grants to begin to address the problem of the uninsured and adoption of antitrust policies that would favor cooperation and collaboration among providers in order to preserve the patient care value system in the healthcare field, is also urged.

In addition to these "macro" measures in healthcare reform, the institute's position is that every effort should be made to use emerging technologies to address specifically the problems of each individual patient, a "micro" approach to healthcare reform that promises improved quality for each person and lowered cost for each encounter.

individual health care account (IHCA) See *Medical Savings Account.*

individually identifiable health information (IIHI) Under the *Privacy Rule*, any *health information* that identifies the individual, or with respect to which there is a reasonable basis to believe the information can be used to identify the individual. See also *de-identification*, *designated record set*, and *protected health information.* 45 C.F.R. § 160.103 (October 1, 2006).

individual mandate See under *mandate.*

individual practice association (IPA) See *independent practice association.*

industrial engineering The designing, installation, maintenance, and improvement of systems that integrate people, equipment, materials, and energy. An industrial engineer is sometimes called an "efficiency expert."

industry screening See *blacklisting.*

INF See *interferon.*

infant care review committee (ICRC) In 1984, the Department of Health and Human Services (HHS) issued regulations under the Rehabilitation Act that hospitals should set up "infant care review committees." These committees were designed to help healthcare providers develop policies and procedures to use when making medical decisions about handicapped infants. These regulations were struck down and presently, under the amendments to the Child Abuse Prevention and Treatment Act, the physician is to use his or her reasonable judgment. See *Child Abuse Amendments.*

infant death See under *death.*

infarction An area of destruction of tissue.

  myocardial infarction (MI) The medical diagnosis for the most frequent form of "heart attack." (Other conditions are also often called "heart attacks" by laypersons.) Some heart muscle (myocardial) tissue is destroyed, caused by interference with the blood supply to the area. In an MI, the infarction is the result of the blockage of one of the arteries supplying blood to the heart muscle. The surgical procedures used to improve circulation to the heart, coronary artery bypass grafts (CABG) and balloon angioplasties, are done to prevent MIs and also the symptoms, such as poor cardiac function and angina, resulting from insufficient oxygen supply to the heart muscle. Sometimes called a "coronary."

infection An illness produced by an *infectious agent* (see under *agent (substance)*).

  community-acquired infection An infection the patient acquired before hospitalization (although it may manifest itself after admission to the hospital).

  cross-infection See *nosocomial infection*, below.

  hospital-acquired infection See *nosocomial infection*, below.

nosocomial infection An infection acquired in the hospital. Such an infection may not become evident until after discharge. Synonyms: cross-infection, hospital-acquired infection.

opportunistic infection An infection caused by an organism that is unable to cause disease (to infect) in an individual (the host) unless the host's resistance has been lowered, usually by drugs or by another infection. Such lowered resistance provides a special "opportunity" for the infection. Opportunistic infections are especially prominent in AIDS patients, and, until 1992, the diagnosis of AIDS was not reported unless a person infected with HIV also had one or more specified opportunistic infections. See **AIDS**.

postoperative infection A nosocomial infection that was acquired during surgery and appeared later.

infection control The policies and procedures used to prevent the transmission of infection from one infected individual to another. The term is used in connection with the protection of the professionals and other employees who may have contact with the infectious patient, and the protection of other patients. Infection-control measures include the use of protective clothing, hand-washing, precautions against needlesticks, decontamination (of the patient's environment, and linen), disposal of wastes, and proper handling of laboratory specimens. The appearance of AIDS and hepatitis B in particular has stimulated increased emphasis on infection-control policies and procedures for all patients. See also **universal precautions** under **precautions**.

infection control professional (ICP) A health professional specializing in infection control. May be a physician, registered nurse, or other health professional.

Certified in Infection Control (CIC) A multidisciplinary credential for health professionals offered by the Certification Board of Infection Control and Epidemiology, Inc. **www.cbic.org**

infectious agent See under **agent**.

infectious disease The study of diseases caused by the growth of pathogenic microorganisms in the body.

infectious waste See **hazardous waste**.

infertile Having reduced or absent capacity to produce offspring, a condition that may sometimes be remedied. See also **sterile (non-reproductive)**.

informatician A person whose special skill or interest is in **informatics**.

nurse informatician See **informatics nursing**.

informatics The science of gathering, storing, manipulating, managing, analyzing, visualizing, and utilizing information. Some define informatics as using computers and statistics to manage information. Informatics may be synonymous with "information science," but "informatics" implies use of technology. See also **bioinformatics**.

medical informatics A discipline that the **American Medical Informatics Association (AMIA)** states is concerned with "all aspects of understanding and promoting the effective organization, analysis, management, and use of information in health care." A major field of interest in medical informatics is the development of the **electronic health record (EHR)**.

informatics nursing A nursing specialty defined by the American Nurses Association (ANA) as integrating "nursing science, computer science, and information science in identifying, collecting, processing and managing data and information to support nursing practice, administration, education, research and the expansion of nursing knowledge." A practitioner is called a **nurse informatician**. Information is available from the American Nursing Informatics Association (ANIA), founded in 1992. **www.ania.org**

Certified Informatics Nurse A registered nurse with a Bachelor of Science in Nursing (BSN) degree who is qualified in informatics nursing and has passed an examination of the American Nurses Credentialing Center (ANCC) (**nursingworld.org/ancc**). The credential is RN, BC (Registered Nurse, Board Certified).

information A term generally used to mean data that have somehow been "digested" (manipulated, summarized, organized, or interpreted) so that inferences may more readily be drawn and decisions made than from "raw" data. The Joint Commission on Accreditation of Healthcare Organizations (JCAHO) defines information as "interpreted set(s) of data that can assist in decision making." See also **data** and **health information**.

information and communication technology (ICT) A replacement term for **information technology (IT)** that takes into account the fact that the Internet, wireless networks, hand-held computers, cell phones, and other telecommunications devices and systems are an integral part of IT today.

information infrastructure The standards, laws, regulations, business practices, and technologies needed to facilitate authorized sharing of electronic data in a safe and secure manner.

Information Infrastructure Standards Panel (IISP) An ANSI-sponsored panel established in 1994 to facilitate the development of standards critical to the Global Information Infrastructure (GII). It became a "maintenance committee" in 1998.

informationist A person who is skilled in obtaining, organizing, analyzing, interpreting, and using information. Davidoff and Florance proposed that an informationist be part of the clinical healthcare team at the point of care, providing the critical link between the vast amounts of medical information available from traditional and electronic sources and the practitioner faced with immediate problems and decisions (and limited time). The clinical informationist would have training in both information science and the essentials of clinical work. Information needs would be referred to informationists, just as EKGs are referred to cardiologists. Informationist time would be billed just like other clinical services. Informationist services would be available to all members of the healthcare team—physicians, nurses, technicians, and administrators—as well as to patients and their families. Synonym: clinical knowledge worker. See also **clinical medical librarian**. (Davidoff, F., & Florance, V. "The Informationist: A New Health Profession?" *Annals of Internal Medicine*, 2000;132(12):996–998.)

InformationLinks A Robert Wood Johnson Foundation (RWJF) program that provides funds to state and local health departments to support and encourage their participation in regional health information organizations (RHIOs). **www.informationlinks.org**

information management department (IM) The department responsible for providing whatever computer services the hospital provides "in house." Its services are often confined to administrative tasks (such as accounting, personnel, medical records, laboratory reporting, and clinic scheduling), with research computer applications handled in some other manner. The IM department is often run by a person known as the manager of information systems (MIS). Previously called data processing department.

information prescription (Ix) See **information therapy**.

information system A poorly defined term used to refer to anything from a pencil and paper to a complex computer system. Usually the term "information system" is modified by words specifying its purpose, such as "hospital information system" (HIS).

case mix management information system (case mix MIS) An information system that combines and correlates, on an individual patient basis, medical data abstracted from the hospital medical record of the patient (discharge abstract) and from the patient's bill. Data analyses and displays relate charges, by DRG, to receipts or allowances for those DRGs for the hospital and for individual physicians. A case mix MIS may be provided in-house, off-site, or through shared services. See also **case mix**.

CLICKS Medical Information System A proprietary integrated electronic medical record (EMR) system developed in Israel. It is used by major healthcare providers in Israel, covering millions of medical files. **www.roshtov.com**

community health integrated management information system (CHIMIS) A set of computer systems and communication devices extending throughout the community in order to facilitate the exchange of clinical, financial, and management information among all parties involved: physicians, hospitals, schools, pharmacies, employers, and others involved in health and health care. The system provides continuous communication linkage among all the components of the entire healthcare system, so that the information for the care of patients is available where it is needed and when it is needed. Cost of care is reduced, as is the cost of information management, the savings in both instances reflecting the minimizing of delays and the elimination of duplication in record-keeping. Synonym: community health information network (CHIN). By the early 2000s, these efforts had evolved to *regional health information organizations* **(RHIOs)**.

healthcare information system (HIS) A term applied to any system in a healthcare facility dealing with information, usually with one or more computers involved. The kinds of data carried in the system will vary from facility to facility; there is no agreement yet on criteria that a system must meet to carry this title. An HIS is one kind of *management information system* (see below).

hospital information system (HIS) A term sometimes used for a hospital's *healthcare information system* (see above).

management information system (MIS) An essentially undefined term, applied to any system set up to provide information to or for management. There is no agreement on the kinds of information to be carried or the technology used. The term "MIS" often implies that a computer is involved—sometimes the hospital's computer system, sometimes shared services with outside computers, and sometimes a hospital discharge abstract system. The information may include data on, for example, patients, finance, personnel, production, or the healthcare industry.

    integrated management information system (IMIS) A management information system that includes in its scope (integrates into a single system) management information from all elements of an enterprise.

nursing information system (NIS) An information system that records all aspects of a patient's nursing care from admission to discharge. Data collected may include nursing diagnoses, nursing plans, dietary information, nursing interventions, and observations. The system may be stand-alone or connected to the hospital's information system (HIS). See also *Nursing Information & Data Set Evaluation Center*.

information technology (IT) The use of computers and computer applications to handle data. Information technology became a popular descriptive label during the 1990s, particularly among universities that wanted a broader label than "computer science" as a name for newly created departments that dealt with the explosion of computer usage. This term is being replaced in some areas by *information and communication technology (ICT)*. See also *electronic health record*, *informatics*, and *telehealth*.

information therapy (IT) The use of Internet-based health information and systems to meet an individual's health knowledge needs. The physician (or other caregiver) writes an **information prescription (Ix)**, recommending a particular web site or sites to the patient. Or the IT may be more customized and be provided by interactive systems and electronic health records, for example. The goal is to get the right information to the patient at the right time to improve health, support decision making, and encourage healthy behaviors.

informed consent Legal permission for treatment or release of information. The consent must be given, voluntarily, by the person involved if legally competent (see *incompetent (legal capacity)*) or, if not, by their legal representative; whoever gives the consent must know the full implications of what they are agreeing to. It is the responsibility of the person obtaining consent to make sure that these legal requirements are met.

    For treatment decisions, the patient must be fully informed, by the physician or other provider proposing the treatment or procedure, of the risks, benefits, and alternatives. The purpose of informed consent is to protect the right of the patient to make his or her own decisions concerning his or her care, and this requires that the patient understand the situation and have the opportunity to ask questions.

    Although it is wise for the physician and hospital to obtain the written consent of the patient prior to a treatment or procedure, the patient's *signature* should not be confused with the consent itself. That is, the piece of paper is evidence of the patient's consent, but the essence of the informed consent is the patient's voluntary agreement based upon the relevant facts that have been communicated to the patient by the physician. Thus, a patient groggy from anesthesia who is asked to "sign this" on the way into the operating suite has not given informed consent.

Biomedical research has very specific requirements for informed consent. Waivers of consent are allowed under certain conditions, and the concepts of **deferred consent** (see below) and **minimal differential risk** have been developed. See also **institutional review board**.

More and more, the issue of informed consent is coming up with regard to disclosure of **health information**. The healthcare system elicits a great deal of information from and about an individual; maintains it in medical records, laboratory reports, electronic systems, and the like; and uses it for a variety of purposes, including treatment of the patient, billing for services, checking quality of care, research, complying with regulatory requirements, and so forth. Basically, the patient has a right of privacy regarding this information and, in most cases, the individual's permission is needed to obtain and use it unless the person's identity is kept confidential (but see also **community consent**, below). Informed consent requires that the patient know what information is to be released, to whom, and the uses to be made of that information. This information is now federally protected; see **Privacy Rule**.

Kinds of information that may be disclosed include demographics, physical characteristics, history, test results, diagnoses, treatments, drugs used, responses to disease and injury, and genetic information. Much of this information is obtained in the course of care, and available from the medical record. However, that obtained from biological samples—especially the genetic information—may be inaccessible and, in fact, the patient may not know of its nature or even of its existence. Genetic information raises serious consent issues:

- Is permission required to acquire the genetic material (biological sample)?
- Is permission required to subject the material to genetic analysis?
- For what, and what kind of studies, may the information be used?

See **community consent**, below. See also **institutional review board**, **Privacy Rule**, **privileged communication**, and **protected health information**.

blanket consent Permission to use information for any purpose. This is sometimes termed a "waiver of consent," and is generally considered unacceptable by institutional review boards.

broad consent Permission to use information for a variety of purposes, not all of which may be specifically known to the person granting consent.

community consent Traditionally, consent of an individual to disclose information is not needed if the information cannot be linked to that individual. Using information collected from medical records or other sources anonymously has been acceptable; consent has been "presumed" according to the norms of our society. But such information can usually be linked to identifiable communities (for example, ethnic or geographic). Data banks in several areas of the world are growing in which genetic information about individuals (genotypes) and also information about the same individuals' physical characteristics and reactions to diseases and other "environmental" factors (phenotypes) is being collected and stored so that studies may be made to correlate specific genotypes and phenotypes.

There is debate on whether consent is required for such information to be assembled and studied, and on who, if anyone, is in a position to grant this consent. "Community consent" implies that someone is authorized to represent the community. Some have suggested that "community consultation" is appropriate, even though specific consent need not be obtained.

Just as with individual consent, the community must be informed about the implications of what is being requested. Genetic research on a population, for example, can have effects in the following areas:

Social. At first glance, such research is of little concern to a community, but the possible labeling of a population as "alcoholic" or "mentally unstable," with resulting prejudice and discrimination, makes the question of community consent a real one. And historically, such labeling, even without genetic studies, has led to eugenic sterilization and euthanasia programs.

Scientific, including potential health benefits. Evidence-based medicine surely benefits from such information gathering.

Financial, especially with the patenting of genetic information and the financial rewards expected from such patenting.

The term "community benefit" has been used to discuss at least the positive implications of research using genetic information.

deferred consent Consent to a therapy after administration of that therapy has already begun. The term was coined (and the concept developed) in connection with resuscitation research, in which an emergency exists (an emergency patient is comatose, for example); any therapy, to be effective, must be administered promptly; and no qualified person is available to give informed consent. Instead of using standard therapy, a therapy under investigation (which has neither proven advantage over standard therapy nor greater risk) may be administered. Then, at the earliest opportunity, the family members or guardian is given full information on the steps taken, and at that time given a choice of granting consent for continuing the therapy under investigation (deferred consent) or having it discontinued. Synonym: ratification.

presumed consent An exception to the usual requirement of obtaining informed consent prior to treatment may be made in an emergency if the patient is unable to consent (is unconscious, for example), there is no one else available to consent, and there is no reason to assume that the patient would not want the treatment. The law presumes that the patient would have consented to the emergency treatment required to save her or his life or protect health.

specific consent Permission granted by an individual to release personal information, after the individual has been informed of the uses to be made of the information (i.e., exactly the questions to be asked of the information and the purpose behind the use of the information).

informed shared decision making (ISDM) An approach to health care in which the patient and the caregiver collaborate in decisions about lifestyle, diagnostic procedures to be undertaken, and treatment to be employed, in contrast with the more traditional authoritarian approach in which the compliant patient simply follows the caregiver's instructions. Shared decision making is not practical unless the patient has enough sound information to collaborate intelligently with the caregiver and, of course, both patient and caregiver must want to share in the decision making. Effective collaboration must take into account not only the clinical benefits of available options, but also the patient's values and preferences.

Clinical information has typically been obtained laboriously (even with the help of the computer) from traditional sources, such as the medical and health consumer literature. But the current trend is to employ a new computer tactic, the use of **electronic clinical guidance tools (ECGT)**. ECGT software, which can reduce the load of biomedical information by increasing its relevance to the particular individual, and which can also take into account that person's own wishes and values, is increasingly available.

The term ISDM is tending to give way to **patient-caregiver collaboration**. See also **patient empowerment**.

infoweaver One who weaves a cohesive web of information from disparate bits of data and other information. This term was coined to extend the usual terms of "writer" and "editor." An infoweaver is a knowledge worker whose skills include the ability to add hypertext links to written text, and to make the presentation of information interactive with its intended consumers. Infoweavers use not only text to present information, but also still and moving pictures, as well as sound, where appropriate. Synonym: multimedia author/editor.

infrastructure See **information infrastructure**.

infusion The administration of a drug or other substance using a device that is inserted through the skin and controls the rate of flow of the drug by gravity, as opposed to being pushed, as in injection. A common device used for infusion is known as a "drip," which controls the volume administered by regulating the frequency of drops passing through the device. See also *injection*.

infusion nursing The nursing specialty concerning intravenous administration of medications, blood products, and parenteral nutrition. Includes initiation, monitoring, maintenance, and termination of the procedure. Formerly called intravenous nursing.

Certified Registered Nurse Infusion (CRNI) A registered nurse who has passed the specialty examination for infusion nursing given by the Infusion Nursing Certification Corporation (INCC) (formerly the Intravenous Nurses Certification Corporation). **ins1.org/ certification**

infusion therapy Administration of medications, blood products, and parenteral nutrition intravenously.

in-home care See *home health care*.

in-house Carried out within the organization, rather than brought in or done outside.

injection The administration of a drug or other substance using a device that is inserted into or through the skin, and out of which the substance is then pushed into the body. There are several routes of administration:

intramuscular (IM): into a muscle
intra-arterial (IA): into an artery
intravenous (IV): into a vein
subcutaneous: under the skin
intradermal: into the skin

Where the rate of flow of the drug is determined by gravity, as opposed to being pushed, it is called *infusion*.

injunction A court order prohibiting someone from doing something or, less commonly, ordering someone to do something. An injunction may be temporary (to preserve the status quo until a lawsuit is finally decided) or permanent (issued as part of the final decision of a lawsuit).

injury (bodily) The damage caused by an external force, as contrasted with an "illness," which simply indicates that the body is not in a healthy condition.

injury (legal) The damage caused by a legal wrong. For example, defamation causes "injury" to a person's reputation; a breach of contract may cause financial injury. See also *damages*.

in-kind services See *donated services*.

i-NMDS See *International Nursing Minimum Data Set* under *data set*.

INMED Partnerships for Children A nonprofit "global development organization dedicated to inspiring communities and fostering their ability to develop healthy, educated children with increased opportunities for the future." INMED works toward this through collaborative public/private sector and community partnerships in Latin America, the Caribbean, Asia, and the United States. One of its programs is *MotherNet*. INMED is derived from INternational MEDical Services for Health. **www.inmed.org**

in-network See *out-of-plan*.

innovator drug See *generic equivalent*.

inpatient A patient who receives care while being lodged in an institution, such as a hospital.

inpatient care Care rendered to patients who are lodged within a healthcare facility.

inpatient care Institution See *inpatient facility*.

inpatient day equivalents See under *day*.

inpatient facility A healthcare institution that provides lodging as well as nursing and continuous medical care for patients within a permanent facility with an organized professional staff (see *staff (group)*). Synonym: inpatient care institution.

inpatient prospective payment system (IPPS) See under *prospective payment system*.

inpatient psychiatric facility (IPF) A facility that provides psychiatric services on an inpatient basis. For Medicare purposes, an IPF may be a freestanding psychiatric hospital, a distinct part psychiatric unit of a general acute care hospital, or a distinct part psychiatric unit of a critical access hospital that provides psychiatric services to Medicare beneficiaries.

inpatient psychiatric facility prospective payment system (IPF-PPS) See under *prospective payment system*.

inpatient rehabilitation facility (IRF) A regulated hospital or other healthcare facility that provides inpatient rehabilitation services, as defined by CMS.

Inpatient Rehabilitation Facility Patient Assessment Instrument (IRF-PAI) A form completed by an inpatient rehabilitation facility (IRF) upon admission and discharge of a patient that provides the basis for classifying that patient for the inpatient rehabilitation facility prospective payment system (IRF-PPS). It includes the Functional Independence Measure (FIM) assessment as well as ICD-9-CM coding and other information.

inpatient rehabilitation facility prospective payment system (IRF-PPS) See under *prospective payment system*.

inpatient service day See under *day*.

in-plan See *out-of-plan*.

in-service Activities, ordinarily education or training, that are carried out without serious interruption of the employees' regular duties.

in-service director The individual responsible for coordinating educational programs for all employees, including training of nursing aides and orderlies, in long-term care facilities.

in-service education See under *education*.

in-service education coordinator See *director of education*.

in-service training See under *training*.

in silico Carried out in the computer by various modeling processes; used in connection with biological investigations. See also *in vitro* and *in vivo*.

inspector general (IG) See *Office of Inspector General*.

Institute for Diversity in Health Management (IDHM) An institute created in 1994 by the American Hospital Association (AHA), the American College of Healthcare Executives (ACHE), and the National Association of Health Services Executives (NAHSE) to inform minority students about opportunities in healthcare management and to assist ethnic minority professionals already in the field. **www.diversityconnection.org**

Institute for Healthcare Improvement (IHI) A nonprofit organization dedicated to leading the improvement of health care throughout the world. Its goals include health care for all with no needless deaths, no needless pain or suffering, no helplessness in those served or serving, no unwanted waiting, and no waste. Two of its initiatives are the *100,000 Lives Campaign* and the *5 Million Lives Campaign*. IHI was founded in 1991 and is based in Cambridge, Massachusetts. **www.ihi.org/ihi**

Institute for Safe Medication Practices (ISMP) A nonprofit organization founded in 1994 dedicated to medication error prevention and safe medication use. **www.ismp.org**

Institute of Electrical and Electronics Engineers (IEEE) See *MEDIX*.

Institute of Medicine (IOM) A body formed by the National Academy of Sciences (NAS) in 1970 to secure the services of eminent members of appointed professions for the examination of policy matters pertaining to the health of the public. The IOM acts under the responsibility given to NAS in 1863 by its charter to be an advisor to the federal government and, upon its own initiative, to study problems of medical care, research, and education. IOM administers the National Research Council (NRC) jointly with the NAS.

Prior to the formation of the IOM, significant work had been done in the medical field by NAS. During World War II, the NRC's Division on Medical Sciences sponsored a research program in many areas of military medicine, including synthesis of penicillin, aviation medicine, work in sanitary engineering, production of drugs and essential supplies, and providing new techniques and therapies for battlefield medicine. The Committee on Food and Nutrition, formed in 1941, published its first "Recommended Dietary Allowances." In 1956, the report of the Committee on Biological Effects of Atomic Radiation was published. In 1969, the NRC drug efficacy study, prepared for the commissioner of the Food and Drug Administration (FDA), was issued.

The IOM charter gave as its purpose "the protection and advancement of the health of the public, including the conduct of study programs relating to the delivery of health care, medical education, and biomedical research and development." Notable medical and health contributions since its formation have been recommendations on *Injury in America* (1985); *Improving the Quality of Care in Nursing Homes* (1986); a series of reports on AIDS; *Mapping and Sequencing the Human Genome* (1988); studies and reports on the status of contraceptive development, on child care in America, on why and how food labeling should be changed, and on how to promote health and prevent disability in Americans over age 50; a report on emerging infections, which led to establishment of a special federal program in disease surveillance; a major study on pesticides in the diets of infants and children; and in 1991 the landmark study *The Computer-Based Patient Record: An Essential Technology for Health Care* (see **computer-based patient record** under **electronic health record**). See also **Institute of Medicine's Health Care Quality Initiative**. www.iom.edu

Institute of Medicine's Health Care Quality Initiative An ongoing effort of the Institute of Medicine to assess and improve the quality of health care in the United States. The initiative has produced a number of extremely influential reports, which are being referred to as "The Quality Chasm Series." The first of these, in 1999, was *Ensuring Quality Cancer Care*, which demonstrated the gap between the expectations for quality cancer care and what was actually being delivered. The second, also in 1999, was *To Err Is Human: Building a Safer Health System*, dealing with the significant number of illnesses and injuries resulting from medical errors by healthcare providers (see **patient safety**). A 2001 report, *Crossing the Quality Chasm*, subtitled "A New Health System for the 21st Century," identified six goals for quality improvement: health care should be safe, timely, effective, efficient, equitable, and patient-centered (STEEEP). Among the IOM's many recommendations was changing current payment methods to encourage higher quality care; see **pay-for-performance**. Seventeen reports had been released as of 2007 (see **www.iom.edu/CMS/8089.aspx**):

Ensuring Quality Cancer Care (1999)

To Err Is Human: Building a Safer Health System (1999)

Crossing the Quality Chasm: A New Health System for the 21st Century (2001)

Envisioning the National Health Care Quality Report (2001)

Leadership by Example: Coordinating Government Roles in Improving Health Care Quality (2002)

Fostering Rapid Advances in Health Care: Learning from System Demonstrations (2002)

Priority Areas for National Action: Transforming Health Care Quality (2003)

Health Professions Education: A Bridge to Quality (2003)

Key Capabilities of an Electronic Health Record System (2003)

Keeping Patients Safe: Transforming the Work Environment of Nurses (2003)

Patient Safety: Achieving a New Standard for Care (2003)

1st Annual Crossing the Quality Chasm Summit: A Focus on Communities (2004)

Quality Through Collaboration: The Future of Rural Health (2004)

Improving the Quality of Health Care for Mental and Substance Use Conditions: Quality Chasm Series (2005)

Performance Measurement: Accelerating Improvement (2005)

Medicare's Quality Improvement Organization Program: Maximizing Potential (2006)

Preventing Medication Errors: Quality Chasm Series (2006)

institutional animal care and use committee (IACUC) A committee in an institution set up to monitor research programs that use live vertebrate animals as subjects. It is the IACUC's responsibility to make sure that the animals are treated humanely in accordance with applicable laws and regulations.

institutional review board (IRB) A committee in an institution set up to monitor research programs that use human subjects and are subject to federal regulations. The IRB is governed by the requirements of the Department of Health and Human Services (HHS) Regulations for Protection of Human Subjects (45 C.F.R. § 46). It is composed of at least five members from varying backgrounds, including both scientists and nonscientists and at least one non-institutional representative. The charge of the IRB is to make sure that the rights and welfare of the human research subjects, as well as the investigator and institution, are protected. The IRB reviews any proposed research, ensures that informed consent is properly obtained, and follows the progress of the research to see that all regulatory and institutional requirements are followed.

institution for mental diseases (IMD) See *IMD exclusion*.

instructional advance directive (IAD) See under *advance directive*.

Instrumental Activities of Daily Living (IADL) scale A "standard scale of function" some-times used to measure severity of illness. It is a portion of the Older American Resources and Services Questionnaire (OARS). The IADL scale measures a person's ability to perform six activities of daily living (ADL): dressing and undressing, walking, taking a bath or shower, going shopping for groceries or clothes, preparing meals, and doing housework. For each activity, a person can perform it either without help, with help, or not at all.

insulin A substance used in the treatment of diabetes.

insurance A method of providing money to pay for specific types of losses that may occur. Insurance is a contract (the insurance policy) between one party (the insured) and another (the insurer). The policy states what types of losses (see *risk (financial)*) are covered, what amounts will be paid for each loss and for all losses, and under what conditions. See *insurance coverage*.

Two types of insurance commonly spoken of in health care are: (1) insurance covering the patient for healthcare services (health insurance, also sometimes called a "third-party payer") (see also *benefits*), and (2) insurance covering the healthcare provider for risks associated with the delivery of health care (liability to a patient for malpractice, for example).

Matters pertaining to insurance are almost always regulated by the government of the state in which the insurance is provided. New York was the first state to enact a general insurance statute in 1849.

catastrophic insurance Insurance intended to protect against the cost of a catastrophic ill-ness, with "catastrophic" defined as exceeding a predetermined cost. Catastrophic insurance comes into play above that cost, in supplement of other insurance, and pays all or a percent-age of the cost above the specified amount. Synonym: major medical insurance.

commercial insurance In health care, traditionally refers to any insurance other than Blue Cross and Blue Shield or Medicare. This term may have a more specific definition in a par-ticular usage, such as in a statute.

Directors' and Officers' (D&O) insurance Insurance that covers an organization's officers and directors for actions (or failures to act) in their official capacity, such as securities fraud or sexual harassment. Whether or not a particular employee is an officer or director for the purposes of this protection is usually determined by the corporate bylaws. Typically the policy covers the individuals, but the corporation may also arrange for its own coverage.

general liability insurance Insurance that covers the risk of loss for most accidents and injuries to third parties (the insured and its employees are not covered) that arise from the actions or negligence of the insured, and for which the insured may have legal liability, except those injuries directly related to the provision of professional healthcare services (the latter risks are covered by professional liability insurance). General liability insurance will pay for slips and falls of visitors on hospital premises, for example.

health insurance Insurance that covers the patient for health care, including physician and hospital services.

indemnity insurance Health insurance based on fee-for-service, in which the carrier reimburses the insured (or pays the provider directly) a percentage of the cost of healthcare services provided. Synonym: indemnity policy. See also *benefits*.

major medical insurance See *catastrophic insurance*, above.

malpractice insurance See *professional liability insurance*, below.

out-of-area insurance Insurance carried by a health plan (such as an HMO) to pay for care for beneficiaries when they are away from home, away from the service area of the plan ("out-of-area").

private insurance Insurance offered by private organizations (Blue Cross and Blue Shield, managed care organizations, insurance companies, employers) rather than by the government (for example, Medicare).

professional liability insurance Insurance that covers the risk of loss from patient injury or illness that results from *professional negligence* (see under *negligence*) or other *professional liability* (see under *liability (legal)*). Professional liability insurance pays malpractice claims. Often, a hospital's professional liability policy will not cover the actions of physicians on the medical staff; those physicians need to obtain their own individual policies. Sometimes called malpractice insurance.

property insurance Insurance that pays for damage to the insured's own property, for example, loss by fire.

reinsurance A type of insurance that insurance companies themselves buy for their own protection. Reinsurance further shares the risk. The entity purchasing the insurance is called the "ceding company" while the insurer selling the reinsurance is called the reinsurer or the "assuming company." Healthcare insurance providers frequently reinsure themselves for specified, rare, and high priced risks, such as heart transplantation. See also *stop-loss insurance*, below.

self-insurance Assumption of risk of loss without an insurance policy. For example, a hospital deciding to "self-insure" would set aside its own funds to protect itself against financial loss, instead of purchasing an insurance policy from an insurance company. In many cases, however, even a so-called "self-insured" hospital will purchase a policy (see *excess coverage* under *insurance coverage*) to protect against very large losses. For example, a hospital might self-insure for losses up to $3 million, then have a policy to cover the next $10 million of loss.

service insurance Health insurance in which the insurer provides services directly rather than just providing the funds to pay for them; see *service benefits* under *benefits*. Synonym: service policy.

stop-loss insurance Insurance carried by a health plan, purchased from an insurance carrier, to reimburse the plan for costs of care for individual patients over a ceiling (for example, $10,000), or for aggregate claims over the course of a year (for example, 125% over the expected amount). This type of insurance is designed to protect the plan from unusually high, catastrophic claims. See also *reinsurance*, above.

insurance benefits See *benefits*.

insurance claim form The form on which a physician or other provider submits the claim for care given. Each insurance company may design and require its own form, as can the federal and state governments. This lack of standardization has at least two negative consequences: (1) everyone has to work much harder to complete and understand the form, and (2) automating this tedious task becomes much more difficult, if not impossible.

insurance clerk See *reimbursement specialist*.

insurance company A private company that provides insurance coverage.

insurance coverage Generally refers to the amount of protection available and the kind of loss that would be paid for under an insurance contract.

claims-made coverage Insurance that will pay for claims that are made during the period of time that the policy is in effect, for events that occur *after* the insurance policy's retroactive date. For example, if a hospital has a claims-made insurance policy in effect for calendar year 2007, with a retroactive date of January 1, 2004, and a patient suffers an injury during a 2005 surgical procedure but does not notify (or sue) the hospital until 2007, the claim will be covered under the 2007 policy. If the surgery was in 2003, it will not be covered. Most medical malpractice insurance today (about 80%) is claims-made coverage. See also *occurrence-based coverage*, below.

excess coverage Extra-high limits of insurance coverage, which will pay amounts over and above the original limits of a specified policy.

first-dollar coverage Insurance that has no copayment or deductible provision; the insured does not have to pay the first dollar—the insurer pays it.

nose coverage See *prior acts coverage*, below.

occurrence-based coverage Insurance that will pay for claims only when the event that gives rise to the claim happens during the period of time that the policy is in effect, regardless of when the claim is made. For example, if a hospital has an occurrence-based insurance policy in effect only for calendar year 2007, and a patient suffers an injury during a 2005 surgical procedure, the claim will not be covered under the 2007 policy because the injury did not occur in 2007. See also *claims-made coverage*, above.

prior acts coverage A special *claims-made* policy (see *claims-made coverage*, above) purchased subsequent to another claims-made policy, which ensures that there is no lapse in coverage between the two policies. Normally, a second claims-made policy would exclude any claims for events that occurred during the term of the first policy, so *tail coverage* (see below) would have to be purchased for those claims. With prior acts coverage, the retroactive date of the new policy goes back to the initial date of the first policy (thus covering claims for events during that time period and making tail coverage unnecessary), with the premium increased as well. For example, if a physician was with the previous insurer for three years, the new policy would begin with third-year-level premiums rather than first-year. Synonyms: nose coverage, retroactive coverage.

retroactive coverage See *prior acts coverage*, above.

tail coverage Insurance purchased to cover events that occurred during the period of a *claims-made* policy (see claims-made coverage, above), but for which no claim was made during that period. That is, to protect the insured in case a claim is made at a future date, after the original claims-made policy has lapsed. A physician typically purchases a "tail" at retirement; however, a physician changing malpractice insurance companies may have to buy one, as may a physician moving from one state to another if his or her insurer does not offer coverage in the new state. Premiums for tail coverage policies often run into hundreds of thousands of dollars, which some insurers require up front. Physicians can sometimes get free tail coverage—for example, if they have purchased claims-made coverage from the same insurer for a certain number of years. See also *prior acts coverage*, above.

umbrella coverage A broad high limit liability policy, usually requiring underlying insurance. For example, a hospital may be insured for $1 million for general liability and $3 million for professional liability, with an umbrella of $10 million. The umbrella will pick up any excess liability over either policy, up to the $10 million additional limit.

wraparound coverage Provides members of basic health plans with coverage for certain services provided by nonplan providers. Beneficiaries of this type of supplemental insurance coverage are frequently members of HMOs or Medicare.

insurance medicine The specialization of physicians who serve as medical directors for insurance companies and use medical science to advise on underwriting and consult on claims and disability management.

insurer See *carrier (insurance)*.

integrated communications A term being used to indicate that public relations, sales literature, employee communications, television advertising, magazine advertising, outdoor displays, direct mail, and other devices should be considered together, because they can contribute to the solution of an organization's positioning efforts.

integrated delivery system (IDS) See *integrated health delivery network*.

integrated health delivery network (IHDN) A group of hospitals, physicians, other providers, insurers, and/or community agencies that work together to coordinate and deliver a broad spectrum of services to their community. This definition is from the *1995–96 AHA Guide to the Healthcare Field*, along with its first-time listing of "integrated health delivery networks." The *Guide* identified networks of "varying organization type," not mutually exclusive of the hospital, healthcare system, or alliance listings.

The amorphousness of the network definition is demonstrated by this caution from the *Guide*: "Networks are very fluid in their composition as goals evolve and partners change. Therefore, some of the networks included in this listing may have dissolved, reformed, or simply been renamed as this section was being produced for publication."

The definition is not any more precise ten years later. Examples of integrated systems include a physician-hospital organization (PHO), management service organization (MSO), and clinic without walls (CWW).

Sometimes called integrated delivery system (IDS), integrated healthcare system (IHS), or integrated health network (IHN). See also *provider service network*.

integrated management information system (IMIS) See under *management information system* under *information system*.

integration Integration is spoken of in health care today in terms of the linking together of components of the healthcare system:

horizontal integration A linkage of hospitals (or other institutions and organizations) that are more or less alike, such as acute general hospitals, to form a multihospital system. The purpose of horizontal integration is to achieve economies of scale in operation, such as greater purchasing power and avoidance of duplication of facilities.

vertical integration A linkage of hospitals (and other institutions and organizations) to form a system providing a range or continuum of care such as preventive, outpatient, acute hospital, long-term, home, and hospice care. The purpose of vertical integration is to keep the patient population within the one system for as many of its healthcare needs as possible.

integrative medicine See *complementary and alternative medicine*.

integrity See *data integrity*.

intellectual property rights A collection of legal rights that may be used to protect an investment of creative effort. In the U.S. legal system, these rights include copyright, patent, trademark, and trade secret protection.

intensive care Care provided to patients with life-threatening conditions who require intensive treatment and continuous monitoring.

intensive care unit (ICU) A hospital patient care unit for patients with life-threatening conditions who require intensive treatment and continuous monitoring. Such units are often set up separately for different kinds of patients, and a hospital may have several ICUs: medical, surgical, pediatric, neonatal, and others. Synonym: critical care unit.

neonatal intensive care unit (NICU) An intensive care unit for infants in the neonatal period. Sometimes shortened to "neonatal ICU."

pediatric intensive care unit (PICU) An intensive care unit for children. The age range for patients deemed to be children will vary from hospital to hospital. Sometimes shortened to "pediatric ICU."

intensivist A physician who specializes in intensive care medicine.

intentional infliction of emotional distress See under *emotional distress*.

intentional tort See under *tort*.

interactive Requiring or allowing a response from the user. In computer and telecommunications usage, interactive refers to a program that assumes the user or viewer will exercise some degree of choice to determine how the program will proceed. Almost all computer programs are interactive in that they present some kind of menu to the user, and then simply wait for the user's input. Almost all television programs now are not interactive, in that they are simply broadcast at a certain time, and the viewer either watches them or not. An interactive television program, for instance, might allow the user to click either of two buttons during the presentation of a movie, one called "Happy Ending" and the other "Sad Ending." You get to watch what you want to see, and the television company instantly knows not only who is watching its program, but also what kind of ending they prefer. There are obviously many ramifications to interactive telecommunications that will need to be sorted out over time.

interactive health communication (IHC) The use of a computer (or telecommunications) to provide health information plus something more—for example, online peer support, decision support, or help with behavior changes. The computer application or web site is interactive with the user—consumer, patient, or physician—who may provide information to and/or query the system to receive information and guidance on a particular disease, condition, or health topic. See also *telehealth*.

interdisciplinary patient care plan (IPCP) A plan required by federal regulations for each patient in a long-term care facility (LTCF). The plan must define the patient's problems and needs, and must also set forth measurable goals, approaches to the care, and the profession (department or service) responsible for the care of the patient. An IPCP is sometimes referred to by the less correct terms interdisciplinary care plan (ICP) or patient care plan.

interest-based bargaining (IBB) Negotiating that takes everyone's interests into account, exploring various solutions and attempting to find an outcome that will, to the greatest extent possible, meet the needs of all parties. Synonyms: joint problem-solving, win-win negotiating.

interferon (INF) A class of chemicals found in the body that provides one of the natural defenses against viral infections and tumors, and that has an effect in regulating immunity. INFs are being investigated for treatment of a number of disorders, and have been approved by the Food and Drug Administration (FDA) for clinical use.

intermediary See *fiscal intermediary*.

intermediate care See under *nursing care*.

intermediate care facility (ICF) A free-standing facility that provides *intermediate care* (see under *nursing care*). Such a facility typically has a *registered nurse (RN)* (see under *nurse*) on-site during at least one nursing shift, rather than for two nursing shifts as in a *skilled nursing facility (SNF)*.

intermediate care facility for the mentally retarded (ICF/MR) A free-standing facility that provides intermediate care for mentally retarded patients. See *intermediate care facility*. Synonym: community residential facility.

intermediate care unit A portion of a *skilled nursing facility (SNF)* that is organized so as to provide "intermediate care" (the other portion of the SNF, that portion giving "skilled nursing care," would be the facility's "skilled nursing unit" (SNU)). Rarely is an intermediate care unit a portion of an acute hospital. The acronym "ICU" for an intermediate care unit should be avoided because ICU is much more likely to be interpreted as "intensive care unit." See *intermediate care* and *skilled nursing care* under *nursing care*.

intermediate life support See under *life support*.

intermediate sanctions rule See *excess benefit transaction rule*.

intermittent care A variety of *home health care* that includes daily care for a two- to three-week period and thereafter under "exceptional circumstances."

intern A person who has already had formal training in a profession who is now obtaining supervised practical training. The term is no longer restricted to physicians; in fact, the physician intern of the past is now called a first-year resident physician.

internal disaster plan See under *disaster preparedness plan*.

internal medicine The study of the diagnosis and medical (nonsurgical) therapy of disorders and diseases of the internal structures of the body. The physician who specializes in internal medicine is an "internist" (not to be confused with "intern," a professional undergoing practical training). See *internist*.

Internal Revenue Code (IRC) The federal legislation (Title 26 of the U.S. Code) that forms the basis for the taxation structure in the United States, and that is constantly revised. Judge Learned Hand, one of the greatest jurists in U.S. history, had the following to say about the IRC:

> The words of the Internal Revenue Code merely dance before my eyes in a meaningless procession: rule upon rule, exception upon exception, cross-reference to cross-reference until my head is spinning—couched in abstract terms that appear to offer no handle to seize hold of. They leave in my mind only a confused sense of some vitally important, yet successfully concealed, purpose which it is my duty to extract, but which is within my power to interpret, if at all, only after the most inordinate expenditure of time.

Internal Revenue Service (IRS) The federal agency responsible for administering the tax laws as set out in the Internal Revenue Code. **www.irs.gov**

International Association of Medical Regulatory Authorities (IAMRA) An international membership organization whose purpose is to support medical regulatory authorities worldwide in protecting the public interest by promoting high standards for physician education, licensure, and regulation, and facilitating the ongoing exchange of information among medical regulatory authorities. IAMRA was established in 2002 with eight founding members, including the Federation of State Medical Boards (FSMB), and in 2007 had a membership of seventy organizations in thirty countries. **www.fsmb.org/iamra.html**

International Classification for Nursing Practice (ICNP) A terminology for nursing practice that includes nursing phenomena (nursing diagnoses), nursing actions, and nursing outcomes, developed by the International Council of Nurses (ICN).

International Classification of Clinical Services (ICCS) A classification and coding system developed by the Commission on Professional and Hospital Activities (CPHA) for certain hospital-provided services in order to standardize patient care data and facilitate computer handling of those data.

International Classification of Diseases (ICD) See *ICD (classification)*.

International Classification of Diseases for Oncology (ICD-O) An extension of the neoplasm chapter (Chapter II) of the *International Statistical Classification of Diseases and Related Health Problems* (see *ICD-10*), published by the World Health Organization, Geneva, 1990. It is now in its Third Revision (ICD-O-3). (The First Edition, although listed as the Second Edition, was an extension of *The International Classification of Diseases, Injuries, and Causes of Death, Ninth Revision* (ICD-9).)

International Classification of Diseases, Ninth Revision (ICD-9) See *ICD-9*.

International Classification of Diseases, Ninth Revision, Clinical Modification (ICD-9-CM) See *ICD-9-CM*.

International Classification of Functioning, Disability, and Health (ICF) A classification used to describe the consequences of disease—how people live with their health conditions. The ICF is structured around three components: (1) body functions and structure, (2) activities (tasks and actions by an individual) and participation (involvement in a life situation), and (3) additional information on severity and environmental factors. ICF was first issued by the World Health Organization (WHO) in 1980 as the *International Classification of Impairments, Disabilities and Handicaps* (ICIDH), and was renamed in 2001. **www3.who.int/icf**

International Classification of Health Interventions (ICHI) A classification of health interventions for international use, developed by the World Health Organization (WHO). It was designed primarily to meet the needs of countries that do not already have a classification system for procedures. ICHI contains 1,420 procedure codes and is based on the Australian Classification of Health Interventions (ACHI).

International Classification of Impairments, Disabilities and Handicaps (ICIDH) See *International Classification of Functioning, Disability, and Health*.

International Conference on Harmonisation See *ICH*.

International Council of Nurses (ICN) A federation of national nurses' associations from over 128 countries, founded in 1899 to ensure quality nursing care for all, sound health policies around the world, the advancement of nursing knowledge, and the presence worldwide of a respected nursing profession and a competent and satisfied nursing work force. **www.icn.ch**

International Food Information Council (IFIC) A nonprofit organization whose mission is to communicate science-based information on food safety and nutrition to health and nutrition professionals, educators, government officials, journalists, and others providing information to consumers. IFIC's support comes primarily from the food, beverage, and agricultural industries. However, IFIC states that it does ". . . not represent any product or company or lobby for legislative or regulatory activities." **www.ific.org**

International Health Regulations (IHR) A set of regulations developed by the World Health Organization (WHO) designed to ensure maximum security against the international spread of diseases with a minimum interference with world trade and travel. The IHR require countries to develop, strengthen, and maintain the capacity to detect, report, and respond to public health threats; WHO provides assistance to countries to help them accomplish this. The IHR also established a single code of procedures and practices for routine public health measures at international airports and ports and some ground crossings.

An important aspect of the IHR is preparedness and responsiveness. Countries are to be vigilant to detect any potential "public health emergency of international concern." This is defined by IHR as an extraordinary public health event that is determined:

1. To constitute a public health risk to other countries through the international spread of disease; and
2. To potentially require a coordinated international response.

These are to be reported immediately to WHO, which makes a "real-time" response to the emergency. WHO recommends measures to be taken by the affected country as well as other countries. Measures could be directed, for example, toward persons, baggage, cargo, containers, ships, aircraft, road vehicles, goods, or postal parcels.

The IHR are legally binding on all WHO Member States who have not rejected them (or have accepted them with approved reservations) and on all non-Member States of WHO that have agreed to be bound by them.

The regulations go back to 1951, when WHO adopted the International Sanitary Regulations. These were replaced by and renamed the International Health Regulations in 1969. The IHR were originally intended to monitor and control just six serious infectious diseases: cholera, plague, yellow fever, smallpox, relapsing fever, and typhus. By the 1990s, however, new infectious agents such as Ebola hemorrhagic fever were appearing. A new set of IHR adopted in 2005, effective in 2007, expanded the regulations to cover any public health emergency of international concern.

International Health Terminology Standards Development Organisation (IHTSDO) An international, nonprofit *standards development organization (SDO)* created in 2007 to own, maintain, and promote *SNOMED Clinical Terms (SNOMED CT)*. The charter member countries are Australia, Canada, Denmark, Lithuania, Netherlands, New Zealand, Sweden, the United Kingdom, and the United States. The goal of the SNOMED SDO is to make

SNOMED CT freely available throughout the world and to encourage international collaboration to produce a global clinical terminology standard.

International Medical Informatics Association (IMIA) An international organization that promotes the use of informatics in health care and biomedical research. Members are government, institutional, academic, and corporate (vendor) organizations. There are four sections: IMIA-LAC (Latin America and the Caribbean), EFMI (Europe), APAMI (Asian and Pacific Region), and Helina (Africa). **www.imia.org**

International Nursing Minimum Data Set (i-NMDS) See under *data set*.

International Organization for Standardization (ISO) See *ISO*.

International Physicians for the Prevention of Nuclear War (IPPNW) A nonpartisan federation of national medical organizations in sixty countries, representing tens of thousands of doctors, medical students, other health workers, and concerned citizens who share the common goal of creating a more peaceful and secure world freed from the threat of nuclear annihilation. It was founded by physicians in the United States and the Soviet Union in 1980 to mobilize efforts to eliminate nuclear weapons throughout the world. IPPNW was given the Nobel Peace Prize in 1985. **www.ippnw.org**

International Society for Infectious Diseases (ISID) An international membership association dedicated to developing partnerships and to finding solutions to the problem of infectious diseases around the world. In 2007 it had individual members from over 155 countries. ISID is the administrator of *ProMED-mail*. **www.isid.org**

International Society for Pharmacoeconomics and Outcomes Research (ISPOR) A nonprofit organization formed in 1995 to promote the practice and science of pharmacoeconomics and health outcomes research. Its members are physicians, pharmacists, economists, nurses and researchers from academia, the pharmaceutical industry, government, managed care, health research organizations, and purchasers of health care. Formerly called the Association for Pharmacoeconomics and Outcomes Research (APOR). **www.ispor.org**

International Society of Technology Assessment in Health Care (ISTAHC) An international membership organization organized in 1985 to encourage research, education, cooperation, and the exchange of information concerning the clinical and social implications of healthcare technologies, and to foster their optimal utilization. The organization published a newsletter (no title) and *The International Journal of Technology Assessment in Health Care* (IJTAHC). ISTAHC's final annual meeting was in 2003; see *Health Technology Assessment International*.

International Standards Organization Common, but incorrect, interpretation of *ISO*.

International Statistical Classification of Diseases and Related Health Problems (ICD-10) See *ICD-10*.

Internet printout syndrome See *cyberchondria*.

internist A physician who practices *internal medicine*. The "internist" is not to be confused with an "intern," a physician (or other professional) in training.

A physician who covers the entire field of internal medicine is a **general internist**; one who specializes usually carries the "-ist" designation for the specialty. Within internal medicine there are a number of specialties, for example, cardiology (diseases of the heart), and the internist specializing in cardiology is a "cardiologist." (For a complete listing of specialties, see *medical specialty*.) A general internist is a "primary care physician" because he or she provides one path of entry to medical care—first evaluating the whole patient, and then obtaining "secondary" (specialist) consultation and care as appropriate. The specialized internist (e.g., the cardiologist) may at times provide primary care but is, generally speaking, a "secondary care physician."

interoperability In the world of computers and informatics, the property that allows one computer system to exchange data with another computer system. It is a measure of compatibility. Frequently, users of these devices and programs have a greater desire for interoperability than their vendors do, so users may choose to work with a standards development organization (SDO) to force the adoption of standards that make certain devices and programs more interoperable. (See **HL7** as an example of such an effort in the healthcare field.) Interoperability is a major concern in the effort to build a **Nationwide Health Information Network (NHIN)**.

There are three levels of interoperability:

"Basic" interoperability allows one computer to receive a message from another, but does not require the receiver to be able to interpret the data.

"Functional" interoperability defines **message format standards** so that messages can be interpreted at the level of data fields. For example, if the first computer has a structured data field for "blood pressure" and transmits the data in that field to a second computer, the second computer could store the information appropriately in a comparably structured field for "blood pressure." Neither computer system, however, would have any understanding of the meaning of the data contained within that field.

"Semantic" interoperability provides the highest level of communication. It means that the receiving computer can interpret the data received. Thus, if the data in the field "blood pressure" showed the value as excessively high, this information could be used to trigger knowledge tools, such as protocols and alerts, in the receiving computer, promoting higher quality care.

See also **data comparability**, **data integrity**, and **data quality**.

interrater reliability See under **reliability**.

interrogatories Written questions sent by one party in a lawsuit to the adverse (opposing) party, in preparation for the trial of the suit. Interrogatories are part of the process of discovery, and must be answered by the adverse party within a certain amount of time.

intersexed An individual whose biological sex is ambiguous. Formerly, the medical term was "hermaphrodite"; this is being rejected as stigmatizing and misleading. Intersex more accurately describes the condition, in which the genitalia have not fully developed into either male or female, but are somewhere along the continuum between the two.

intervening cause See under **cause**.

intervention (clinical) An action or actions intended to interrupt the course of events that are in progress; an illness or bleeding, for example.

crisis intervention An intervention by mental health professionals to assist an individual through a crisis.

nursing intervention An action performed by a nurse to prevent illness or its complications and to promote, maintain, or restore health. Intervention is defined in the Nursing Interventions Classification (NIC) as "any treatment, based upon clinical judgment and knowledge, that a nurse performs to enhance patient/client outcomes."

surgical intervention An intervention performed by surgery (treatment). For example, a surgeon intervenes in appendicitis by operating and removing the appendix (performing an appendectomy).

intervention (supportive) An organized approach to helping an addict (an alcoholic, for example) by having family members, friends, and professionals meet with the troubled individual, help them to see the existence of the problem, and offer support in getting the person into and through treatment.

interventionist A physician, such as a cardiologist or gastroenterologist, whose specialty requires performance of interventions, such as placement of cardiac pacemakers or procedures through a gastroscope.

intra-arterial (IA) Given into a patient's artery (for example, via a needle). For some purposes, the injection is given into a vein rather than an artery, and is then intravenous (IV). The injection may be made for the administration of medication or as a part of a diagnostic procedure.

intramuscular (IM) A method of administration of medication or nourishment, in which an injection is given into a patient's muscle.

intraoperative See *operative*.

intraoperative monitoring (IM) Electroneurodiagnostic testing that is done during the course of surgery.

intraoperative monitoring technologist (IMT) An electroneurodiagnostic technologist with special training in intraoperative monitoring.

> **Certified Neurophysiologic Intraoperative Monitoring Technologist (CNIM)** An electroneurodiagnostic technologist who passed an examination in intraoperative monitoring given by the American Board of Registration of Electroencephalographic and Evoked Potential Technologists (ABRET). **www.abret.org**

intrapreneur A person within an organization who creates a new venture or "product" for the organization. See also *entrepreneur*.

intrarater reliability See under *reliability*.

intravenous (IV) An injection given into a patient's vein (for example, via a needle). For some purposes, the injection is given into an artery rather than a vein, and is then intra-arterial (IA). The injection may be made for the administration of medication, blood products, or nourishment, or as a part of a diagnostic procedure.

intravenous nursing See *infusion nursing*.

inurement Private gain from corporate activities. A nonprofit corporation cannot keep its tax-exempt status if there is "inurement" to individuals or proprietary (for-profit) interests. One common area in which inurement issues arise is physician recruitment. Hospitals often provide incentives to attract physicians in needed specialties. If the hospital contracts to pay the physician a salary in excess of reasonable compensation for services, or provides an interest-free loan to the physician, these incentives may be considered by the Internal Revenue Service (IRS) to be inurement and thus jeopardize the hospital's tax-exempt status. The hospital must show that it (and the community) receives measurable value for the incentives provided. Inurement issues are also sometimes raised by hospital joint ventures. See also *excess benefit transaction rule*.

invasion of privacy See *privacy*.

invasive A term describing a diagnostic or therapeutic procedure or technique that requires penetration of the skin or mucous membrane, either by incision (cutting) or insertion of a needle or other device. A biopsy (removing a portion of tissue for examination and analysis) is invasive, as is the removal of a specimen of blood. See also *noninvasive*.

investigation An inquiry undertaken officially as a result of a legal or other requirement. In a hospital, for example, investigations may be conducted into the qualifications or performance of physicians and other health professionals. Circumstances requiring investigations and outlines of the procedures to be followed should be included in the hospital's official documents.

Application by a physician for membership on a hospital's medical staff, and the awarding of privileges, both require rigorous investigations. As to staff membership, for example, pre-application starts the process in order to determine if there is an opening on the medical staff for the skill offered (e.g., in pediatrics or internal medicine). Only if there is an opening may an actual application be submitted, usually on forms supplied by the hospital. The application must be complete in every respect, including education, specific references, teaching experience, all hospital affiliations, board certifications, and licensures. The National Practitioner Data Bank (NPDB) is consulted for any malpractice claims.

Any time gaps are queried and resolved. Medicare's Office of the Inspector General (OIG) is queried for any Medicare sanctions. A criminal background check is made. Such an investigation, with satisfactory resolution of any ambiguities, precedes any consideration by the hospital's credentials committee, the first step toward awarding of membership.

A performance investigation is triggered by a specific allegation—for example, sexual harassment—and the reason must be stated in the documentation. The scope of the investigation must be determined, the subject notified, the investigating individuals or body designated, documents obtained, and witnesses interviewed, and there must be proper documentation and dissemination of the resulting report. The hospital then follows up with any appropriate action. See also *credentialing*.

investigator In health care, "investigator" means an individual who is carrying out a clinical trial or other medical research. Sometimes called clinical investigator. Under federal regulation, he or she must meet certain standards of informed consent of subjects, peer review, reporting, and accounting. See also *institutional review board*.

physician investigator A physician who designs, monitors, or conducts clinical trials and is responsible for the safety and ethical conduct of the trial.

Certified Physician Investigator (CPI) A physician investigator who has been certified by the Academy of Pharmaceutical Physicians and Investigators (APPI). **appinet.org**

in vitro Carried out in an artificial environment such as a test tube or culture media; used in connection with biological investigations. See also *in silico* and *in vivo*.

in vivo Carried out in living tissue; used in connection with biological investigations. See also *in silico* and *in vitro*.

involuntary commitment See under *commitment*.

involuntary smoking Inhaling air containing tobacco smoke produced by other persons who are smoking. Synonym: passive smoking.

IOM See *Institute of Medicine*.

iontophoresis See *electrotransport*.

IPA See *independent practice association*.

IPCP See *interdisciplinary patient care plan*.

IPF See *inpatient psychiatric facility*.

IPF-PPS See *inpatient psychiatric facility prospective payment system* under *prospective payment system*.

IPIA See *Improper Payments Information Act of 2002*.

IPPNW See *International Physicians for the Prevention of Nuclear War*.

IPPS See *inpatient prospective payment system* under *prospective payment system*.

IPS See *ICU physician staffing*.

IRB See *institutional review board*.

IR-DRG See *International-Refined DRG* under *DRG*.

IRF See *inpatient rehabilitation facility*.

IRF-PAI See *Inpatient Rehabilitation Facility Patient Assessment Instrument*.

IRF-PPS See *inpatient rehabilitation facility prospective payment system* under *prospective payment system*.

irrigation Flushing by use of a liquid.

ISBN International Standard Book Number. A thirteen-digit code (prior to 2007, it was ten digits) used to permanently and uniquely identify individual books and other media forms. In the United States, the ISBN system is administered by R.R. Bowker, a private company. Any publisher can buy a block of ISBN numbers that are then permanently linked to that publisher. The publisher then assigns individual ISBNs to each specific book or other work, making sure to never re-use a previously used number. The ISBN itself should not be confused with the familiar *bar code* symbol found on the back of books, which is an encoded symbol representing the ISBN, but that includes other numbers, plus a check digit. **www.isbn.org**

ISDM See *informed shared decision making*.

ISID See *International Society for Infectious Diseases*.

ISMP See *Institute for Safe Medication Practices*.

ISO International Organization for Standardization (frequently but incorrectly referred to as the International Standards Organization). The ISO is a worldwide, private federation of national standards groups from over 150 countries, one from each country. ISO's work results in international agreements that are published as **International Standards**. For example, the format of the common credit card is derived from an ISO International Standard. Cards that adhere to that standard, which defines such features as an optimal thickness (0.76 mm), can be used worldwide.

Established in 1947, the mission of the ISO is to promote the development of standardization and related activities in the world with a view to facilitating the international exchange of goods and services, and to developing cooperation in the spheres of intellectual, scientific, technological, and economic activity. Each member in the ISO is the national body most representative of standardization in its country. The member from the United States is *ANSI* (American National Standards Institute), a founding member of ISO. In 2001, there were eighty-eight countries represented in ISO; by 2007, there were 157.

Confusion about the fact that the official name doesn't match the sequence of letters is explained by the fact that ISO is *not* an acronym. In this context, ISO is used as a word, derived from the Greek "isos," meaning equal. Used as a prefix, iso- occurs in such other words as isometric, meaning of equal measure or dimensions. This line of reasoning led to the choice of ISO as the name of the organization. Also, the name ISO is valid in each of the organization's three official languages (English, French, and Russian), and so avoids the confusion that would arise through the use of an acronym. The ISO is headquartered in Geneva, Switzerland. **www.iso.ch**

isobar See under *nuclide*.

isolation Arrangements made so that (as completely as possible) an individual is neither able to contaminate others nor able to be contaminated by them. Isolation may be applied to an individual patient or person or to a group. A patient highly susceptible to infection, such as a premature infant, may be isolated from other patients and from hospital and medical personnel for his or her own protection. (In some instances such isolation systems result in entire "clean rooms" being set up.) A person with a contagious disease may be isolated from those who are not ill for the protection of others. A physician or hospital employee may also use isolation techniques when he or she has a cold, for example, in order to protect patients and other hospital personnel. Depending on the situation, the isolation may attempt to prevent direct physical contact, transfer of infectious material by air (air currents, sneezing, and so on), contamination of water supply or sewage, or contamination of objects, such as linen and dishes. See also *quarantine*.

isomer See nuclear isomers under *nuclide*.

ISO 9000 A family of process (vs. product) standards for quality management and quality assurance promulgated by the *ISO*. The ISO 9000 standards represent an international consensus on the essential features of a quality system, used by manufacturing or service businesses, to ensure their own effective operation. The ISO 9000 core series was first published in 1987. By 2007, more than 161 countries had adopted the ISO 9000 series as national standards for a wide range of economic activities, including manufacturing, financial services, retailing, government, and agriculture, as well as health care. There have also been two large regional adoptions, by *CEN* (European Committee for Standardization) and *COPANT* (the Pan-American Standards Commission).

Standards in this series originally fell into two categories: guidance (9000 and 9004) and requirements (9001, 9002, 9003). The 9002 and 9003 standards have since been discontinued, leaving the ISO 9001 requirements standard.

An organization may voluntarily seek "certification" (also called "registration") from a third party known as an **accredited registrar**. If the organization meets the requirements of a specific ISO standard, the organization's *quality system* (not the organization itself) is said to be certified. Over 8,500 companies in the United States are **ISO 9000 certified**. **www.iso.org**

ISO/TC 215 A "technical committee" established in January 1998 by the ISO Technical Management Board to address the subject of health informatics. Its main purpose is to ensure standardization in the use of health, health information, and communications technology. The United States is providing input via the *US TAG*. There are eight ISO/TC 215 "working groups" (WGs):

1. Data structure
2. Data interchange
3. Semantic content
4. Security
5. Health cards
6. Pharmacy and medicines business
7. Devices
8. Business requirements for electronic health records

isotope See under *nuclide*.

ISPOR See *International Society for Pharmacoeconomics and Outcomes Research*.

IT See *information technology* and *information therapy*.

IV See *intravenous*.

Ix Information prescription. See *information therapy*.

J

Jackson Hole Group An informal healthcare "think tank" founded by Paul Elwood, MD, in the early 1970s. Elwood periodically convenes a small group of people interested in the problems they perceive in the healthcare system at his home in Jackson Hole, Wyoming, and leads informal discussions on possible solutions to the problems. In the 1970s, the group spearheaded the concept of health maintenance organizations (HMOs). In 1991, it gained national attention with the release of a "white paper" entitled "The 21st Century American Health System: The Jackson Hole Group Proposals for Health Care Reform Through Managed Competition." Meetings fell off in the mid 1990s, but the group reactivated in 2002 to look again at ways to improve the healthcare system. Areas of focus include improving quality of care, the role of the consumer, restraining the growth of healthcare costs, and expanding coverage to the uninsured.

JAMA See *Journal of the American Medical Association*.

JCAH See *Joint Commission on Accreditation of Hospitals*.

JCAHO See *Joint Commission on Accreditation of Healthcare Organizations*.

JD Juris Doctor. The basic general law degree. Generally, in order to practice law, people must earn their JD and then pass the bar exam in the state in which they are going to practice. In most jurisdictions the JD replaced the Bachelor of Laws (LLB) in the 1960s. The two other academic degrees in law are the Master of Laws (LLM) and the Doctor of Laws (LLD). Many law school professors obtain LLMs in addition to the JD, especially within specialty practices such as taxation.

Jehovah's Witnesses A religious group holding a belief that prohibits any member to receive a blood transfusion. Although it has been established that any adult can refuse treatment for him- or herself, courts generally will not uphold a parent's wish, based on religious beliefs, that medical intervention be withheld from their child if a reasonable parent would want that intervention. Because health professionals are required to report suspected child abuse or neglect (which includes lack of medical care), members of this religion may avoid contact between their sick children and healthcare providers.

JNPP See *Joint Notice of Privacy Practice* under *Notice of Privacy Practice*.

job lock Remaining in employment for fear of losing one's health insurance coverage. This is caused by waiting periods for pre-existing conditions, high rates, and outright denials of coverage. See *portability*.

jocko A common pronunciation of the acronym JCAHO. See *Joint Commission on Accreditation of Healthcare Organizations*.

John E. Fogarty International Center (FIC) See under *National Institutes of Health*.

Joint Commission on Accreditation of Healthcare Organizations (JCAHO) An independent, nonprofit, voluntary organization that develops standards and provides accreditation and certification to hospitals and to other healthcare organizations, such as psychiatric facilities, long-term care facilities, and ambulatory care. It also offers education programs, consultation, and publications. See also *accreditation manual* and *certification manual*.

JCAHO (often referred to simply as "the Joint Commission") is sponsored by the American College of Physicians (ACP), the American College of Surgeons (ACS), the American Hospital Association (AHA), the American Medical Association (AMA), and other medical, dental, and healthcare organizations. It is based in Chicago, Illinois. Governance is by a board of commissioners designated by the sponsoring organizations. JCAHO is the successor to the Hospital Standardization Program (HSP) of the ACS. It was formerly (until 1987) called the Joint Commission on Accreditation of Hospitals (JCAH). **www.jointcommission.org**

Joint Commission on Accreditation of Hospitals (JCAH) The former (until 1987) name of the Joint Commission on Accreditation of Healthcare Organizations.

joint conference committee A hospital committee with members from the governing body, the medical staff, and the hospital management (administration). Its purpose is to facilitate understanding and communication, not to introduce a channel of management that competes with the line channels of the hospital administration and the medical staff.

Joint Notice of Privacy Practice (JNPP) See under *Notice of Privacy Practice*.

joint planning See under *planning*.

joint venture A business arrangement between two or more parties to share profits, losses, and control. In health care, the term usually indicates a formalized cooperative effort between the hospital and its medical staff (or physicians from its medical staff), as opposed to a relationship in which the two, hospital and physicians, are in competition with one another. For example, a joint venture may be established in order to set up a diagnostic facility.

The legal form of the joint venture may be a partnership (general or limited), lease arrangement, corporation, or other form suited to the requirements of the venture. Sometimes the term "joint venture" is used synonymously with "partnership"; however, although a partnership may be a joint venture, not all joint ventures are partnerships. "Joint venture" may also have a specific legal meaning under state law.

Joint ventures may raise legal concerns for hospitals; see *antitrust*, *fraud and abuse*, *inurement*, and *safe harbor regulations*.

integrated joint venture A joint venture arrangement to provide prepaid health services in which providers who would otherwise be competitors pool their capital to finance the venture by themselves, or together with others, and share the substantial risk of adverse financial results caused by unexpectedly high utilization or costs of healthcare services.

Journal of the American Medical Association (JAMA) The weekly clinical publication of the American Medical Association (AMA).

judgment proof A defendant in a civil suit for money damages who is insolvent or protected by statutes that exempt property and wages from execution. Even if the plaintiff proves the defendant's liability (obtains a judgment), the plaintiff will not be able to collect any money. To get around this, the plaintiff tries to name as many defendants as possible, especially defendants with *deep pockets*, so even if one defendant turns out to be judgment proof, the other defendants may be able to pay the judgment. See also *joint and several liability* under *liability (legal)*.

judicial law See *common law*.

judicial notice A legal concept that allows obvious facts into evidence during litigation, without requiring them to be proved. Generally, before any fact in a court of law is considered to be true, it must be held to be true by a fact finder, who may be either a judge or a jury. If a fact is accepted under the standard of judicial notice, it is deemed to be true for the purposes of the litigation. A commonly given example for this is the well-known fact that the earth is round—from which you can draw your own conclusions. This term should not be confused with *legal notice*.

Juran Institute An educational organization (originally called Juran Enterprises) formed in 1979 by Joseph M. Juran, a distinguished independent consultant, lecturer, and the author of *Quality Control Handbook* and other volumes on quality management. The institute has been key in the Total Quality Management (TQM) movement, self-directed work teams, improvement of information on quality and its analysis, Six Sigma, and other cutting-edge quality initiatives. **www.juran.com**

K

Kaiser Family Foundation One of the nation's largest private foundations devoted exclusively to health, created in 1948 by industrialist Henry J. Kaiser. Its areas of focus include Medicaid, State Children's Health Insurance Program (SCHIP), Medicare, health costs and insurance, the uninsured, prescription drugs, HIV/AIDS, minority health, women's health policy, entertainment media studies, and health and development in South Africa. In 1991 the foundation established the Kaiser Commission on the Future of Medicaid (now called the Kaiser Commission on Medicaid and the Uninsured) to function as a Medicaid policy institute and serve as a forum for analyzing, debating, and evaluating future directions for Medicaid and other health reforms with the primary goal of improving access to care for low-income Americans.

The foundation also supports programs relating to health policy and innovation in its home state of California. It is not related to the Kaiser hospitals or the Kaiser-Permanente Medical Care Program. **www.kff.org**

Kaiser-Permanente Short for Kaiser-Permanente Medical Care Program, the United States' largest nonprofit health maintenance organization, serving 8.4 million members in nine states and the District of Columbia (**www.kaiserpermanente.org**). Considered to be a pioneer in comprehensive prepayment systems, Kaiser-Permanente includes the following three components:

Kaiser Foundation Health Plan The health maintenance organization (HMO) under which the members are organized. The San Francisco HMO was started in 1945.

Kaiser Foundation Hospitals A nonprofit corporation that provides hospital services to the HMO members.

Permanente Medical Groups The physician partnerships and professional corporations that provide the actual medical services to the HMO.

kaizen The Japanese word for continuous improvement. See *continuous quality improvement* under *quality improvement*.

KDB Knowledge database; see *knowledgebase*.

KDD Knowledge discovery in databases; see *data mining*.

Kefauver-Harris Drug Amendments of 1962 Federal legislation passed to ensure drug efficacy and safety. For the first time, drug manufacturers were required to prove to the Food and Drug Administration (FDA) the safety and effectiveness of their products before marketing them. These amendments are also known as the Drug Efficacy Amendment of 1962 or the "1962 drug effectiveness law." See also *Federal Food, Drug, and Cosmetic Act of 1938* and *Safe Medical Devices Act of 1990*. Public Law 87-781, 76 Stat. 780 (1962).

Kellogg Foundation See *W.K. Kellogg Foundation*.

Kendra's Law A law passed in New York in 1999 that provides for *assisted outpatient treatment (AOT)* for individuals with mental illness who, in view of their treatment history and circumstances, are unlikely to survive safely in the community without supervision. The law also established the Medication Grant Program to ensure that individuals moving from hospitals or correctional facilities to the community receive necessary psychiatric medications without interruption. The law was named for Kendra Webdale, a young woman who died in January 1999 after being pushed in front of a New York City subway train by a person who had failed to take the medication prescribed for his mental illness. New York Mental Hygiene Law § 9.60 (1999).

Kennedy-Kassebaum bill See *HIPAA*.

Kevorkian See *Doctor Death*.

key See *public key* and *public key infrastructure*.

keyhole surgery See *laparoscopic surgery* under *surgery (treatment)*.

kinesiology The study of human movement, including anatomy and mechanical principles.

kinesiotherapist (KT) A health professional who provides kinesiotherapy services under the direction of a physician.

  Registered Kinesiotherapist (RKT) A kinesiotherapist with at least a bachelor's degree with a major in exercise science or related field, who has met the requirements of the Council on Professional Standards for Kinesiotherapy (COPS-KT). **www.akta.org**

kinesiotherapy (KT) The use of therapeutic exercise and education to treat the effects of disease, injury, and congenital disorders. The slogan of the American Kinesiotherapy Association (**www.akta.org**) is "improvement through movement." Formerly called corrective therapy.

kininase See *angiotensin-converting enzyme*.

kiosk Pronunciation of QIOSC. See *quality improvement organization support center*.

Kirklin system A method of staging tumors. See *staging (tumors)*.

knowledge No clear distinction exists between "information" and "knowledge," although the term "knowledge" has become fashionable in usages for which information would, at an earlier date, have sufficed. Dictionaries typically define information more narrowly than knowledge, and as more likely to be based on data, whereas knowledge is defined more broadly. Knowledge perhaps adds its owner's interpretation and biases to the information. A newer term, *knowledge-based information*, also has appeared. See also *knowledgebase* and *knowledge-based management*.

knowledge asymmetry The situation that exists when two individuals are attempting to come to a decision and the amount of information each has on the subject is very different. For example, until recent developments, physicians have had far more information on diseases and their treatment than patients, and attempts to empower patients to participate in decision making on their own care have been largely futile. See *decision-support software*, *Health Commons Institute*, *informed shared decision making*, *patient empowerment*, and *Problem Knowledge Couplers*.

knowledgebase A special kind of *database*. The knowledgebase is not as structured as the traditional database (which consists of tables made up of rows and columns), and would probably not be normalized, nor have a data dictionary. This also distinguishes the knowledgebase from the *data warehouse* and *data mart*.

  A knowledgebase is typically a free-form collection of records that may themselves be of various formats, such as text, pictures, hypertext links, or multimedia "objects." The hallmark of an effective knowledgebase is that it is an easily accessible repository of information about a certain subject. Accessibility depends not only on the search and navigation features of the viewer (software program) used to access the knowledgebase, but also on the skill and effort of the knowledgebase's authors and creators.

  A promising use of knowledgebases is to supplement (or even replace) paper-based workflows. In the information age, the knowledgebase can be the workspace where shared information is continually being added, modified, deleted, and accessed. It can be simultaneously accessed by any number of knowledge workers, all working smarter because each has instant access to the combined knowledge of all the others. Someday each individual will have a personal knowledgebase dedicated just to his or her health and health care—possibly called something like the *electronic health record (EHR)*.

knowledge-based information A term used by the Joint Commission on Accreditation of Healthcare Organizations (JCAHO) to mean "a collection of stored facts, models, and information found in the clinical, scientific, and management literature that can be used for designing and redesigning processes and for problem solving." So in this context, "knowledge-based" is confined to "library" information. The meaning has been considerably broadened in other contexts; see, for example, *knowledge-based management*.

knowledge-based management Management supported by valid data about a specific population, such as a geographic or ethnic community. In health care, information about a patient population, combined with data accumulated through their care, can serve as a powerful tool for providers (for example, a physician or managed care organization responsible for their care). Information is of two kinds: demographic data and performance data.

The demographic data include the size of the population and its age and sex distribution, vital statistics including mortality and morbidity, and data about the population's special health and environmental characteristics, ethnic makeup, and sources of payment for health care.

The provider can add data on the health care received to the knowledge base. This requires a management information system that carries the necessary detail about diagnoses, procedures, and patient care management to permit compilations of statistical patterns on such items as immunizations given, use of hospital days, surgical and other treatments, use of prescription drugs, and so on. The data can be used to develop report cards for individual physicians and other caregivers and institutions. Comparisons of these patterns against recognized standards and the performance of peers are useful in managing and improving practices.

A knowledge-based management system can even provide contemporaneous patient safeguards, in addition to retrospective analysis and future planning. In the more sophisticated systems, which employ Online Analytical Processing (OLAP), rules are developed (rudimentary artificial intelligence) by which one component of the computer processing is a continuous monitoring of performance. Warning alarms can be sounded in "real time" for individual patients when predetermined signal events are detected. For example, it is common to have a warning sound when an order is issued for a drug incompatible with another already being given, or for a drug for which dietary restrictions should be invoked.

knowledge discovery in databases (KDD) The process of taking the raw results of *data mining* and transforming them into potentially useful information.

Kona Architecture See *Patient Record Architecture*.

KT See *kinesiotherapist* and *kinesiotherapy*.

K2 Kennedy-Kassebaum bill. See *HIPAA*.

Kyl-Archer Amendment Formally known as "The Medicare Beneficiary Freedom to Contract Act." Introduced in 1997 by Senator Jon Kyl (Republican, AZ) and Representative Bill Archer (Republican, TX), this bill was proposed as an amendment to the *Balanced Budget Act of 1997 (BBA)*. The controversial amendment generated an extraordinary amount of interest and debate, which tended to fall along partisan lines.

It was introduced to give Medicare beneficiaries a more flexible way to enter into a *private contract* (see under *contract*) with any healthcare provider, in addition to or instead of receiving the usual Medicare benefits. The amendment's sponsors argued that under the unamended BBA, beneficiaries would be "trapped" by the Medicare provisions and could not contract for any medical services outside of Medicare.

The Democrats and others opposing the amendment argued that it would allow providers to bypass balance billing and charge more for services than if they were provided under Medicare. Opponents of the amendment also feared abuses by providers, such as rejecting Medicare coverage and pressuring beneficiaries to pay the higher "private contract" rates, as well as the possibility of "double-dipping"—charging beneficiaries fees under the private contract, then also getting reimbursed under the Medicare claim.

Threatening a veto of the entire budget, President Clinton, a Democrat, managed to insert Section 4507 into the BBA, which effectively countered the effects of the Kyl-Archer amendment. Section 4507 of the BBA allows a private contract between a provider and a Medicare beneficiary, but neither may receive any Medicare funds for the contracted service. Section 4507 also prohibits providers from entering into any private contract with a person eligible for Medicare unless that provider also agrees to not participate in the Medicare program for the following two years. Not having the votes to override the veto, Congress passed the BBA with Section 4507 intact.

L

Labeler Identification Code (LIC) See *Health Industry Business Communications Council*.

laboratory A facility where testing, research, experimentation, and sometimes preparation of scientific equipment and substances are carried out. In a hospital, when the word "laboratory" is used alone, it refers to the *clinical laboratory* (see below).

> **clinical laboratory** A laboratory for examining materials from the human body. The examinations typically fall under headings such as hematology, cytology, bacteriology, histology, biochemistry, toxicology, and serology.

> **forensic laboratory** The specialized laboratory of the forensic pathologist, who deals with legal issues, particularly crime. Included in the scope are determining the cause of violent or mysterious death, the time of death, and toxicology.

> **pathology laboratory** A laboratory used in anatomic pathology (see *pathology*). Pathology, the study of the structures, organs, and tissues of the body in disease, is divided into several major specialties, including anatomic pathology, which deals with tissues removed in surgery and with autopsy material. It is in the pathology laboratory that organs removed in surgery and biopsy specimens are studied for the presence of disease and its nature (such as infections, cancer, and the like). This laboratory is also the place where autopsies are performed.

> Other major divisions of pathology include clinical pathology and forensic pathology. Clinical pathology is concerned with analysis of materials obtained from the body, such as blood and urine. The laboratory for this service is called the clinical laboratory (see above). Every hospital will have both a pathology laboratory for anatomic pathology and a clinical laboratory, or will make arrangements for laboratory services, both anatomic and clinical, that are acceptable to the accrediting and licensing agencies.

> Forensic pathology, dealing with crime, typically has its laboratory in a municipal hospital or with a law enforcement organization.

laboratory information management system (LIMS) A system used in pharmaceutical manufacturing and for other chemical measurements. A LIMS is subject to the ASTM E-1578 standard. It is distinguished from the **laboratory information system (LIS)**, which focuses on the day-to-day production side of clinical laboratory data management. Increasingly, LISs are becoming known as **clinical laboratory information management systems (CLIMS)**.

> It is the CLIMS that handles the information related to laboratory procedures (tests) ordered by caregivers, the delivery of the results, and storage of the information for future use. It has been estimated that approximately 80% of numerical data generated in a medical facility comes from the laboratory. The CLIMS, unlike the LIMS, is also moving toward integration with the *electronic health record (EHR)*.

labor room A room for maternity patients who are in labor. A labor room is not to be confused with the delivery room, where actual birth takes place.

lactation consultant A health professional who provides breastfeeding assistance to babies and mothers.

> **International Board Certified Lactation Consultant (IBCLC)** An interdisciplinary credential available to qualified lactation consultants from the International Board of Lactation Consultant Examiners. **www.iblce.org**

Landscape See *HealthCare Standards Landscape*.

language See *natural language*.

laparascopic surgery See under *surgery (treatment)*.

laser A device that emits intense energy and heat by converting light of a spectrum of frequencies into light of a single frequency (wavelength) in a narrow, focused beam. The term comes from *Light Amplification by Stimulated Emission of Radiation*. See also **laser surgery** under **surgery**.

LBW See **low birth weight**.

LCCE See **Lamaze Certified Childbirth Educator** under **childbirth educator**.

LCP See **life care plan**.

Leading Health Indicators A set of ten key determinants, defined in **Healthy People 2010**, that influence health and are used to measure the health of the nation. The indicators were chosen to reflect the major health concerns in the United States at the beginning of the twenty-first century. Each of the indicators has one or more objectives from Healthy People 2010 associated with it. They were selected on the basis of their ability to motivate action, the availability of data to measure progress, and their importance as public health issues. The indicators are:

- Physical Activity
- Overweight and Obesity
- Tobacco Use
- Substance Abuse
- Responsible Sexual Behavior
- Mental Health
- Injury and Violence
- Environmental Quality
- Immunization
- Access to Health Care

See also **health status indicator**.

Leapfrog Group A group of *Fortune 500* companies and other large healthcare purchasers whose aim is to initiate breakthroughs in the safety and quality of health care in the United States by harnessing their purchasing power. Sponsored by the Business Roundtable, the group was formed in response to the 1999 Institute of Medicine report, *To Err Is Human: Building a Safer Health System* (see **patient safety**). The group initially pushed for three methods to improve patient safety: **computerized physician order entry (CPOE)**, **evidence-based hospital referral (EHR)**, and **ICU physician staffing (IPS)**. In 2004, it added the "Leapfrog Safe Practices Score," based on hospitals' progress meeting the National Quality Forum (NQF)-endorsed **30 Safe Practices**, which, if utilized, reduce the risk of harm in certain processes, systems, or environments of care (these practices include the original three Leapfrog "leaps"). **www.leapfroggroup.org**

learned intermediary A legal defense used by manufacturers of prescription drugs and medical devices that grants them immunity from product liability for design defects or "failure to warn" if they properly warned the physician who prescribed the treatment or medical intervention. The physician is considered the "learned intermediary." The manufacturer's duty to warn the patient is relieved if the physician was properly warned.

The theory of this defense is that drugs and devices are by their nature dangerous, but the value to society outweighs the danger, so manufacturers must be protected from suit. This protection is designed to serve as an incentive to do more research in the medical field and introduce new devices and drugs for the good of society.

There are three recognized exceptions: vaccines, birth control pills, and intrauterine devices. In these areas the manufacturer has a duty to directly warn the ultimate users of the products.

leave of absence (LOA) A predetermined period of time during a hospital stay when the patient is permitted to be away from the hospital, with the understanding that the patient will return at the end of the period. An LOA may be for a few hours, a day, or several days. A leave is granted by the attending physician, who has satisfied her- or himself that the patient's condition warrants the absence. The patient's departure is not a discharge, and the return is not an admission. There is debate as to whether the absent days are a part of the patient's length of stay (LOS). Questions also arise as to responsibility for the patient on LOA, that is, whether the hospital or patient is liable if the patient's condition worsens or there is an accident.

legacy system A computer term referring to an inherited set of independent computer systems within an organization (enterprise). The term comes into use as enterprises seek to consolidate the systems of the past into a single information source, either by somehow linking them so that they can communicate with each other (and with the inquirer) or, more likely, by replacing them with an *integrated management information system (IMIS)* (see under *management information system*, under *information system*).

Hospitals commonly have installed, at different times, independent computer systems for laboratory, x-ray, business office, and admitting, for example. Unless this legacy system is replaced by an IMIS, (1) it is impossible to obtain a comprehensive view of the hospital's activities; (2) because much of the same information is found in each system, such as patient demographic data, there is a much higher likelihood of error than if there were a single entry for each piece of information; and (3) there is duplication of cost.

"Legacy system" is also frequently used to describe *any* previously existing computer system that is considered to be now obsolete and ready for replacement or incorporation into a new system.

legal health record (LHR) See *legal medical record* under *medical record*.

legal medical record See under *medical record*.

legal medicine The discipline that focuses on issues where law and medicine converge. Topics include, for example, informed consent, assisted suicide, malpractice, governance, fraud and abuse, antitrust, and credentialing.

legal notice A specific kind of notification that must be given by someone to satisfy a legal requirement. The requirement may arise from a private agreement between two or more parties, or from governmental laws or regulations. The requirement typically spells out the details of the notification, such as whether it need be in writing, be personally delivered and signed for, be published in a legal newspaper for a certain number of issues, or be given a certain period of time before some other event is allowed to happen. This term should not be confused with *judicial notice*.

legal nurse consulting The area of nursing focusing on the information and knowledge needs of attorneys, patients, and health professionals within the context of medical-legal matters and litigation. The legal nurse consultant serves as a liaison between the legal and medical disciplines.

Legal Nurse Consultant Certified (LNCC) A specialist in legal nurse consulting who has passed an examination of the American Legal Nurse Consultant Certification Board (ALNCCB). **www.aalnc.org/lncc**

LEIE See *List of Excluded Individuals/Entities*.

length of stay (LOS) See *average length of stay*.

LEP See *limited English proficient*.

leukoreduction A filtering process that removes more than 99.9% of the white blood cells (leukocytes) from blood to be used for transfusion, leaving only the red blood cells and platelets, and a residual white cell content of less than 5 million white blood cells (WBC) per cubic millimeter. The result is "leukoreduced blood," which is preferred over "natural" blood to (1) prevent recurrent fever and chill reactions with blood transfusions, (2) prevent or delay rejection of transplanted bone marrow or other organs by removing most of the *human leukocyte antigens (HLA)* that are responsible for rejection, and (3) reduce the risk of *cytomegalovirus (CMV)* infection transmitted by the transfusion.

level of care The amount (intensity) and kind of professional *nursing care* required for a patient in order to achieve the desired medical and nursing care objectives for the patient, that is, to carry out the orders of the attending physician and to meet the patient's nursing care needs. The term "level of care" is primarily used outside the acute hospital, where three levels of care are recognized: skilled nursing care (the highest level), intermediate care, and rest home care (custodial care, the lowest level).

Levels of care (and facilities to provide them) have specific definitions in Medicare, Medicaid, and other payment programs, and also under statutes and regulations of the various states. The determination of the level of care to be provided to a given patient is a serious matter; on the one hand, the patient should be placed at the lowest level of care commensurate with his or her needs as a matter both of appropriate care and of economy, while, on the other hand, payment is greater for each succeeding higher level of care.

leverage Financing by borrowing.

> **capital leverage** See *financial leverage*, below.

> **financial leverage** The ratio of total debt to total assets (in a stock corporation, the ratio of long-term debt to shareholders' equity). An institution uses financial leverage (it "trades on its equity") when it believes it has **positive leverage**, that is, that it can use the money obtained by debt financing (see *financing (finance)*) to earn more money than it costs to borrow the money (interest and taxes). Should the cost of borrowing exceed the added revenue, the situation is one of **negative leverage**. Synonym: capital leverage.

> **negative leverage** See *financial leverage*, above.

> **operating leverage** The ratio of fixed costs to variable costs (see *cost*). When it takes very little added labor or materials to provide added units of service or products, the operating leverage is high (and the marginal cost of added units is low); a greater volume brings accelerated profits, once the break-even point is reached. The higher the proportion of the costs that are variable (that is, the lower the operating leverage) the greater an increase in units of service or products will be required to increase profits.

> **positive leverage** See *financial leverage*, above.

leveraged Financed largely by borrowed funds. See *leverage*.

LGBT Lesbian, gay, bisexual, and transgender.

LHEG See *local healthcare executive group*.

LHII See *local health information infrastructure*.

LHR Legal health record. See *legal medical record* under *medical record*.

LHS See *London Handicap Scale* under *quality of life scale*.

liability (financial) In finance, an obligation to pay. Liabilities are shown on an institution's balance sheet under such headings as "accounts payable" (money owed to vendors and others), "accrued salaries" (when a statement is drawn before checks have been issued for a given pay period), and the like.

> **current liability** A liability due in less than one year.

liability (legal) An actual or potential responsibility to do something, pay something, or refrain from doing something. Liability is used to refer to a legal duty or other obligation, often one that must be enforced by a lawsuit. When liability is of the "potential responsibility" type, it is often thought of as "exposure" or "risk." If a hospital, for instance, is liable for the negligent acts of its physicians, the hospital is not really obligated to do anything unless and until one of its physicians commits a negligent act. A separate legal duty may arise in this situation, however, such as the obligation to obtain malpractice insurance. See also *duty (legal)*, *accountability (governance)*, and *negligence*.

> **corporate liability** Legal responsibility of a corporation, rather than of an individual. In the healthcare context, the term is often used to denote a specific type of responsibility: that of the hospital as an institution (corporation) to exercise reasonable care in selecting, retaining, and granting privileges to members of its medical staff.

> A hospital may be liable to a patient injured by a physician (or other health professional) if the hospital knew or should have known that the physician was not competent to perform the procedure involved (or to otherwise treat the patient), and did not reasonably act to pro-

tect the patient (for example, by restricting that physician's privileges or by requiring supervision). "Knew" means that the hospital may not "look the other way" if it learns of problems with a physician that could endanger patients; "should have known" means that the hospital must diligently investigate a physician's credentials prior to granting staff privileges, *and* that the hospital must systematically monitor the care provided by that physician, once on the staff. See also *compliance*.

enterprise liability A system under which individual healthcare providers are relieved of liability for medical malpractice, and healthcare organizations such as hospitals and health maintenance organizations bear liability for malpractice committed by their affiliated care providers, whether or not those providers are employees of the organization. The system was proposed by Kenneth S. Abraham, JD. Sometimes called organizational liability.

joint and several liability The responsibility of more than one defendant to share in legal liability to a plaintiff. If the defendants (for example, the hospital and a physician) are jointly and severally liable, each is responsible to pay the entire judgment to the plaintiff (although the plaintiff cannot collect more than the amount of the judgment).

product liability An area of law that imposes legal responsibility on manufacturers (and in some cases distributors and retailers) of goods that leave the factory in an unreasonably dangerous condition, and that in fact cause harm to someone because of that condition. Product liability does not require proof that the manufacturer was negligent (careless) in designing or producing the item.

professional liability A legal duty that is the result of performing (or failing to perform) something that one does (or should have done) as a professional. A physician who drives a car carelessly and injures another will be simply "liable" for that person's injuries; the fact that she is a physician is not relevant to the fact that she injured the other person. If that same physician carelessly misses a diagnosis and again injures another, the legal responsibility is called "professional liability," because her actions as a physician caused the injury. Sometimes the phrase "professional liability" is used interchangeably with "professional negligence," but that usage is inaccurate because a professional can become liable for reasons other than negligence (for example, by improperly disclosing a patient's confidences, operating without informed consent, or abandoning a patient).

strict liability Legal responsibility for injury, which is imposed regardless of any fault or lack of fault. A plaintiff suing under strict liability does not need to show that the defendant was negligent, reckless, or malicious. The plaintiff does, however, still need to prove the existence of a defect (such as in a product) or an action (such as selling liquor to an intoxicated person), and that the defect or action caused the plaintiff's injuries.

Libby Zion case A 1986 legal case involving the death in 1984 of an 18-year-old woman, Libby Zion, in New York. The woman died a few hours after treatment in a hospital emergency department. Ms. Zion's father claimed that her care had been inadequate, and a grand jury investigation later followed. Although the grand jury did not return a criminal indictment, it did make a number of recommendations regarding emergency room staffing, supervision of physicians in training, regulation of work hours for interns and junior resident physicians, restraint of patients (and the care of patients under restraint), and protection of patients from contraindicated combinations of drugs. Each recommendation—particularly that of limiting the number of hours a physician in training may work consecutively—attracted a good deal of attention in New York and nationally.

libel Written words that injure the reputation of another; written defamation. Oral defamation is called "slander." See *defamation*.

LIC Labeler Identification Code. See *Health Industry Business Communications Council*.

license A legal term that represents a specific right to do or use something, or to refrain from it. Although a license is often associated with a written or other object that represents the license, such as a "driver's license," it need not be. A license is often also a contract.

When a healthcare facility or provider is described as being "licensed," it means it has a legal right, granted by a government agency, in compliance with a statute governing a profession (such as medicine or nursing), occupation, or the operation of an activity (such as a hospital). See also *licensure*.

licensed beds See under *bed capacity*.

licensed independent practitioner (LIP) See under *allied health professional*.

licensure A method used by most states to ensure that persons who provide health (and other) services are adequately qualified. The licensure law will also define the scope of practice for that profession, and anyone performing services within that scope must first have a license to do so.

life care A *long-term care* alternative in which all care required for the lifetime of the participant is provided. A retirement home that agrees to provide not only facilities for independent living, but also nursing care and hospitalization to residents as needed, is a "life care community."

life care plan (LCP) A formal document prepared for a person who has chronic healthcare and/or other needs due to illness, injury, or disability, delineating present and future needs and their expected costs. It covers such items as frequency and type of services (physician, home health, diagnostic evaluations, therapies, rehabilitation), equipment and transportation, housing, activities, education, vocational training, and so forth. The life care plan is utilized by insurers, attorneys, treatment teams, economists, and trustees, as well as by patients and their families.

life care planning The process of developing a *life care plan*. This has become a specialized area, engaged in by health professionals with extensive training in this field. Qualified life care planners often have backgrounds in case management, nursing, rehabilitation counseling, and related fields.

Certified Life Care Planner (CLCP) A specialist in life care planning who has passed an examination of the Commission on Health Care Certification (CHCC). **www.cdec1.com**

Certified Nurse Life Care Planner (CNLCP) A nurse specializing in life care planning who has passed an examination of the American Association of Nurse Life Care Planners (AANLCP). **aanlcp.org**

life expectancy A statistically derived estimate as to how much longer a given individual may be expected to live. Reference tables for life expectancy have been produced by insurance companies and public health statisticians for many years. The earliest such tables took into account age- and sex-specific death rates compiled for the general population, usually by governmental offices of vital statistics. The tables are periodically updated as these offices publish new data, and the more recent tables have been refined as data have become available permitting adjustments for other factors, such as smoking habits, occupation, and family history.

Lifeline A program to help low-income consumers pay the cost of monthly telephone service. See *Universal Service Fund*.

Life Safety Code A code of construction and operation for buildings, intended to maximize fire safety, issued and periodically revised by the National Fire Protection Association (NFPA). Compliance with this code (also known as NFPA 101) is required of hospitals seeking accreditation by the Joint Commission on Accreditation of Healthcare Organizations (JCAHO).

life signs See *vital signs*.

life support Maintenance of vital body functions (e.g., breathing and heartbeat) to sustain life. See also *emergency medical technician*.

Advanced Cardiovascular Life Support (ACLS) A program of standardized instruction and certification offered by the American Heart Association for medical provider evaluation and treatment of patients with symptoms and signs suggestive of heart and vascular problems. It includes *Basic Life Support* (see *basic life support*, below). The course is designed for physicians, nurses, emergency medical technicians, paramedics, respiratory therapists, and other professionals who may respond to a cardiovascular emergency.

advanced life support (ALS) A term used in emergency medical services that usually refers to the administration of intravenous medications and the use of defibrillation (heart starting) equipment. This term may have a specific definition in a state's statutes or regulations governing emergency medical care. For example, the Illinois Emergency Medical Services Systems Act states:

"Advanced Life Support (ALS) Services" means an advanced level of pre-hospital and inter-hospital emergency care . . . that includes basic life support care, cardiac monitoring, cardiac defibrillation, electrocardiography, intravenous therapy, administration of medications, drugs and solutions, use of adjunctive medical devices, trauma care, and other authorized techniques and procedures, as outlined in the Advanced Life Support national curriculum of the U.S. Department of Transportation. 210 Ill. Comp. Stat. § 50/3.10(a) (2006).

advanced trauma life support (ATLS) Emergency medical care provided on-site or near a disaster within "a few hours" of the occurrence of the injuries. It is usually provided by *emergency medical technicians (EMTs)*.

basic life support (BLS) Medically accepted noninvasive procedures to sustain life. The American Heart Association offers a Basic Life Support (BLS) course that includes training in *cardiopulmonary resuscitation (CPR)*, use of an *automated external defibrillator (AED)* (see under *external defibrillator*, under *defibrillator*), and relief of choking.

intermediate life support (ILS) A term used in emergency services with particular reference to the prevention and treatment of shock. This term may have a specific definition in a state's statutes or regulations concerning emergency medical care. For example, the Illinois Emergency Medical Services Systems Act states:

"Intermediate Life Support (ILS) Services" means an intermediate level of pre-hospital and inter-hospital emergency care and non-emergency medical services care that includes basic life support care plus intravenous cannulation and fluid therapy, invasive airway management, trauma care, and other authorized techniques and procedures, as outlined in the Intermediate Life Support national curriculum of the U.S. Department of Transportation 210 Ill. Comp. Stat. § 50/3.10(b) (2006).

Pediatric Advanced Life Support (PALS) A course of instruction offered by the American Heart Association to provide healthcare professionals with information and strategies needed to recognize, prevent, and provide advanced life support services for cardiopulmonary arrest in infants and children.

life support system Equipment and services, including administration of nutrition and fluids, that support one or more of the life-sustaining functions of circulation (heart), respiration (breathing), nutrition, and kidney function. When a patient is completely dependent on artificial (mechanical) means for maintenance of one or more of these functions, stopping or removing the equipment will cause death, and the stopping or removal is referred to as "termination of life support systems."

lifetime reserve A Medicare term referring to the pool of sixty days of hospital care upon which a patient may draw after he or she has used up the maximum Medicare benefit for a single *spell of illness*.

Likert scale A scale developed by Rensis Likert, a social psychologist, to quantify a person's response to a particular statement. A typical application, for instance, might be a survey on healthcare costs that includes the following statement: "Doctors earn too much money," and then asks whether you "strongly agree, have no opinion, or strongly disagree." The respondent's choice is then scaled—for example, as either a zero, a five, or a ten, depending on the construction of the scale. This type of scale is very commonly used in survey research where researchers attempt to quantify human attitudes and feelings.

limited-access facility See *limited-service hospital* under *hospital*.

limited English proficient (LEP) A person who may need help or an interpreter to understand the English language.

limited liability company (LLC) A form of business organization that allows all owners and managers to have limited liability for the debts of the company, but also favorable tax treatment. These companies are taxed like partnerships, with flow-through taxation (also called conduit taxation), which avoids the traditional corporate "double taxation" (taxes are levied at both the corporate level and the individual dividend level). Most states that have adopted this new form also allow professionals to use it. Some states have adopted **professional limited liability companies** (also known as professional limited companies) that blend together the features of the LLC and the *professional corporation (PC)* (see under *corporation*).

limited-service hospital See under *hospital*.

LIMS See *laboratory information management system*.

line A term used in the context of line and staff, which refers to authority in an organization. Line authority is hierarchical: a floor nurse reports to a head nurse, who in turn reports to the chief of nursing, who in turn reports to the chief executive officer of the hospital who, finally, reports to the governing body. Only a person higher in this series is authorized to "give orders" to a person lower in the series.

    The contrast is with "staff," which refers to persons who assist in the operation of the organization by furnishing services to line personnel. Staff personnel do not have authority to "give orders" (except within the narrow limits of the staff group itself). The chief of nursing is a line person. The controller is a staff person, although the controller may also have line authority for the business office, for example.

line and staff A phrase used in organizations describing the two kinds of roles played by personnel. "Line" pertains to positions in the "chain of command" in which superiors direct subordinates at a series of levels, and "staff" refers to positions in which individuals (or components of the organization) are not in the "chain of command" but are employed to provide assistance to those in line positions.

linear regression See *regression*.

linkage See *genetic linkage*.

Link Up A program to help low income consumers pay the cost of telephone installation and other one-time charges. See *Universal Service Fund*.

Linnaean System A system for classifying plants and animals, based on a hierarchy: kingdom, phylum, class, order, family, genus, and species. It was developed by an eighteenth-century Swedish botanist and medical doctor named Karl von Linné (better known as Carolus Linnaeus, the Latinized form he chose for his name). The Linnaean System is still the most widely used biologic taxonomy. See also *PhyloCode*.

LIP See *licensed independent practitioner* under *allied health professional*.

liquidity The ability to turn assets into cash.

LIS Laboratory information system. See *laboratory information management system*.

List of Excluded Individuals/Entities (LEIE) A database of the Department of Health and Human Services (HHS) Office of Inspector General (OIG) of providers who are currently excluded from participation in Medicare, Medicaid, and all federal healthcare programs. Individuals and entities who have been reinstated are removed from the LEIE. There are many bases for an exclusion, including a conviction related to the Medicare or Medicaid program, a conviction related to patient abuse, or an action taken by a state licensing authority. The LEIE only reports exclusion actions taken by the OIG; it does not report actions taken by other agencies. Synonym: Exclusions List. **oig.hhs.gov/fraud/exclusions.html**

lithotripsy Fragmentation (shattering) of stones (kidney, urinary tract, and bladder stones, as well as gallstones). Several methods are in use or under development: electrohydraulic lithotripsy (EHL), which produces shock waves at or near the stone through the use of a probe;

ultrasonic lithotripsy (UL), which produces a drilling effect; and extracorporeal shock wave lithotripsy (ESWL), in which shock waves are generated in a bath in which the patient is placed. The latter method is the most widespread in current use. Lithotripsy is noninvasive; the patient is spared surgery requiring invasion of his or her body.

lithotriptor A device for fragmenting stones in the process of *lithotripsy*.

living-in unit A hospital room where a mother can assume care of her newborn infant under the supervision of the hospital's nursing personnel. This term may also apply to relatives or others assisting in the care of a chronically ill or other type of patient.

living will See under *advance directive*.

LLB Bachelor of Laws. See *JD*.

LNCC See *Legal Nurse Consultant Certified* under *legal nurse consulting*.

LOA See *leave of absence*.

loan closet A collection of articles to be drawn on, without charge, when needed. Usually a loan closet is a volunteer operation, stocked with donated articles. In a health loan closet one would find hospital beds, wheelchairs, crutches, canes, bed pans, and other items that are borrowed during illness and then returned when the need is past.

lobbying Attempts to influence the passage or defeat of legislation. There are limits on such activities, and certain other political activities, by tax-exempt organizations, such as 501(c)(3) corporations. Hospitals are often 501(c)(3) organizations, and thus are limited in their lobbying (and campaigning) efforts.

local healthcare executive group (LHEG) Any association of healthcare executives in a local area, either formal or informal, designed to provide networking opportunities. A variety of such groups exist under many names, the earliest perhaps being "young administrators' groups."

local health department A unit of local government that is the action arm of national and state public health agencies. It typically carries out some clinical services, environmental services, and support services. Clinical services may include, for example, dental health, occupational health, nursing, maternal and child health, family planning, communicable disease, and Women, Infants and Children (WIC) programs. Environmental services may include general environment, vector control, animal control, and pollution control. Support services may include, in addition to administration, vital statistics, laboratory, and health education.

local health information infrastructure (LHII) The former term for the r*egional health information organization (RHIO)*.

locality rule A legal doctrine that states that the *standard of care (legal)* in a malpractice lawsuit will be measured by the degree of care exercised by similar professionals within the same geographic area (locality), rather than within the world, nation, state, or profession at large. Some states use this rule; others do not. See also *school rule*.

local public health agency (LPHA) A unit of local or state government with public health responsibilities, covering an area smaller than the state (for example, a city or county).

locum tenens physician See under *physician*.

Logical Observation Identifiers Names and Codes (LOINC) A database of universal names and codes to identify laboratory and clinical observations and test results. The laboratory portion of the LOINC database contains the categories of chemistry, hematology, serology, microbiology (including parasitology and virology), and toxicology, as well as categories for drugs and the cell counts from a complete blood count or a cerebrospinal fluid cell count. The clinical portion of LOINC includes entries for vital signs, hemodynamics, intake/output, EKG, obstetric ultrasound, cardiac echo, urologic imaging, gastroendoscopic procedures, pulmonary ventilator management, selected survey instruments, and other clinical observations. It was developed by a group of clinical pathologists, chemists, and laboratory service vendors with support from the Hartford Foundation, the National Library of Medicine (NLM), and the Agency for Health Care Policy and Research (AHCPR). The codes are designed to be used in the context of ASTM E1238 and HL7 Version 2.2 laboratory results and observation messages. **www.regenstrief.org/loinc**

LOINC See *Logical Observation Identifiers Names and Codes*.

London Handicap Scale See under *quality of life scale*.

long-term acute care (LTAC) A CMS designation for an acute care hospital with an average Medicare inpatient length of stay of more than twenty-five days. The level of care is greater than that provided in a skilled nursing facility (SNF). Synonym: long-term care hospital (LTCH).

long-term care (LTC) Care for patients, regardless of age, who have chronic diseases or disabilities, and who require preventive, diagnostic, therapeutic, and supportive services over long periods of time. LTC may call on a variety of health professionals (such as physicians, nurses, physical therapists, and social workers) as well as nonprofessionals (family, others), and may be delivered in a healthcare or other institution or in the home.

Long-term care customarily refers to those for whom the care is thought to be necessary for the rest of their lives (i.e., for whom the disability is thought not to be reversible). When the prediction is that the person can be returned to a more independent mode of living, the person is placed under skilled nursing or intermediate care (under "extended care" rather than "long-term care"); see *nursing care*. Rehabilitation efforts are made for persons in long-term care, however, and some of them do recover sufficiently to become less dependent.

long-term care alternatives (LTC alternatives) Alternatives to the traditional nursing home.

long-term care facility (LTCF) A facility that provides lodging and healthcare services to patients with chronic healthcare needs; see *long-term care*. See also *nursing home*.

long-term care hospital (LTCH) See *long-term acute care*.

long-term care hospital prospective payment system (LTCH-PPS) See under *prospective payment system*.

LOS Length of stay. See *average length of stay*.

loss (financial) Excess of expense over income. Actually means a decrease in assets. The defining phrase "negative fund balance" is often used in nonprofit corporations as a substitute for the word "loss."

loss (insurance) The amount an insurance company is obligated to pay under an insurance contract, usually due to physical damage or injury to the property or person of the insured or a third party.

loss ratio Total incurred claims for a given insurance plan divided by the total premiums.

Lou Gehrig's disease See *amyotrophic lateral sclerosis*.

low birth weight (LBW) A weight of 2,500 grams (5 pounds, 8.2 ounces) or less at birth. **Very low birth weight (VLBW)** is 1,500 grams (3 pounds, 4.5 ounces) or less. **Ultralow birth weight (ULBW)** is 1,000 grams (2 pounds, 3.0 ounces) or less.

low vision A level of vision (sometimes defined as 20/70 or worse), not correctible with glasses, contacts, medicine, or surgery, that interferes with the ability to perform everyday activities, such as reading or driving. Conditions causing low vision include macular degeneration, diabetic retinopathy, glaucoma, cataract, other diseases, injury, and genetic birth defects. A person with low vision may have a limited visual field, loss of contrast sensitivity, distortion, loss of color vision, loss of depth perception, reduced visual acuity, or other difficulty. See also *blind* and *visually impaired*.

low vision therapist A health professional who provides low vision therapy.

Certified Low Vision Therapist (CLVT) A low vision therapist who has passed a certification examination of the Academy for Certification of Vision Rehabilitation and Education Professionals (ACVREP) (**www.acvrep.org**). CLVTs must have at least a bachelor's degree in education, rehabilitation, or health care.

low vision therapy (LVT) Methods to assist people with low vision to make the most of their visual ability. This may include training of visual motor and perceptual skills, and training in the use of low vision assistance devices such as large print, magnifiers, software, electronic devices, lighting, writing implements, reading stands, and so forth. Low vision therapy can also involve modification of the person's environment, and training in techniques to maximize available vision.

LPHA See *local public health agency*.

LPN See *licensed practical nurse* under *nurse*.

LTAC See *long-term acute care*.

LTACH Long-term acute care hospital. See *long-term acute care*.

LTC See *long-term care*.

LTC alternatives See *long-term care alternatives*.

LTC-DRG See under *DRG*.

LTCF See *long-term care facility*.

LTCH Long-term care hospital. See *long-term acute care*.

LTCH-PPS See *long-term care hospital prospective payment system* under *prospective payment system*.

lumpectomy See *mastectomy*.

LVN Licensed vocational nurse. See *licensed practical nurse* under *nurse*.

LVT See *low vision therapy*.

M

M See *Microbiology Technologist* under *clinical laboratory technologist*, and *MUMPS*.

MA See *market administration* under *administration (management)*, and *medical assistant*. Also *Medicare Advantage* and *medical audit*; see *patient care audit* under *audit*.

MAB See *monoclonal antibody*.

MAC See *Medicare Administrative Contractor*. Also maximum allowable cost (see *generic equivalent*) and *Master Addiction Counselor* (see under *addiction counselor*).

MacArthur Foundation The John D. and Catherine T. MacArthur Foundation is a private, independent grantmaking institution dedicated to helping groups and individuals foster lasting improvement in the human condition. The foundation is perhaps best known for its so-called "genius grants," given to individuals with exceptional creativity and originality. **www.macfound.org**

macrobiotics A primarily vegetarian diet developed by George Ohsawa, and now promulgated by Michio Kushi of the Kushi Institute. It has been advocated for relief of cancer and other illnesses. Critical studies, however, have shown that cancer patients on the diet are actually deprived of essential nutrients and undergo serious weight loss, and that Dutch children fed the macrobiotic diet were smaller and weighed less than children fed normal diets.

macro measures In health care, refers to steps taken to improve the healthcare system at the community level (for example, local, state, or national) with respect to such problems as insurance, financing, tort reform, access, and the like, rather than to improve care for individual patients. See also *micro measures*.

macular degeneration (MD) A group of diseases that cause the cells in the "macular zone" of the retina to lose function. Adult MD is the major cause of blindness of those over fifty-five years old in the United States. Recent studies have suggested a possible genetic link.

mad cow disease Bovine spongiform encephalopathy (BSE). A degenerative brain disease affecting cattle first reported in England in 1986. It is believed that eating the meat from cattle infected with BSE can lead to a fatal neurological condition in humans called Creutzfeldt-Jakob disease (CJD). Synonym: chronic wasting disease. See also *prion*.

maggot therapy (MT) See *biosurgery*.

magnetic resonance imaging (MRI) A diagnostic technique for creating cross-sectional images of the body by the use of *nuclear magnetic resonance*. MRI can also provide information on tissue biochemical activity. The procedure is noninvasive. The device used is called an MRI scanner. Synonyms: nuclear magnetic resonance imaging (NMRI), zeugmatography, spin density.

> **functional MRI** The use of magnetic resonance imaging to detect increases or decreases of blood flow in the brain, which reflect changes in neural activity.

magnetic resonance imaging technologist A health professional trained in performing nuclear magnetic resonance imaging examinations.

> **Registered Technologist—Magnetic Resonance Imaging (RT(MR))** A *Registered Technologist (RT)* (see under *radiologic technologist*) with advanced qualifications in nuclear magnetic resonance imaging from the American Registry of Radiologic Technologists (ARRT). **www.arrt.org**

magnetic sitter An electronic system similar to that used in clothing stores to detect removal of a magnetically tagged garment past a sensor at the exit. Similar magnetic "sitters" are used to keep track of patients who, because of confusion, may wander away or enter a dangerous area. Such patients, who would otherwise have to be restrained, may be granted freedom of movement, with assurance that sensors placed near exits, windows, and other areas denied to patients will inform the nursing staff if the patient goes out of bounds.

magnetic surgery system (MSS) A method of directing a surgical instrument within the body with the use of a computer-controlled magnet, guided by the surgeon. The device lets the surgeon see the body structures and send the tiny magnet along a path that can follow curves and thus avoid blood vessels and other sensitive areas. The magnet carries a tiny tube (catheter). When the destination has been reached, the magnet is withdrawn and the catheter remains, through which the surgeon can insert biopsy and other instruments. The device was first used in a human in 1999 at Washington University in St. Louis in neurosurgery.

Magnet Recognition Program (MRP) A program of the American Nurses Credentialing Center (ANCC) to recognize healthcare organizations with outstanding nursing services. Organizations are judged on quality indicators and standards of nursing practice as defined in the American Nurses Association's *Scope and Standards for Nurse Administrators*. A recipient of the recognition has achieved **Magnet Status**. This lasts for four years, after which it must be renewed following a new evaluation.

Magnet Status See *Magnet Recognition Program*.

mainstreaming A policy of providing services to special classes of individuals within the organizational structure that serves the general population. For example, handicapped children, often educated in special classrooms, are "mainstreamed" when they are educated in the regular classroom.

> **gender mainstreaming** In health care, the term is being used to promote equality in the provision of services, education, and resources for both men and women. The aim is to articulate and then mainstream—integrate—gender issues into public policy, financing, delivery of services, and so forth, to eliminate disparities of treatment.

Major Diagnostic Category (MDC) A term used in the *prospective payment system (PPS)*. All patients are ultimately classified into one of the 468 DRG categories. On the way to that classification, each patient first falls into one of twenty-three MDCs on the basis of her or his *principal diagnosis* (see under *diagnosis*); the patient is then further classified according to age, complications, whether an operating room procedure was performed, and so forth.

major medical insurance See *catastrophic insurance* under *insurance*.

Malcolm Baldrige National Quality Award See *Baldrige National Quality Program*.

malice A legal term that describes the state of mind of someone doing a wrongful act intentionally, with the purpose of doing injury or with reckless disregard as to whether the act will result in injury.

malicious prosecution Legal grounds upon which a defendant may countersue a plaintiff if the plaintiff's lawsuit was totally frivolous and without any merit, and was brought simply to harass the defendant. To prove a case of malicious prosecution, the plaintiff's case must have been decided in favor of the defendant, and the defendant must show that there was no probable cause to believe that the defendant was liable and that the plaintiff (or plaintiff's attorney) acted with malice in bringing the suit. Given those restrictions, physicians have had very limited success in suing malpractice plaintiffs for malicious prosecution.

malignant As applied to a tumor, one that is subject to unlimited growth and extension or dispersal within the body, often leading to death. If it is not malignant, it is "benign."

malpractice A failure of care or skill by a professional, which causes loss or injury and results in legal liability. This narrow definition means the same as *professional negligence* (see under *negligence*). Some use the term "malpractice" more broadly to describe all acts by a health professional in the course of providing health care—including breach of contract—that may result in legal liability.

> **malpractice crisis** In the 1970s, insurance providers and physicians declared a "malpractice crisis," basing it on rising jury verdicts in medical malpractice litigation and the rise in the number of those claims generally. A number of states have since enacted measures addressing these problems, for example, prelitigation screening panels, caps (ceilings) on the amount of punitive damages allowed, and the development of clinical practice guidelines

(see *guidelines*). See also *prelitigation screening panel*, *damages*, *Medical Injury Compensation Reform Act*, and *tort reform*.

malpractice reform See *tort reform*.

mammogram The picture produced by the process of *mammography*.

mammographer A health professional trained to do mammography procedures.

Registered Technologist—Mammography (RT(M)) A *Registered Technologist (RT)* (see under *radiologic technologist*) with advanced qualifications in mammography from the American Registry of Radiologic Technologists (ARRT). **www.arrt.org**

mammography The diagnostic use of x-rays to visualize the breast and surrounding tissue.

managed behavioral healthcare organization (MBHO) A managed care organization (MCO) that specializes in the management, administration, and/or provision of behavioral healthcare benefits. An MBHO may serve members of HMOs or other managed care organizations in respect to mental health and substance abuse benefits; this is known as a behavioral health "carve-out."

managed care Any arrangement for health care in which someone is interposed between the patient and physician and has authority to place restraints on how and from whom the patient may obtain medical and health services, and what services are to be provided in a given situation. Under the terms of a prepaid health plan, for example, the payer may require: that except in an emergency, a designated person (usually a physician; see *gatekeeper (health care)*) be the patient's first contact with the healthcare services; that all care be authorized and coordinated by the gatekeeper rather than permitting the patient to go directly to specialists; that only certain physicians and facilities be used (if the prepayment plan is to pay for the services); that preadmission certification (PAC) precede hospitalization; that second opinions be obtained for elective surgery; and that certain care be delivered in the outpatient setting.

Managed care was originally designed to control costs, encourage efficient use of resources, and ensure that care given is appropriate. However, there is increasing interest in trying to see that each patient *gets* the care indicated and is spared unnecessary or ill-advised care.

managed care nursing The nursing specialty that focuses on the needs of members of a managed care health plan, especially wellness and prevention, disease management, and demand management programs.

Certified Managed Care Nurse (CMCN) A specialist in managed care nursing who has passed an examination of the American Board of Managed Care Nursing (ABMCN). **www.abmcn.org**

managed care organization (MCO) A term applied to a variety of organizations that contract to provide management services for the reduction and control of healthcare costs to corporations, insurers, and third-party administrators. MCOs employ such methods as making decisions as to what care is to be given individual patients and where it will be provided, negotiating contracts with providers as to quantities of and prices for services (often discounts), and auditing and approving the bills for the services the patients receive. Sometimes the MCO offers a stipulated care package for a prearranged capitation fee. Typically such organizations do not themselves provide care and do not operate hospitals or other healthcare facilities. They would, however, have legal duties similar to those of *managed care plans (MCP)*.

managed care plan (MCP) An organization providing managed care. A managed care plan has a defined group of providers and an identified group of enrollees to be served. Forward-looking plans develop explicit standards of care to be required of its providers, and are concerned not only with treatment and amelioration of disease, but also with prevention. The plan may or may not operate its own hospitals or other healthcare facilities. The financing is typically prearranged by capitation.

There are different purposes for managed care plans. One is for-profit, to make money for shareholders of a corporation. Another is a nonprofit plan set up by hospitals, physicians, insurers, or others, to control rising healthcare costs—to save money. Yet another may have as its primary purpose the preservation and improvement of the health of its members. A community may use managed care, for example, as a strategy to (1) benefit the individuals served by the plan; (2) benefit the health of the entire community; and (3) provide services in the most efficient, effective, and economic manner in view of the finite resources available.

Perhaps the biggest concern about managed care is that people will not get the medical care they need. In fact, some plans are more concerned about patient care than others. However, it is becoming clear that a managed care plan—whether owned by an insurance company, hospital, or another entity—is in a fiduciary relationship with respect to the enrollees, and may not act in a manner that jeopardizes their welfare. For example, a hospital was held liable because it had a policy to discharge patients when their insurance ran out. The court ruled that this interfered with the medical judgment of the physician, and that this resulted in the premature discharge of a psychiatric patient who later committed suicide. (Even though a managed care plan was not involved, the principles would be the same.)

managed competition (MC) A proposed strategy for purchasing health care in a manner intended to obtain maximum value for the price for the purchasers of the health care and the recipients. The concept was developed primarily by Alain Enthoven (Stanford University) and was promulgated in the early 1990s by the Jackson Hole Group.

The strategy depends on the existence of "sponsors" and acceptable providers, under government regulation. Sponsors for certain groups exist in the form of large employers, state governments, and similar institutions. For smaller and less well-organized groups, an organization called a "health alliance" (HA) is envisioned as the sponsor. The HA would be a non-profit corporation established by appropriate employer and community groups. The sponsor would act as an intermediary between the population to be insured and the competing provider groups (accountable health plans (AHPs)) that take care of both financing and delivery of care. (For competition to occur, of course, there would need to be more than one supplier.)

The "competition" would be price competition among annual premiums for a defined, standardized benefit package rather than for individual services. The competition would be "informed" in that the sponsor has data and expertise to guide it, along with an informed, critical population of subscribers being served. Presumably the AHP that convinces both the sponsor and the consumers that it can provide the highest quality of care, at the lowest cost, and with the most satisfied patients (beneficiaries), will flourish because of increased business.

The sponsor would (1) select participating AHPs; (2) make sure that the eligible providers (AHPs) cannot evade price competition; (3) take care of the enrollment process; (4) insist on equity, which includes such considerations as availability of the plan to every applicant (even though subsidy may be required), continuous coverage, community rating, and no exclusion for preexisting conditions; (5) make sure that the premium is adjusted on the basis of the risks presented by the covered population so that surcharges or subsidies, as may be required, are applied and result in equal premiums among the AHPs; and (6) make sure that the demand is price-elastic (that is, the more subscribers, the lower the cost).

Managed competition proponents make the following contentions: (1) MC is expected to work because it depends on the application of proven microeconomic principles; (2) pluralism is ensured because of the existence of a choice of providers; (3) individuals are made responsible for their own health; and (4) all citizens are covered (although financing is not a component of the MC process). Proponents insist that managed competition is *not*: free market, a voucher system, deregulation, more of the present system, mandatory enrollment in HMOs or large clinics, lower quality care, a blind experiment, a "buzzword" without definition, a panacea, or a process that is difficult to implement, requiring a long time to put in place.

management (Mx) (case) The plan and course of action for the care of the patient, often shown in the shorthand "Mx," similar to "Dx" for diagnosis and "Rx," which is used for "treatment" as well as for "prescription."

management (organization) In an organization, the task of getting things done systematically by, through, or with people with the necessary tools and facilities. See also *knowledge-based management* and *medical management*.

contract management An arrangement under which an "employing" institution obtains ongoing management services from a "managing" organization under a contract. The employing institution retains full ownership of and final responsibility for the institution. The services to be rendered by the contracting organization are spelled out in the management contract. If the contractual services are for department management, the contracting organization reports to the employing institution exactly as though its manager were the employing institution's own employee, that is, at the same point in the hierarchy. If the contractual services are for the management of the entire institution, the contracting organization furnishes a chief executive officer (CEO) who reports to the governing body of the employing institution as though he or she were employed by the governing body as its CEO. Contract management is one variety of relationship found in some multihospital systems.

product line management (PLM) A type of management in which the organization is considered to be a cluster or assemblage of strategic business units (SBUs). Each SBU has a separate product with a distinct market. In a hospital, a specific operation or class of operations (for example, eye surgery) could be considered an SBU, as could an alcoholism rehabilitation service. Each SBU has its specific resource requirements, information system needs, and management demands. Hospitals try to determine which product lines are "saleable" in their service areas, that they have appropriate resources for, and that they feel put them in advantageous competitive positions, and concentrate on those product lines.

service management A philosophy of management that emphasizes "service" to mean satisfaction of the demands and wishes of the customer and attention to his or her perceptions, rather than paying primary attention to the "products" provided or satisfying the provider (the hospital or physician, for example).

management information system (MIS) See under *information system*.

management service organization (MSO) A central service, created by a hospital for its physicians, or by one or more medical groups, that provides administrative services such as insurance and other billing; scheduling of consultations, referrals, hospitalizations, facilities, equipment, and personnel; and so forth. It may also provide group purchasing as a service. Only one staff, that of the MSO, needs to become expert in the requirements of the various insurance carriers, and a single computer system is used, with terminals in the physicians' offices. Synonym: medical service organization.

manager Any individual who is responsible for directing the activities of an organization or one of its components. In the hospital field, however, the title of "manager" is rarely given to high ranking persons, particularly in the professions; the chief executive officer (CEO) and the chief of nursing are not called "managers." The title is more likely to be used in such areas of the hospital as housekeeping, maintenance, and the like.

M&A Mergers and acquisitions. A flurry of these in recent years in the healthcare industry have resulted in a smaller number of larger healthcare organizations. See *antitrust* and *physician-hospital organization*.

mandate To require, or a requirement. In health care, the term is being used to refer to federal- or state-imposed requirements on insurance companies, employers, and so forth, to pay for health care or to provide specific benefits:

employer mandate A requirement that employers must provide coverage for their employees or be penalized. Synonym: play or else. See *Hawaii plan*.

individual mandate A requirement that all individuals must purchase health insurance or be penalized. See *Healthy Americans Act* and *Massachusetts plan*.

play or pay A slang phrase describing a proposed employer mandate that would require the employer to either participate in the health plan offered or pay for an acceptable alternative, such as a tax that would go to a public plan to provide for the employed uninsured and the unemployed. Synonym: pay or play.

state mandate State laws that mandate private healthcare insurers to cover a wide variety of services, including well baby care and so forth, sometimes resulting in premiums out of reach of small employers. See also *bare-bones health plan*.

mandated choice A requirement that competent adults make prospective choices as to what should be done under specified circumstances. This procedure has been suggested with regard to organ donation, because it has been found that most adults have not really considered whether they want to make their organs available for donation. Furthermore, a study has found that a much higher percentage of adults would donate if they were personally faced with the decision, than when the decision is made by the next of kin or the family.

mandated reporter A person required by law to report to child protection authorities any suspected case of abuse, neglect, or at-risk situations involving children or vulnerable adults. This group, mandated by state law, typically includes physicians, nurses, psychologists, dentists, other health professionals, teachers, police officers, social workers, clergy, counselors, marital and family therapists, and child care providers.

mandatory assignment A requirement for physicians to accept Medicare reimbursement as payment in full for their services; they would not be allowed to bill the patient for any difference between their fees and the amount that Medicare will pay.

manual arts therapist A health professional who provides manual arts therapy.

manual arts therapy (MAT) The use of manual arts to help prevent deconditioning and to develop, maintain, or improve work skills. Sometimes called industrial arts, the manual arts include woodworking, photography, metalworking, agriculture, graphic arts, and so forth.

MAP See *Medical Audit Program*.

mapping (genetic) See *genetic mapping*.

marginal worker See *contingent worker*.

marker (genetics) A gene with a known location on a chromosome that can be readily identified so it can be used as a point of reference in the mapping of other loci.

market The characteristics of the buyers of health services; also can mean the geographical area to which services are to be provided.

market administration (MA) See under *administration*.

market-based approach See *consumer choice*.

market basket update See *consumer price index* under *index (numerical)*.

market-driven system See under *economic system*.

market forces The economic forces of supply and demand.

marketing Activity to publicize a hospital or service, and to increase its use. See also *demarketing*.

Markle Foundation A philanthropic organization whose mission is to accelerate the use of emerging information and communication technologies to address critical public needs, particularly in the areas of health and national security. One effort is *Connecting for Health*. **www.markle.org**

Mark O. Hatfield Clinical Research Center See *Clinical Center* under *National Institutes of Health*.

marriage and family counselor A counselor specializing in working with married couples and families.

marriage and family therapist (MFT) A health professional with a master's or doctoral degree in marriage and family therapy. At least forty-six states require licensure, for which the MFT must pass an examination conducted by the Association of Marital and Family Therapy Regulatory Boards (AMFTRB). **www.amftrb.org/**

MAS See *medical administrative specialist* and *medical audit study*.

MASH unit See *surge capacity unit*.

Massachusetts plan A law enacted in Massachusetts in 2006 aimed at attaining "near universal" healthcare insurance coverage. It requires everyone in the state to purchase health insurance, and imposes a financial penalty of up to 50% of the cost of a plan (via income tax filings) on those who do not. This is sometimes called the "individual mandate" (as opposed to employer mandate) or "personal responsibility provision." To make it affordable, the law created the Commonwealth Health Insurance Connector, a private marketplace offering personal, portable health insurance products. The Connector operates as a clearinghouse to match buyers and sellers. Employers with fifty or fewer employees may designate the Connector as their group insurance plan, allowing employees to choose among the many products offered and to pay premiums with pretax dollars. Individuals may purchase insurance directly through the Connector. Employees and individuals may switch coverage during an annual open season, and may take their coverage with them as they move from job to job.

The state also provides subsidies for low-income individuals to purchase insurance. The money for the subsidies is to come from money previously used to pay for care for the uninsured. In addition, the law expanded the Massachusetts Medicaid program to cover more children and adults.

The law also requires employers with more than ten employees who do not provide health insurance coverage to pay up to $295 per employee annually into the uncompensated care pool. Also called the Massachusetts Health Care Reform Plan. See also *Healthy Americans Act*.

massage therapist A health professional specializing in massage therapy.

  Nationally Certified in Therapeutic Massage (NCTM) A massage therapist with a required amount of training and experience who has passed a certifying examination of the National Certification Board for Therapeutic Massage and Bodywork (NCBTMB). **www.ncbtmb.com**

  Nationally Certified in Therapeutic Massage and Bodywork (NCTMB) A massage therapist with a required amount of training and experience who has passed an advanced certifying examination of the National Certification Board for Therapeutic Massage and Bodywork (NCBTMB). **www.ncbtmb.com**

massage therapy The use of pressure, friction, kneading, and manipulation of the body to improve health and well-being. See also *bodywork therapy*.

  abhiyanga massage An ayurvedic therapy that incorporates herbal oil.

  shiatsu massage An Oriental medicine technique that uses pressure and assisted stretching.

mass disaster See under *disaster*.

mass number See under *nuclide*.

mastectomy The surgical removal of an entire breast. Typically done as part of the treatment of breast cancer. When just the cancerous lump is removed, the operation is referred to as a **lumpectomy**.

mastectomy fitter A health professional specializing in the fitting of breast prostheses and mastectomy products and services.

  Certified Fitter-Mastectomy (CFm) A mastectomy fitter who has been certified by the American Board for Certification in Orthotics and Prosthetics (ABC). **www.abcop.org**

  Certified Mastectomy Fitter (CMF) A mastectomy fitter who has been certified by the Board for Orthotist/Prosthetist Certification (BOC). **www.bocusa.org**

master file See *AMA Physician Masterfile*.

master's degree An advanced postgraduate academic degree that usually comes before, and requires less education than, a doctorate degree. In some fields, the master's is the highest degree that can be obtained.

MAT See *manual arts therapy*.

materiel The tools, equipment, and supplies necessary to do any given work, as contrasted with the personnel needed to do the work.

Maternal and Child Health Bureau (MCHB) One of the key program areas of the Health Resources and Services Administration (HRSA). It is charged with promoting and improving the health of the nation's mothers and children. **mchb.hrsa.gov**

maternal and child health (MCH) program A program providing preventive and treatment services for pregnant women, mothers, and children. The services may include health education (often with particular attention to nutrition) and family planning. Funding may be from federal, state, or local sources.

maternal death See under *death*.

maternal newborn nursing The area of nursing focusing on the needs of new mothers and their babies.

   Maternal Newborn Nurse (RNC) A registered nurse specializing in maternal newborn nursing who has passed an examination of the National Certification Corporation (NCC) and received the credential Registered Nurse Certified (RNC). **www.nccnet.org**

maternity patient A patient who is under medical or hospital care because she is pregnant. Synonym: obstetric patient.

maximum allowable cost (MAC) See *generic equivalent*.

Maxsys A proprietary system for carrying out *occurrence screening* (see under *screening (quality)*) to detect cases in which there was a possible quality problem. It was authored by Joyce W. Craddick, MD, and developed by Landacorp. Formerly called Medical Management Analysis (MMA).

MBHO See *managed behavioral healthcare organization*.

MBO See *Medicare Beneficiary Ombudsman*.

MC See *managed competition* and *menopause clinician*.

MCAT See *Medical College Admission Test*.

McCarran-Ferguson Act A 1945 act that declared that the insurance industry was not affected by federal laws regulating interstate commerce, unless the laws specifically applied to the "business of insurance." As a result, healthcare insurers have not been subject to federal antitrust laws. The Supreme Court has interpreted this exemption strictly, holding that spreading policyholders' risk is insurance. Some propose that the antitrust exemption for healthcare insurers should be repealed. 15 U.S.C. § 1011 et seq. (2005).

MCE See *Medicare Code Editor*.

MCES Medical care evaluation study. See *patient care audit* under *audit*.

MCH See *maternal and child health program*.

MCHB See *Maternal and Child Health Bureau*.

McKinney Homeless Assistance Act (MHAA) A federal act passed in 1987 to fund health and social services for the homeless. Programs include physical and mental health care, substance abuse treatment, housing, shelter, outreach, education, job training, and social services. 42 U.S.C. § 11301 et seq. (2004).

MCM See *medical countermeasure*.

MCP See *Medicare Cost Plan* and *middle care provider*.

MCR Medical care ratio and medical cost ratio; see *medical loss ratio*.

MD Doctor of Medicine (MD). The degree awarded to an individual upon graduation from a school of allopathic medicine (or, formerly, homeopathic medicine). A recipient of this degree is frequently referred to as a "medical doctor." See *physician* and *allopathy* (under *medicine (system)*). See also *macular degeneration*.

MDC See *Major Diagnostic Category*.

MDF Message Development Framework. See *HL7*.

MDH See *Medicare Dependent Hospital Program*.

MDRG See *Medicare DRG* under *DRG*.

MDS Minimum Data Set; see *Resident Assessment Instrument*.

MDSR See *Medical Device Safety Reports*.

mean By itself, this term usually means *arithmetic mean* (see below).

arithmetic mean The simple *average*. It is the sum of a set of quantities, divided by the number of quantities in the set. (In this term, the first and third syllables of "arithmetic" are accented.) See also *median*.

geometric mean The *n*th root of the product of *n* items. For example, the geometric mean of 2 and 8 is 4, because 4 is the second root (square root) of 2 × 8, or 16. Geometric means of hospital lengths of stay (see *average length of stay*), compiled from reference data, are sometimes used as standards in LOS comparisons.

MEC See *medical executive committee*.

med See *medication*.

MedBiquitous Consortium An international group of professional medical and healthcare associations, universities, and commercial and governmental organizations, accredited by ANSI to develop information technology standards for healthcare education and competence assessment. MedBiquitous also provides a forum to exchange ideas about innovative uses of web technologies for healthcare education and communities of practice. **www.medbiquitous.org**

MEDCIN A proprietary, clinical *nomenclature*. MEDCIN appeared in the public eye in early 1997 with the publication by Springer-Verlag of a book entitled *Medcin—A New Nomenclature for Clinical Medicine*, authored by Peter Goltra, president and founder of Medicomp Systems, Inc. MEDCIN had been developed (beginning in 1978) by Medicomp Systems for use in the electronic medical record (EMR). The structure of the nomenclature is hierarchical in such a fashion that each element inherits the characteristics of the higher levels of that hierarchy. Between each two levels there is a parent-child relationship; elements of equal level within a given hierarchy are called siblings. The publication of *Medcin* put the nomenclature itself in its hierarchical form into public view. In 2007, MEDCIN was advertised as "an electronic medical record engine, which allows rapid entry, retrieval and correlation of relevant clinical information at the point of care." **www.medicomp.com**

MedDRA Medical Dictionary for Regulatory Activities. An international terminology being developed under the auspices of *ICH* for electronic transmission of adverse drug event reporting and coding of clinical trial data.

Medem An Internet web site founded in 1999 to provide a "physician-patient communications network." Medem provides tools and "secure technologies for physicians to provide patients access to trusted health information via their doctor's own Web site." Founding societies include the American Academy of Ophthalmology; American Academy of Pediatrics; American College of Allergy, Asthma & Immunology; American College of Obstetricians and Gynecologists; American Medical Association; American Psychiatric Association; and American Society of Plastic Surgeons. Many more national and state societies now participate.

In 2007, over 80,000 doctors were participating. Patients can create their own *personal health records (PHRs)* (see under *electronic health record*), called an "iHealthRecord" by Medem, on the system. There are also programs for disease management and medication adherence, along with other information and tools for both physicians and patients. **www.medem.com**

med error Medication error; see *adverse drug event*.

median A statistical term. The middle point in a series of quantities arranged in order of size. The median for the series 7, 8, 9, 10, and 51 is 9, the third of the five items. For the same series, the simple average (arithmetic mean), for that series would be 17 (the sum, 85, divided by the number of quantities, 5). When the series of quantities has an even number of items, the median is customarily calculated as the average of the two middle items. See also *average*.

mediation See under *alternative dispute resolution*.

Medicaid The federal program that provides health care to indigent and medically indigent persons. Although partially federally funded (and managed by CMS), the Medicaid program is administered by the states, in accordance with an approved plan for each state. Each state has considerable flexibility in designing its plan and operating its Medicaid program, but still must comply with federal requirements. This is in contrast with *Medicare*, which is federally funded and administered at the federal level by CMS. The Medicaid program was established in 1965 by amendment to the Social Security Act, under a provision entitled "Title XIX—Medical Assistance."

Medicaid buy-in A program that permits uninsured individuals to enroll in Medicaid by paying premiums on a sliding scale. As of June 2006, thirty-three states were operating Medicaid buy-in programs.

Medicaid Psychiatric Hospital Fairness Act (MPHFA) See *IMD exclusion*.

Medi-Cal Medicaid in California. Because each state administers Medicaid, the program in California is unique (as are the programs in the other states).

medical When applied as an adjective, as in "medical treatment," this term means "nonsurgical," that is, the avoidance of the surgical methods of operation and manipulation. However, specialties within surgery are technically considered "medical" specialties (see *medical specialty*).

medical administrative specialist (MAS) A health professional trained in all aspects of "front office" medical practice administration, including medical records, insurance forms, coding and billing, reception of patients, information processing, and the like.

> **Certified Medical Administrative Specialist (CMAS)** A medical administrative specialist who has been certified by the American Medical Technologists (AMT). **www.amt1.com**

Medical Assistance See *Medicaid*.

medical assistant (MA) A health professional who, under supervision of a physician, performs clinical procedures and administrative tasks. An MA will usually have completed a medical assistant program and have a certificate or diploma (one-year program) or an associate degree (two-year program). Not the same as a *physician assistant (PA)*.

> **Certified Medical Assistant (CMA)** A medical assistant who has graduated from an accredited medical assisting program and passed the certification examination of the American Association of Medical Assistants (AAMA). **www.aama-ntl.org**

> **Registered Medical Assistant (RMA)** A medical assistant with training and experience who has been certified by the American Medical Technologists (AMT). **www.amt1.com**

medical association See *medical society*.

medical audit (MA) See *patient care audit* under *audit*.

Medical Audit Program (MAP) A specific program of data display formerly offered as part of the *Professional Activity Study (PAS)* system. Clinical data on patient condition and diagnostic procedures, along with diagnoses and therapy, were used to show patterns of care useful in the evaluation of care. See *patient care audit* under *audit*.

medical audit study (MAS) The operational unit of a medical audit. See *patient care audit* under *audit*.

medical care The totality of diagnostic efforts and treatment involved in the care of patients. The term "medical care" may be interpreted as only those portions of the care provided directly or personally by a physician. Modern caregiving, however, requires many other professionals and elements in the care process (such as nursing, rehabilitation, patient transportation, and the like). So the term "patient care" was introduced to encompass the totality. For example, "evaluation of medical care" was replaced in most usage by "evaluation of patient care"; the latter term not only focuses on the patient, but also ensures that all components of the care—not just what the physician does—are included.

What is considered "medical care" will also vary, of course, depending on the context. For example, state laws regulating the "practice of medicine" will have specific definitions of what that entails. In Minnesota, a person is practicing medicine if, among other things, he or she does one of the following:

offers or undertakes to prescribe, give, or administer any drug or medicine for the use of another . . . offers or undertakes to prevent or to diagnose, correct, or treat in any manner or by any means, methods, devices, or instrumentalities, any disease, illness, pain, wound, fracture, infirmity, deformity or defect of any person . . . offers or undertakes to perform any surgical operation including any invasive or noninvasive procedures involving the use of a laser or laser assisted device, upon any person . . . offers to undertake to use hypnosis for the treatment or relief of any wound, fracture, or bodily injury, infirmity, or disease." Minn. Stat. § 147.081(3) (2006).

Other laws may have a broader definition. For example, Minnesota's statute regarding medical assistance for needy persons defines "medical care" to include "medical, surgical, hospital, ambulatory surgical center services, optical, visual, dental and nursing services; drugs and medical supplies; appliances; laboratory, diagnostic, and therapeutic services; nursing home and convalescent care; screening and health assessment services provided by public health nurses"; and much more. Minn. Stat. § 256B.02(7)(a) (2006). See also **patient care**.

medical care evaluation Usually refers to the patient care audit (medical audit), which is a retrospective review of the quality of care of a group of patients, ordinarily a group with the same diagnosis or therapy. See **patient care audit** under **audit**.

medical care evaluation study (MCES) See **patient care audit** under **audit**.

medical care hotel A hotel for patients who need certain hospital services, but who can live in hotel surroundings, that is, without round-the-clock nursing. This is not a hotel for the families of patients.

hospital medical care hotel A medical care hotel operated by a hospital.

medical care ratio (MCR) See **medical loss ratio**.

medical center An essentially undefined term that may refer to a single institution, but is usually taken to mean that there is more to the institution than merely a single hospital—perhaps several hospitals in a complex, or perhaps a wider range of facilities and services than an ordinary hospital is likely to offer. The term does not automatically imply that the institution is an academic center, nor is there any licensure requirement before the term may be used.

academic medical center A medical center that ordinarily consists of a university hospital and medical school, often along with other teaching hospitals, research organizations and their laboratories, outpatient clinics, libraries, and related facilities.

Medical College Admission Test (MCAT) A national examination, similar to the Scholastic Aptitude Test (SAT), that most medical schools require of individuals seeking admission to medical school. The test was developed by the Association of American Medical Colleges (AAMC).

medical cost ratio (MCR) See **medical loss ratio**.

medical countermeasure (MCM) A biological or chemical defense—such as a drug or vaccine—against public health threats, including chemical, biological, radiological, or nuclear (CBRN) attack, as well as pandemics. See **Project Bioshield**.

medical device A machine, instrument, apparatus, or item used for diagnosis, treatment, or prevention of disease, which does not achieve its purpose through chemical action on or within the body (to distinguish it from a drug). Examples of medical devices include artificial heart valves, cardiac pacemakers, prostheses, hearing aids, crutches, and wheelchairs.

Since the passage of the Federal Food, Drug, and Cosmetic Act of 1938, the Food and Drug Administration (FDA) has been charged with the task of regulating medical devices to assure that they are safe and effective. The FDA states that because medical devices vary widely in their complexity and their degree of risk, they don't all need the same degree of regulation. Because of this, the FDA places all medical devices into one of three regulatory classes based on the level of control necessary to assure safety and effectiveness. Examples of

Class I devices (the least stringent regulations) include elastic bandages, examination gloves, and hand-held surgical instruments. Examples of Class II devices include powered wheelchairs, infusion pumps, and surgical drapes. Class III devices are usually those that support or sustain human life, are of substantial importance in preventing impairment of human health, or present a potential, unreasonable risk of illness or injury.

Also, the safety and quality of medical devices have long been monitored by a private, independent, nonprofit organization called *ECRI*.

Medical Device Safety Reports (MDSR) A repository of information about medical devices independently maintained by a private, independent, nonprofit organization called *ECRI*. It is periodically updated and reviews the types of problems that have occurred with medical devices and "lessons learned" since the mid 1960s. MDSR focuses on things that medical device users can do to prevent or reduce safety risks. ECRI has made some of this information available free to the public at **www.mdsr.ecri.org**.

medical direction At the specific order of or under the supervision of a physician. In the context of an emergency medical services system (EMS or EMSS), medical direction means physician responsibility for the development, implementation, and evaluation of the clinical aspects of the system.

Medical Directive, The See under *advance directive*.

medical director (health plan) A physician who contracts with or is employed by a health plan (or other managed care organization) to provide medical direction. Responsibilities will include review of authorizations for referrals and admissions; review of cases for quality and utilization issues; formulation of clinical policies, criteria, and standards; and so forth.

medical director (hospital) A physician, usually employed by the hospital, who serves as the administrative head of the medical staff. "Medical director" tends to be the title for the chief of staff when that person is a paid hospital employee. The title may also be "vice president for medical affairs" or something similar. This term is discussed further under *chief of staff*.

medical director (long-term care facility) A physician, in a long-term care facility (LTCF), retained to coordinate the medical care in the facility, to ensure adequacy and appropriateness of the medical services provided to each patient, and to maintain surveillance of the health status of employees. An LTCF is required to have a medical director.

medical doctor A physician with a Doctor of Medicine (MD) degree.

medical dosimetrist A health professional who, under the supervision of a medical physicist, calculates and generates radiation doses for treating cancer.

Certified Medical Dosimetrist (CMD) A medical dosimetrist who has passed an examination of the Medical Dosimetrist Certification Board (MDCB). **www.mdcb.org**

medical education See under *education*.

medical education number A unique, permanent number assigned by the American Medical Association (AMA) to each medical student in the United States, regardless of their membership status in the AMA. The number is used to track the medical students throughout their careers, and is a "key" to individual physicians in the *AMA Physician Masterfile* database.

medical examiner A physician who investigates certain kinds of deaths (e.g., accidental, suspicious, or not within a healthcare facility) to determine the cause of death; this often requires an *autopsy*. The medical examiner is a public official, usually appointed to the position, and is often a specialist in *forensic pathology* (see under *pathology*). See also *coroner*.

Do not confuse this term with the state's organization that administers medical examinations for physician licensing (see *state medical board* under *board (credentialing)*).

medical executive committee (MEC) The executive committee of the *medical staff* of a hospital. It has the power to act on behalf of the medical staff organization in all matters, except those specifically withheld by the medical staff bylaws, when the full medical staff is not in session. Among its typical functions are reviewing credentials, committee reports, and making recommendations to the governing body. Synonym: medical staff executive committee.

Medical Expenditure Panel Survey (MEPS) A national survey of families and individuals, their medical providers, and employers across the United States regarding the utilization and costs of healthcare services and how they are paid for. It has been conducted by the Agency for Healthcare Research and Quality (AHRQ) since 1996 in conjunction with the National Center for Health Statistics (NCHS). The MEPS updates information from 1987, the date of the previous such survey (entitled the National Medical Expenditure Survey (NMES)). The first such survey was the National Medical Care Expenditure Survey in 1977. MEPS is now conducted annually rather than once every ten years. **www.meps.ahrq.gov**

medical futility See *futile care* and *futility policy*.

medical genetics See under *genetics*.

medical geology The study of connections between geologic materials (minerals and trace elements) and processes and the health of humans and animals. It focuses on both short-term relationships, such as acute exposure to toxic substances, and the long-term health effects of the geologic environment. Medical geology is interdisciplinary, involving geoscientists and medical, public health, veterinary, agricultural, environmental, and biological scientists. See also *conservation medicine*.

Medical Group Management Association (MGMA) The national association of business managers of medical group practices. Founded in 1926 as the National Association of Clinic Managers; the name was changed in 1963. **www.mgma.com**

medical harm Defined by the Institute for Healthcare Improvement (IHI) as unintended physical injury that results from or is contributed to by medical care (including the absence of indicated medical care) and that requires additional monitoring, treatment, or hospitalization, or results in death. IHI is working to shift efforts in *patient safety* away from counting errors to focusing on patient harm, much of which results from flawed systems rather than faulty performance.

medical history See under *history*.

Medical Illness Severity Grouping System (MedisGroups) A proprietary system for classifying hospital patients by severity of illness using objective data specially abstracted from the patients' medical records (see *abstract* and *abstracting*). It was developed by MediQual Systems, Inc.

medical illustrator (MI) A professional artist who specializes in creating visual material to help record and disseminate knowledge of medicine and related subjects. Most MIs have a master's degree in medical illustration.

> **Certified Medical Illustrator (CMI)** A medical illustrator who has met the requirements for certification of the Medical Illustrators Board of Certification (MIBC). **www.medical-illustrators.org**

medical indigence See *medically indigent* under *indigent*.

medical informatics See under *informatics*.

Medical Injury Compensation Reform Act (MICRA) A California law enacted in 1975 that has been proposed as a model for malpractice reform. Its provisions include caps on noneconomic damages; elimination of joint and several liability, and instead holding defendants liable only in proportion to their degree of fault; offsets by awards from collateral sources; limits on statutes of limitations; and limits on attorney contingency fees.

medical interpreter (MI) A health professional who provides translation services for patients who do not speak English. An MI must have cultural sensitivity and knowledge of both medical and colloquial terminology.

medical IRA See *Medical Savings Account*.

medicalization The process by which a health-related condition, natural life process, behavior, or lifestyle is identified as appropriate for intervention by healthcare professionals. Examples include alcoholism, sexual preference, birth, menopause, and aging.

Medicalizing a condition may be beneficial (e.g., making medical care available for alcoholism) or it may have undesired results (e.g., relieving the individual of responsibility). It may also result in adding or removing *stigmas* associated with the condition.

Demedicalization is, of course, the reverse, that is, the shifting of a condition considered to be medical back to one of personal responsibility, or classifying behavior once thought deviant as normal.

medical knowledge Medical information that has been evaluated by experts and converted into useful medical concepts and options.

Medical Laboratory Technician (MLT) See under *clinical laboratory technician*.

medical librarian See *health science librarian*.

Medical Literature Analysis and Retrieval System (MEDLARS) See *MEDLINE*.

Medical Logic Module (MLM) See *Arden Syntax*.

medical loss ratio (MLR) The percentage of the insurance premium that must be paid out to care for patients. The obverse of the administrative costs plus profit (in for-profit insurances). In the view of those in health care, the higher the medical loss ratio the better, because health care is what the premium was intended to buy, and a high loss ratio reflects parsimonious administration. (In a for-profit insurance company, the incentive is to keep this number low in order to reward the investors.) Synonyms: medical cost ratio (MCR), medical care ratio.

medically indicated See *indicated*.

medically indigent See under *indigent*.

medically necessary A drug, item, procedure, or other medical service that a physician or other provider has determined to be medically required, or *indicated*, for a patient in a particular instance. Most health insurers will only pay for services that are "medically necessary" (and, of course, whether a service is medically necessary is sometimes open to debate).

Medicare will only pay for medically necessary services, defined as: "Services or supplies that: are proper and needed for the diagnosis or treatment of your medical condition, are provided for the diagnosis, direct care, and treatment of your medical condition, meet the standards of good medical practice in the local area, and aren't mainly for the convenience of you or your doctor."

Medically Underserved Area (MUA) A rural or urban area that does not have enough healthcare resources to meet the needs of its population or whose population has relatively low health status. The term is defined in the Public Health Service Act and used to determine which areas have priority for assistance.

Medically Underserved Population (MUP) A population group that does not have enough healthcare resources to meet its needs. The group may reside in a Medically Underserved Area, or may be a population group with certain attributes; for example, migrant workers, Native Americans, and prison inmates may constitute Medically Underserved Populations. The term is defined in the Public Health Service Act and used to determine which groups have priority for assistance.

medical management The field of practice engaged in by physicians who are in management roles. These physicians are referred to as "physician executives."

The term also is used sometimes to describe the course of care being rendered by a physician (and other health professionals) to an individual patient for a given episode of illness or for a health problem. Some are now using medical management to include, for individuals, preventive measures in well persons, and managed care case management decisions and approval of services. Sometimes the term refers broadly to quality improvement activities and "management" of specific populations. Thus the term has lost its specificity and can only be understood in context. See also *case management* and *medical practice management*.

Medical Management Analysis (MMA) The former name of *Maxsys*.

medical necessity See *medically necessary*.

medical neglect See under *neglect*.

medical nutrition therapy The American Dietetic Association (ADA) defines this as the assessment of patient nutritional status followed by therapy, ranging from diet modification to administration of specialized nutrition therapies such as intravenous or tube feeding.

Medical Outcomes Study (MOS) A two-year study in the 1980s of patients with chronic conditions, designed to determine whether variations in patient outcomes were related to physician specialty, technical and interpersonal style, or the system of care, and to develop tools for the routine monitoring of patient outcomes. Outcomes measured included clinical end points; physical, social, and role functioning in everyday living; patients' perceptions of their general health and well-being; and satisfaction with treatment. An important result of the study was the development of the *SF-36 Health Survey*; see under *quality of life scale*.

medical practice act A state statute governing the practice of medicine within the state.

medical practice management (MPM) The administration and management of medical group practices.

Certified Medical Practice Executive (CMPE) A specialist in medical practice management who has been board certified by the American College of Medical Practice Executives (ACMPE) (**www.mgma.com**). A CMPE who meets additional criteria may become a **Fellow of the ACMPE (FACMPE)**.

medical practice plan In a medical school setting, an official document setting forth the policies under which patient services are rendered by medical school faculty physicians, the method of obtaining reimbursement, and the disposition of the funds obtained for such services. The detail of procedures is usually covered in the document. Synonyms: clinical practice plan, faculty practice plan.

medical procedure patent See *method or process patent* under *patent*.

medical-process patent See *method or process patent* under *patent*.

medical record A file kept for each patient, maintained by the hospital (physicians also maintain medical records in their own practices), which documents the patient's problems, diagnostic procedures, treatment, and outcome. Related documents, such as written consent for surgery and other procedures, are also included in the record. The Joint Commission on Accreditation of Healthcare Organizations (JCAHO) places great importance on the medical record in the accreditation process, and its *Comprehensive Accreditation Manual for Hospitals (CAMH)* contains an extensive description of the desired and required contents of the medical record. At a minimum, JCAHO requires sufficient information to identify the patient, support the diagnosis, justify the treatment, document the course of treatment, document the results of treatment, and promote continuity of care among providers.

Ordinarily the record is kept on paper, but it is increasingly being kept in computer (electronic) media as an electronic medical record (EMR). Some hospitals keep a separate medical record for each hospitalization (hospital admission); the better practice is to use the "unit record system," that is, keep a "unit record" for each patient, with all records of the patient's successive hospitalizations in the patient's unit file. In a physician's office or clinic, each patient typically has just one medical record.

The record itself is usually organized in either the "traditional" or "problem-oriented" method (see below). Synonyms: health record, clinical record, patient's chart, chart. See also *charting, Patient Medical Record Information, electronic health record*, and *health information*.

computerized medical record (CMR) See under *electronic health record*.

digital medical record (DMR) See under *electronic health record*.

electronic medical record (EMR) See under *electronic health record*.

legal medical record There is no uniform definition of what constitutes a medical record (also called health record) for legal purposes. As with most things legal, the definition varies with the purpose in question. However, the American Health Information Management Association (AHIMA) has formulated guidelines to assist its members and the healthcare industry in developing policies and procedures for the creation, retention, and release of information in a medical record. These guidelines break down the medical record into four categories:

1. *Legal health record (LHR):* The basic medical record, defined as the documentation of the healthcare services provided to an individual in any aspect of healthcare delivery by a healthcare provider organization. This is a legal business record to the extent that documentation is made in the normal course of business, at or near the time of the matter recorded, and by the person with knowledge of the facts or opinions recorded.
2. *Patient-identifiable source data:* Dictation, diagnostic images, electrocardiogram tracings, and the like.
3. *Administrative data:* Patient-identifiable data used for administrative, regulatory, healthcare operations, and payment (financial) purposes. Examples: claims, release of information authorizations, data reviewed for quality assurance.
4. *Derived data:* Data derived from patient records that are aggregated so that there are no means to identify patients. Examples: accreditation reports, research data, ORYX reports, statistical reports.

AHIMA recommends that the information in category one (and sometimes two, if there is no interpretation or summary in the LHR) be considered the legal health record. Categories three and four would be provided the same level of confidentiality, but would not be considered part of the LHR for the purposes of responding to a subpoena for a medical record. See also *designated record set*.

online medical record (OMR) See under *electronic health record*.

problem-oriented medical record (POMR) A medical record organized around the problems presented by the patient (see *problem*). The POMR is organized so that the reader can find out *why* the steps in investigation and management were done. In the traditionally organized medical record (see below), the reader can only find out *what* was done. A common form of organization of the POMR is "SOAP": Subjective (complaints), Objective (observations, test results), Assessment, and Plan for each problem. The same principle is increasingly used for nursing information and that of other professionals in the medical record; that is, nursing and other information is recorded in connection with the problem(s) to which it pertains. See also *systems review*.

traditionally organized medical record A medical record organized according to "presenting complaint," "history," "review of systems" (such as cardiovascular and respiratory), "physical examination," and the like. The traditional organization tells only "what was done," whereas the problem-oriented medical record (POMR; see above) tells "why it was done." The nursing record is traditionally organized chronologically. See also *charting*.

medical record abstracter A person who extracts a specific predetermined array of information from a medical record, usually on a precoded form to be used as input into a hospital discharge abstract system. See *abstract* and *abstracting*.

medical record administrator (MRA) See *health information administrator*.

medical record analyst (MRA) See *health record analyst*.

medical record department A special area in the hospital (or other healthcare facility) dedicated to processing, keeping, maintaining, retrieving information from, and safeguarding medical records. This is where the records are physically created, dictation is transcribed, cases are abstracted, information is obtained, and reports are made for medical staff, administration, and others.

medical record designee The individual in a long-term care facility (LTCF) assigned the responsibility of maintaining medical records on all patients. Note that this term applies to the duty, not to the qualifications, of the individual.

medical record entry Something written in the medical record. Certain members of the healthcare team, such as physicians, nurses, respiratory therapists, and physical therapists, are authorized by the hospital to write in the medical record. Each person doing so follows a certain protocol, which includes dating the written information and authenticating (signing) it (see **authentication**). Customarily, a notation made by one person at one time is called an entry. "Written" may include computer and audio entries, or any type of recording approved for that hospital's medical record system.

medical record index See under **index (list)**.

medical record librarian (MRL) An obsolete term for **health information administrator**.

medical record professional See **coding specialist**, **health information administrator**, **health information technician**, and **medical transcriptionist**.

Medical Records Institute (MRI) An independent organization promoting electronic health records as a part of a seamless, patient-centered information system. MRI provides educational programs and publications in the field. For a number of years MRI has been sponsoring conferences entitled TEPR (Toward an Electronic Patient Record). It is also affiliated with the Mobile Healthcare Alliance (MoHCA) and the Continuity of Care Record (CCR) project. **www.medrecinst.com**

medical record technician (MRT) See **health information technician**.

Medical Reserve Corps (MRC) A program, founded in 2002 and administered by the Office of the U.S. Surgeon General, to organize local groups of volunteer medical personnel to respond to medical and public health emergencies. MRC volunteers—physicians, nurses, pharmacists, dentists, veterinarians, epidemiologists, and others—supplement existing emergency and public health resources. **www.medicalreservecorps.gov**

medical review agency An agency established under the prospective payment system (PPS) to carry out certain surveillance functions with respect to hospital and physician performance and detection of fraud.

medical review officer (MRO) A physician who is an expert in drug and alcohol testing and the application of federal regulations to the process. MROs are employed by business, industry, and government agencies to help achieve a "drug-free workplace." Certification is available from the Medical Review Officer Certification Council (MROCC) of the American Society of Addiction Medicine (ASAM).

Medical Savings Account (MSA) A mechanism created in 1996 by **HIPAA** to help individuals with a high-deductible health plan (HDHP) provide funds for health care. It was a savings account set up for an individual under regulations and tax treatment similar to an individual retirement account (IRA). Synonyms: health IRA, individual health care account (IHCA), medical IRA, medisave. Replaced in 2004 by the **Health Savings Account**.

medical screening exam See **Emergency Medical Treatment and Labor Act**.

medical service organization (MSO) See **management service organization**.

medical society A term generally used with reference to a geographically defined association of physicians, for example, a city, county, state, or national medical society. The medical staff of a hospital is not a medical society. Synonym: medical association. See also **specialty society**.

medical sociology The discipline concerned with the relationship between social factors and health, and with the application of sociological theory and research techniques to questions related to health, the healthcare system, and public policy. Areas of study include the influence of ethnicity, gender, age, or socioeconomic status on the access to and quality of health care; health and risk-taking behaviors; social constructs of illness; health beliefs and perceptions; health effects of sociocultural changes; the role of health institutions and health professionals in society; and other sociological aspects of medical organization and practice.

medical specialty A branch of allopathic or osteopathic medicine in which physicians specialize (includes surgical specialties). The physician usually completes an approved residency in the specialty, and may also become certified by an appropriate credentialing board; however, a physician does not have to be board certified to be qualified to practice a specialty. In fact, there are many medical specialties and subspecialties for which certification is not available. For example, an ophthalmologist might be trained in and specialize in glaucoma, or a surgeon in trauma surgery, yet no board presently certifies those specialties.

The two major multispecialty certifying bodies for both allopathic and osteopathic physicians are the American Board of Medical Specialties (ABMS) and the American Board of Physician Specialties (ABPS). The Bureau of Osteopathic Specialists (BOS) certifies a number of osteopathic specialties. There are also a few "stand-alone" certifying bodies.

The ABMS requires a physician to first be certified in a *general* specialty, such as internal medicine, before being certified in a subspecialty, such as cardiovascular disease. Another type of credential, called a certificate of added qualifications (CAQ), is offered in some subspecialty areas. The ABMS certifies the following specialties and subspecialties (* denotes a general certificate):

addiction psychiatry
adolescent medicine
aerospace medicine*
allergy and immunology*
anatomic pathology*
anatomic pathology and clinical pathology*
anesthesiology*
blood banking/transfusion medicine
cardiovascular disease
chemical pathology
child and adolescent psychiatry
clinical and laboratory dermatological immunology
clinical and laboratory immunology
clinical biochemical genetics*
clinical cardiac electrophysiology
clinical cytogenetics*
clinical genetics (MD)*
clinical molecular genetics*
clinical neurophysiology
clinical pathology*
colon and rectal surgery*
critical care medicine
cytopathology
dermatology*
dermatopathology
developmental-behavioral pediatrics
diagnostic radiologic physics
diagnostic radiology*
emergency medicine*
endocrinology, diabetes, and metabolism
family medicine*
forensic pathology
forensic psychiatry
gastroenterology
geriatric medicine
geriatric psychiatry
gynecologic oncology
hematology
hospice and palliative medicine
hyperbaric medicine—see **undersea** and **hyperbaric medicine**

infectious disease
internal medicine*
interventional cardiology
maternal-fetal medicine
medical microbiology
medical nuclear physics
medical oncology
medical toxicology
molecular genetic pathology
neonatal-perinatal medicine
nephrology
neurodevelopmental disabilities
neurological surgery*
neurology*
neurology with special qualifications in child neurology*
neuropathology
neuroradiology
neurotology
nuclear medicine*
nuclear radiology
obstetrics and gynecology*
occupational medicine*
ophthalmology*
orthopaedic sports medicine
orthopaedic surgery*
otolaryngology—head and neck surgery*
pain medicine
pediatric cardiology
pediatric critical care medicine
pediatric dermatology
pediatric emergency medicine
pediatric endocrinology
pediatric gastroenterology
pediatric hematology-oncology
pediatric infectious diseases
pediatric nephrology
pediatric otolaryngology
pediatric pathology
pediatric pulmonology
pediatric radiology
pediatric rehabilitation medicine
pediatric rheumatology
pediatrics*
pediatric surgery
pediatric transplant hepatology
physical medicine and rehabilitation*
plastic surgery*
plastic surgery within the head and neck
psychiatry*
psychosomatic medicine
public health and general preventive medicine*

    pulmonary disease
radiation oncology*
radiologic physics*
reproductive endocrinology and infertility
rheumatology
sleep medicine
spinal cord injury medicine
sports medicine
surgery*
surgery of the hand
surgical critical care
therapeutic radiologic physics
thoracic surgery*
transplant hepatology
undersea and hyperbaric medicine
urology*
vascular and interventional radiology
vascular neurology
vascular surgery*

The ABPS provides certification in the following areas for both allopathic and osteopathic physicians:

    anesthesiology
dermatology
diagnostic radiology
disaster medicine
emergency medicine
family practice
geriatric medicine
internal medicine
obstetrics and gynecology
ophthalmology
orthopaedic surgery
plastic and reconstructive surgery
psychiatry
radiation oncology
surgery

Osteopathic physicians can be certified under the preceding specialty programs, but there are also a number of osteopathic specialties. A general certificate is required before a subspecialty certificate may be obtained. Certificates of added qualifications are offered in some areas. The BOS certifies the following specialties and subspecialties (* denotes a general certificate):

    addiction medicine
adolescent/young adult medicine
allergy/immunology
anatomic pathology*
anatomic pathology and laboratory medicine*
anesthesiology
blood banking/transfusion medicine
body imaging
cardiology
chemical pathology

child/adolescent psychiatry
child neurology
cytopathology
dermatology*
dermatopathology
diagnostic radiology*
emergency medical services
emergency medicine*
endocrinology
family practice*
forensic pathology
gastroenterology
general surgery
geriatric medicine
geropsychiatry
gynecologic oncology
hand surgery
hematology
immunopathology
infectious disease
internal medicine*
interventional cardiology
in vivo and in vitro nuclear medicine
laboratory medicine*
maternal and fetal medicine
medical microbiology
medical toxicology
Mohs-micrographic surgery
neonatology
nephrology
neurological surgery
neurology*
neuromusculoskeletal medicine and osteopathic manipulative medicine*
neuropathology
neurophysiology
neuroradiology
nuclear cardiology
nuclear imaging and therapy
nuclear medicine*
nuclear radiology
obstetrics and gynecology*
occupational medicine
oncology
ophthalmology*
orthopaedic surgery*
otolaryngic allergy
otolaryngology*
otolaryngology/facial plastic surgery*
pain management
pediatric allergy/immunology
pediatric endocrinology

pediatric pulmonology
pediatric radiology
pediatrics*
physical medicine and rehabilitation*
plastic and reconstructive surgery
preventive medicine/aerospace medicine*
preventive medicine/occupational-environmental medicine*
preventive medicine/public health-community medicine*
proctology*
psychiatry*
pulmonary diseases
radiation oncology*
reproductive endocrinology
rheumatology
sports medicine
thoracic cardiovascular surgery
urological surgery
vascular and interventional radiology
vascular surgery

In addition, boards operating independently offer certification in the following areas:

addiction medicine (American Society of Addiction Medicine)
bariatric medicine (American Board of Bariatric Medicine)
clinical pharmacology (American Board of Clinical Pharmacology)
facial plastic and reconstructive surgery (American Board of Facial Plastic and Reconstructive Surgery)
hospice and palliative medicine (American Board of Hospice and Palliative Medicine)

There are a few specialty areas that do not involve a branch of medical science:

insurance medicine (Board of Insurance Medicine)
legal medicine
pharmaceutical medicine

medical staff An organization of a hospital's *medical staff members* formed to carry out two functions: (1) to provide the management structure through which the hospital policies that pertain to the medical staff members are carried out, with particular attention to the quality of care; and (2) to serve as the spokesperson for the physicians to the governing body. This organization is variously referred to as the "medical staff," the "organized medical staff," the "medical staff organization," or simply the "MSO."

closed medical staff A medical staff in a hospital that has a formal plan describing its desired medical staff size and specialty needs. Such medical staff is "closed" except where a vacancy exists (or is anticipated) under its plan. The fact that a hospital has one or more exclusive contracts (contracts that give a physician or physician group the exclusive privilege of furnishing certain administrative or clinical services) does not make that hospital a closed medical staff hospital.

open medical staff A medical staff in a hospital that has no formal plan describing its desired medical staff size and specialty needs, and which, therefore, accepts new applications for medical staff membership and clinical privileges at any time. Also called simply "open staff."

medical staff activities A term used to include both the rights and duties of medical staff members. The rights include, primarily, the right to vote in medical staff meetings. The duties include carrying out the functions that devolve on members under the *medical staff bylaws* (see under *bylaws*), including committee membership and participation, and accepting the supervision and sanctions laid out in the bylaws. All medical staff members are governed by the medical staff bylaws, which contain some provisions that affect all classes of members, such as those dealing with professional and personal conduct and completion of medical records.

medical staff bylaws See under *bylaws*.

medical staff corporation See under *corporation*.

medical staff executive committee See *medical executive committee*.

medical staff member A physician or allied health professional who is permitted to care for patients independently in the hospital. Each medical staff member must be formally appointed to the *medical staff* by the governing body, and be authorized by that body to treat patients, independently, in the hospital. This appointment to the medical staff must be based on the individual being licensed and meeting the hospital's own requirements. Members are granted specific privileges by the governing body, delineating what they are permitted to do within the hospital, and are subject to the medical staff bylaws and rules and regulations and to review under the hospital's quality management program. In addition, all members must be reappointed periodically, and their privileges reaffirmed.

Physician practitioners on the medical staff are usually authorized to admit patients. Nonphysician practitioners usually do not have admitting privileges. For a discussion of the procedures for appointing physicians and other professionals to the medical staff, see *credentialing*; for more detail regarding admitting and clinical privileges, see *privileges*.

Members of the medical staff are often erroneously referred to as "hospital staff" or merely "staff"; in fact, members are usually in private or group practices. Generally, "hospital staff" refers to hospital employees, whereas "staff" alone is ambiguous unless taken in context.

active medical staff Medical staff members with full clinical privileges (according to their abilities, as awarded by the governing body; see *privileges*), and with full responsibilities with respect to medical staff activities, such as committee membership.

associate medical staff Persons eligible to apply for medical staff membership, who have applied for membership, who have been awarded limited privileges on an interim basis, and whose participation in medical staff activities is somewhat limited. New medical staff members may be appointed to the associate medical staff for the first year, for example. Sometimes called the provisional medical staff.

courtesy medical staff Medical staff members who admit patients only occasionally, or who only consult, and so are granted limited privileges (less than those of active staff members) and are not required to participate in medical staff activities.

honorary medical staff Persons whose professional qualifications make them eligible for medical staff membership, but who do not have admitting privileges (see *privileges*) and do not participate in medical staff activities. Typically, honorary medical staff are retired members of the medical staff. Sometimes called emeritus staff.

provisional medical staff See *associate medical staff*, above.

medical staff services professional A health professional who provides credentialing, privileging, and other administrative services for physicians and other health professionals; typically employed by a hospital or other healthcare organization. See also *provider credentialing specialist*.

Certified Professional Medical Services Management (CPMSM) A medical staff services professional who has been certified by the National Association Medical Staff Services (NAMSS). **www.namss.org**

Medical Subject Headings (MeSH) The authorized list for the subject analysis of the biomedical literature in the National Library of Medicine (NLM). See *tree structure*. **www.nlm.nih.gov/mesh**

medical-surgical nursing The area of nursing concerning the needs of adult medical and surgical patients.

Board Certified Medical-Surgical Nurse A registered nurse with a Bachelor of Science in Nursing (BSN) degree who is qualified in medical-surgical nursing and has passed an examination of the American Nurses Credentialing Center (ANCC) (**nursingworld.org/ancc**). The credential is RN,BC (Registered Nurse, Board Certified).

Certified Medical-Surgical Nurse A registered nurse with an associate degree or diploma who is qualified in medical-surgical nursing and has passed an examination of the American Nurses Credentialing Center (ANCC) (**nursingworld.org/ancc**). The credential is RN,C (Registered Nurse, Certified).

Certified Medical-Surgical Registered Nurse (CMSRN) A registered nurse who is qualified in medical-surgical nursing and has passed an examination of the Medical-Surgical Nursing Certification Board (MSNCB). **www.medsurgnurse.org**

Medical Technologist (MT) See under *clinical laboratory technologist*.

medical telemetry device (MTD) A machine, such as a cardiac monitor, that monitors a patient's vital signs and transmits the information via radio to a remote location. For example, an MTD may be used by paramedics at an accident site, with the information sent to a hospital emergency room, or by a patient at home, with data transmitted to a doctor's office. The devices use broadcasting bandwidth and are regulated by the Federal Communications Commission (FCC). See also *telemedicine*.

medical transcriptionist (MT) A person who listens to and transcribes clinical reports dictated by physicians and other health professionals. As the quality of computer-based speech recognition improves, an increasing amount of medical transcription is done with computer assistance. An MT is typically an employee of a healthcare provider, an independent contractor, or a member ("subcontractor") of a medical transcription service organization (MTSO).

Certified Medical Transcriptionist (CMT) A medical transcriptionist who has at least two years of transcription experience in the acute care (or equivalent) setting and has passed the certification examination of the American Association for Medical Transcription (AAMT). **www.aamt.org**

Registered Medical Transcriptionist (RMT) A medical transcriptionist who has passed the Registered Medical Transcriptionist examination of the American Association for Medical Transcription (AAMT). **www.aamt.org**

medical transcription service organization (MTSO) An organization providing medical transcription services to healthcare providers. It employs or contracts with *medical transcriptionists (MTs)* to provide these services. Because such an organization handles and stores *protected health information (PHI)*, it is subject to the requirements of HIPAA as a *business associate (BA)*, not a *covered entity (CE)*. Primarily, MTSOs must be able to ensure the security and confidentiality of the patient's PHI, and maintain an audit trail of all who have had access to the PHI.

medical underwriting See under *underwriting*.

medical waste See *hazardous waste*.

Medicare The federal program that provides payment for health care for persons sixty-five years of age and older and other qualified individuals (see Medicare Part A, below). In 2007, over 41 million Americans were covered by Medicare. The program is administered at the federal level by the Centers for Medicare and Medicaid Services (CMS), as contrasted with Medicaid, which is administered by the states.

Medicare was established in 1965 by amendment to the Social Security Act (Public Law 89-97), the pertinent section of the amendment being "Title XVIII—Health Insurance for the Aged." It has been affected by a significant amount of federal legislation since 1965, including the Balanced Budget Act of 1997 (BBA); the Balanced Budget Refinement Act of 1999 (BBRA); the Medicare, Medicaid and SCHIP Benefits Improvement and Protection Act of 2000 (BIPA); and the Medicare Modernization Act of 2003 (MMA). For a discussion of how payments to providers are determined under Medicare, see *Omnibus Budget Reconciliation Act of 1989*. **www.medicare.gov**

Medicare Part A The Medicare program that pays for hospital services, as well as for skilled nursing facility care, home health care, and hospice care following a covered hospital stay. Individuals who are age sixty-five and over and who qualify for the Social Security "Old Age, Survivors, Disability and Health Insurance Program," or who are entitled to railroad retirement benefits, or who are under age sixty-five but (1) have been receiving Social Security Disability Insurance (SSDI) for more than two years, (2) qualify for the end stage renal disease (ESRD) program, or (3) have been diagnosed with amyotrophic lateral sclerosis (ALS) (commonly known as Lou Gehrig's disease) are automatically enrolled in Medicare Part A. Synonym: Hospital Insurance (HI).

Medicare Part B The Medicare program through which persons entitled to Medicare Part A may obtain assistance with payment for physicians' services, diagnostic tests, and other professional and outpatient services. Individuals participate voluntarily through enrollment and payment of a monthly fee and annual deductible. Sometimes called Medical Insurance (MI).

Medicare Part C Formerly Medicare+Choice, now *Medicare Advantage*.

Medicare Part D The Medicare program that pays for prescription drugs. Introduced in 2003 by the Medicare Modernization Act, the program is voluntary for Medicare beneficiaries, who may enroll in a choice of plans and pay an extra premium each month for the coverage. There is also a deductible. See *prescription drug plan* and *doughnut hole*.

Original Medicare Plan The term used by CMS to describe the basic, "fee-for-service" Medicare plan, offered by the federal government and available nationwide. Unless the beneficiary chooses a Medicare Advantage plan, the Original plan will be the one in effect. To help meet the costs of services not provided in the Original plan, the beneficiary may purchase *Medigap* insurance. See also *Medicare Select*.

Medicare Administrative Contractor (MAC) An entity that has been awarded a contract by CMS to administer the Medicare fee-for-service program and perform the tasks previously handled by carriers and fiscal intermediaries. The Medicare Modernization Act of 2003 required that full and open competitions be held for all Medicare contracts, as part of Medicare contracting reform, to ensure the best value in cost and quality. Beginning in 2005, CMS established fifteen "primary" A/B MACs (to administer both Part A and Part B programs), four specialty MACs servicing home health and hospice providers (HH MACs), and four MACs servicing suppliers of durable medical equipment (DME MACs).

Medicare Advantage (MA) A program that permits those with Medicare Part A and Part B to choose among several types of health plans, including health maintenance organizations (HMOs), preferred provider organizations (PPOs), provider-sponsored organizations (PSOs), private fee-for-service plans (PFFS), and Medicare Special Needs Plans (MSNPs). These plans, which cover more than Original Medicare, usually eliminate the need for a Medigap policy.

Medicare Beneficiary Ombudsman (MBO) A person within the Department of Health and Human Services (HHS) who provides Medicare beneficiaries with information upon request, provides assistance as needed, and receives and responds to complaints and grievances. The position was established by the Medicare Modernization Act (MMA).

Medicare Code Editor (MCE) Software published by CMS to assist providers in processing claims under the *prospective payment system (PPS)*. It detects and reports errors in the coding of Medicare claims data.

Medicare Cost Plan (MCP) A health plan option open to Medicare beneficiaries in some areas, in which the services are provided by physicians and hospitals within the plan's network. If an out-of-network provider is used, the services are covered under the *Original Medicare Plan* (see under *Medicare*).

Medicare Dependent Hospital (MDH) Program A federal program originally created in 1989 to strengthen rural hospitals, ensuring that vital health care remains accessible for seniors in rural areas. (Rural areas have traditionally had a higher percentage of seniors, and therefore a higher percentage of Medicare beneficiaries.) The program provides higher reimbursement for rural facilities that are not already classified as a *Sole Community Hospital (SCH)* (see under *hospital*). To qualify as an MDH, the facility must have fewer than 100 beds and serve large numbers of Medicare beneficiaries (typically 60% or more of inpatient stays). See also *Critical Access Hospital Program*.

Medicare fraud and abuse See *fraud and abuse*.

Medicare Geographic Classification Review Board (MGCRB) The board, advisory to CMS, that reviews applications from hospitals for their classification into one of the three tiers of reimbursement levels available to hospitals under Medicare.

Medicare Hospital Insurance Trust Fund See *Medicare Trust Fund*.

Medicare Insured Group (MIG) An organizational concept allowing businesses or labor unions to distribute Medicare funds to retired employees. By targeting a specific group of retirees, it was hoped that costs could be lowered through the use of managed care.

Medicare Integrity Program (MIP) A program created by HIPAA in which CMS contracts with private sector entities to carry out Medicare fraud and abuse investigations and perform other functions to protect the integrity of Medicare and preserve the Medicare Trust Fund. Sometimes called fraud prevention program. See *Program Safeguard Contractor*.

Medicare, Medicaid, and SCHIP Benefits Improvement and Protection Act of 2000 (BIPA) Federal legislation enacted in 2000 to increase the benefits available to Medicare, Medicaid, and State Children's Health Insurance Program (SCHIP) beneficiaries. The law provides $35 billion over five years to offset what many refer to as "the unintended consequences" of the Balanced Budget Act of 1997 (BBA), and adds another $9 billion give-back in the Balanced Budget Refinement Act of 1999 (BBRA). Among the improved benefits are expanded coverage for Medicare Pap tests from once every three years to once every two years. BIPA was part of the Consolidated Appropriations Act. Pub. L. No. 106-554, Sec. 1(a)(6), 114 Stat. 2763, 2763A-463 (2000).

Medicare Modernization Act (MMA) Federal legislation enacted in 2003 that notably added prescription drug coverage (*Medicare Part D*, see under *Medicare*) to Medicare; previously there was none. The act also for the first time introduced variations in premiums, cost sharing, and coverage—prior to this, all beneficiaries paid the same amounts and received the same benefits. The new law instituted "means tests" to determine payment levels for drug coverage.

The MMA also implemented the *Medicare Advantage* program, made changes in the FDA approval process to bring lower cost generic drugs to the market sooner, and established *Health Savings Accounts (HSAs)*. It expanded Medicare benefits for preventive care by adding a "welcome to Medicare" physical examination for new enrollees and covering screening tests for cardiovascular disease and diabetes. Other provisions included measures to combat waste, fraud, and abuse and to improve quality of care and contain costs. The full title is the Medicare Prescription Drug, Improvement, and Modernization Act of 2003. Pub. L. No. 108-173, 117 Stat. 2066 (2003).

Medicare Payment Advisory Commission (MedPAC) Approved by Congress in the summer of 1997, this fifteen-member group assumed many of the duties of the *Prospective Payment Assessment Commission (ProPAC)* and the *Physician Payment Review Commission (PPRC)*.

Medicare+Choice This program was created by the Balanced Budget Act of 1997 to allow direct contracting between Medicare and provider-sponsored organizations (PSOs). Synonym: Medicare Part C. This has become the *Medicare Advantage* program.

Medicare Prescription Drug Plan (MPDP) See *prescription drug plan*.

Medicare Preservation Act of 1995 A Republican-sponsored bill introduced in 1995 to "amend title XVIII of the Social Security Act to preserve and reform the Medicare program" and to "reform the Medicare program, in order to preserve and protect the financial stability of the program." See *provider service organization* and *provider-sponsored organization*.

Medicare Provider Analysis and Review (MEDPAR) A database file maintained by CMS containing post-payment information on inpatient hospital and skilled nursing facility (SNF) Medicare stays. Both clinical and financial data are maintained and can be retrieved via personal identifiers for both providers and beneficiaries.

Medicare Quality Improvement Community See *MedQIC*.

Medicare Rural Hospital Flexibility Program (MRHFP) See *Critical Access Hospital Program*.

Medicare Secondary Payer (MSP) Rules Rules that grant "secondary payer" status to Medicare when a Medicare beneficiary is also eligible for healthcare benefits from another specific health insurance plan that is the "primary payer." The rules for which health insurance plans are considered to be primary payers were defined in the 1982 Tax Equity and Fiscal Responsibility Act (TEFRA). Typically, Medicare is the secondary payer (pays only the remaining portion left after the primary payer pays) in cases where the beneficiary is an employee with dual coverage because of age (sixty-five to sixty-nine years old), or has end stage renal disease (ESRD), or the beneficiary also qualifies under some other federal health insurance program such as the Veteran's Administration (VA).

MSP Rules also apply where automobile, liability, or no-fault insurance; workers' compensation; or other insurance is primarily liable to the beneficiary. CMS will not recognize a settlement between the primary payer and the beneficiary that does not protect Medicare's interests as the secondary payer. Medicare has the right to recover any payments it has made from the primary payer, or from anyone who has received proceeds of a settlement. This right is not subject to any statutes of limitations. See also *Medicare Set-Aside*.

Medicare Select A Medicare option, available in some states, consisting of the *Original Medicare Plan* (see under *Medicare*) plus one of the standardized *Medigap* plans (A through L). With a Medicare Select plan, generally the beneficiary must use specific hospitals, and in some cases specific doctors, to get full insurance benefits (except in an emergency). For this reason, Medicare Select plans usually cost less. If the beneficiary uses a non-Medicare Select hospital or doctor for nonemergency services, she or he will have to pay what the Original Medicare Plan doesn't pay. The Original Medicare Plan will pay its share of approved charges no matter what hospital or doctor is chosen.

Medicare Set-Aside (MSA) An arrangement to provide a funding mechanism for future medical expenses that would otherwise be paid by Medicare. Medicare Secondary Payer (MSP) Rules give Medicare the right to recover proceeds from insurance or workers' compensation settlements. The Medicare Set-Aside assures that funds will be available when the time comes to pay medical expenses covered by Medicare. It applies when the beneficiary is already a Medicare beneficiary, or has a "reasonable expectation" of enrollment within thirty months of the settlement date. CMS must approve MSA funding arrangements, including structured settlement annuities.

Medicare Set-Aside Consultant Certified (MSCC) A specialist in Medicare Set-Aside arrangements who has passed an examination of the Commission on Health Care Certification (CHCC). www.cdec1.com

Medicare special needs plan (MSNP) See *special needs plan*.

Medicare supplement insurance See *Medigap*.

Medicare Transaction System (MTS) A single, centralized computer-based claims and payment system intended for use by HCFA (now CMS) to process Medicare claims. Planning and development for the new system began in 1991. At that time, HCFA managed the Medicare program with fourteen systems at sixty sites operated by more than seventy contractors. The new MTS system was designed to replace them, at an estimated cost of $1 billion or more. By 1997, reportedly about $50 million had been spent on the project, which was soon after abandoned.

Medicare Trust Fund The money that funds the Medicare Part A program (see under **Medicare**). It is financed by payroll taxes from employers and employees. Part B and Part D are funded by premiums from beneficiaries and general revenues, apart from the trust fund. Synonym: Medicare Hospital Insurance Trust Fund.

Medicare Value Purchasing (MVP) Act of 2005 Proposed legislation that would give the Department of Health and Human Services (HHS) the authority to develop and implement *value-based purchasing* programs for hospitals, physician and nonphysician practitioners, Medicare Advantage plans, end stage renal disease providers, and home health agencies, based on the *pay-for-performance (P4P)* model. It did not become law.

Medicare Volume Performance Standards (MVPS) A type of expenditure target that was one element of the physician payment reform introduced by the Omnibus Budget Reconciliation Act of 1989 (OBRA 89).

medication A term used in health care to cover both prescription and nonprescription drugs. Often shortened to "med" or "meds."

medication administration The giving of a single dose of a medication (drug) to a patient. See *adverse drug event* for more information. See also *injection* and *infusion* for an explanation of commonly used methods of administration.

medication error Not synonymous with, but defined and discussed under, *adverse drug event*.

medication order A written order by a physician, dentist, or other authorized provider for a medication (either a prescription drug or a nonprescription drug) to be given to a specific *inpatient*. A similar order written for a prescription drug for an outpatient or outside the hospital is a *drug prescription*. For a nonprescription drug (an over-the-counter drug), no similar paperwork is required outside the hospital.

medication reconciliation A process performed at admission, transfer, or discharge of a patient, or any time a patient changes care providers, to reduce the chances of adverse drug events. The process has three steps: (1) A complete list is made of the medications the patient is currently taking, including prescription medications, over-the-counter medications, vitamins, herbals, nutraceuticals, and others. The patient or the patient's family provides essential information for this step. (2) A list is made of medications that might be prescribed for the patient. (3) The lists are compared (reconciled) to avoid medication errors such as omissions, duplications, dosing errors, or drug interactions. A complete list of current medications should follow the patient upon discharge, and from provider to provider.

medication therapy management services (MTMS) Services designed to optimize therapeutic outcomes and reduce the cost of medication therapy, as well as reduce the incidence of adverse drug events. A wide range of patient-specific services, provided primarily by pharmacists, include performing or obtaining an assessment of the patient's health status, formulating a medication treatment plan, performing a drug utilization review (DUR), interviewing the patient, reviewing medication therapy, educating the patient, monitoring and evaluating the patient's response to therapy, disease management, communicating with other care providers, and more, depending on the patient's needs. These services are distinct from the dispensing services of the pharmacist, and may or may not be connected to the provision of a medication product.

The Medicare Modernization Act requires that Medicare Advantage-Prescription Drug Plans (MA-PDs) and Prescription Drug Plans (PDPs) provide Medicare MTMS to "targeted beneficiaries," defined as patients with multiple chronic diseases, those taking multiple covered Part D drugs, and those with high drug costs. Some plans offer MTMS to all beneficiaries. CMS has said that MTMS must "evolve and become a cornerstone of the Medicare Prescription Drug Benefit."

medicine (science) The science and art of the diagnosis and treatment of disease and the maintenance of health.

medicine (substance) A substance administered to treat disease.

medicine (system) A system of diagnosis, and particularly treatment, based upon a specific theory of disease and healing. See also *complementary and alternative medicine*.

allopathy A system of medicine based on the theory that successful therapy depends on creating a condition antagonistic to or incompatible with the condition to be treated. Thus drugs such as antibiotics are given to combat diseases caused by the organisms to which they are antagonistic. Allopathy is the predominant system in the United States, and its practitioners are Doctors of Medicine (MDs).

ayurvedic medicine The traditional natural system of medicine of India based on lifestyle interventions and natural therapies. Mental techniques such as meditation are employed for prevention and treatment, as are individually prescribed dietary, sleeping, bodily posture, and exercise programs. Herbal preparations are prescribed as well as various methods to eliminate toxic products in the body. A healthy social life is encouraged. Formal education programs in ayurvedic medicine, providing continuing education credit, are available for medical practitioners in the United States. Synonym: ayurveda.

chiropractic A system of medicine based on the theory that disease is caused by malfunction of the nerve system, and that normal function of the nerve system can be achieved by manipulation and other treatment of the structures of the body, primarily the spinal column. A practitioner is a chiropractor.

homeopathy A system of medicine based on the theory that diseases should be combated (1) by giving drugs that, in healthy persons, can produce the same symptoms from which the patient is suffering; and (2) by giving these drugs in minute doses.

naturopathy The system of medicine where only natural medicines are used. Examples are manual manipulation, using food science and nutrition, hygiene, and immunization. A practitioner is called a naturopathic physician (ND or NMD).

Oriental medicine Traditional Oriental medicine emphasizes the proper balance of the body's vital energy, called qi (pronounced chi). Disturbance of qi can cause disease. Therapies such as acupuncture, herbal medicine, bodywork therapy, and qi gong are used to restore balance.

osteopathy A system of medicine that emphasizes the theory that the body can make its own remedies, given normal structural relationships, environmental conditions, and nutrition. It differs from allopathy primarily in its greater attention to body mechanics and manipulative methods in diagnosis and therapy. Dr. Andrew Taylor Still, founder of osteopathic medicine, wrote "to find health should be the object of the doctor. Anyone can find disease."

Six percent of physicians in the United States today are osteopaths. Osteopathic physicians are granted the Doctor of Osteopathy (DO) degree. ("OD" stands for "optometric doctor.")

medicine (treatment) A general method of treatment of disease by means other than surgical; that is to say, "medical treatment" is treatment without surgery (without operation or manipulation), although a number of diagnostic procedures, some of them invasive, are used in medical (as opposed to surgical) treatment. See also *medical care*.

Medicine Equity and Drug Safety Act of 2000 (MEDS Act) A federal law to allow drugs manufactured in the United States, but exported to other countries, to be reimported by pharmacies and drug wholesalers for resale in the United States. This would presumably save consumers money on drugs. (People were already traveling to Mexico and Canada to buy prescription drugs at lower prices.) The law was passed in response to increasing drug prices and the fact that many people could no longer afford their medications. The act was never implemented because the Department of Health and Human Services (HHS) determined that the safety of reimported drugs could not be assured. The Secretary of HHS said that "[o]pening our borders as required under this program would increase the likelihood that the shelves of pharmacies in towns and communities across the nation would include counterfeit drugs, cheap foreign copies of FDA-approved drugs, expired drugs, contaminated drugs, and drugs stored under inappropriate and unsafe conditions." Pub. L. 106-387, Sec. 1(a), 114 Stat. 1549, 1549A-35 (2000).

Medigap Insurance that may be purchased by an individual to add to the benefits provided under *Medicare*. Intelligent purchase of such insurance was virtually impossible until 1992, when uniform benefit packages, which standardized benefits for Medicare supplement insurance, were mandated by the federal government. A total of twelve standard plans (A through L) are specified. Each standardized Medigap policy must cover "basic benefits." Medigap Plans A through J have one set of basic benefits, and Plans K and L have a different set of basic benefits. There are exceptions in Massachusetts, Minnesota, and Wisconsin, which have their own standardized Medigap plans. Synonym: Medicare supplement insurance. See also *Medicare Select*. **www.medicare.gov/medigap**

medisave See *Medical Savings Account*.

MedisGroups See *Medical Illness Severity Grouping System*.

MEDIX Standards for the exchange of data between hospital computer systems. A project of the Institute of Electrical and Electronics Engineers (IEEE) Engineering in Medicine and Biology Society (EMBS), it is formally known as IEEE P1157 Medical Data Interchange. See also *HL7*.

MEDLARS Medical Literature Analysis and Retrieval System. See *MEDLINE*.

MEDLINE Medical Literature Analysis and Retrieval System Online. A biomedical database containing bibliographic material from over 5,000 medical journals (over 15 million references), from 1966 to the present. It was developed and is maintained by the National Library of Medicine (NLM), and is available to individuals and medical libraries. Searches are carried out through NLM's **Medical Literature Analysis and Retrieval System (MEDLARS)**. See also *NLM Gateway*. **www.nlm.nih.gov/pubs/factsheets/medline.html**

MedlinePlus An online service of the National Library of Medicine (NLM) that provides health information for consumers. **medlineplus.gov**

MEDMARX A national, Internet-accessible database that hospitals and healthcare systems voluntarily use to report, track, and trend adverse drug reactions and medication errors. Sponsored by the United States Pharmacopeia (USP). **www.usp.org/patientSafety/medmarx**

MedPAC See *Medicare Payment Advisory Commission*.

MEDPAR See *Medicare Provider Analysis and Review*.

MedQIC Medicare Quality Improvement Community. An online resource on quality improvement for quality improvement organizations (QIOs) and providers, sponsored by CMS. Pronounced "med-quick." **www.medqic.org**

meds Short for *medications*.

MEDS Act See *Medicine Equity and Drug Safety Act of 2000*.

Medstat A health information company based in Ann Arbor, Michigan, that provides decision support systems, market intelligence, benchmark databases, and research for managing the purchase, administration, and delivery of health services and benefits. It serves nearly 1,000 organizations including employers, providers, pharmaceutical companies, government organizations, and health plans and insurance companies. It is assisting the *Leapfrog Group* in its health initiatives by providing data collection, analysis, and support services. Medstat is a division of Thomson. **www.medstat.com**

MedWatch A postmarketing surveillance program of the Food and Drug Administration (FDA) in which physicians and other health professionals, and consumers, report on the adverse effects of and product problems with drugs and other medical products after they have been put on the market. See also *Adverse Event Reporting System*. **www.fda.gov/medwatch**

member See *enrollee*.

member month A measurement unit that is equal to one member enrolled in a managed care plan (MCP), such as a health maintenance organization (HMO), for one month. Two "member months" could equal one member enrolled for two months, or two members enrolled for one month. See also *enrollee*.

meme An idea, behavior, style, or usage that spreads from person to person within a culture. Pronounced "meem." Examples are hugging as a greeting, catchy tunes, or attending church. Ideas competing for attention in our society may be called memes, and there is a theory that they spread by contagion, like a virus, rather than other reasons (such as validity). It's being speculated that in humans, cultural evolution by selection of adaptive ideas (memes) has superseded biological evolution by selection of hereditary traits. The term is credited to Richard Dawkins, a zoologist at Oxford who published a book on the concept in 1976, *The Selfish Gene* (Oxford University Press, 1989).

memetics The study of *memes*.

menopause clinician A clinical health professional who focuses practice on menopause management.

> **Certificate of Added Qualification—Menopause Clinician** A certificate of added qualification available to physicians, pharmacists, nurse practitioners, nurse midwives, and physician assistants who pass an examination of the National Certification Corporation (NCC). **www.nccnet.org**

menopause nursing The area of nursing focusing on the needs of women in their menarchal years.

mental distress See *emotional distress*.

mental health The state of being of the individual with respect to emotional, social, and behavioral maturity. Although the term is often used to mean "good mental health," mental health is a relative state, varying from time to time in the individual, and from individual to individual.

> The National Mental Health Information Center at the Substance Abuse and Mental Health Services Administration (SAMHSA) defines mental health as "[h]ow a person thinks, feels, and acts when faced with life's situations. Mental health is how people look at themselves, their lives, and the other people in their lives; evaluate their challenges and problems; and explore choices. This includes handling stress, relating to other people, and making decisions."

mental health counselor A counselor specially trained in mental health care.

> **Certified Clinical Mental Health Counselor (CCMHC)** A mental health counselor who has met the certification requirements of the National Board for Certified Counselors (NBCC). **www.nbcc.org**

Mental Health Parity Act (MHPA) A federal law requiring that health plan dollar limits on annual or lifetime mental health benefits be no lower than on medical and surgical benefits. Benefits for substance abuse and chemical dependency are excluded, as are small employers (less than fifty employees). A plan is also exempt if it can show that its costs would be raised by 1% or more by compliance with the act. The MHPA took effect in January 1998, but had a "sunset" provision so that it would cease to apply to services and benefits provided after September 30, 2001; this was extended to December 31, 2007. See also *parity*. Pub. L. No. 104-204, title VII, 110 Stat. 2944 (1996).

mentally retarded/developmentally disabled (MRDD) A term defined in legislation to designate people who qualify for certain rights or benefits.

mentor A trusted and experienced advisor or teacher. In Greek legend, Mentor, a loyal friend of Odysseus, served as teacher and guide of Odysseus' son, Telemachus. Recently, the word has been used in health care in the term "telementoring," using telecommunications to advise or guide. See *telemedicine*.

MEPS See *Medical Expenditure Panel Survey*.

Merck Manual A widely used reference on diagnosis and treatment of disease, published by Merck & Co., Inc. First published in 1899 as a small 192-page book titled *Merck's Manual of* *the Materia Medica*, it was carried by Albert Schweitzer to Africa in 1913 and by Admiral Byrd to the South Pole in 1929. The full name now is *The Merck Manual of Diagnosis and Therapy*. **www.merck.com**

Merck Manual of Geriatrics A companion volume to the *Merck Manual*, concerning the diagnosis and treatment of disease in aging patients, published by Merck & Co., Inc.

mercy killing See *euthanasia*.

merger The formal union of two or more corporations (such as hospitals) into a single corporation. In a merger, one of the original corporations retains its identity and continues to exist, while the other corporations are merged into it and lose their former identities. The surviving corporation acquires the assets and assumes the liabilities of the former corporations. See also *consolidation* and *virtual merger*.

MeSH See *Medical Subject Headings*.

Message Development Framework (MDF) See *HL7*.

message format standards (MFS) Standards for the electronic exchange of information between computer systems so that the exchange is efficient, unambiguous, and secure. These are essential to permit full *interoperability*.

messenger ribonucleic acid (mRNA) See under *ribonucleic acid*, under *DNA*.

MET See *metabolic equivalents*. Also multiple employer trust; see *multiple employer welfare arrangement*.

meta-analysis A research method that entails taking several studies on a given topic and analyzing those studies together, thus making a large study out of them. The method is of relatively recent development, and much attention is being given to improving the methodology itself. The study resulting from using meta-analysis is also called a "meta-analysis."

metabolic equivalents (MET) A clinical measure of exercise tolerance or exercise capacity. An individual's MET is a score that is the result of clinical exercise testing, usually on a treadmill. One MET is defined as the amount of energy expended in sitting quietly (about 3.5 ml of oxygen consumed per kilogram of body weight per minute for an average adult). Thus a MET of 5 means that the person can tolerate exercise that is five times as strenuous as sitting quietly. A study in 2002 reported that individuals with MET scores of 8 or more had half the mortality as those with MET scores of 5 or less, indicating that physical fitness is highly important in preventing untimely death.

metabolism The biochemical processes that sustain a living organism or a living cell.

metadata registry A place where facts about the characteristics of data are kept, which are necessary to clearly describe, inventory, analyze, and classify the data. See *United States Health Information Knowledgebase*.

Metathesaurus See *UMLS Metathesaurus*.

method A technique or procedure for doing something. Compare with *modality*.

method effectiveness When a treatment fails to achieve its intended results, the failure may be due to the method employed or its use. For example, a contraceptive failure may occur because the method was inadequate, because it really was not used, or because it was used improperly. Thus either the **method effectiveness** or the **use effectiveness** of the contraceptive may have been at fault, and the failure may have been either a **method failure** or a **use failure**.

method failure See *method effectiveness*.

method or process patent See under *patent*.

MEWA See *multiple employer welfare arrangement*.

MFS See *message format standards*.

MFT See *marriage and family therapist*.

MGCRB See *Medicare Geographic Classification Review Board*.

MGMA See *Medical Group Management Association*.

MHAA See *McKinney Homeless Assistance Act*.

MHC See *Migrant Health Center.*

MI See *medical illustrator*, *medical interpreter*, and *myocardial infarction* (under *infarction*). Also Medical Insurance; see *Medicare Part B* under *Medicare.*

MICRA See *Medical Injury Compensation Reform Act.*

microbicide A substance that can kill or disable disease-causing organisms such as viruses and bacteria. Topical microbicides (such as creams, gels, or foams) are being developed that, when applied to the vagina or rectum, would help prevent sexually transmitted diseases such as HIV/AIDS.

microbiology The science dealing with microbes (microscopic—and smaller—organisms).

Microbiology Technologist (M) See under *clinical laboratory technologist.*

micro measures In health care, refers to steps taken to improve the health care provided to individual patients, rather than the healthcare system. See *macro measures.*

microorganism A microscopic plant or animal. Not all microorganisms cause disease, although germs and viruses are microorganisms that get a lot of attention.

microregulation Regulation of the health care of patients at the level of the individual institution, physician, and patient. Not only does microregulation interfere with the freedom of all three, but it also significantly increases administrative costs and paperwork, because of the oversight system required to monitor the "behavior" of the physician, patient, and institution.

microscopic anatomy See *histology* under *anatomy.*

middle care provider (MCP) A health professional who is not a physician, dentist, or pharmacist, but has training and experience exceeding those of a basic technician, technologist, or other professional in a health science discipline. Used to distinguish between those who must work under the supervision of a physician or other health professional, and those permitted to perform certain functions autonomously. May be thought of as someone "between" a paramedic and a doctor. Examples are *nurse practitioners* and *physician assistants*. See also *midlevel practitioner.*

midlevel practitioner (MP) Under CMS rules, a midlevel practitioner is a nurse practitioner, physician assistant (PA), or certified nurse midwife. Synonym: mid level practitioner (MLP). See also *Rural Health Clinic.*

midwifery The practice of assisting a woman in childbirth. The midwife, as a health professional, has been around since ancient times. States vary in their acceptance of, and requirements for, midwives practicing independently.

Certified Midwife (CM) A practitioner of midwifery (not necessarily a nurse) who has been qualified by and passed an examination of the American Midwifery Certification Board (AMCB). **www.amcbmidwife.org**

Certified Nurse-Midwife (CNM) A registered nurse who has been qualified by and passed an examination of the American Midwifery Certification Board (AMCB). **www.amcbmidwife.org**

Certified Professional Midwife (CPM) A practitioner of midwifery (not necessarily a nurse) who has been qualified by and passed an examination of the North American Registry of Midwives (NARM). **www.narm.org**

MIG See *Medicare Insured Group.*

Migrant Health Center (MHC) A federal program to provide healthcare services to migrant farm workers and their families. See also *Federally Qualified Health Center.*

Milbank Memorial Fund An endowed national foundation committed to nonpartisan analysis, study, research, and communication on significant issues in health policy. Established in 1905, its mission is to improve health by helping decision makers in the public and private sectors acquire and use the best available evidence to inform policy for health care and population health. It publishes the *Milbank Quarterly*. **www.milbank.org**

Milliman Care Guidelines *Clinical practice guidelines* (see under *guidelines*) used by a number of managed care organizations and insurance companies to detail the care physicians are expected to provide to beneficiaries. Also used by hospitals, physician groups, health plans, and other healthcare managers. Published by Milliman Care Guidelines LLC, A Milliman Company. Formerly called Milliman & Robertson Care Guidelines. **www.mnr.com**

mind-body medicine A philosophy of medical practice in which the major focus is on the whole person rather than on a physiological system. Attention is given to patient empowerment, emotional connections, families, and cultural and language barriers. Patients are encouraged to use support groups, and are taught such techniques as meditation, yoga, stretching, nutrition, and relaxation exercises. An increasing number of hospitals are establishing Centers for Mind-Body Health. See also *complementary and alternative medicine* and *holistic medicine.*

minimal differential risk A concept applied to evaluate the difference in risk between two treatments or procedures, particularly in research, when there is very little difference in risk of an undesirable outcome between standard, commonly accepted therapy used for the condition and the experimental therapy under study.

minimally invasive surgery (MIS) See under *surgery (treatment).*

Minimum Data Set (MDS) See *Resident Assessment Instrument.*

Minnesota Model An approach to the treatment of alcoholism and drug dependence based on a system developed by the Hazelden Foundation (located in Minnesota) and the Betty Ford Center. The Model is a residential program that includes abstinence from drugs and alcohol, individual and group therapy, participation in Alcoholics Anonymous (AA), classes, family involvement, work assignments, activity therapy, and use of counselors—many of whom are recovering alcoholics—and multiprofessional staff.

Minnesota plan Healthcare reform legislation enacted by Minnesota in 1992, known as "HealthRight" (later renamed the MinnesotaCare Act). The law (1) established a commission whose goal was at least a 10% decrease in the annual rate of increase in healthcare costs; (2) established a voluntary, state-subsidized insurance called MinnesotaCare to be available to low-income persons on a sliding scale proportional to income, with a maximum premium; (3) placed reform regulations on insurance companies to prevent such practices as exclusion of pre-existing conditions and to provide portability of benefits and work toward standardization of rates across contracts; and (4) gave special attention to the unique problems of rural communities. The stipulation that physicians practicing within state-approved guidelines are given defense thereby in malpractice litigation attracted considerable attention. Minnesotans point out that the law outlines a state's responsibility to provide a healthcare system rather than approaching the problem from the citizen's right to health care.

minor A person who has not yet reached the age required by law for a particular purpose. The age may vary from state to state; however, in most states, for most purposes (such as voting or making contracts) the age of majority is eighteen years.

A minor is usually legally incompetent to give consent for treatment. However, in many states a minor may give valid consent if he or she is married, emancipated (living away from home and supporting him- or herself), or sufficiently mature (emotionally and intellectually capable of understanding his or her disease, need for treatment, and so forth). In addition, many states have specific ages at which even a (otherwise incompetent) minor can consent; for example, to testing and treatment for venereal disease or for drug or alcohol abuse, or to make a decision whether to remain in a psychiatric hospital.

Minority Medical Education Program (MMEP) Former name of the *Summer Medical and Dental Education Program (SMDEP).*

minutes The written record of the proceedings of a body or group. In health care, such bodies include the governing body, the medical staff, and committees of the hospital and medical staff. Minutes should include the date of the meeting, who was present, and who wrote the minutes. Topics should be listed separately for ease of reading and retrieval of information, and all significant actions taken by the body should be noted. Minutes need not (and should not) include "minute" detail of discussions (usually, the fact that a topic was discussed, and whether action was taken, is sufficient), who said what, who made or seconded a motion, or who voted for what (unless a request is made to note names of voters). Excessive detail can inhibit the free speech necessary for intelligent decision making. Minutes may in some instances become evidence in a lawsuit or other legal proceeding, so their accuracy and conciseness are important.

MIP See *Medicare Integrity Program*.

MIS See *management information system* under *information system*. Sometimes used for "manager of information systems." See also *minimally invasive surgery*, under *surgery (treatment)*.

mission-critical See *critical (essential)*.

MLM Medical Logic Module. See *Arden Syntax*.

MLP Mid level practitioner; see *midlevel practitioner*.

MLR See *medical loss ratio*.

MLT See *Medical Laboratory Technician* under *clinical laboratory technician*.

MMA See *Medical Management Analysis* and *Medicare Modernization Act*.

MMEP See *Minority Medical Education Program*.

MND See *motoneuron disease*.

Mobile Healthcare Alliance (MoHCA) An independent, nonprofit organization whose mission is to promote the adoption of mobile technologies to support the delivery of higher quality health. One initiative is the *Consumer Health Manager (CHM)* project.

modality A therapeutic (treatment) method employing electrical or physical (as contrasted with chemical or other) means. "Modality" is often used incorrectly as a synonym for method.

Model HMO Act Regulatory guidelines first issued in 1972 by the National Association of Insurance Commissioners (NAIC), who along with the National Association of Managed Care Regulators (NAMCR) now update the Model Act. The act is used by many states to regulate their HMOs, ensuring the delivery of basic healthcare services according to the appropriate standards of care.

modified diet See under *diet*.

modifier A two-digit or letter code that "modifies" the *CPT* code system. Typically a modifier is used to reflect an unusual circumstance surrounding the use of the code in identifying the service that was provided, or an additional detail affecting the amount of payment required for that service.

For example, for federal Medicare payment purposes using *HCPCS* codes, the global CPT code may be split into the two following components, each being identified by a "26" or "TC" in the modifier field:

26 (PC) professional component

TC technical component

A global CPT code's relative value unit (RVU) values will be equal to the sum of the professional (26) and technical (TC) components. Other modifier values may also be used to represent variations of the service or product that code identifies.

For instance, a "bilateral modifier" (value of 50) reflects a type of "quantity discount" concept applied to fees for provided services where the human body has two or more parts, such as arms, legs, or ears. For example, the repair of a protruding ear (CPT code 69300) is for one ear only. If both ears were repaired in the same operation, CPT code 69300 should be listed with a bilateral modifier, resulting in a fee at 150% of a single ear operation, instead of 200%.

modular certification An earlier credential from the American Nurses Credentialing Center (ANCC) (**nursingworld.org/ancc**) for registered nurses who passed an advanced examination in a specialty area. The designation was RN,Cm. Two were offered: ambulatory care nursing and nursing case management.

modular language See the diagram at *natural language*.

MoHCA See *Mobile Healthcare Alliance*.

Mohs-micrographic surgery A specialized, microscopic treatment for the removal of skin cancer cells.

molecular Pertaining to a *molecule*.

molecular biology The study of the makeup, structure, and function of biological molecules such as DNA, RNA, and proteins.

molecular diagnostics Tests and methods used to identify a disease or the predisposition for a disease by analyzing *DNA* or *RNA* (see *ribonucleic acid* under *DNA*).

molecular genetics See under *genetics*.

molecular pathology See under *pathology*.

Molecular Pathology Technologist (MP) See under *clinical laboratory technologist*.

molecule A combination of two or more atoms that make up a specific chemical compound. The molecule is the smallest quantity into which any substance can be divided and still keep its identifiable characteristics. A molecule of water, for instance, consists of two hydrogen atoms and one oxygen atom. If any one of the atoms were removed from the molecule, you would no longer have water.

monitoring Keeping track of events in a systematic fashion. The term is applied to monitoring the quality of medical care, monitoring the performance of physicians, and monitoring patient condition and response to care.

  admission pattern monitoring (APM) The monitoring of the distribution of kinds of patients admitted to a hospital (that is, of the admission case mix) in order to detect changing needs for services, displacement of patients to other institutions, or other changes.

monoclonal antibody (MAB) A class of diagnostic and therapeutic agents (substance) that is produced biologically (grown) in a laboratory using a clone of a single special kind of cell (hybridoma) that has the ability to produce a continuous supply of identical antibodies. Each kind of MAB recognizes only one kind of antibody. MABs are used in identifying bacteria, viruses, certain tumors, and hormones; in diagnosing infectious diseases; and in blood typing. They are also used to treat certain infections, and are being studied for treatment of cancer. See *biotechnology product*.

monogamous A relationship between a doctor and a hospital in which a doctor does all her or his hospital work in a single hospital.

monopoly suicide An economic phenomenon referring to the observation that any monopoly enterprise that succeeds in raising its prices to the point where "windfall" profits occur will attract such competition into the field that the monopoly will be destroyed.

monopsonistic From monopsony, a market in which there is only one buyer, and that buyer exerts a disproportionate influence on the market; a special type of oligopsony, in which there are a few buyers with such influence.

moral A belief system in which we judge actions and people to be "right" or "wrong," good or bad. Also morals, morality. See also *ethics (moral)*.

moral hazard A term derived from the fire insurance industry describing the phenomenon that insured buildings are more likely to burn than uninsured ones. This has significance for the healthcare industry because the same phenomenon applies to utilization of healthcare benefits—patients are more likely to use a service if they pay for it with "somebody else's money" (SEM). Any delivery system with a high moral hazard component is likely to cost more because there is no incentive built into the system to encourage the reduction of costs.

morbidity Illness, injury, or other than normal health. This term is often used in describing a rate (a statistical term). One type of hospital morbidity rate, for example, is the postoperative infection rate; it is the number of patients with infections following surgery, expressed as a proportion of those undergoing surgery, within a given period of time.

  comorbidity As used in the prospective payment system (PPS), a diagnosis present *before* hospitalization that is thought to extend the hospital stay at least one day for roughly 75%

or more of the patients with a given principal diagnosis. The presence of a comorbidity is reported in the PPS by placing, as a secondary ICD-9-CM diagnosis code in the patient's bill, a condition defined by PPS as a comorbidity. See also *complication*.

compression of morbidity The situation that results if persons are healthier until later in life than at present, that is, if disability is postponed more than death, so that an individual's period of disability preceding death is shorter, and the older population is both "older and healthier." The converse could be called "expansion of morbidity," so that the population becomes "older and sicker." Which will occur is not known; guesses about this aspect of the aging of the population are critical in planning for long-term care.

mortality A term that applies to death, or the state of being mortal. This term is often used in the phrase "mortality rate," which means the number of patients who died expressed as a proportion of those at risk. Same as *death rate*.

Mortality Medical Data System (MMDS) A system of the National Center for Health Statistics (NCHS) that automates the entry, classification, and retrieval of cause of death information reported on death certificates. The system was first developed in 1967.

mortality rate See *death rate*.

MOS See *Medical Outcomes Study*.

MotherNet A community health outreach program to provide critically needed health, education, and support services to at-risk children and families in the United States, with an emphasis on underserved minority communities. It originated as the Resource Mothers Development Project (RMDP), initiated by the National Commission to Prevent Infant Mortality (NCPIM). RMDP promoted the use of lay home visitors called "resource mothers" to guide pregnant and parenting women through birth and child care and also through the healthcare system. The range of services provided by MotherNet has greatly expanded since late 1993, when it came under the auspices of INMED Partnerships for Children. **www.inmed.org/programs/mothernet.htm**

motoneuron disease (MND) A class of degenerative muscle disorders, which includes *amyotrophic lateral sclerosis (ALS)* (Lou Gehrig's disease) and *multiple sclerosis (MS)*. The diseases in the class all result in increasing muscular weakness and lack of muscle control. The causes of MND are not known.

MP See *midlevel practitioner* and *Molecular Pathology Technologist* (under *clinical laboratory technologist*).

MPDP Medicare prescription drug plan; see *prescription drug plan*.

MPHFA Medicaid Psychiatric Hospital Fairness Act. See *IMD exclusion*.

MPKC See *management problem knowledge coupler* under *Problem Knowledge Couplers*.

MPM See *medical practice management*.

MQIO Medicare *quality improvement organization*.

MRA Medical record administrator; see *health information administrator*. Also medical record analyst; see *health record analyst*.

MRC See *Medical Reserve Corps*.

MRDD See *mentally retarded/developmentally disabled*.

MRHFP Medicare Rural Hospital Flexibility Program. See *Critical Access Hospital Program*.

MRI See *magnetic resonance imaging* and *Medical Records Institute*.

MRL See *medical record librarian*.

MRO See *medical review officer*.

MRP See *Magnet Recognition Program*.

MRT Medical record technician. See *health information technician*.

MS See *multiple sclerosis*.

MSA See *Medical Savings Account* and *Medicare Set-Aside*.

MSCC See *Medicare Set-Aside Consultant Certified* under *Medicare Set-Aside*.

MSN Master of Science in Nursing.

MSNP Medicare *special needs plan*.

MSO See *management service organization* and *medical staff*.

MSO activities See *medical staff activities*.

MSP See *Medicare Secondary Payer Rules*.

MSS See *magnetic surgery system*.

MT See *medical transcriptionist* and *music therapist*. Also maggot therapy; see *biosurgery*.

MT(ASCP) See *medical technologist* under *clinical laboratory technologist*.

MT-BC See *Board Certified Music Therapist* under *music therapist*.

MTD See *medical telemetry device*.

MTMS See *medication therapy management services*.

MTP See *myofascial trigger point*.

MTPT See *myofascial trigger point therapist*.

MTS See *Medicare Transaction System*.

MTSO See *medical transcription service organization*.

MUA See *Medically Underserved Area*.

multicasualty accident See under *disaster*.

multidisciplinary Made up of individuals from different fields. In the hospital, a committee on patient care that has members who are physicians, nurses, and managers, for example, is a multidisciplinary committee.

multihospital system A term that technically pertains to two or more hospitals under a single governing body. In current usage, "multihospital system" also applies to a number of formal and informal arrangements among hospitals, varying from sharing of one or two services, through a variety of leasing, sponsoring, and contract-managing schemes, to full-blown single ownership of two or more facilities. Synonyms: chain organization, hospital chain.

multihospital system code A number that identifies the specific multihospital system to which a given hospital belongs. This code is used by the American Hospital Association in its listing of hospitals in its annual *AHA Guide to the Health Care Field*.

multipayer system A healthcare reform approach that uses a number of payers, usually both private and public. The *German-style system* is a multipayer system. See also *single-payer plan*.

multiple employer trust (MET) See *multiple employer welfare arrangement*.

multiple employer welfare arrangement (MEWA) An employee welfare benefit plan (EWBP) or other arrangement established to provide healthcare coverage to the employees (and/or their dependents) of two or more employers (including one or more self-employed individuals), by direct payment, reimbursement, or otherwise. Excluded from the definition are collective bargaining agreements and rural electric cooperatives. An MEWA can take various forms, such as an insurance company, health maintenance organization, or other health plan. The term is fully defined in the Employee Retirement Income Security Act (ERISA) (29 U.S.C. § 1002(40)(A) (2005)). Formerly multiple employer trust (MET). See also *association health plan*.

multiple sclerosis (MS) A chronic, often disabling disease of the central nervous system, diagnosed most often in people between the ages of twenty and forty. Symptoms may be mild, such as numbness in the limbs, or severe, such as paralysis or loss of vision. The effects are unpredictable and can be lifelong. Information is available from the National Multiple Sclerosis Society. **www.nmss.org**

multiskilling See *upskilling*.

MUMPS A computer programming language developed at Massachusetts General Hospital in the late 1960s and 1970s. It is now sometimes referred to simply as "M," and is used in many different industries in addition to health care. It has no relationship to the common contagious disease known as "mumps," which is characterized by swollen parotid and other salivary glands (in front of and below the ears). MUMPS stands for Massachusetts General Hospital Utility Multiprogramming System.

MUP See *Medically Underserved Population*.

musculoskeletal Pertaining to the muscles and the skeleton.

music therapist (MT) A health professional qualified to practice music therapy.

> **Board Certified Music Therapist (MT-BC)** A music therapist who has completed an accredited college program in music therapy and an internship and passed a national examination offered by the Certification Board for Music Therapists (CBMT). **www.cbmt.com**

music therapy The use of music to improve the psychological, physical, cognitive, or social functioning of people with health or educational problems.

mutagen Any chemical or physical agent (such as x-rays) that causes changes in DNA.

mutation Any change in the sequence of DNA in the *genome*.

mutual aid The furnishing of resources, from one individual or agency to another individual or agency, including but not limited to facilities, personnel, equipment, and services, pursuant to an agreement with the individual or agency, for use within the jurisdiction of the individual or agency requesting assistance. An example would be an agreement among fire departments or emergency medical systems.

MVP See *Medicare Value Purchasing Act of 2005*.

MVPS See *Medicare Volume Performance Standards*.

Mx See *management (case)*.

MyMedicare.gov See *Medicare Beneficiary Portal* under *portal*.

MyNDMA See *Citizens Health Portal* under *portal*.

myocardial infarction (MI) See under *infarction*.

myofascial trigger point (MTP) A place in a muscle that is a focus of hyper-irritability, which when compressed may cause pain, tenderness, and other symptoms in other places. The fascia is a fibrous membrane that covers, supports, and separates muscles.

myofascial trigger point therapist (MTPT) A health professional specially trained in the treatment of pain caused by a myofascial trigger point.

> **Certified Myofascial Trigger Point Therapist (CMTPT)** An MTPT who has passed an examination of the Certification Board for Myofascial Trigger Point Therapists (CBMTPT). **www.myofascialtherapy.org**

N

NACCHO See *National Association of County and City Health Officials*.

NAHDO See *National Association of Health Data Organizations*.

NAHIT See *National Alliance for Health Information Technology*.

NAHMOR National Association of HMO Regulators. See *National Association of Managed Care Regulators*.

NAHQ See *National Association for Healthcare Quality*.

NAHSE See *National Association of Health Services Executives*.

NAIC See *National Association of Insurance Commissioners*.

NAMCR See *National Association of Managed Care Regulators*.

NAMSS See *National Association Medical Staff Services*.

NANDA International (NANDA-I) An organization founded in 1982 committed to developing and classifying nursing diagnoses. It periodically publishes *Nursing Diagnoses: Definitions and Classification*, commonly referred to as "NANDA" (or "NANDA International"). Formerly called the North American Nursing Diagnosis Association (NANDA). **www.nanda.org**

naprapathy A treatment method focusing on the manipulation of connective tissue, including ligaments, tendons, and muscles, to release tension and restore balance. From the Czech "napravit" (to correct) and the Greek "pathos" (suffering). Some states license its practitioners, called naprapaths.

Naranjo algorithm See under *algorithm*.

NARL See *no adverse response level*.

NASM-CPT See *Certified Personal Trainer* under *personal trainer*.

National Academies See *National Academy of Sciences*, *National Research Council*, *National Academy of Engineering*, and *Institute of Medicine*.

National Academy of Engineering (NAE) Established in 1964 under the charter of the National Academy of Sciences (NAS) as a parallel organization of outstanding engineers. It is autonomous in its administration and in the selection of its members, sharing with NAS the responsibility for advising the federal government. NAE also sponsors engineering programs aimed at meeting national needs, encourages education and research, and recognizes the superior achievements of engineers. **www.nae.edu**

National Academy of Sciences (NAS) A private, nonprofit, self-perpetuating society of distinguished scholars engaged in scientific and engineering research, dedicated to the furtherance of science and technology and to their use for the general welfare. Upon the authority of the charter granted to it by the Congress when it was formed in 1863, the NAS has a mandate that requires it to advise the federal government on scientific and technical matters. Under the NAS charter, the National Research Council (NRC) was established in 1916, the National Academy of Engineering (NAE) in 1964, and the Institute of Medicine (IOM) in 1970. **www.nasonline.org**

National Alliance for Health Information Technology (NAHIT) A national organization committed to accelerating the implementation of world-class, standards-based information technology to improve health care. The alliance comprises over 100 member organizations from all industry sectors: providers, payers, health plans, information technology suppliers, and other relevant nonhealthcare organizations. **www.nahit.org**

National Association for Healthcare Quality (NAHQ) A national organization, founded in 1976, committed to improving the quality of health care and to supporting the development of healthcare quality management professionals. Its Healthcare Quality Certification Board (HQCB) provides certification (Certified Professional in Healthcare Quality (CPHQ)). **www.nahq.org**

National Association Medical Staff Services (NAMSS) The national organization of medical staff services professionals. **www.namss.org**

National Association of Area Agencies on Aging (N4A) An umbrella organization for the 655 *area agencies on aging (AAAs)* and more than 230 *Title VI programs* for Native Americans in the United States. Based in Washington, DC, N4A advocates on behalf of and provides support to the local agencies to ensure that needed resources and services are available to older Americans. **www.n4a.org**

National Association of County and City Health Officials (NACCHO) The national nonprofit organization representing local public health agencies (including city, county, metro, district, and tribal agencies) **www.naccho.org**

National Association of Health Data Organizations (NAHDO) A nonprofit organization committed to improving health care through the collection, analysis, dissemination, public availability, and use of health data. **www.nahdo.org**

National Association of Health Services Executives (NAHSE) A "non-profit association of Black health care executives founded in 1968 for the purpose of promoting the advancement and development of Black health care leaders, and elevating the quality of health care services rendered to minority and underserved communities." **www.nahse.org**

National Association of HMO Regulators (NAHMOR) See *National Association of Managed Care Regulators*.

National Association of Inpatient Physicians Former name of the *Society of Hospital Medicine*.

National Association of Insurance Commissioners (NAIC) An organization of state insurance commissioners that works toward development of uniformity in insurance regulation. NAIC develops and publishes model laws, regulations, and guidelines for insurance companies, prepaid managed care plans, and state legislatures. Other NAIC activities include maintaining market-based information systems, monitoring legislative activity, conducting research, and providing consumer information. It also offers an accreditation program. **www.naic.org**

National Association of Managed Care Regulators (NAMCR) An organization formed in 1975 to work with the National Association of Insurance Commissioners (NAIC) in the area of health maintenance organization (HMO) regulation. NAMCR is composed of both regulator members and associate industry members. NAMCR provides expertise and a forum for discussion to state regulators and managed care companies about current issues facing managed care. Formerly called the National Association of HMO Regulators (NAHMOR). **www.namcr.org**

National Bipartisan Commission on the Future of Medicare Created by Congress in the Balanced Budget Act of 1997 (BBA), it was charged with reviewing the Medicare program and making recommendations to strengthen and improve it in time for the retirement of the "baby boomers." The commission worked with the following assumptions: (1) The Medicare program is solvent for the next ten years, but then faces problems; (2) Medicare's future financial problems are real; and (3) Medicare's future is important to all Americans because they either benefit from it now or pay taxes for it now to get benefits when they retire. The commission issued its final proposal in March 1999 in three parts: (1) the design of a premium support system, (2) improvements to the current Medicare program, and (3) financing and solvency of the Medicare program. This proposal was also known as the Final **Breaux-Thomas Medicare Reform Proposal**. **medicare.commission.gov/medicare**

National Board of Medical Examiners (NBME) An independent nonprofit organization that tests and provides certification for students and graduates of U.S. and Canadian medical schools. **www.nbme.org**

National Business Coalition on Health (NBCH) A national, nonprofit membership organization of employer-based health coalitions (containing over 7,000 mid- and large-sized employers, both public and private). It promotes *value-based purchasing* and reform measures to improve the quality of care provided by employer-sponsored health plans, as well as the overall health of the community. See also *Bridges to Excellence*. **www.nbch.org**

National Cancer Institute (NCI) See under *National Institutes of Health*.

National Center for Chronic Disease Prevention and Health Promotion (NCCDPHP) See under *Coordinating Center for Health Promotion*, under *Centers for Disease Control and Prevention*.

National Center for Complementary and Alternative Medicine (NCCAM) See under *National Institutes of Health*.

National Center for Environmental Health (NCEH) See *National Center for Environmental Health/Agency for Toxic Substances and Disease Registry* under *Coordinating Center for Environmental and Occupational Health and Injury Prevention*, under *Centers for Disease Control and Prevention*.

National Center for Health Marketing (NCHM) See under *Coordinating Center for Health Information Service*, under *Centers for Disease Control and Prevention*.

National Center for Health Statistics (NCHS) See under *Coordinating Center for Health Information Service*, under *Centers for Disease Control and Prevention*.

National Center for HIV/AIDS, Viral Hepatitis, STD, and TB Prevention (NCHHSTP) See under *Coordinating Center for Infectious Diseases*, under *Centers for Disease Control and Prevention*.

National Center for Human Genome Research (NCHGR) See *National Human Genome Research Institute* under *National Institutes of Health*.

National Center for Immunization and Respiratory Diseases (NCIRD) See under *Coordinating Center for Infectious Diseases*, under *Centers for Disease Control and Prevention*.

National Center for Injury Prevention and Control (NCIPC) See under *Coordinating Center for Environmental and Occupational Health and Injury Prevention*, under *Centers for Disease Control and Prevention*.

National Center for Nursing Research See *National Institute of Nursing Research* under *National Institutes of Health*.

National Center for Preparedness, Detection, and Control of Infectious Diseases (NCP-DCID) See under *Coordinating Center for Infectious Diseases*, under *Centers for Disease Control and Prevention*.

National Center for Public Health Informatics (NCPHI) See under *Coordinating Center for Health Information Service*, under *Centers for Disease Control and Prevention*.

National Center for Research Resources (NCRR) See under *National Institutes of Health*.

National Center for Toxicological Research (NCTR) The division of the Food and Drug Administration (FDA) with the responsibility to conduct scientific research that supports and anticipates the FDA's current and future regulatory needs. This includes research aimed at understanding biological mechanisms of action underlying the toxicity of products regulated by the FDA, and developing methods to improve assessment of human exposure, susceptibility, and risk. **www.fda.gov/nctr**

National Center for Zoonotic, Vector-Borne and Enteric Diseases (NCZVED) See under *Coordinating Center for Infectious Diseases*, under *Centers for Disease Control and Prevention*.

National Center on Birth Defects and Developmental Disabilities (NCBDDD) See under *Coordinating Center for Health Promotion*, under *Centers for Disease Control and Prevention*.

National Center on Minority Health and Health Disparities (NCMHD) See under *National Institutes of Health*.

National Certification Commission for Acupuncture and Oriental Medicine (NCCAOM) A nonprofit organization established in 1982 to set standards for and certify practitioners in acupuncture and Oriental medicine. Certificates are granted in Oriental medicine, acupuncture, Chinese herbology, and Asian bodywork therapy; those certified receive the title "Diplomate." **www.nccaom.org**

National Commission for Certifying Agencies (NCCA) See *National Organization for Competency Assurance*.

National Commission to Prevent Infant Mortality (NCPIM) A Washington, DC–based organization that in the early 1990s initiated the Resource Mothers Development Project. See *MotherNet*.

National Committee for Quality Assurance (NCQA) An independent, nonprofit organization whose mission is to improve healthcare quality in managed care. It serves as an accrediting agency for managed care organizations (MCOs), preferred provider organizations (PPOs), and other organizations and programs. Accrediting and certification programs address quality, credentialing, members' rights and duties, utilization, preventive health services, and clinical records. Report cards are available at its web site to compare health plans. NCQA has a number of educational, performance measurement, and other quality improvement initiatives, including HEDIS. **www.ncqa.org**

National Committee on Vital and Health Statistics (NCVHS) An independent, nonprofit organization that serves as the statutory public advisory body to the Department of Health and Human Services (HHS) on health data, statistics, and national health information policy. Its mandate includes being a national forum on health data and information systems. It was restructured in 1996 under HIPAA to meet expanded responsibilities regarding standards for health data. **www.ncvhs.hhs.gov**

National Community Care Network Demonstration Program See *community care network*.

National Council for Prescription Drug Programs (NCPDP) A nonprofit, standards development organization (SDO) working to promote pharmacy data interchange and processing standards in the healthcare industry. Members include drug manufacturers, drug distributors, insurance carriers, prescription benefit managers, independent pharmacies, chain pharmacies, federal and state government agencies, computer companies, and consultants. The NCPDP is frequently, but erroneously, referred to as the "National Council *of* Prescription Drug Programs." It is recognized as an SDO by ANSI, and also as a Designated Standard Maintenance Organization (DSMO) by the Department of Health and Human Services (HHS) under HIPAA. See also *HCIdea and NCPDP SCRIPT*. **www.ncpdp.org**

National Council of Community Hospitals (NCCH) An association of over 150 nonprofit community hospitals and healthcare systems dedicated to the survival and increasing efficiency of community hospitals, which deliver 80% of the hospital services provided to patients in the United States. NCCH began in the mid 1970s and ended operation in the early 2000s. It was a respected source of information, drafted legislation, and had an effect on a number of legislative and regulatory activities.

National Credentialing Agency for Laboratory Personnel (NCA) A credentialing body for clinical laboratory professionals. **www.nca-info.org**

National Digital Mammography Archive (NDMA) The former name (until 2005) of the *National Digital Medical Archive*.

National Digital Medical Archive (NDMA) A system used by healthcare providers around the world to securely collect, retrieve, distribute and store digital medical images and data. NDMA provides an intelligent infrastructure platform for data management and communications, enabling the sharing of healthcare information among physicians, patients, and researchers, and providing on-demand access, visualization, and distribution of diagnostic-quality images and related clinical data, regardless of the source.

NDMA originated as the National Digital Mammography Archive, a federally funded, collaborative effort between the University of Pennsylvania, IBM, and a group at Tennessee's Oak Ridge National Laboratory to establish a computer network serving North American hospitals in an effort to foster breast cancer research. The effort utilized a technology called "grid computing," which allows widely distributed computers to work together intelligently over a very fast and reliable network (in this case the second iteration of the Internet). Going "live" in 2002, the project connected hospitals at the University of Pennsylvania, the University of Chicago, the University of North Carolina at Chapel Hill, and the Sunnybrook and Women's Hospital in Toronto, Canada. The project fostered research by allowing the sharing and analysis of digitized versions of traditional film-based x-rays. This remains something of a technical challenge, given the fact that an average digital mammogram file requires about 100 to 200 MB (megabytes) of storage space. By 2005, twenty-four hospitals could access the database, which contained over 1 million mammography images. The name was changed to more accurately describe the breadth of its breast imaging services, which extend beyond mammography to include ultrasound and breast MRI. See also *Citizens Health Portal (myNDMA)* under *portal*. **www.i3archive.com**

National Disaster Medical System (NDMS) A section within the Federal Emergency Management Agency (FEMA) that responds when a mass disaster occurs that overwhelms or destroys the disaster response resources of a local region. The NDMS includes (1) rapid medical response, (2) patient evacuation, and (3) definitive hospital care. The NDMS has several components, described below. **www.oep-ndms.dhhs.gov**

Disaster Medical Assistance Team (DMAT) A group of professional and paraprofessional medical personnel (supported by a cadre of logistical and administrative staff) organized to provide medical care during a disaster or other event. Each team has a sponsoring organization, such as a major medical center, public health or safety agency, or other nonprofit, public, or private organization that signs a Memorandum of Agreement (MOA) with the Department of Health and Human Services (HHS). The DMAT sponsor organizes the team and recruits members, arranges training, and coordinates the dispatch of the team. In addition to "standard" DMATs, there are highly specialized DMATs that deal with specific medical conditions such as crush injuries, burns, and mental health emergencies.

Once a team has been activated for response during an emergency, the U.S. Public Health Service (PHS) appoints the team members as temporary federal employees. This eliminates problems regarding interstate licensure or certification, and provides professional liability coverage for team members. The PHS provides transportation, food, supplies, shelter, and logistic support to the DMAT; compensates team members for services and expenses; and returns them to their sponsor when their work is completed.

Disaster Mortuary Operational Response Team (DMORT) Similar in operation to a *Disaster Medical Assistance Team (DMAT)* (see above), a DMORT is a group of professionals who, in a mass disaster or other emergency, provide technical assistance and personnel to recover, identify, and process deceased victims. Team members include funeral directors, medical examiners, coroners, pathologists, forensic anthropologists, medical records technicians and transcribers, fingerprint specialists, forensic odontologists, dental assistants, x-ray technicians, mental health specialists, computer professionals, administrative support staff, and security and investigative personnel.

In support of the DMORT program, the Federal Emergency Management Agency (FEMA) maintains two **Disaster Portable Morgue Units (DPMUs)** staged at FEMA Logistics Centers, one in Rockville, Maryland, and the other in San Jose, California. The DPMU is a depository of equipment and supplies for deployment to a disaster site. It contains a complete morgue with designated workstations for each processing element and prepackaged equipment and supplies.

Federal Coordinating Center (FCC) Each FCC recruits hospitals and maintains local non-federal hospital participation in the NDMS; assists in the recruitment, training, and support of DMATs; coordinates exercise development and emergency plans with participating hospitals and other local authorities in order to develop patient reception, transportation, and communication plans; and, during NDMS activation, coordinates the reception and distribution of patients being evacuated to the area.

National Nurse Response Team (NNRT) A specialty *Disaster Medical Assistance Team (DMAT)* (see above) composed of nurses who receive special training, which is used "in any scenario requiring hundreds of nurses to assist in chemoprophylaxis, a mass vaccination program, or a scenario that overwhelms the nation's supply of nurses in responding to a weapon of mass destruction event."

National Pharmacy Response Team (NPRT) A specialty *Disaster Medical Assistance Team (DMAT)* (see above) composed of pharmacists, pharmacy technicians, and students of pharmacy. NPRTs respond to assist in chemoprophylaxis or the vaccination of hundreds of thousands, or even millions of Americans, in case of emergency, or in other situations requiring their assistance.

Veterinary Medical Assistance Team (VMAT) A specialty *Disaster Medical Assistance Team (DMAT)* (see above) composed of clinical veterinarians, veterinary pathologists, animal health technicians (veterinary technicians), microbiologist/virologists, epidemiologists, toxicologists, and various scientific and support personnel. VMATs may be called upon to assist in the medical treatment and stabilization of animals in an emergency, animal disease surveillance, zoonotic disease surveillance and public health assessments, technical assistance to assure food and water quality, hazard mitigation, animal decontamination, and biological and chemical terrorism surveillance.

National Drug Code (NDC) A code maintained by the Food and Drug Administration (FDA) for identifying drugs and medications for humans. Because the NDC system was originally developed to enable reimbursement under Medicare, NDC codes are not limited to prescription drugs. The NDC is a unique ten-digit, three-segment number that identifies the labeler or vendor, the product, and the trade package size. See *identifier*. The FDA keeps an FAQ covering the directory of NDC codes at **www.fda.gov/cder/ndc**, as well as links to downloadable files containing the codes and related information. See also *unique device identifier* and *Universal Product Number* for nondrug products used in health care.

National Electronic Disease Surveillance System (NEDSS) An initiative within the Centers for Disease Control and Prevention (CDC) to promote the use of data and information system standards to advance the development of efficient, integrated, and interoperable surveillance systems at federal, state, and local levels. It is a major component of the Public Health Information Network (PHIN). The goals of NEDSS are to build systems to detect outbreaks rapidly and to monitor the health of the nation, facilitate the electronic transfer of clinical information from the healthcare system to public health departments, reduce the provider's burden in the provision of information, and enhance both the timeliness and quality of information provided. **www.cdc.gov/nedss**

National Eye Institute (NEI) See under *National Institutes of Health*.

National Fire Protection Association (NFPA) An international nonprofit organization whose mission is to reduce the worldwide burden of fire and other hazards on the quality of life by providing and advocating consensus codes and standards, research, training, and education. NFPA membership totals more than 79,000 individuals from around the world and more than 80 national trade and professional organizations. One of its efforts is the *Life Safety Code*. **www.nfpa.org**

National Formulary (NF) A publication of the United States Pharmacopeia (USP) containing recipes for the standard preparation (compounding) of medicinal drugs. See *United States Pharmacopeia—National Formulary (USP-NF)*.

National Health and Nutrition Examination Survey (NHANES) An annual national survey conducted by the National Center for Health Statistics (NCHS) for data on the health and nutritional status of the American people. It is noted for the data it provides on the prevalence of obesity.

national health care Some use this term to describe an approach to healthcare reform in which the government pays for and delivers health care. Sometimes used (inaccurately) as a synonym for the *Canadian-style system*.

National Health Corps See *National Health Service Corps*.

national health expenditures (NHE) An economic indicator to show what the United States spends on health care each year. It is usually expressed as a percentage of the *gross domestic product (GDP)*. The NHE is the sum total of all healthcare expenditures, including physician and hospital services, drugs, home nursing care, eyeglasses, dental services, and so forth, as well as administrative costs, construction, and research. The NHE for 1993 was $940 billion, equal to about 14% of the GDP. In 2004 total spending was $1.9 trillion, or $6,280 per person, amounting to 16% of the GDP.

National Health Information Center (NHIC) A health information referral service that puts health professionals and consumers who have health questions in touch with those organizations that are best able to provide answers. NHIC also provides key support for *healthfinder*. NHIC was established in 1979 by the Office of Disease Prevention and Health Promotion (ODPHP). **www.health.gov/nhic**

National Health Information Infrastructure (NHII) The framework required to facilitate the secure exchange of health information throughout the United States. This concept evolved to the *Nationwide Health Information Network (NHIN)*.

National Health Information Network (NHIN) Original name of the *Nationwide Health Information Network*.

national health insurance A federally established and operated system of healthcare financing encompassing all (or nearly all) citizens. Such a system, not in effect in the United States, would provide uniform benefits to all and be paid for via taxes. Distinguish this from *national health service*, in which the government is not only the payer, as here, but also the provider. This term encompasses "socialized medicine."

National Health Interview Survey (NHIS) A survey conducted annually by the National Center for Health Statistics (NCHS) to obtain information on access to health care, insurance, incidence of illness and injury, disability, utilization of services, health-related behaviors, and so forth. Sample households are selected, and face-to-face interviews conducted. It is the principal source of information on the health of the civilian noninstitutionalized population of the United States and is one of the major data collection programs of the NCHS. The interview instrument is revised every ten to fifteen years, most recently in 1997. It has been conducted since established by the National Health Survey Act in 1957. **www.cdc.gov/nchs/nhis.htm**

National Health Plan Identifier (NPlanID) A unique identifier, similar to the *National Provider Identifier (NPI)*, required by HIPAA to identify *health plans* that are *covered entities*.

national health service An approach to healthcare reform in which the government actually *owns* the hospitals and employs the physicians, thereby becoming the provider of health services. This is distinguished from national health insurance, in which the government is the sole payer, but not provider. Sometimes called nationalized health care.

National Health Service (NHS) An organization created by the United Kingdom in 1948 to provide health care for all of its citizens. Its core principles are the "provision of quality care that: (1) meets the needs of everyone, (2) is free at the point of need, and (3) is based on a patient's clinical need not their ability to pay." The NHS has been in place since 1948. It is funded by the taxpayers and is accountable to Parliament. **www.nhs.uk**

National Health Service Corps (NHSC) A federal program to provide financial assistance for persons who are preparing for health professions (medical, dental, and nursing), and in return obligating them to serve in areas where there is a shortage of health professionals. They are placed by the U.S. Public Health Service. Also known as the "National Health Corps" or simply "The Corps." Financial assistance to students is available via the National

Health Service Corps Scholarship Program. The program was established in 1970 by the Emergency Health Personnel Act (Pub. L. No. 91-623, 84 Stat. 1868). **nhsc.bhpr.hrsa.gov**

National Health Survey See *National Health Interview Survey*.

National Heart, Lung, and Blood Institute (NHLBI) See under *National Institutes of Health*.

National Highway Transportation Safety Administration (NHTSA) The federal agency, within the Department of Transportation (DOT), that is responsible for reducing deaths, injuries, and economic losses resulting from motor vehicle crashes. NHTSA sets and enforces safety standards for motor vehicle equipment, and funds efforts by local and state governments to improve highway safety. In recent years NHTSA has been active with such automotive safety issues as drunk driving, seat belt usage, air bags, child restraints, and the sometimes well-publicized automotive "recalls." Established by the Highway Safety Act of 1970 as the successor to the National Highway Safety Bureau. Often referred to by its acronym sounded out like "nitsa." **www.nhtsa.gov**

National Hospital Discharge Survey (NHDS) An annual national survey conducted by the National Center for Health Statistics (NCHS) for data on the characteristics of inpatients discharged from nonfederal short-stay hospitals in the United States.

National Hospital Indicator Survey (NHIS) A quarterly nationally representative panel survey to evaluate hospital financial and utilization data, for use in national policy making. The survey was commissioned by CMS and the Medicare Payment Advisory Commission (MedPAC), and is conducted by the American Hospital Association (AHA) in collaboration with The Lewin Group, a national healthcare and human services consulting firm. NHIS surveys nearly 1,900 community (for-profit and nonprofit) hospitals throughout the United States.

National Hospital Quality Measures (NHQM) A set of *performance measures*, adopted by the *Hospital Quality Alliance (HQA)*, used by hospitals to voluntarily report their performance to CMS. By 2007, about twenty standardized measures had been approved by HQA and endorsed by the National Quality Forum (NQF). These measures are identical to the National Quality Improvement Goals (NQIGs) (see *performance measure*) developed by the Joint Commission on Accreditation of Healthcare Organizations (JCAHO). They include ten "starter set" indicators initiated in 2004. The measures have gone through years of extensive testing for validity and reliability by CMS and its quality improvement organizations (QIOs), JCAHO, HQA, and researchers. The goal is for the NHQMs to eventually be reported by all hospitals and accepted by all purchasers, oversight and accrediting entities, payers, and providers.

Examples of measures include aspirin on arrival for acute myocardial infarction (AMI) patients, beta blocker on arrival for those same patients, left ventricular function assessment for heart failure patients, initial antibiotic received within four hours of hospital arrival for patients with pneumonia, smoking cessation counseling for all of these patients, and prophylactic antibiotic received within one hour prior to surgical incision for all surgical patients to prevent surgical infections.

A current use of the NHQMs is to inform consumers about hospital quality via the *Hospital Compare* web site. Also, the Medicare Modernization Act (MMA) required hospitals paid under the inpatient prospective payment system (IPPS) to submit NHQM data to CMS to receive their full Medicare payment updates. Synonym: Hospital Quality Measures (HQMs). See also *National Patient Safety Goals*, *pay-for-performance*, and *transparency initiative*.

National Human Genome Research Institute (NHGRI) See under *National Institutes of Health*.

National Information Center for Health Services Administration (NICHSA) A special resource, based in Chicago, created to support the information needs of its participating members: the American College of Healthcare Executives (ACHE), the American Health Information Management Association (AHIMA), and the American Hospital Association (AHA). The NICHSA ceased operations in 2003.

National Institute for Occupational Safety and Health (NIOSH) See under *Centers for Disease Control and Prevention*.

National Institute of Standards and Technology (NIST) An agency of the U.S. Department of Commerce (DOC), founded in 1901 as the nation's first federal physical science research laboratory. Examples of NIST's research and development areas include image processing, DNA diagnostic "chips," smoke detectors, atomic clocks, x-ray standards for mammography, scanning tunneling microscopy, pollution-control technology, and high-speed dental drills. NIST's Advanced Technology Program (ATP) involves partnerships with the private sector to accelerate development of "innovative technologies that promise significant commercial payoffs and widespread benefits for the nation." One major ATP is aimed at building an "Information Infrastructure for Healthcare." NIST is the sponsor of the *HealthCare Standards Landscape (HCSL)*. **www.nist.gov**

National Institutes of Health (NIH) The nation's premier biomedical research organization, the NIH is an agency within the Department of Health and Human Services (HHS). Based in Bethesda, Maryland, NIH is composed of twenty-eight separate institutes and centers. The institutes carry out research and programs related to certain specific types of diseases, such as mental and neurological disease, arthritis, cancer, and heart disease. There is an institute for each of the categories of disease for which NIH has programs, and a number of other components not specific to any disease categories (see individual listings below). **www.nih.gov**

Center for Information Technology (CIT) A non-disease-specific component of NIH concerned with incorporating modern computer technology into the biomedical research and administrative procedures of the NIH. CIT also serves as a technological resource for the Public Health Service and other federal agencies with biomedical and computing needs. **www.cit.nih.gov**

Center for Scientific Review (CSR) A non-disease-specific component of NIH concerned with the receipt, referral, review, award, and administration of grant applications and research contracts in areas covered by the NIH. CSR also assigns NIH applications to supporting institutes and centers and to CSR integrated review groups, and provides for scientific review of most NIH research grants and Individual National Research Service Awards (Fellowships). CSR receives over 80,000 grant applications per year. Formerly called the Division of Research Grants (DRG). **www.csr.nih.gov**

Clinical Center (CC) The research hospital for the NIH, designed to bring facilities for patient care right next to research labs so that newly developed knowledge and technology could be quickly applied to the treatment of real patients (translational research or "bench-to-bedside"). The Clinical Center consists of two main facilities. The original facility is the **Warren Grant Magnuson Clinical Center**, opened in 1953. It has 14 stories and 7 million bricks, more than 5,000 rooms, 9 miles of corridor, 2.5 million square feet, 15 outpatient clinics, and a Laboratory Medicine Department housed in a space the size of a football field. The **Mark O. Hatfield Clinical Research Center**, finished in 2004, has 870,000 square feet, 242 inpatient beds, and 90 day-hospital stations. The Clinical Center has over 1,600 laboratories that conduct basic and clinical research. In the mid-2000s, the Clinical Center had approximately 7,000 inpatient admissions and over 100,000 outpatient visits annually.

All patients must be referred by their physicians, and must have the precise kind or stage of illness under investigation. There are no labor and delivery services, and no other services common to community hospitals. Areas of clinical study include aging; alcohol abuse and alcoholism; allergy, arthritis, and musculoskeletal and skin diseases; cancer; child health; chronic pain; deafness and other communication disorders; dental and orofacial disorders; diabetes; digestive and kidney diseases; eye disorders; heart, lung, and blood diseases; infectious diseases; medical genetics; mental health; neurological disorders; and stroke. **www.cc.nih.gov**

John E. Fogarty International Center (FIC) A non-disease-specific component of NIH concerned with promoting international cooperation in all aspects of the health sciences.

It serves as the liaison to the World Health Organization (WHO), Pan American Health Organization, European Medical Research Councils, and other organizations. The center was created in 1968 and named after the late Congressman from Rhode Island. Its full name is the John E. Fogarty International Center for Advanced Study in the Health Sciences. **www.fic.nih.gov**

Mark O. Hatfield Clinical Research Center See *Clinical Center*, above.

National Cancer Institute (NCI) The first NIH institute to be created for dealing with a specific illness or disease. The NCI was established by the National Cancer Act of 1937 and has had its scope broadened by subsequent legislation. The NCI now supports a national network of cancer centers, funds its own and others' research and training, and helps incorporate state-of-the-art cancer treatment into clinical practice. Also, the NCI provides information about cancer and its treatment to the public through its web site. **www.cancer.gov**

National Center for Complementary and Alternative Medicine (NCCAM) The NIH institute concerned with scientific research into and dissemination of information on *complementary and alternative medicine (CAM)*. Congress established NCCAM in 1998 to investigate CAM and support research into which CAM practices work, which do not, and why. Its mission is to give the U.S. public reliable information about the safety and effectiveness of CAM practices. **nccam.nih.gov**

National Center for Research Resources (NCRR) A non-disease-specific component of NIH that creates, develops, and provides a comprehensive range of human, animal, technological, and other resources to enable biomedical research advances. Its support is concentrated in four areas: clinical research, biomedical technology, comparative medicine, and research infrastructure. **www.ncrr.nih.gov**

National Center on Minority Health and Health Disparities (NCMHD) A non-disease-specific component of NIH that works to promote minority health and eliminate health disparities. The NCMHD conducts and supports research, fosters emerging programs, disseminates information, and offers support to minority and other health disparity communities. The NCMHD was established in 2000; its predecessor was the Office of Research on Minority Health (ORMH), established in 1990. **ncmhd.nih.gov**

National Eye Institute (NEI) The NIH institute concerned with blinding eye diseases, visual disorders, and the special health needs of the visually impaired or blind. Begun in 1968, NEI supports vision research through approximately 1,600 research grants and training awards made to scientists at more than 250 medical centers, hospitals, universities, and other institutions across the country and around the world. The NEI also conducts laboratory and patient-oriented research at its own facilities located on the NIH campus in Bethesda, Maryland. **www.nei.nih.gov**

National Heart, Lung, and Blood Institute (NHLBI) The NIH institute concerned with diseases of the heart, blood vessels, lungs, blood and blood resources, and sleep disorders. This institute, the second oldest, came into being as the National Heart Institute with the passage of the National Health Act of 1948. It administers the *Framingham Heart Study*. From October 1997 until 2006, the NHLBI also had administrative responsibility for the NIH Woman's Health Initiative, a 15-year study beginning in 1991 that focused on the major causes of death, disability, and frailty in postmenopausal women. **www.nhlbi.nih.gov**

National Human Genome Research Institute (NHGRI) A non-disease-specific NIH institute concerned with the structure and function of the human genome and its role in health and disease. NHGRI was originally established in 1989 as the National Center for Human Genome Research (NCHGR), with the original mission of heading the NIH contribution to the *Human Genome Project (HGP)*. In 1993, NCHGR expanded its role by establishing the Division of Intramural Research (DIR) to apply genome technologies to the study of specific diseases. In 1996, the Center for Inherited Disease Research (CIDR) was established (co-funded by eight NIH institutes and centers) to study the genetic components of complex disorders. In 1997, the center received the new name and status as an institute. **www.genome.gov**

National Institute of Allergy and Infectious Diseases (NIAID) The NIH institute concerned with developing better ways to diagnose, treat, and prevent infectious, immunologic, and allergic diseases. **www3.niaid.nih.gov**

National Institute of Arthritis and Musculoskeletal and Skin Diseases (NIAMS) The NIH institute that supports research into the causes, treatment, and prevention of diseases of the bones, joints, skin, and muscle. **www.niams.nih.gov**

National Institute of Biomedical Imaging and Bioengineering (NIBIB) A non-disease-specific NIH institute devoted to merging the physical and biological sciences to develop new technologies that improve health. **www.nibib.nih.gov**

National Institute of Child Health and Human Development (NICHD) The NIH institute concerned with the reproductive, neurobiologic, developmental, social, and behavioral processes that determine and maintain the health of children, adults, families, and populations. Among its activities, the NICHD funds and coordinates the U.S. component of an international study, "Health Behavior in School-Aged Children." This study, released every four years by the World Health Organization (WHO), compares such behaviors as alcohol and tobacco consumption, exercise, and general eating habits. **www.nichd.nih.gov**

National Institute of Dental and Craniofacial Research (NIDCR) The NIH institute concerned with oral, dental, and craniofacial health. **www.nidcr.nih.gov**

National Institute of Diabetes and Digestive and Kidney Diseases (NIDDK) The NIH institute supporting research encompassing the broad spectrum of metabolic diseases such as diabetes, inborn errors of metabolism, endocrine disorders, mineral metabolism, digestive diseases, nutrition, urology and renal disease, and hematology. **www2.niddk.nih.gov**

National Institute of Environmental Health Sciences (NIEHS) The NIH institute whose mission is to reduce illness and dysfunction resulting from environmental causes. This institute conducts multidisciplinary biomedical research aimed at increasing the understanding of how environmental factors, individual susceptibility, and age interact to result in human illness. **www.niehs.nih.gov**

NIEHS also houses the **National Toxicology Program (NTP)** of the Department of Health and Human Services (HHS). NTP works with other federal agencies, including the Food and Drug Administration's (FDA's) National Center for Toxicological Research, and the Centers for Disease Control and Prevention's (CDC's) National Institute for Occupational Safety and Health (NIOSH). The NTP coordinates toxicology research and testing, and provides information to health and regulatory agencies and to the public. **ntp.niehs.nih.gov**

National Institute of General Medical Sciences (NIGMS) The NIH institute concerned with basic biomedical research that is not targeted to specific diseases, but to a better understanding of life processes and how this can result in better disease diagnosis, treatment, and prevention. **www.nigms.nih.gov**

National Institute of Mental Health (NIMH) The NIH institute dedicated to research focused on understanding, treatment, and prevention of mental disorders and the promotion of mental health. **www.nimh.nih.gov**

National Institute of Neurological Disorders and Stroke (NINDS) The NIH institute concerned with biomedical research on disorders of the brain and nervous system. **www.ninds.nih.gov**

National Institute of Nursing Research (NINR) A non-disease-specific component of NIH that supports nursing research. Areas of research include chronic and acute diseases, health promotion and maintenance, symptom management, health disparities, caregiving, self-management, and the end of life. Formerly the National Center for Nursing Research. **www.ninr.nih.gov**

National Institute on Aging (NIA) The NIH institute concerned with geriatrics and all issues related to the aging process. Congress has designated the NIA as the primary federal agency on Alzheimer's disease research. **www.nia.nih.gov**

National Institute on Alcohol Abuse and Alcoholism (NIAAA) The NIH institute concerned with the causes, consequences, treatment, and prevention of alcoholism and alcohol-related problems. **www.niaaa.nih.gov**

National Institute on Deafness and Other Communication Disorders (NIDCD) The NIH institute concerned with the special health needs of the hearing impaired and those with other communication disorders, other than vision. NIDCD supports research in the normal and disordered processes of hearing, balance, smell, taste, voice, speech, and language. **www.nidcd.nih.gov**

National Institute on Drug Abuse (NIDA) The NIH institute that supports research on drug abuse and addiction. NIDA research extends from the molecule to managed care, and from DNA to community outreach research. Established in 1974, NIDA became part of NIH in 1992. **www.nida.nih.gov**

National Library of Medicine (NLM) A non-disease-specific component of NIH, located on the NIH campus in Bethesda, Maryland, that is the world's largest library dealing with a single scientific topic. As of 2007, the NLM contained more than 2.5 million volumes and more than 6 million other physical items, including manuscripts, microforms, pictures, audiovisuals, and electronic media. NLM has extensive information available online via services such as *MEDLINE*. The NLM is, among other things, concerned with improving the nation's medical library system; it is the hub of the *National Network of Libraries of Medicine (NN/LM)*. The NLM also maintains the *Unified Medical Language System (UMLS)*. See also *NLM Gateway*. **www.nlm.nih.gov**

Office of the Director (OD) The central administrative and management office within the NIH. The OD is also the umbrella for many other departments, including the NIH Office of Disease Prevention (ODP), Office of AIDS Research (OAR), Office of Research Services (ORS), Office of Technology Transfer (OTT), Office of Legislative Policy and Analysis (OLPA), and many others. **www.nih.gov/icd/od**

Warren Grant Magnuson Clinical Center (CC) See *Clinical Center*, above.

National Institutes of Health Consensus Development Program A program operated since 1977 by the NIH Office of Medical Applications of Research (OMAR) to produce evidence-based consensus statements addressing controversial issues in medicine. Topics must meet three criteria: (1) public health importance, (2) controversy or a gap between current knowledge and practice, and (3) an adequately defined and available base of scientific information. Some recent topics are tobacco use, cesarean delivery on maternal request, management of menopause-related symptoms, improving end-of-life care, preventing violence and related health-risking social behaviors in adolescents, and total knee replacements.

OMAR, along with one or more NIH institutes or centers, sponsors a conference bringing together a panel of experts that is independent, non-Department of Health and Human Services (non-HHS) related, broad based, and having no scientific or financial conflicts of interest. There are two types of conferences. "Consensus Conferences" are held when there is a strong body of higher-quality evidence (randomized trials, well-designed observational studies) and it is reasonable to expect that the panel will be able to give clinical direction. "State-of-the-Science" conferences are held when the evidence base is weaker and the sponsoring NIH institute or center is seeking the panel's opinion on future research and priorities.

OMAR prepares a number of questions on the topic, and the Agency for Healthcare Research and Quality (AHRQ) prepares a systematic literature review for use by the panel. During the first day and a half of the conference, the panel listens to scientific data presented by invited experts and comments from the general public. It then prepares a statement addressing the questions. This is called a "Consensus Statement" or "State-of-the-Science Statement" (formerly known as a "Technology Assessment Statement"), and is circulated on the third day of the conference for comment from the audience. The revised statement is released at the end of the conference, and disseminated widely to healthcare practitioners, policymakers, the media, and the general public. The statement is an independent report and is not a policy statement of the NIH or the federal government. **consensus.nih.gov**

National Institutes of Health Technology Assessment Statements See *National Institutes of Health Consensus Development Program*.

nationalized health care See *national health service*.

nationalized health insurance See *national health insurance*.

National League for Nursing (NLN) A national organization whose purpose is to advance excellence in nursing education that prepares the nursing work force to meet the needs of diverse populations in an ever-changing healthcare environment. It is a membership organization of individuals and of agencies, and includes nurses, related professionals, and consumers. NLN's subsidiary, the National League for Nursing Accrediting Commission (NLNAC), is the official accrediting agency for schools of nursing (professional and vocational). **www.nln.org**

National Library of Medicine (NLM) See under *National Institutes of Health*.

National Medical Association (NMA) A national nonprofit professional and scientific organization, founded in 1895, representing over 25,000 African American physicians and their patients in the United States. The NMA is committed to (1) preventing the diseases, disabilities, and adverse health conditions that disproportionately or differentially impact persons of African descent and underserved populations; (2) supporting efforts that improve the quality and availability of health care to underserved populations; and (3) increasing the representation, preservation, and contribution(s) of persons of African descent in medicine. **www.nmanet.org**

National Network of Libraries of Medicine (NN/LM) A program directed by the National Library of Medicine (NLM) to provide equal access to biomedical information to all U.S. health professionals and improve the public's access to health information. The NN/LM consists of a nationwide network of health science libraries and information centers, including approximately 4,762 primary access libraries (PALs) (mostly in hospitals), 159 resource libraries (at medical schools), and eight regional medical libraries (RMLs) (major institutions under contract with the NLM). Formerly the Regional Medical Library Program. **www.nnlm.gov**

National Nurse Response Team (NNRT) See under *National Disaster Medical System*.

National Nutrient Database See *USDA National Nutrient Database for Standard Reference*.

National Office of Public Health Genomics (NOPHG) See under *Coordinating Center for Health Promotion*, under *Centers for Disease Control and Prevention*.

National Organization for Competency Assurance (NOCA) A national organization established in 1977 that sets quality standards for organizations that grant credentials. Its accrediting body is the National Commission for Certifying Agencies (NCCA). **www.noca.org**

National Patient Identifier (NPI) A concept that was proposed in the original HIPAA objectives, similar to the National Provider Identifier (also NPI), in which patients would be given, in essence, a national identification number for use in electronic health information networks. The idea has been rejected so far, due in part to concerns about privacy and identity theft. Instead, patient indexing systems have been developed and used in which a combination of identifying elements—such as name, date of birth, gender, and address—are linked to establish and authenticate a patient's identity. As of 2007, a national standard for patient authentication has yet to be developed. See also *record locator service*.

National Patient Safety Goals (NPSGs) Recommendations developed by the Joint Commission on Accreditation of Healthcare Organizations (JCAHO) for accredited healthcare organizations to implement to reduce errors and accidents in patient care. Hospitals are required by JCAHO to report on their progress in addressing issues of communication among caregivers, misidentification of patients, surgery on the wrong body part, and so forth. Each year, some goals may be "retired" (actually, they usually remain as accreditation standards) if compliance has been good, and others put on the NPSG list so that the most important safety goals are spotlighted. Results of hospitals' compliance are published online at Quality Check; see **Quality Reports**. See also **National Hospital Quality Measures** and **patient safety**.

National Payer ID An *identifier* assigned by CMS to an organization that pays for healthcare services. Synonyms: Health Plan ID, Plan ID; formerly called PAYERID. A payer that is also a provider, such as a managed care organization (MCO), is additionally assigned another, but different, identifier known as a **National Provider Identifier (NPI)**.

National Pharmacy Response Team (NPRT) See under **National Disaster Medical System**.

National Plan and Provider Enumeration System (NPPES) See **National Provider Identifier**.

National Practitioner Data Bank (NPDB) A clearinghouse for information on disciplinary and malpractice actions against physicians created by the Health Care Quality Improvement Act (HCQIA) of 1986, which went into operation in 1990. The act requires that the following actions must be reported to the data bank (NPDB): (1) an insurance company (or other entity) that makes a payment on a malpractice claim (whether in settlement or pursuant to a court decision), (2) a state board of medical examiners that imposes a sanction on a physician, and (3) a healthcare entity (such as a hospital) that takes a professional review action adversely affecting a physician's privileges for more than thirty days. Eligible parties may then inquire of the NPDB for information about a particular physician; for example, a hospital may inquire prior to granting privileges. If a hospital fails to comply with the reporting requirements, it loses for three years the protection it would otherwise have under the act. **www.npdb-hipdb.com**

National Provider File (NPF) An early name for the database created by the National Plan and Provider Enumeration System (NPPES). See **National Provider Identifier**.

National Provider Identifier (NPI) A unique ten-digit number permanently assigned to a healthcare provider. HIPAA requires that NPIs be implemented as part of the standards for electronic transactions. All covered entities (providers that transmit electronic health information) must have an NPI. All other providers including individuals (such as physicians, dentists, pharmacists) and organizations (e.g., hospitals, pharmacies, group practices, laboratories, ambulatory care facilities, nursing homes) may obtain an NPI if they wish. Some entities who are not covered entities may need an NPI if they are referred to in electronic transactions of covered entities.

The NPI number is "intelligence-free," meaning that it does not carry information about the provider, such as its location (state) or specialty. It is assigned to providers by the **NPI Enumerator**, a company (Fox Systems, Inc.) with whom CMS has contracted to provide this service. A provider who has been assigned an NPI is said to be **enumerated**. Application for an NPI can be made on paper and sent by mail, done online through a web-based process, or submitted electronically. CMS calls the administrative system the **National Plan and Provider Enumeration System (NPPES)** (**nppes.cms.hhs.gov**). See also **National Health Plan Identifier**.

The NPI came about as a result of efforts begun in 1993 by HCFA (now CMS) to develop a provider identification system to meet Medicare and Medicaid needs. A workgroup learned that some existing identifiers, such as the Employer Identification Number (EIN), the Social Security Number (SSN), and the Drug Enforcement Administration (DEA) number, were not appropriate for identification of *all* healthcare providers. Other identifiers, such as the National Supplier Clearinghouse number and the Unique Physician Identification Number (UPIN), applied only to some providers, while others, such as the Medicare provider number assigned to certified (typically institutional) providers, had a format that would not accommodate enough healthcare providers. Additionally, some existing identifiers, such as the Health Industry Number (HIN) (see Health Industry Business Communications Council) could not be used because they were proprietary. The Final Rule about NPIs was issued by CMS in 2004.

National Provider Registry (NPR) An early name for the NPI Enumerator. See **National Provider Identifier**.

National Provider System (NPS) An early name for the National Plan and Provider Enumeration System (NPPES). See *National Provider Identifier*.

National Quality Alliance Steering Committee (NQASC) See *Quality Alliance Steering Committee*.

National Quality Forum (NQF) A private, nonprofit membership organization created to develop and implement a national strategy for healthcare quality measurement and reporting. The NQF attempts to bring about national change to improve patient outcomes, increase workforce productivity, and reduce healthcare costs.

The NQF is a voluntary consensus standards–setting organization and has a formal process by which it achieves consensus on standards that it endorses. Through 2006, NQF had endorsed more than 300 measures, indicators, events, practices, and other products to help assess and improve quality across the healthcare continuum. See, for example, *AQA*, *30 Safe Practices*, and *National Hospital Quality Measures*. NQF endorsement is considered the "gold standard" for the measurement of healthcare quality.

The NQF is governed by a twenty-five-member board of directors representing healthcare consumers, purchasers, providers, health plans, and experts in health services research. The board also includes representatives from two federal agencies, CMS and the Agency for Healthcare Research and Quality (AHRQ). Formerly called the National Forum for Health Care Quality Measurement and Reporting. **www.qualityforum.org**

National Quality Improvement Goals (NQIGs) See *performance measure*.

National Quality Measures Clearinghouse (NQMC) A public repository for evidence-based performance measures and measure sets, sponsored by the Agency for Healthcare Research and Quality (AHRQ). The database includes structured, standardized abstracts (summaries) containing information about measures and their development; a utility for comparing attributes of two or more measures in a side-by-side comparison; and links to full-text measures (when available) and/or ordering details for the full measure. **www.qualitymeasures.ahrq.gov**

National Research Corporation (NRC) A major provider of survey-based, healthcare performance measurement services, established in 1981 and headquartered in Lincoln, Nebraska. **www.nationalresearch.com**

National Research Council (NRC) One of the four organizations in the U.S. National Academies, the NRC carries out research for the National Academy of Sciences (NAS) and the National Academy of Engineering (NAE). It is administered jointly by NAS, NAE, and the Institute of Medicine (IOM). **www.nas.edu/nrc**

National Resident Matching Program (NRMP) A private, nonprofit corporation that matches medical students to residency programs. Results are announced in the third week of March. Sponsored by the American Board of Medical Specialties (ABMS), American Medical Association (AMA), Association of American Medical Colleges (AAMC), American Hospital Association (AHA), and Council of Medical Specialty Societies (CMSS). **www.nrmp.org**

National Response Plan (NRP) See *Federal Emergency Management Agency*.

National Science Foundation (NSF) An independent federal agency created in 1950 to promote the progress of science; advance the national health, prosperity, and welfare; and secure the national defense. The NSF is dedicated to the support of education and fundamental research in all scientific and engineering disciplines. Its mission is to ensure that the United States maintains leadership in scientific discovery and the development of new technologies. The NSF is the funding source for approximately 20% of all federally supported basic research conducted by the nation's colleges and universities. **www.nsf.gov**

National Technical Information Service (NTIS) An agency of the U.S. Department of Commerce that is the central source of scientific, technical, engineering, and related business information produced by or for the federal government. Related and complementary material from international sources is also available. In 2007, the NTIS had information on more than 600,000 information products covering over 350 subject areas from over 200 federal agencies. **www.ntis.gov**

National Toxicology Program (NTP) See *National Institute of Environmental Health Sciences* under *National Institutes of Health*.

National Uniform Billing Committee (NUBC) A consortium of healthcare providers, payers, administrative agencies, and other interested parties that seeks uniformity and standards in the way that healthcare services and products are billed by institutional (hospital) providers. The NUBC developed the Uniform Billing Code of 1982 (UB-82), Uniform Billing Code of 1992 (UB-92), and UB-04 billing form. These are government-approved forms for institutional use in submitting bills to a third-party payer. The forms provide sufficient information on each patient admission to allow a detailed review of what healthcare services and products were provided to the patient; see *UB-04*. **www.nubc.org**

National Uniform Claim Committee (NUCC) An organization that includes representatives from key provider and payer organizations, as well as standards development organizations, state and federal regulators, and the National Uniform Billing Committee (NUBC). It is chaired by the American Medical Association (AMA) and includes CMS as an important partner. This organization develops and supports the *National Uniform Claim Committee Data Set (NUCC-DS)* (see under *data set*).

The NUCC was designated in the administrative simplification section of HIPAA as one of the organizations to be consulted by the *ANSI* accredited standards development organizations, and the Secretary of the Department of Health and Human Services (HHS) as they develop, adopt, or modify national standards for healthcare transactions. **www.nucc.org**

National Uniform Claim Committee Data Set (NUCC-DS) See under *data set*.

National Vital Statistics System (NVSS) A system of the National Center for Health Statistics (NCHS) that contains the nation's official *vital statistics*. **www.cdc.gov/nchs/nvss.htm**

National Voluntary Hospital Reporting Initiative (NVHRI) The former name of the *Hospital Quality Alliance*.

National Wellness Institute (NWI) A self-supporting, nonprofit organization founded in 1977 to provide services and resources to health promotion and wellness professionals (not consumers). Two major NWI programs are the National Wellness Conference (held annually in Stevens Point, Wisconsin) and the TestWell Wellness Assessments (information at **www.testwell.org**). **www.nationalwellness.org**

Nationwide Health Information Network (NHIN) A national network to link disparate healthcare information systems to allow patients, physicians, hospitals, public health agencies, and other authorized users to share clinical and other healthcare information in real-time under stringent security, privacy, and other protections. The NHIN would not involve a central database of information, but rather allow appropriate access to information stored in a variety of locations, such as providers' offices, hospitals, organizational and government web sites, and population health databases (see also *independent health record bank*). The network requires nationwide interoperability among electronic health record systems (EHRS) and other healthcare information sources, such as public health databases (see *Patient Medical Record Information*). Such a system would make critical patient information instantly available to any emergency department or doctor's office anywhere in the United States, and would facilitate telemedicine.

The "building blocks" of the NHIN are the *regional health information organizations (RHIOs)*. The initiative is under the direction of the Office of the National Coordinator for Health Information Technology (ONC). It was originally called the National Health Information Network (and in earlier discussions, the National Health Information Infrastructure (NHII)). **www.os.dhhs.gov/healthit/nhin.html**

natural death act Legislation governing procedures by which a competent person can execute an ***advance directive*** concerning the withholding or withdrawal of life-sustaining treatment, in case of incompetence. Most states have such a law. See also ***right to die***.

natural history See under *history*.

natural language The spoken or written words actually used by people in health care—by both those treating and those being treated. They will draw these words from their "native" language (e.g., English, Spanish, Estonian), the "common" language (English in most U.S. hospitals), their learning, their culture, their experiences, and their beliefs.

Natural language is how people express themselves, every day, as a natural part of who they are. When health professionals record information in the medical record (whether directly in writing or by dictation), they will use their natural language to the extent possible. This is how they have learned to express themselves. Health professionals will use, in addition to natural language, special language learned in studying health care. Patients will use their own natural language, which may include a vast vocabulary, or be very limited in ways, to express their feelings and symptoms. They will not necessarily "speak the same language" as the caregiver.

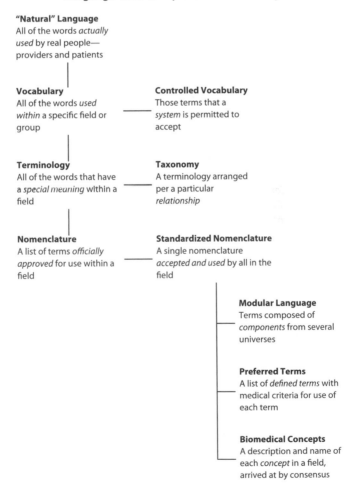

NATURAL LANGUAGE
Language Used to Express Clinical Concepts

"Natural" Language
All of the words *actually used* by real people—providers and patients

Vocabulary
All of the words *used within* a specific field or group

Controlled Vocabulary
Those terms that a *system* is permitted to accept

Terminology
All of the words that have a *special meaning* within a field

Taxonomy
A terminology arranged per a particular *relationship*

Nomenclature
A list of terms *officially approved* for use within a field

Standardized Nomenclature
A single nomenclature *accepted and used* by all in the field

Modular Language
Terms composed of *components* from several universes

Preferred Terms
A list of *defined terms* with medical criteria for use of each term

Biomedical Concepts
A description and name of each *concept* in a field, arrived at by consensus

natural language processing (NLP) The use of computer programs to analyze free-form text and determine its meaning. In health care, such programs are being developed to assist in identifying and coding of such data as diagnoses and elements of physicians' notes. A word search program can find words and terms (sets of words taken together), but cannot take into account the meanings of the words or terms in context and the sentence structure—functions attempted by NLP software. For example, NLP should be able to detect whether a diagnostic term, such as "shortness of breath," was a statement made by the patient or a conclusion of the physician. In one study, NLP software currently in development, although not identifying precisely the diagnosis entity in most cases, succeeded in placing 60% to 70% of the diagnoses in the categories of ICD-9-CM where a human would have placed them. Thus, for billing coding, NLP would have been satisfactory 60% to 70% of the time.

naturally occurring retirement community (NORC) Basically, an area where "a lot of older people are living." In connection with the concept of *aging in place*, the term was coined in the 1980s by researchers at the University of Wisconsin-Madison to refer to areas that attracted, but had not been planned for, older immigrants. NORC has come to mean any building or neighborhood where a disproportionate number of residents are over age sixty.

naturopathic physician (ND or NMD) A health professional who has completed a certifying program in naturopathy. Some states require licensure.

naturopathy See under *medicine (system)*.

NBCH See *National Business Coalition on Health*.

NBME See *National Board of Medical Examiners*.

NCA See *National Credentialing Agency for Laboratory Personnel*.

NCAC See *National Certified Addiction Counselor* under *addiction counselor*.

NCBDDD See *National Center on Birth Defects and Developmental Disabilities* under *Coordinating Center for Health Promotion*, under *Centers for Disease Control and Prevention*.

NCC See *National Certified Counselor* under *counselor*.

NCCA National Commission for Certifying Agencies. See *National Organization for Competency Assurance*.

NCCAM See *National Center for Complementary and Alternative Medicine* under *National Institutes of Health*.

NCCAOM See *National Certification Commission for Acupuncture and Oriental Medicine*.

NCCDPHP See *National Center for Chronic Disease Prevention and Health Promotion* under *Coordinating Center for Health Promotion*, under *Centers for Disease Control and Prevention*.

NCCH See *National Council of Community Hospitals*.

NCEH See *National Center for Environmental Health/Agency for Toxic Substances and Disease Registry* under *Coordinating Center for Environmental Health and Injury Prevention*, under *Centers for Disease Control and Prevention*.

NCGC See *National Certified Gambling Counselor* under *gambling counselor*.

NCHGR National Center for Human Genome Research. See *National Human Genome Research Institute* under *National Institutes of Health*.

NCHHSTP See *National Center for HIV/AIDS, Viral Hepatitis, STD, and TB Prevention* under *Coordinating Center for Infectious Diseases*, under *Centers for Disease Control and Prevention*.

NCHM See *National Center for Health Marketing* under *Coordinating Center for Health Information Service*, under *Centers for Disease Control and Prevention*.

NCHS See *National Center for Health Statistics* under *Coordinating Center for Health Information Service*, under *Centers for Disease Control and Prevention*.

NCI See *National Cancer Institute* under *National Institutes of Health*.

NCIPC See *National Center for Injury Prevention and Control* under *Coordinating Center for Environmental Health and Injury Prevention*, under *Centers for Disease Control and Prevention*.

NCIRD See *National Center for Immunization and Respiratory Diseases* under *Coordinating Center for Infectious Diseases*, under *Centers for Disease Control and Prevention*.

NCLC See *Board Certified Contact Lens Technician* under *contact lens technician*.

NCLC-AC See *Board Certified Contact Lens Technician—Advanced Certification* under *contact lens technician*.

NCMHD See *National Center on Minority Health and Health Disparities* under *National Institutes of Health*.

NCPDCIP See *National Center for Preparedness, Detection, and Control of Infectious Diseases* under *Coordinating Center for Infectious Diseases*, under *Centers for Disease Control and Prevention*.

NCPDP See *National Council for Prescription Drug Programs*.

NCPDP SCRIPT Messaging standards for the electronic transfer of prescription data between retail pharmacies and prescribers. It was developed by the *National Council for Prescription Drug Programs (NCPDP)*.

NCPHI See *National Center for Public Health Informatics* under *Coordinating Center for Health Information Service*, under *Centers for Disease Control and Prevention*.

NCPIM See *National Commission to Prevent Infant Mortality*.

NCQA See *National Committee for Quality Assurance*.

NCRR See *National Center for Research Resources* under *National Institutes of Health*.

NCS See *Neurologic Certified Specialist* under *physical therapist*. See also *nerve conduction studies*.

NCSC See *National Certified School Counselor* under *school counselor*.

NCSF-CPT See *NCSF Certified Personal Trainer* under *personal trainer*.

NCSN See *National Certified School Nurse* under *school nursing*.

NCT See *nerve conduction technologist*.

NCTM See *Nationally Certified in Therapeutic Massage* under *massage therapist*.

NCTMB See *Nationally Certified in Therapeutic Massage and Bodywork* under *massage therapist*.

NCTR See *National Center for Toxicological Research*.

NCVHS See *National Committee on Vital and Health Statistics*.

ND Doctor of naturopathy. See *naturopathic physician*.

NDC See *National Drug Code*.

NDF-RT National Drug File Reference Terminology. A terminology developed by the Department of Veterans Affairs (VA) that classifies drugs by mechanism of action and physiologic effect.

NDMA See *National Digital Medical Archive*.

NDMS See *National Disaster Medical System*.

near-patient testing See *point-of-care*.

necropsy See *autopsy*.

NEDEL See *no epidemiologically detectable exposure level*.

NEDSS See *National Electronic Disease Surveillance System*.

needleless intravenous infusion system A technology that replaces a needle in transferring substances into blood vessels. Such devices have been developed in an effort to reduce the incidence of needlesticks, a source of danger and infection to healthcare workers. See also *infusion*.

needlestick An accident in which a used hypodermic needle pierces the skin of an individual other than the patient. This is a serious cause of injury and infection for health professionals, especially because such diseases as hepatitis B, hepatitis C, and AIDS can be spread this way. Thus special precautions (see *universal precautions* under *precautions*), such as hard-sided, disposable needle waste units, have become almost universal in the United States. See also *sharp*.

negative incentive See *disincentive.*

neglect A legal term for failure to provide the necessary care for a dependent person.

  medical neglect Withholding medically indicated treatment from a child, a form of child abuse and neglect. See *Child Abuse Amendments.*

negligence The failure to exercise reasonable care. In addition to its ordinary meaning, negligence has a specific legal meaning; it is one kind of *tort* that results in legal liability. The tort of negligence requires (1) a duty to exercise reasonable care, (2) a failure to exercise such care, and (3) an injury that was proximately caused by that failure. One may commit a careless act, but if no one is injured as a result, there is no "negligence" as far as legal liability is concerned. See also *duty (legal)* and *liability (legal).*

  corporate negligence The failure of a corporation to exercise care. A hospital, for example, has a duty to perform in a manner to ensure the health and safety of its patients, employees, and visitors. If it does not properly screen the credentials of a physician, for example, who is then granted privileges and injures a patient, and if the screening would have revealed that this physician was not qualified for those privileges, the hospital may be liable for corporate negligence.

  gross negligence Acting with reckless or willful disregard for the safety of others.

  professional negligence In the context of health care, professional negligence is the failure of a professional to exercise that degree of care and skill practiced by other professionals of similar skill and training (and, in some states, in the same geographic locality) under similar circumstances (see *standard of care (legal)*). Such lack of care alone, however, will not result in legal liability; there must be an injury to the patient, and the injury must have been caused by the negligent act. This is one type of *malpractice.*

negligence per se Legal liability, based on negligence, that is established in a lawsuit by showing that a law (statute) was violated. Violation of a law, by itself, does not prove negligence. For example, driving without the current automobile registration required by state law will not make a driver liable for hitting a pedestrian, in the absence of any carelessness or fault of the driver. To establish negligence per se, a plaintiff must prove that: (1) the law was violated by the defendant; (2) the plaintiff was injured as a result of the violation; (3) the plaintiff was a person whom the law was intended to protect; and (4) the harm that resulted was the type of harm to be avoided by the law.

  An example of negligence per se in health care would be the failure of a physician to report a case of suspected child abuse to the child protection authorities (a requirement commonly imposed by state law), where the child is further injured because no one intervened to protect him or her.

negligent credentialing See *negligence* and *credentialing.*

negligent infliction of emotional distress See under *emotional distress.*

negotiated fee schedule See under *fee schedule.*

negotiated payment schedule See *negotiated fee schedule* under *fee schedule.*

negotiated underwriting See under *underwriting.*

NEI See *National Eye Institute* under *National Institutes of Health.*

neighborhood health center A facility, located where it will be easy for patients to go, that provides various services short of inpatient care. See also *Federally Qualified Health Center.*

NEJM See *New England Journal of Medicine.*

neonatal A term pertaining to the infant's first four weeks (twenty-eight days) after birth. Synonym: newborn.

neonatal nursing The area of nursing focused on the needs of newborns.

  Low Risk Neonatal Nurse (RNC) A registered nurse specializing in low risk neonatal nursing, who has passed an examination of the National Certification Corporation (NCC) and received the credential Registered Nurse Certified (RNC). **www.nccnet.org**

  Neonatal Care Nurse Practitioner A nurse practitioner specializing in neonatal nursing, who has passed an examination of the National Certification Corporation (NCC) and received the credential Registered Nurse Certified (RNC). **www.nccnet.org**

Neonatal Intensive Care Nurse (RNC) A registered nurse specializing in intensive care neonatal nursing, who has passed an examination of the National Certification Corporation (NCC) and received the credential Registered Nurse Certified (RNC). **www.nccnet.org**

neonatal-perinatal medicine The medical specialty within pediatrics that deals with the newborn infant at and around the time of birth.

neonatology The science and art of diagnosis and treatment of disorders of the infant in the neonatal period—the first four weeks (twenty-eight days) after birth.

neo-no-fault compensation See *patients' compensation* under *compensation*.

nephrology The study of diseases and disorders of the urinary system and kidney function.

nephrology nursing The nursing specialty focusing on the needs of patients with *end stage renal disease (ESRD)* and their families. See also *dialysis nursing*.

Certified Nephrology Nurse (CNN) A nephrology nursing specialist who has passed an examination of the Nephrology Nursing Certification Commission (NNCC). **www.nncc-exam.org**

Certified Nephrology Nurse—Nurse Practitioner (CNN-NP) A nurse practitioner specializing in nephrology nursing who has passed an examination of the Nephrology Nursing Certification Commission (NNCC). **www.nncc-exam.org**

nerve conduction studies (NCS) The use of electroneurodiagnostic procedures to record and evaluate electrical activity of the peripheral nervous system.

nerve conduction technologist (NCT) An electroneurodiagnostic technologist who has special training in performing nerve conduction studies.

Registered Nerve Conduction Studies Technologist (R.NCS.T.) An electroneurodiagnostic technologist who has been certified in performing nerve conduction studies by the American Association of Electrodiagnostic Technologists (AAET). **www.aaet.info**

network (health care) An entity that provides, or provides for, integrated health services to a defined population of individuals. A network offers comprehensive or specialty services and has a centralized structure that coordinates and integrates services provided by components and practitioners participating in the network. The term broadly covers a wide variety of arrangements, including health maintenance organizations (HMOs), preferred provider organizations (PPOs), vertically integrated hospital delivery systems, home care networks, behavioral health networks, and physician-hospital organizations (PHOs), or any group of providers or insurers who contract to provide health services.

The amorphousness of the "network" definition is demonstrated by this caution from the *1995–96 AHA Guide*, which had for the first time a listing of "integrated health delivery networks." The *Guide* noted that "[n]etworks are very fluid in their composition as goals evolve and partners change. Therefore, some of the networks included in this listing may have dissolved, reformed, or simply been renamed as this section was being produced for publication."

Examples of arrangements that might be classified as networks include:

- Individual practice associations (IPAs) in which physicians and/or other health professionals provide their services through the IPA to a given prepayment plan. This model has no direct integration of the physicians with the hospital; that link is provided by the prepayment plan.
- Medical service organizations (MSOs) in which the hospital provides a single point through which many physicians can have such tasks as their billings to various insurance companies and their scheduling handled. Only one staff needs to become expert in all the insurance policies; only one call can schedule consultations, referrals, and hospitalizations.
- Contracts between individual physicians and hospitals.

- Hospitals employing physicians.
- Hospitals contracting with physicians. The purchaser deals with the hospital. The hospital often pays the primary care physicians by capitation, and the specialists by fee-for-service.
- Health maintenance organizations (HMOs) that contract with both physicians and hospitals, and which offer prepayment contracts.
- "Foundations" in which the physicians and hospital(s) are members. The purchaser deals with the foundation, who may have a variety of arrangements with physicians and with hospitals.
- "Health systems" in which all physicians are employed by the system, which also operates the hospital. Thus the purchaser can simply deal with the system.
- "Care management organizations," which interpose a care manager between the patient and physician to administer the provision of services within the defined benefit package.
- "Fully integrated" arrangements, which offer prepayment plans with defined benefit packages (i.e., they offer insurance packages to employers and other purchasers). Such plans typically manage the care as well. The philosophy of both the benefit package construction and the care management will vary from plan to plan.

  See also **gateway (organization)** and **integrated health delivery network**.

network accreditation See **Health Care Network Accreditation Program**.

net worth Assets minus liabilities; also called "equity."

neural network As used in computers and informatics, the (artificial) neural network is a group of simple software-based processors connected in parallel. As such, the artificial neural network is superficially comparable to a biological (real) neural network, such as the human brain. Because the network connections can be given different weights (bias) depending on data inputs, the neural network can be "trained" and can also acquire "experience." In this respect it differs from the computer-based "expert system," which is a computer program with "hard-coded" rules and no training component. The expert system contains a fixed knowledgebase of accumulated experience and a set of rules for applying that knowledge to a particular problem presented to it. The expert system cannot "learn," requiring an outsider to modify either the knowledgebase or the rule set.

The neural network, on the other hand, can learn—it can change its outputs over time, based on large quantities of input. Given enough input data, the neural network is capable of recognizing patterns. This is often described in terms of knowledge layers, in which learned relationships between data inputs can "feed forward" to other knowledge layers.

neurology The study of the nervous system, its functions, diseases, and disorders.

neuropathology See under **pathology**.

neurophysiological monitoring Assessment of the functional integrity of the peripheral or central nervous system. See also **electroneurodiagnostics**.

neuroscience nursing The nursing specialty focusing on the needs of patients with dysfunction of the central nervous system such as changes in consciousness, cognition, communication, mobility, sensation, and so forth, which may be due to head or spinal cord trauma, cancer, or stroke.

  Certified Neuroscience Registered Nurse (CNRN) A specialist in neuroscience nursing who has passed an examination of the American Board of Neuroscience Nursing (ABNN). www.aann.org/credential

neurotology The study of the inner ear, especially the nerves. Synonym: otoneurology.

never list See **serious reportable event**.

newborn A baby from the time of birth through the first twenty-eight days of life. Synonym: neonate. See also **neonatal**.

Newborns' and Mothers' Health Protection Act (NMHPA) A federal law requiring health plans that provide maternity coverage to pay for at least a forty-eight-hour hospital stay following childbirth (ninety-six hours for cesarean section). Also called simply the Newborns' Act. Pub. L. No. 104-204, 110 Stat. 2935 (1996).

New England Journal of Medicine (NEJM) The weekly clinical journal published by the Massachusetts Medical Society. **content.nejm.org**

NF See *National Formulary*.

N4A See *National Association of Area Agencies on Aging*.

NFPA See *National Fire Protection Association*.

NFPA 101 See *Life Safety Code*.

NFPT-CPT See *NFPT Certified Personal Trainer* under *personal trainer*.

NGT See *Nominal Group Technique*.

NGT process See *Nominal Group Technique*.

NHANES See *National Health and Nutrition Examination Survey*.

NHDS See *National Hospital Discharge Survey*.

NHE See *national health expenditures*.

NHGRI See *National Human Genome Research Institute* under *National Institutes of Health*.

NHIC See *National Health Information Center*.

NHII See *National Health Information Infrastructure*.

NHIN See *Nationwide Health Information Network*.

NHIS See *National Health Interview Survey* and *National Hospital Indicator Survey*.

NHLBI See *National Heart, Lung, and Blood Institute* under *National Institutes of Health*.

NHQI Nursing Home Quality Initiative. See *Quality Initiative*.

NHQM See *National Hospital Quality Measures*.

NHRA See *Nursing Home Reform Act*.

NHS See *National Health Service*.

NHSC See *National Health Service Corps*.

NHS Clinical Terms See *Clinical Terms Version 3*.

NHS Codes See *Clinical Terms Version 3*.

NHTSA See *National Highway Transportation Safety Administration*.

NIA See *National Institute on Aging* under *National Institutes of Health*.

NIAAA See *National Institute on Alcohol Abuse and Alcoholism* under *National Institutes of Health*.

NIAID See *National Institute of Allergy and Infectious Diseases* under *National Institutes of Health*.

NIAMS See *National Institute of Arthritis and Musculoskeletal and Skin Diseases* under *National Institutes of Health*.

NIBIB See *National Institute of Biomedical Imaging and Bioengineering* under *National Institutes of Health*.

NIC See *Nursing Interventions Classification*.

NICHD See *National Institute of Child Health and Human Development* under *National Institutes of Health*.

NICHSA See *National Information Center for Health Services Administration*.

NICU See *neonatal intensive care unit* under *intensive care unit*.

NIDA See *National Institute on Drug Abuse* under *National Institutes of Health*.

NIDCD See *National Institute on Deafness and Other Communication Disorders* under *National Institutes of Health*.

NIDCR See *National Institute of Dental and Craniofacial Research* under *National Institutes of Health*.

NIDDK See *National Institute of Diabetes and Digestive and Kidney Diseases* under *National Institutes of Health*.

NIDSEC See *Nursing Information & Data Set Evaluation Center*.

NIEHS See *National Institute of Environmental Health Sciences* under *National Institutes of Health*.

NIGMS See *National Institute of General Medical Sciences* under *National Institutes of Health*.

NIH See *National Institutes of Health*.

NIH Consensus Development Program See *National Institutes of Health Consensus Development Program*.

NIMH See *National Institute of Mental Health* under *National Institutes of Health*.

NINDS See *National Institute of Neurological Disorders and Stroke* under *National Institutes of Health*.

NINR See *National Institute of Nursing Research* under *National Institutes of Health*.

NIOSH See *National Institute for Occupational Safety and Health* under *Centers for Disease Control and Prevention*.

NIS See *nursing information system* under *information system*.

NIST See *National Institute of Standards and Technology*.

nitsa Common pronunciation of *National Highway Transportation Safety Administration (NHTSA)*.

NLIP Nonphysician licensed independent practitioner. A term used by the Joint Commission on Accreditation of Healthcare Organizations (JCAHO) in its accreditation manuals. See *allied health professional*.

NLM See *National Library of Medicine* under *National Institutes of Health*.

NLM Gateway An Internet-based system that lets users search simultaneously in multiple retrieval systems of the U.S. National Library of Medicine (NLM). Users may initiate searches from a single site, providing "one-stop searching" for many of NLM's information resources and databases, including MEDLINE, PubMed, and many others. **gateway.nlm.nih.gov**

NLN See *National League for Nursing*.

NLP See *natural language processing*.

NMA See *National Medical Association*.

NMD Doctor of naturopathic medicine. See *naturopathic physician*.

NMDS See *Nursing Minimum Data Set* under *data set*.

NMES National Medical Expenditure Survey. See *Medical Expenditure Panel Survey*.

NMHPA See *Newborns' and Mothers' Health Protection Act*.

NMMDS See *Nursing Management Minimum Data Set* under *data set*.

NMR See *nuclear magnetic resonance*.

NMRI Nuclear magnetic resonance imaging. See *magnetic resonance imaging*.

NMT See *nuclear medicine technologist*.

NN/LM See *National Network of Libraries of Medicine*.

NNRT See *National Nurse Response Team* under *National Disaster Medical System*.

no adverse response level (NARL) A measure, derived from animal studies, of the level of contamination in a soil below which there is no hazard to the animals. In some instances the NARL has been extrapolated as applicable to humans.

NOC See *Nursing Outcomes Classification*.

NOCA See *National Organization for Competency Assurance*.

nocebo effect The occurrence of adverse "side effects" after a patient has taken a *placebo*, unrelated to the substance in the placebo. This confounds clinical studies that compare a drug with a placebo. From the Latin, meaning "I shall harm."

no-code order See *do not resuscitate*.

NODMAR See *notice of discharge and Medicare appeal rights*.

no epidemiologically detectable exposure level (NEDEL) One of several measures used to advise on the hazards of environmental exposure to toxic substances in the soil. The NEDEL is calculated by making studies of appropriate populations of humans exposed to the toxic agent in the soil, and determining whether the persons show significantly elevated levels of the toxic agent, symptoms of toxicity, or both. The measure was developed by the Centers for Disease Control and Prevention (CDC) and the Montana Department of Health and Environmental Sciences. Other measures have been developed from studies of laboratory animals: the no observable effect level (NOEL), the *no adverse response level (NARL)*, and the *acceptable daily intake (ADI)*.

Noerr-Pennington Doctrine   A legal doctrine that grants immunity from antitrust liability to organizations or entities who get together to influence the government, even though they may otherwise be competitors. The Supreme Court stated that "Noerr shields from the Sherman Act a concerted effort to influence public officials regardless of intent or purpose. . . . Joint efforts to influence public officials do not violate the antitrust laws even though intended to eliminate competition." *United Mine Workers of America v. Pennington*, 381 U.S. 657, 670 (1965).

noetic   Originating or existing in the intellect or the spiritual world. An increasing number of healthcare organizations are emphasizing the integration of science and spirituality in order to enhance the "healing force," joining scientific medicine with a spiritual or noetic dimension, to create whole person and whole community health care. See also *holistic health*.

no-fault   See *no-fault compensation* under *compensation*.

nomenclature   A subset of the *terminology* for a given domain, discipline, or universe. It consists of names for the terms (or groups of terms) in a terminology. Each name is called a "nomen" (from the Latin for name). A nomenclature is created not by chance or usage, but by an official body or publisher of some kind that is seeking to organize (and/or standardize) this particular terminology.

A nomenclature is like a classification of the contents of a terminology—every term in a terminology must find its home under one of the nomens of the nomenclature. The nomenclature cannot ignore any of the terms in use as though they did not exist. In most classifications, this problem is handled by categories labeled "other." That solution won't work in a nomenclature, because a meaningless nomen would be created.

A nomenclature is a much more stable set of terms than a terminology, but it can change from time to time. There can be a number of nomenclatures within a given terminology, even if only one nomenclature is allowed in an individual setting for a given universe (such as diagnoses or procedures). There can also be two or more lists of words and phrases, advertised as nomenclatures, competing for the same universe. For example, today both *SNOMED Clinical Terms (SNOMED CT)* and *MEDCIN* are advertised (and sold) as nomenclatures for clinical medicine. Perhaps the closest to an official nomenclature in the United States is that used in the *Unified Medical Language System (UMLS)* of the National Library of Medicine (NLM).

Distinguish from *vocabulary*, and see the diagram at *natural language*.

Nominal Group Technique (NGT)   A process developed by Delbecq, Van de Ven, and Gustafson for "increasing the creative productivity of group action, facilitating group decisions . . . and saving human effort and energy." A **nominal group** is a group "in name only," a type of group in which individuals are together but do not talk or interact until late in the **NGT process**.

NOMNC   See *notice of Medicare non-coverage*.

noncompete clause   See *covenant not to compete*.

noncompliance   Failure or refusal to follow directions or rules. In health care, noncompliance usually refers to a patient not taking medications according to instructions, or not following through on recommended or prescribed therapy. Reasons for noncompliance vary, and may or may not be within the control of the patient, who is called "noncompliant."

nonexempt distinct part unit   A term used in Medicare, apparently to mean a part of the hospital considered by Medicare to qualify for a different pay rate than another part. For transfer in or transfer out purposes, Medicare considers a nonexempt distinct part equivalent to another hospital.

noninvasive A diagnostic or therapeutic procedure or technique that does not require penetration of the skin or mucous membrane by a needle or surgical instrument. The various imaging scanners, for instance, are noninvasive, as is lithotripsy.

nonprofit An entity whose profits (excess of income over expenses) are used for its own purposes rather than returned to its members (shareholders, investors, owners) as dividends. To qualify for tax exemption, no portion of the profits of the entity may "inure" to the benefit of an individual. See *inurement*. "Nonprofit" does not necessarily mean "tax-exempt"; see *tax-exempt* and *501(c)(3)* (under *501(c)(*)*). Also see *nonprofit corporation* under *corporation*, and *nonprofit hospital* under *hospital*. Distinguish from *for-profit*. Synonym: not-for-profit.

nonproprietary drug See *generic equivalent*.

nonrepudiation An assurance, provided as a result of an *authentication* process, that the apparent person linked to an activity (for example, the sender of a message or creator of a document) is in fact that person. This assurance is critical for certain healthcare transactions, where trusted individuals engage in activities that have immediate life or death consequences.

nonsurgical See *medical*.

nonviable (cannot live) Not capable of living, as a baby born below a certain birth weight.

nonviable (cannot succeed) Not capable of being carried out or of succeeding, for example, "nonviable plans."

NOPHG See *National Office of Public Health Genomics* under *Coordinating Center for Health Promotion*, under *Centers for Disease Control and Prevention*.

NORC See *naturally occurring retirement community*.

North American Nursing Diagnosis Association (NANDA) Former name of *NANDA International*.

nosocomial Originating in a hospital. See also *iatrogenic*.

nosohusial Originating in the home. See also *nosocomial*.

nosology The branch of medical science that deals with the *classification (scheme)* of diseases.

not-for-profit See *nonprofit*.

notice of discharge and Medicare appeal rights (NODMAR) A notice that must be given to a Medicare HMO beneficiary when that patient is discharged from the hospital because the hospital believes that a continued stay will not be covered by Medicare. See also *hospital-issued notice of non-coverage*.

notice of Medicare non-coverage (NOMNC) A notice that must be given by a skilled nursing facility (SNF), home health agency (HHA), comprehensive outpatient rehabilitation facility (CORF), or hospice when the provider determines that the services will no longer be covered by Medicare. The NOMNC must include the rights of the beneficiary to appeal the decision. Synonym: notice of Medicare provider non-coverage. See also *hospital-issued notice of non-coverage*.

Notice of Privacy Practice (NPP) A written notice that must be given to every patient by a *covered entity*, describing how that entity will protect the patient's privacy rights under HIPAA.

Joint Notice of Privacy Practice (JNPP) A Notice of Privacy Practice prepared by the two or more covered entities in an Organized Health Care Arrangement (OHCA). The JNPP discloses the identities of the entities and the service delivery sites.

Notice of Proposed Rulemaking (NPRM) A formal announcement in the *Federal Register* that administrative rules are under consideration, and soliciting comments on those rules.

not to be coded See *do not resuscitate*.

NP See *nurse practitioner*.

NP-C See *Nurse Practitioner, Certified* under *nurse practitioner*.

NPDB See *National Practitioner Data Bank*.

NPF See *National Provider File*.

NPI See *National Patient Identifier* and *National Provider Identifier*.

NPI Enumerator See *National Provider Identifier*.

NPlanID See *National Health Plan Identifier*.

NPP Non-physician practitioners. Also *Notice of Privacy Practice*.

NPPES National Plan and Provider Enumeration System. See *National Provider Identifier*.

NPR See *National Provider Registry*.

NPRM See *Notice of Proposed Rulemaking*.

NPRT See *National Pharmacy Response Team* under *National Disaster Medical System*.

NPS See *National Provider System* and *Neonatal/Pediatric Respiratory Care Specialist* (under *respiratory therapist*).

NPSG See *National Patient Safety Goals*.

NQASC National Quality Alliance Steering Committee. See *Quality Alliance Steering Committee*.

NQF See *National Quality Forum*.

NQIGs See *National Quality Improvement Goals*.

NQMC See *National Quality Measures Clearinghouse*.

NR See *nursing services*.

NRC See *National Research Corporation* and *National Research Council*.

NRMP See *National Resident Matching Program*.

NRP National Response Plan. See *Federal Emergency Management Agency*.

NSCA-CPT See *NSCA-Certified Personal Trainer* under *personal trainer*.

NSF See *National Science Foundation*.

NTIS See *National Technical Information Service*.

NTP National Toxicology Program. See *National Institute of Environmental Health Sciences* under *National Institutes of Health*.

NUBC See *National Uniform Billing Committee*.

NUCC See *National Uniform Claim Committee*.

NUCC-DS See *National Uniform Claim Committee Data Set* under *data set*.

nuclear isomer See under *nuclide*.

nuclear isotope See under *isotopes* under *nuclide*.

nuclear magnetic resonance (NMR) A physical phenomenon brought about in the body by subjecting the body to radio frequency fields in a strong magnetic field. It does not use radioactive materials or x-rays. NMR is used in nuclear magnetic resonance imaging (NMRI) and the study of certain biochemical activity.

nuclear magnetic resonance imaging (NMRI) See *magnetic resonance imaging*.

nuclear medicine A medical specialty that involves the use of radioactive materials to diagnose and treat diseases, especially neurological conditions, cancers, and cardiovascular problems.

Diagnostic uses in the body (in vivo) involve the "tracer" principle. Several hundred radioactive chemicals called radionuclides (radiopharmaceuticals) have been developed, each with the ability to seek out specific organs or tissues, where they emit radiation that can be detected from outside the body. In nuclear medicine, instruments detect the function of the organ or tissue, whereas x-rays and ultrasound detect the anatomic structure. The radioactive chemicals used have limited half-lives, varying from a few seconds to several hours, so that their radioactivity will not persist. A small amount of an appropriate radionuclide, for instance one targeting the lung, is given to the patient (by injection, orally, or inhaled) and the function of the tissue where it accumulates is studied by one of two methods:

Single Photon Emission Computer Tomography (SPECT) uses a rotating nuclear camera or cameras (gamma cameras) to detect the location of the tracer that has been injected and, using a computer, to draw "function pictures" of the organ or tissue that has absorbed the tracer.

Positron Emission Tomography (PET) uses an array of stationary detectors around the patient's body to detect gamma rays produced by the interaction of previously administered radionuclides with the body tissue. PET is especially useful in detecting biochemical processes. GCPET (gamma camera PET) is being developed to use gamma cameras instead of stationary detectors to obtain PET images. Sometimes called positron tomography.

The necessity of using radionuclides with short half-lives introduces a constraint on these technologies, because the imaging site must have rapid access to sources of the chemicals. PET scanners originally could only function in conjunction with large cyclotrons, which produced the radionuclides on site.

Diagnostic uses outside the body (in vitro) involve the removal of blood samples from the body and the examination of the samples by such techniques as radioimmunoassay (RIA) or immunoradiometric assay (IRMA). With these techniques, the patient is not subjected to any radiation.

Therapeutic uses of radiation typically use both external sources of radiation, which are not thought of as nuclear medicine, and radioactive substances introduced into the body. Recently, radionuclides have been successfully attached to monoclonal antibodies (disease-fighting proteins that can seek out and attach themselves to specific cells or tissues). By this method, radiation can be given directly to the specific cells.

nuclear medicine science The field of science concerned with the diagnostic, therapeutic (exclusive of sealed radiation sources), and investigative uses of *radionuclides* (see under *nuclide*). See also *medical physics* under *physics*.

nuclear medicine physics and instrumentation The area of nuclear medicine science that deals with diagnostic and therapeutic applications of radionuclides and the equipment associated with their production and use.

radiation protection The area of nuclear medicine science that deals with protective measures for ionizing radiation from radionuclides.

radiopharmaceutical science The area of nuclear medicine science that deals with preparation and use of radiopharmaceuticals for use in nuclear medicine, and radiolabeled chemicals for investigative studies.

nuclear medicine scientist A health professional with at least a master's degree who specializes in nuclear medicine science. See also *medical health physicist* and *medical physicist* (both under *physicist*).

Nuclear Medicine Physics and Instrumentation A certificate awarded to a nuclear medicine scientist who has met the requirements of the American Board of Science in Nuclear Medicine (ABSNM) in the specialty area of nuclear medicine physics and instrumentation. **www.snm.org/absnm**

Radiation Protection A certificate awarded to a nuclear medicine scientist who has met the requirements of the American Board of Science in Nuclear Medicine (ABSNM) in the specialty area of radiation protection. **www.snm.org/absnm**

Radiopharmaceutical Science A certificate awarded to a nuclear medicine scientist who has met the requirements of the American Board of Science in Nuclear Medicine (ABSNM) in the specialty area of radiopharmaceutical science. **www.snm.org/absnm**

nuclear medicine technologist (NMT) A health professional specially trained to work closely with a nuclear medicine physician before, during, and after an imaging procedure. Many states require licensure.

Certified Nuclear Medicine Technologist (CNMT) A nuclear medicine technologist who has met the requirements of the Nuclear Medicine Technology Certification Board (NMTCB). **www.nmtcb.org**

Registered Technologist—Nuclear Medicine Technology (RT(N)) A *Registered Technologist (RT)* (see under *radiologic technologist*) who has been certified in nuclear medicine by the American Registry of Radiologic Technologists (ARRT). **www.arrt.org**

nuclease A class of enzymes used to split DNA and RNA molecules.

nucleic acid The class of molecules to which DNA and RNA belong.

nucleoside A specific type of chemical compound found in DNA and RNA. Similar to a nucleotide.

nucleotide A specific type of a chemical compound found in DNA, portions of which are nucleosides.

nuclide A term used in atomic physics, meaning a species of atoms having a specific mass number and a specific atomic number. It has become the custom to refer to "radioactive nuclides" rather than "radioactive isotopes" in nuclear medicine, hence the brief discussion of the terms below (see also *atom*).

atomic number Each atom (the smallest particle of matter that exhibits unique chemical properties) has a nucleus surrounded by electrons. The chemical properties of the atom are determined by the number of protons in its nucleus. The number of protons in the nucleus also determines the atomic number of the element. (The term "element" is applied to a collection of atoms of one chemical type.) For example, the element carbon, which has six protons, has the atomic number "6."

isobars When the mass number of two or more different nuclides is the same, but the atomic number is different, the nuclides are called isobars. For example, some atoms of titanium, vanadium, and chromium all have a mass number of 50: ^{50}Ti (titanium-50), ^{50}V (vanadium-50), and ^{50}Cr (chromium-50). These three elements are called isobars (not isotopes).

isotopes When two or more atoms have the same atomic number but different atomic mass, they are different nuclides, but they are called isotopes (of the element in question). In the case of carbon, for example, seven different masses have been found—atoms that all have the six protons making the element carbon, but with between four and ten neutrons, producing the seven carbon isotopes: carbon-10, carbon-11, carbon-12, carbon-13, carbon-14, carbon-15, and carbon-16.

mass number The nucleus of an atom contains one or more neutrons. Adding together the numbers of protons and neutrons in an atom's nucleus gives its atomic mass, known as its mass number. A given element, while retaining its chemical properties, can have atoms of different masses, depending on the number of neutrons in their nuclei. As a matter of fact, most elements occur in nature as mixtures of atoms with the same atomic number but different mass numbers. The most common form of carbon (over 98% of it in nature), for example, has six protons and six neutrons, therefore its atomic mass is 12; a rare form of carbon, which has the same chemical properties (but is radioactive), has six protons and eight neutrons; its atomic mass is 14.

notation When one describes an atom, one must give both its atomic mass and its name or atomic number (sometimes both name *and* atomic number). This is done in one (or both) of two ways: (1) give the full chemical name and the atomic mass (the two separated by a hyphen), or (2) give first the mass (number of protons + number of neutrons) as a superscript followed by the abbreviation for the element's chemical name. Carbon (atomic number 6) with the most common atomic mass, 12 (six protons plus six neutrons) would be given as carbon-12 or ^{12}C. Sometimes for safety, the expression would be ^{12}C (carbon-12). Radioactive carbon, with six protons and eight neutrons, would be given as carbon-14 or ^{14}C. An alternative notation would give the atomic mass as a leading superscript, and the atomic number as a leading subscript, thus carbon-14 could be given as $^{14}_{6}$C.

nuclear isomers Not all radioactive nuclides have the same "half-life" or "degree" of radioactivity. Bromine, atomic number 35, for example, has a nuclide with mass number 80 that is found to exist as a mixture of nuclides with different half-lives, known as different metastable states. These are expressed as bromine-80 and bromine-80m, or ^{80}Br and ^{80}mBr. When, as in this example, two or more of the same nuclides differ in some physical respect, they are called isomers.

radioactivity In general, the greater the difference between the numbers of protons and neutrons in a given nuclide, the more "unstable" the nuclide, and the more likely it is to be radioactive, that is, for its nucleus to disintegrate spontaneously, and for it to give off ionizing radiation in the process. Two of the nuclides (isotopes) of carbon, carbon-12 and carbon-13, are stable; the other four, including carbon-14, are radioactive.

radionuclide A nuclide that emits nuclear radiation (see *radioactivity*, above); used in nuclear medicine.

numeric A string of numerals, with no alphabetic characters. The term is employed to describe codes, which are typically either numeric or alphanumeric.

nurse A health professional specializing in *nursing*. A nurse must be qualified by accredited formal training at an academic or diploma school of nursing. See also *nursing specialty*.

associate nurse Usually, a nurse who is responsible for carrying out a primary nurse's care plans, although in some states the term is used for a diploma nurse or a nurse with an associate degree (AD).

charge nurse A registered nurse "in charge of" nursing in a patient care unit during a given work period.

circulating nurse A registered nurse who functions as a *circulator* in the *operating room*.

degree nurse A nurse whose nursing education was obtained in an educational institution that granted an academic degree. The degree referred to is usually Bachelor of Science in Nursing (BSN).

diploma nurse A nurse whose nursing education was obtained in a hospital school of nursing that granted a diploma rather than an academic degree.

float nurse A nurse assigned to various patient care units of the hospital depending on their staffing needs, rather than regularly assigned to the same unit; thus, such a nurse "floats." Synonym: prn nurse.

floor nurse A nurse working on, but not in charge of, a patient care unit.

general duty nurse A registered nurse whose duties do not require specialty preparation. The term is ordinarily used with hospital nursing.

graduate nurse Ordinarily, a nurse who has graduated from a professional nursing education program but who does not hold a valid state license. Although a registered nurse logically could be called a "graduate nurse," because he or she has "graduated" from a nursing program, that term instead refers to the lack of a license.

head nurse A registered nurse whose duty is to be in charge of a patient care unit on an ongoing basis. This nurse is the charge nurse's superior, because the head nurse's responsibility continues through all work shifts, whereas the charge nurse's responsibility is only for the shift when the charge nurse is present. The title and the management system vary from hospital to hospital.

licensed practical nurse (LPN) A person licensed by the state to carry out specified nursing duties under the direction of a registered nurse. He or she must have had formal training in a practical or vocational nursing education program. Synonym: licensed vocational nurse (LVN).

licensed vocational nurse (LVN) See *licensed practical nurse*.

pool nurse A registered nurse or licensed practical nurse (LPN) who is not a member of the nursing staff of an institution but who is hired through an agency to provide patient care on a temporary basis (for example, one shift) when sufficient regular nursing staff are not available to provide such care.

practical nurse A person who has had formal training in a practical or vocational nursing education program. When a practical nurse has been licensed by the state to carry out specified nursing duties under the direction of a head nurse or nursing team leader, that person may assume the title of licensed practical nurse (LPN). Synonym: vocational nurse.

primary nurse A nurse who is responsible around the clock for planning, supervising, and, when present, giving nursing care to an assigned group of patients. This approach to nursing care is replacing team nursing (see under *nursing*), in which a "committee" rather than an individual carries out these functions.

private-duty nurse A registered nurse who is employed by the patient.

prn nurse See *float nurse*.

registered nurse (RN) A nurse who has been granted a "registered nurse" license by the state. Nurses educated in state-approved baccalaureate programs in nursing or in associate degree programs in nursing (in degree-granting institutions), and those trained in hospital schools of nursing, are eligible to sit for registration (credentials) licensing examinations given by state boards of nursing. The registration license is intended to ensure minimum levels of competence and thus protect the public, not to indicate the educational background of the nurse. Registration typically requires periodic renewal.

team nurse A nurse who is a member of a nursing team. A nursing team is a group of registered nurses and ancillary personnel who provide nursing services, under a team leader, for a designated group of inpatients during a single nursing shift. See also *primary nurse* (above).

technical level nurse A proposed term for a nurse whose education was in an associate degree (AD) program in nursing (in a degree-granting institution) or in a diploma program in nursing.

vocational nurse See *practical nurse*.

nurse assistant See *nursing assistant*.

nurse clinical instructor A registered nurse who carries out clinical teaching, with patients, for nursing students.

nurse clinician An imprecise term, sometimes used as a job title. More context is needed. See *nursing specialty*.

nurse informatician See *informatics nursing*.

nurse midwife See *Certified Nurse-Midwife* under *midwifery*.

nurse practice act A state law governing the practice of nursing within the state.

nurse practitioner (NP) A registered nurse who has completed a nurse practitioner program at the master's degree level or higher. NPs have qualifications that permit them to carry out expanded healthcare evaluation and decision making regarding patient care, with focus on primary care and patient education. A nurse practitioner has a degree of independence from the supervision of a physician, with the boundaries of this independence set by state law. In most states, NPs may prescribe medication. There are many specialty areas of nurse practitioners; see *nursing specialty*. Compare with *physician assistant*. See also *advanced practice nurse* and *clinical nurse specialist*.

Nurse Practitioner, Certified (NP-C) A registered nurse, usually with a Bachelor of Science in Nursing degree, who is qualified in adult nursing or family nursing and has passed an examination of the American Academy of Nurse Practitioners (AANP). **www.aanp.org**

nursing The American Nurses Association (ANA) defines nursing as "the protection, promotion, and optimization of health and abilities, prevention of illness and injury, alleviation of suffering through the diagnosis and treatment of human response, and advocacy in the care of individuals, families, communities, and populations." See also *nursing diagnosis*, *nursing intervention* (under *intervention (clinical)*), and *nursing services*.

primary nursing A system of nursing care in which one registered nurse (RN) is responsible around the clock for planning, supervising, and, when present, giving nursing care to an assigned individual or group of patients. This approach to nursing care is replacing *team nursing* (see below).

team nursing A type of organization of nursing services in which a team headed by a registered nurse, and with other registered nurses and ancillary personnel, cares for an assigned group of patients in a patient care unit. A team of four to six members gives care to from fifteen to twenty-five patients. Each duty shift has its own team, with a team leader who assigns patients to team members for care according to the complexity of need and the team members' capability. See also *primary nursing* (above).

nursing administration The area of nursing concerning the management of nursing services.

Board Certified Nursing Administrator A registered nurse with a Bachelor of Science in Nursing (BSN) degree who is qualified in nursing administration and has passed an examination of the American Nurses Credentialing Center (ANCC) (**nursingworld.org/ancc**). The credential is RN,CNA,BC (Registered Nurse, Certified in Nursing Administration, Board Certified). The former certificate credential was CNA.

Board Certified Nursing Administrator, Advanced A registered nurse with a graduate degree who is qualified in nursing administration and has passed an advanced examination of the American Nurses Credentialing Center (ANCC) (**nursingworld.org/ancc**). The credential is RN,CNAA,BC (Registered Nurse, Certified in Nursing Administration, Advanced, Board Certified). The former certificate credential was CNAA.

Certified Director of Nursing Administration (CDONA) A director of nursing or assistant director of nursing in long-term care who has passed an examination given by the National Association of Directors of Nursing Administration in Long Term Care (NADONA/LTC). **www.nadona.org**

nursing aide See under *aide*.

nursing assistant An unlicensed health professional who provides nursing and/or personal care under the supervision of a nurse. May have no training, on-the-job training, or have completed a training course. Sometimes called nurse aide. See also *aide*.

Certified Nursing Assistant (CNA) A nursing assistant who has completed a state-approved course of training, usually at a community college or medical facility, and received a certificate upon its completion.

nursing care Provision of those services and procedures that fall under the heading of *nursing*. Nursing care is defined at several levels, as discussed below; see also *level of care*.

basic nursing care See *intermediate care* (below).

custodial care See *rest home care* (below).

extended care See *skilled nursing care* (below).

hospital nursing care Round-the-clock nursing care supervised at all times by a registered nurse, with the bedside care provided by both licensed nurses (registered nurses and licensed practical nurses (LPNs)) and auxiliary nursing personnel as appropriate for the patient.

intermediate care The second highest level of nursing care provided outside the acute hospital setting (the highest level is "skilled nursing care"): nursing care for a patient whose professional nursing needs are less demanding than for skilled nursing care, but are of a nature to require overall supervision by a registered nurse. This supervision requirement is ordinarily met by having an RN in charge for one shift each day. Intermediate care patients typically can participate to some extent in the activities of daily living (ADLs).

The payer (a government program such as Medicare and Medicaid, insurance, or another prepayment plan) typically has its own definition of the term, under which specific procedures and services are included as intermediate care, while others are excluded. It is wise to consult the regulations governing the program, such as Medicare, or the terms of the insurance contract, for specific inclusions and exclusions. Sometimes called basic nursing care. See also *skilled nursing care* (below).

rest home care Care for a patient who is unable to live independently, that is, who needs assistance with the activities of daily living (ADLs), and who may need occasional assistance from a professional nurse. Such nursing service is obtained from a visiting nurse. The setting for rest home care (formerly called custodial care) is, understandably, a rest home.

skilled nursing care The highest level of nursing care recognized outside the acute hospital setting: nursing care for a patient whose professional nursing needs are not so demanding as to require acute hospital nursing care, but are of a nature to need inpatient supervision by a *registered nurse* (see under *nurse*). Patients require skilled nursing care either because the procedures prescribed for them are those that must be given by a professional nurse or because the amount of nursing care necessary is considerable ("heavy care"), or both. The term "skilled nursing care" is not used for regular nursing care in an acute hospital, but rather for care given in a skilled nursing facility (SNF), in a skilled nursing unit (SNU) (a portion of another facility), or in a home healthcare (in-home care) program.

The payer (a government program such as Medicare and Medicaid, insurance, or another prepayment plan) often has its own definition of the term, under which specific procedures and services are included as skilled nursing care, while others are excluded. Although "skilled nursing care" has some general meaning, it is wise to consult the regulations governing the program, such as Medicare, or the terms of the insurance contract for specific inclusions and exclusions.

Formerly called "extended care." See also *intermediate care* (the immediately lower level of care), above.

nursing care objectives One item of content of a nursing care plan giving the specific aims of the nurse with respect to reducing the patient's stress and improving the patient's ability to adapt to the situation.

nursing care plan A formal written plan of care and activities for a patient. Typically, the physician's activities are not part of the plan; the plan pertains to nursing and to other services, and is part of the nursing record. See also *nursing process*. Synonym: care plan.

nursing classification See *nursing language*.

nursing continuing education See under *continuing education*.

nursing data set See *nursing language*.

nursing department See *nursing service*.

nursing diagnosis A judgment made by a nurse describing an individual's actual or potential health needs that are amenable to *nursing intervention* (see under *intervention*). The focus of the nursing diagnosis is on the individual's response to illness or other factors that may adversely affect the attainment or maintenance of wellness. These diagnostic acts are distinct from those of medical and dental diagnoses. To illustrate, the physician's diagnosis may be "hypertension" (high blood pressure). Certain nursing diagnoses commonly are found for patients with hypertension; for example, "nutrition, alteration in, more than body requirements," because obesity may aggravate hypertension. The nursing intervention would therefore include patient education to reduce intake of salt, fats, and sugar. Synonym: nursing phenomenon. See also *NANDA International*.

nursing differential An allowance originally added to payments for Medicare patients in recognition of the greater cost of providing nursing services to elderly patients.

nursing diploma A credential given an individual on successful completion of the course of instruction in nursing given by a hospital school of nursing. An individual completing the nursing course in an academic program, that is, one offered by an educational institution, usually receives a nursing degree rather than a nursing diploma. Both degree and diploma holders are eligible to be licensed as a registered nurse (see *nurse*).

nursing director See *nursing service administrator*.

nursing home An institution that provides continuous nursing and other services to patients who are not acutely ill, but who need nursing and personal services as inpatients. A nursing home has permanent facilities and a professional staff. Some use this term interchangeably with *long-term care facility*; others see nursing homes as one type of long-term care facility. State and federal laws should be consulted for current legal definitions.

For example, Minnesota defines "nursing home" as "a facility or that part of a facility which provides nursing care to five or more persons" (Minn. Stat. § 144A.01(5) (2006)). In a federal statute, the definition of "long-term care facility" includes one providing skilled nursing care, or rehabilitation services, or "on a regular basis, health-related care and services to individuals who because of their mental or physical condition require care and services (above the level of room and board) which can be made available to them only through institutional facilities, and is not primarily for the care and treatment of mental diseases . . ." or another "adult care home similar to" these (42 U.S.C. § 3002(32) (January 3, 2005)). So when determining whether a given facility is a nursing home or long-term care facility (or both), the purpose for the determination is relevant for financing, state regulation, payment for Medicaid services, and other factors.

academic nursing home A nursing home affiliated with or operated by an institution providing medical residency, with goals of research and the education of health professionals in addition to the provision of patient care. The education programs may include medicine, nursing, social work, psychology, speech pathology, audiology, pharmacy, gerodentistry, occupational therapy, and other disciplines.

Nursing Home Compare An interactive CMS web site that allows the user to obtain "detailed information about the past performance of every Medicare and Medicaid certified nursing home in the country." **www.medicare.gov/NHCompare**

Nursing Home Reform Act (NHRA) A 1987 federal law that instituted significant regulations for long-term care facilities. It required upgrading in the physical facilities of nursing homes and increased enforcement in several areas including discrimination against Medicaid recipients, licensed nurse coverage, and federal standards for nursing home administrators. Substantial reduction in antipsychotic drug use in nursing homes after the implementation of this act has been reported.

The NHRA was aimed at improving care for Medicare and Medicaid nursing home residents, with rehabilitation as the goal for the residents. Specifically addressed were such issues as comprehensive assessment of newly admitted residents (within fourteen days of admission, annually after that; see *Resident Assessment Instrument*), restrictions on the use of chemical or physical restraints, absolute right to refuse medical treatment, and the number and qualifications of staff.

Passed as part of the Omnibus Budget Reconciliation Act of 1987 (OBRA 87) (Pub. L. No. 100-203, 101 Stat. 1330), the NHRA was the result of a 1986 report of the Institute of Medicine (IOM), *Improving the Quality of Care in Nursing Homes*, which included extensive recommendations, most of which were incorporated into the act.

nursing informatics See *informatics nursing*.

Nursing Information & Data Set Evaluation Center (NIDSEC) An organization established by the American Nurses Association (ANA) to review, evaluate against defined criteria, and recognize information systems from developers and manufacturers that support documentation of nursing care within electronic health records or nursing information systems (**www.nursingworld.org/nidsec**). The following had been approved as "supporting nursing practice" as of 2007:

ABC Codes
Clinical Care Classification (CCC)
International Classification for Nursing Practice (ICNP)
Logical Observation Identifiers Names and Codes (LOINC)
NANDA International
Nursing Interventions Classification (NIC)
Nursing Management Minimum Data Set (NMMDS) (see under *data set*)
Nursing Minimum Data Set (NMDS) (see under *data set*)
Nursing Outcomes Classification (NOC)

Omaha System
Patient Care Data Set (PCDS) (see under *data set*)
Perioperative Nursing Data Set (PNDS) (see under *data set*)
SNOMED Clinical Terms (SNOMED CT)

nursing information system (NIS) See under *information system*.

nursing intervention See under *intervention*.

Nursing Interventions Classification (NIC) A comprehensive, standardized classification and description of nursing interventions, for use in clinical documentation, communication of care across settings, integration of data across systems and settings, effectiveness research, productivity measurement, competency evaluation, reimbursement, and curricular design. The NIC can be used in all care settings and by all specialties. It can also be used by non-nurse providers to describe treatments performed. Maintained and updated by the Center for Nursing Classification & Clinical Effectiveness at the University of Iowa, **www.nursing.uiowa.edu/centers/cncce**. See also *Nursing Outcomes Classification*.

nursing language A standardized vocabulary used in nursing to describe what nurses do, so that it may be communicated, measured, evaluated, used in electronic health records, and so forth. Not exactly synonyms, but often used interchangeably: nursing classification, nursing data set, nursing terminology, nursing vocabulary. See also *Clinical Care Classification*, *data set*, and *Nursing Information & Data Set Evaluation Center*.

Nursing Management Minimum Data Set (NMMDS) See under *data set*.

Nursing Minimum Data Set (NMDS) See under *data set*.

nursing order A statement written by the nurse that specifies the nursing interventions (see *intervention*) that all nurses caring for the patient should follow.

nursing outcome The Nursing Outcomes Classification (NOC) defines a nursing outcome as "a measurable individual, family, or community state, behavior or perception that is measured along a continuum and is responsive to nursing interventions."

Nursing Outcomes Classification (NOC) A comprehensive, standardized classification of patient/client outcomes developed to evaluate the effects of nursing interventions. The NOC may be used in all settings and across the care continuum to follow patient outcomes throughout an illness episode or over an extended period of care. Because the outcomes describe patient/client status, they can also be used by non-nurses to evaluate their interventions. Maintained and updated by the Center for Nursing Classification & Clinical Effectiveness at the University of Iowa, **www.nursing.uiowa.edu/centers/cncce**. See also *Nursing Interventions Classification*.

nursing phenomenon See *nursing diagnosis*.

nursing process A systematic manner for determining the client's problems, making plans to solve them, initiating the plan or assigning others to implement it, and evaluating the extent to which the plan was effective in resolving the problems identified. The five steps in the process are assessment, diagnosis, planning, implementation, and evaluation.

nursing professional development The continuing education (nonacademic) of professional nurses and others involved in providing nursing care.

Board Certified in Nursing Professional Development A registered nurse with a Bachelor of Science in Nursing (BSN) degree who is qualified in nursing professional development and has passed an examination of the American Nurses Credentialing Center (ANCC) (**nursingworld.org/ancc**). The credential is RN,BC (Registered Nurse, Board Certified).

nursing record That portion of the *medical record* that is the responsibility of the nurse. It contains the nursing care plan, nursing orders, and "nurse's notes" regarding the patient's response. It provides a sequential record of all nursing activities on behalf of the patient as well as accountability and validation of orders (physician and nurse) being carried out.

nursing service The department of the hospital that provides nursing services. Synonym: nursing department.

nursing service administrator A registered nurse responsible for the overall administration and management of nursing services in a hospital. It is the highest nursing position in the hospital. The nursing service administrator may have the title "vice president for nursing" or some similar title. The former title was "nursing director." Synonyms: nursing director, nursing service director, chief of nursing. See also *nursing administration*.

nursing services Those services normally provided by nurses, including personal care, administration of drugs and other medications and treatments, assessment of patients' needs and care requirements, and preparation of care plans for individual patients. Nurse practice acts (laws) in the various states place limitations on the tasks (for example, administration of intravenous medication) that can be performed by registered nurses (RNs), licensed practical nurses (LPNs), and allied personnel, with and without supervision.

nursing specialty An area of nursing practice that is recognized as requiring experience, education, and/or training beyond the basic minimum for licensure. See also *advanced practice nurse*, *certified nurse*, *clinical nurse specialist*, *nurse*, and *nurse practitioner*. The following list is not exhaustive, because new specialties emerge continually (see individual listings for details):

>*acute care nursing*
>*addictions nursing*
>*adult nursing*
>*ambulatory care nursing*
>*anesthetist*
>*baromedical nursing*
>*breastfeeding nursing*
>*cardiac/vascular nursing*
>*case management*
>*coding specialist*
>*college health nursing*
>*community health nursing* (see *public health nursing*)
>*continuing nursing education* (see under *continuing education*)
>*correctional nursing*
>*critical care nursing*
>*developmental disabilities nursing*
>*diabetes nursing*
>*dialysis nursing*
>*electronic fetal monitoring*
>*emergency nursing*
>*family nursing*
>*first assistant*
>*flight nursing*
>*forensic nursing*
>*gastroenterology nursing*
>*general nursing*
>*genetic nursing*
>*gerontological nursing*
>*gynecologic/reproductive health care nursing*
>*HIV/AIDS nursing*
>*holistic nursing*
>*home health nursing*
>*hospice and palliative nursing*
>*informatics nursing*
>*infusion nursing*

legal nurse consulting
life care planning
managed care nursing
maternal newborn nursing
medical-surgical nursing
menopause nursing
midwifery
neonatal nursing
nephrology nursing
neuroscience nursing
nursing administration
nursing professional development
nutrition support
obstetric nursing
occupational health nursing
oncology nursing
ophthalmic nursing
orthopedic nursing
otorhinolaryngology and head-neck nursing
pain management
pediatric nursing
perianesthesia nursing
perinatal nursing
perioperative nursing
plastic surgical nursing
post anesthesia nursing
progressive care nursing
psychiatric and mental health nursing
public health nursing
radiology nursing
rehabilitation nursing
school nursing
telephone nursing practice
transport nursing
urologic nursing
women's health care nursing
wound, ostomy, and continence nursing

nursing staff Those persons employed by a nursing service (nursing department). The nursing staff may include not only registered nurses (RNs), practical nurses, and nurses' aides, but also clerical and other support persons.

nursing team A group of registered nurses (RNs) and auxiliary nursing personnel who provide nursing services, under a nursing team leader, for a designated group of patients.

nursing team leader A registered nurse in charge of a nursing team.

nursing terminology See *nursing language*.

nursing unit See *patient care unit*.

nursing vocabulary See *nursing language*.

nurturing The provision of nourishment. In health care, the nourishment under consideration is that required for the mental, spiritual, emotional, and social well-being of the patient and family as well as their physical well-being. The topic is getting increasing attention as hospital stays are becoming shorter and hospitalization is often being avoided altogether; the nurturing formerly provided by the hospital is proportionately reduced. The situation is compounded in today's society by many factors, including family members' diminished acceptance of responsibility for nurturing one another. Healthcare organizations, community and church support groups, and others are increasing their efforts to assist with nurturing in the home and other settings.

nutraceutical A food or part of a food that is proven to be active in preventing or treating disease, or otherwise beneficial to human health. It was coined in 1989 by Dr. Stephen DeFelice who combined "nutrition" and "pharmaceutical." Some apply the term to foods or food supplements that are alleged (but not proven) to be beneficial. Synonym: functional food.

Nutrient Database for Standard Reference (SR) See *USDA National Nutrient Database for Standard Reference*.

Nutrient Data Laboratory (NDL) The division of the Agricultural Research Service of the U.S. Department of Agriculture (USDA) that is responsible for providing information on the nutrient content of foods consumed in the United States. NDL develops and maintains a number of different databases including the *USDA National Nutrient Database for Standard Reference (SR)*. SR nutrient data serve as the core for most commercial and many foreign databases containing food information.

NDL and its precursors at the USDA have been collecting and managing data about the nutrient content of the U.S. food supply for over 100 years. The first food composition tables were published in 1891 by W.O. Atwater and C.D. Woods, who analyzed the refuse, water, fat, protein, ash, and carbohydrate content of approximately 200 different foods. **www.ars.usda.gov**

nutrition A field of science dealing with the relationships of food products and eating patterns to the development, growth, maintenance, and repair of living organisms. See also *dietetics*.

nutrition assessment Determining the nutritional status of an individual or a group through physical, biochemical, or dietary intake indicators.

anthropometric assessment Measurement of an individual's height, weight, skin fat folds, arm circumference, elbow breadth, or other body measures for the purpose of assessing nutritional status, growth, and development. Synonym: anthropometry.

biochemical assessment The use of laboratory tests on urine, blood, blood fractions, and other tissue to describe an individual's nutritional status. For example, sodium excretion (in urine) can be used to measure compliance with a low sodium diet in hypertensive patients.

dietary assessment Analysis of the nutrient constituents of foods as recorded in a food history. The histories are compiled by trained interviewers doing dietary recalls, by individuals keeping food diaries, or through checking off the frequency of foods consumed, to arrive at a food frequency pattern. Analyses of nutrient constituents can be done using a number of specially developed computer programs or by using printed reference materials such as the U.S. Department of Agriculture (USDA) *Handbook 8* (AH-8) series. See also *USDA Nutrient Database for Standard Reference*.

The assumption is made that consuming amounts of nutrients meeting a standard such as the U.S. National Academy of Sciences' Recommended Dietary Allowances (RDAs) ensures better health through a good nutritional status.

nutritionist A health professional who works in the area of nutrition for either animals or humans. A nutritionist in the field of human nutrition has usually had training that includes chemistry, biochemistry, human physiology and psychology, as well as food science and nutrition.

The term is not definite; there is no consensus among national groups about minimum qualifications—currently, anyone who wishes to do so may call him or herself a nutritionist unless the state's licensure laws have defined the term. Some states require licensure. A nutritionist may be a *dietitian* or *dietetic technician* or neither. The American Hospital Association uses the term as a job classification for registered dietitians. See also *dietetics* and *public health nutritionist*.

Certified Clinical Nutritionist (CCN) A nutritionist with a bachelor's or graduate degree (if bachelor's, a 900-hour internship is required) who has met all requirements for certification by the Clinical Nutrition Certification Board (CNCB). **www.cncb.org**

Certified Nutritionist (CN) This credential designates a graduate of a distance-learning program of the American Health Science University (AHSU) and the National Institute of Nutritional Education (NINE) (**www.ahsu.edu**). This is *not* a national credentialing body, but rather a private institution.

Some states, such as New York, certify qualified nutritionists, in which case they may call themselves "certified nutritionists." State laws vary on qualifications and whether licensure is required.

Certified Nutrition Specialist (CNS) A nutritionist with an advanced degree (master's or doctorate) in nutrition or a related field and professional experience who has passed an examination of the Certification Board for Nutrition Specialists (CBNS), the credentialing arm of the American College of Nutrition (ACN). **www.cert-nutrition.org**

nutrition support The application of nutritional interventions to individuals whose ability to eat, digest, or absorb nutrients has been compromised. This may involve, for example, enteral nutrition (use of a feeding tube into the stomach or intestine) and/or parenteral nutrition (intravenous feeding of special solutions into the large veins).

Certified Nutrition Support Dietitian (CNSD) A registered dietitian who has passed an examination for nutrition support dietitians given by the National Board of Nutrition Support Certification (NBNSC). **www.nutritioncertify.org**

Certified Nutrition Support Nurse (CNSN) A registered nurse who has passed an examination in nutrition support nursing given by the National Board of Nutrition Support Certification (NBNSC). **www.nutritioncertify.org**

Certified Nutrition Support Physician (CNSP) A physician who has passed an examination for nutrition support physicians given by the National Board of Nutrition Support Certification (NBNSC). **www.nutritioncertify.org**

NVHRI See *National Voluntary Hospital Reporting Initiative*.

NVSS See *National Vital Statistics System*.

O

OAM See *Office of Alternative Medicine.*

O&M See *orientation and mobility specialist.*

OAS Office of Applied Studies. See *Substance Abuse and Mental Health Services Administration.*

OASH *Office of the Assistant Secretary for Health.* See *Assistant Secretary for Health.*

OASIS See *Organization for the Advancement of Structured Information Standards* and *Outcome and Assessment Information Set* (under *data set*).

OAT See *Office for the Advancement of Telehealth.*

obesity The condition of being obese, or significantly overweight. Determining a person's "ideal" body weight is now typically done by calculating the *body mass index (BMI)*, a number that takes into account an individual's height and weight. People with a BMI of 25 to 29.9 are considered simply "overweight." Those with a BMI of 30 and above are considered "obese."

In a 1999 study, researchers from the Centers for Disease Control and Prevention (CDC) reported that more than half of all U.S. adults were overweight or obese. By 2004, that percentage had grown to 66% (with an estimated 30% of adults being obese). Several studies note that obesity has become a major cause of death in the United States (approximately 280,000 people annually) and a major public health problem.

Ob/Gyn See *obstetrics-gynecology.*

OBHSA Oregon Basic Health Services Act. See *Oregon Health Plan.*

OBQI See *outcome based quality improvement.*

OBRA 80 See *Omnibus Budget Reconciliation Act of 1980.*

OBRA 81 See *Omnibus Budget Reconciliation Act of 1981.*

OBRA 87 See *Omnibus Budget Reconciliation Act of 1987.*

OBRA 89 See *Omnibus Budget Reconciliation Act of 1989.*

OBRA 90 See *Omnibus Budget Reconciliation Act of 1990.*

OBRA 93 See *Omnibus Budget Reconciliation Act of 1993.*

observation bed See under *bed.*

obstetric nursing The area of nursing focusing on the needs of women during pregnancy and childbirth.

   Inpatient Obstetric Nurse (RNC) A registered nurse specializing in inpatient obstetric nursing, who has passed an examination of the National Certification Corporation (NCC) and received the credential Registered Nurse Certified (RNC). **www.nccnet.org**

obstetric patient See *maternity patient.*

obstetrics The branch of medicine dealing with pregnancy and the delivery of babies.

obstetrics-gynecology (Ob/Gyn) The study of disorders of the female reproductive system, pregnancy, and the delivery of babies.

occasion of service A specific act of service provided a patient, such as a test or procedure.

occupancy rate See under *rate (ratio).*

occupational health An area of specialization in health care that concerns the factors (such as working conditions and exposure to hazardous materials) in an occupation that influence the health of workers in that occupation, and which is concerned generally with the prevention of disease and injury and the maintenance of fitness (because these factors are important in maintaining a stable work force).

occupational health nursing The nursing specialty that focuses on the needs of employees in the work setting, including accident prevention, counseling, and health education.

   Certified Occupational Health Nurse (COHN) An occupational health nursing specialist who has passed an examination of the American Board for Occupational Health Nurses

(ABOHN). See also *Certified Occupational Health Nurse/Case Manager* under *case manager*. www.abohn.org

Certified Occupational Health Nurse—Specialist (COHN-S) An occupational health nursing specialist with a bachelor's degree or higher who has passed an advanced examination of the American Board for Occupational Health Nurses (ABOHN). See also *Certified Occupational Health Nurse—Specialist/Case Manager* under *case manager*. www.abohn.org

occupational medicine The medical specialty within preventive medicine that deals with occupational health.

Occupational Safety and Health Administration (OSHA) A federal agency responsible for developing and enforcing regulations regarding safety and health among workers in the United States. OSHA was created by the Occupational Safety and Health Act of 1970, along with the National Institute for Occupational Safety and Health (NIOSH). See also *Voluntary Protection Program*. www.osha.gov

occupational therapist (OT) A health professional who practices occupational therapy. Requires a minimum of a bachelor's degree in OT and state licensure.

Occupational Therapist Registered (OTR) An occupational therapist who has passed a national certification examination. Beginning in 2007, a master's degree is required. National Board for Certification in Occupational Therapy (NBCOT). www.nbcot.org

occupational therapy (OT) Treatment by means of activities to assist a person who is disabled, for example due to illness, accident, aging, or emotional problems. The purpose is to help the person develop or improve the skills necessary for an independent, productive, and satisfying life. Treatment may address psychological, social, and environmental factors that impede successful functioning. It may also help compensate for a permanent loss of function, such as with use of special equipment.

occupational therapy assistant (OTA) A health professional who provides occupational therapy treatment under the direction of an occupational therapist (OT). At least an associate's degree or certificate is required.

Certified Occupational Therapy Assistant (COTA) An occupational therapy assistant who has passed a national examination given by the National Board for Certification in Occupational Therapy (NBCOT). www.nbcot.org

occurrence-based coverage See under *insurance coverage*.

occurrence reporting A system of reporting cases that have been detected in *occurrence screening* (see under *screening*) and then, in the judgment of reviewers, merit further study within the hospital.

occurrence screening See under *screening (quality)*.

OCE See *Outpatient Code Editor*.

OCN See *Oncology Certified Nurse* under *oncology nursing*.

OCS See *Orthopaedic Certified Specialist* under *physical therapist*.

ocularist A health professional who specializes in the fabrication and fitting of artificial eyes, called ocular prosthetics.

Board Certified Ocularist (BCO) An ocularist certified by the National Examining Board of Ocularists (NEBO). www.neboboard.org

OD Doctor of Optometry; see *optometrist*. See also *Office of the Director*, under both *Centers for Disease Control and Prevention* and *National Institutes of Health*.

odontology See *dentistry*.

ODPHP See *Office of Disease Prevention and Health Promotion*.

office audit system A technique reported from Canada in which a review team goes into the offices of physicians whose practice is outside the hospital and examines patient records (medical records) for the purpose of determining the quality of care.

Office for Human Research Protection (OHRP) A division of the Department of Health and Human Services (HHS) established in 2000 to make sure that institutions are complying with regulations concerning research using human subjects. See also *institutional review board*. **www.hhs.gov/ohrp**

Office for the Advancement of Telehealth (OAT) A division of the Health Resources and Services Administration (HRSA) dedicated to supporting and promoting the use of *telehealth* technologies, especially to meet the needs of underserved populations. **www.hrsa.gov/telehealth**

Office of Alternative Medicine (OAM) An agency within the National Institutes of Health (NIH) established by an act of Congress in 1991. NIH has since created the *National Center for Complementary and Alternative Medicine (NCCAM)* (see under *National Institutes of Health*) to replace it.

Office of Disease Prevention and Health Promotion (ODPHP) An agency within the Department of Health and Human Services (HHS) charged with developing and coordinating national disease prevention and health promotion strategies. Among its many projects are the *Dietary Guidelines for Americans*, published every five years; *healthfinder*, a health information web site; and *Healthy People 2010*. **odphp.osophs.dhhs.gov**

Office of Genetics and Disease Prevention (OGDP) See *National Office of Public Health Genomics* under *Coordinating Center for Health Promotion*, under *Centers for Disease Control and Prevention*.

Office of Health Technology Assessment (OHTA) A former component of the Agency for Healthcare Research and Quality (AHRQ) that evaluated, on request from CMS, the risks, benefits, and clinical effectiveness of new or unestablished medical technologies that were being considered for coverage under Medicare. The assessments of OHTA formed the basis for recommendations to CMS as to coverage policy decisions under Medicare. OHTA reports were called Health Technology Assessment Reports (HTARs). AHRQ continues to provide this service to CMS through its "technology assessment program." See also *Office of Technology Assessment (OTA)*. **www.ahrq.gov/clinic/techix.htm**

Office of Inspector General (OIG) A federal official who reports to Congress and to certain heads of administrative agencies on the activities of those agencies. This "watchdog" post is typically created by statute. Agencies also have their own inspector generals (IGs) who carry out similar functions with respect to the internal functions of the agency and outside programs that the agency funds.

In the Department of Health and Human Services (HHS), the OIG is responsible for conducting and supervising audits, investigations, and inspections relating to programs and operations of the HHS. The OIG's efforts are to improve HHS efficiency as well as prevent fraud and abuse. This position came into being in 1976 largely as a result of congressional concerns about fraud and abuse in Medicare and Medicaid.

In an effort at coordinating the efforts of different governmental agencies, the online resource called "IGNet" provides information on Inspector General functions throughout the executive branch. **www.ignet.gov**

Office of Management and Budget (OMB) The agency in the federal executive branch that prepares and monitors the budget. **www.whitehouse.gov/omb**

Office of Medical Applications of Research (OMAR) An agency of the National Institutes of Health (NIH) whose mission is to study and evaluate research as to its applicability in medicine, and to promulgate its findings. A major responsibility of OMAR is the coordination of the *National Institutes of Health Consensus Development Program*. **odp.od.nih.gov/omar**

Office of Minority Health (OMH) An agency within the Department of Health and Human Services (HHS), under the direction of the Deputy Assistant Secretary for Minority Health, that advises the Secretary of HHS and the Office of Public Health and Science (OPHS) on public health program activities affecting American Indians and Alaska Natives, Asian Americans, Blacks/African Americans, Hispanics/Latinos, Native Hawaiians, and other Pacific Islanders. **www.omhrc.gov**

Office of Personnel Management (OPM) The office that purchases health services for the federal government through the Federal Employees Health Benefits Program (FEHBP, FEP), Federal Employees Dental and Vision Insurance Program (FEDVIP), and other programs. **www.opm.gov**

Office of Public Health and Science (OPHS) An agency within the Department of Health and Human Services (HHS), under the direction of the Assistant Secretary for Health (ASH) (**www.osophs.dhhs.gov/ophs**). The OPHS includes a number of divisions:

> Office of Disease Prevention & Health Promotion
> Office of Global Health Affairs
> Office of HIV/AIDS Policy
> Office of Human Research Protections
> Office of Minority Health
> Office of Population Affairs
> Office of Research Integrity
> Office of the Surgeon General
> Office on Women's Health
> President's Council on Physical Fitness and Sports
> Regional Health Administrators

Office of Technology Assessment (OTA) A congressional investigative body established in 1972 whose duties had to do with assessing the merits and applications of technology. OTA ceased functioning in September 1995 due to budget cuts. However, some archived documents and other information are still available. See also *Office of Health Technology Assessment*. **www.gpo.gov/ota**

Office of Terrorism Preparedness and Emergency Response (OTPER) See *Coordinating Office for Terrorism Preparedness and Emergency Response* under *Centers for Disease Control and Prevention*.

Office of the Assistant Secretary for Health (OASH) See *Assistant Secretary for Health*.

Office of the Director (OD) See *Office of the Director* under both *Centers for Disease Control and Prevention* and *National Institutes of Health*.

Office of the National Coordinator for Health Information Technology (ONC/ ONCHIT) A division of the U.S. Department of Health and Human Services (HHS), created in 2004, whose mission is to support and promote the widespread adoption of interoperable electronic health records (EHRs) (see *Nationwide Health Information Network*) and provide leadership to achieve the goals of the *Strategic Framework*. The ONC also provides management of and logistical support for the *American Health Information Community (AHIC)*. **www.hhs.gov/healthit**

Office of the Secretary of Health and Human Services (OS) The agency within the Department of Health and Human Services (HHS) that supports the work of the secretary, which is to advise the president on federal health, welfare, and income security plans, policies, and programs. It includes the *Office of Disease Prevention and Health Promotion (ODPHP)* and the *Office of Public Health and Science (OPHS)*. **www.hhs.gov/secretaryspage.html**

Office of Women's Health (OWH) A division of the Food and Drug Administration (FDA) dedicated to issues especially concerning women. **www.fda.gov/womens**

Office on Women's Health (OWH) A division of the Department of Health and Human Services (HHS) that focuses on women's health issues, and works to redress inequities in research, healthcare services, and education that have historically placed the health of women at risk. **www.4woman.gov/owh**

officer A person holding a position of authority, either by election or appointment, in an organization. In a corporation, the officers are appointed by the corporate directors to manage the day-to-day affairs of the corporation, and have specific authority and responsibilities given to them by the directors and by law.

office visit See under *visit*.

off-label use Use of a drug for conditions other than those approved by the Food and Drug Administration (FDA). At least one in five prescriptions is written for an off-label use.

OGDP See *National Office of Public Health Genomics* under *Coordinating Center for Health Promotion*, under *Centers for Disease Control and Prevention*.

OHCA See *Organized Health Care Arrangement*.

OHP See *Oregon Health Plan*.

OHRP See *Office for Human Research Protection*.

OHS Online healthcare services; see *telehealth*.

OHTA See *Office of Health Technology Assessment*.

OIG See *Office of Inspector General*.

OLAP See *Online Analytical Processing*.

Older Americans Act (OAA) A federal statute enacted in 1965 that defines the national policy on aging. The OAA also established the Administration on Aging (AoA) as the federal focal point and advocate agency for older Americans (sixty years of age or older). The objectives of the OAA are implemented with joint efforts among the federal, state, and local agencies dealing with aging, and include such programs as congregate and home-delivered meals. The OAA was amended in 1992 to give state agencies greater powers in protecting the rights of vulnerable older Americans via Title VII, the "Vulnerable Elder Rights Protection Title." See also *area agency on aging* and *vulnerable adult*. 42 U.S.C. § 3001 et seq. (2004).

oligopsony A market in which there are only a few buyers, who exert great influence on the market. A special case of oligopsony is a monopsony, where there is only one buyer.

OLT See *ophthalmic laboratory technician*.

OLTP Online Transaction Processing. See *Online Analytical Processing*.

OMA See *ophthalmic medical assistant*.

Omaha System A standardized classification for use by nurses and other healthcare professionals in any setting from the time of patient/client admission to discharge. The system has three components: an assessment component (Problem Classification Scheme), an intervention component (Intervention Scheme), and an outcomes component (Problem Rating Scale for Outcomes). The Omaha System was originally developed in the early 1970s by the Visiting Nurses Association (VNA) of Omaha, Nebraska. An extensive revision of terms, codes, and definitions was published in 2005. **www.omahasystem.org**

OMB See *Office of Management and Budget*.

ombudsperson See *patient advocate*. See also *Medicare Beneficiary Ombudsman*.

OMD Doctor of *Oriental medicine* (see under *medicine (system)*).

OMH See *Office of Minority Health*.

OMM Osteopathic manipulative medicine. See *osteopathy* under *medicine (system)*.

Omnibus Budget Reconciliation Act of 1980 (OBRA 80) Federal legislation that included the creation of *ambulatory surgical center (ASC)* payment benefits. It also made a significant change in the provision of the Medicaid law that governs payment for long-term care facility (LTCF) services. See also *Omnibus Budget Reconciliation Act of 1981*. Pub. L. No. 96-499, 94 Stat. 2599.

Omnibus Budget Reconciliation Act of 1981 (OBRA 81) Federal legislation that made several significant changes in the provisions of the Medicaid law that govern payments for inpatient hospital services. OBRA 81 made these payments comparable to those for long-term care facility (LTCF) services, as had been done in the previous OBRA 80. Previously, payments made by the states for Medicaid services were based on a reasonable cost calculation, whereas under OBRA 80 and OBRA 81 the states were given more administrative and fiscal discretion to set payment rates. The resulting rates needed only to be "reasonable and adequate." Collectively these two acts were referred to as the **Boren Amendment**. Pub. L. No. 97-35 (1981).

Omnibus Budget Reconciliation Act of 1987 (OBRA 87) A federal act that included the *Nursing Home Reform Act (NHRA)*. Pub. L. No. 100-203, 101 Stat. 1330 (1987).

Omnibus Budget Reconciliation Act of 1989 (OBRA 89) Federal legislation that, among other things, called for significant physician payment reform and increased funding for effectiveness research. The act amended Title XVIII of the Social Security Act by adding section 1848, "Payment for Physician Services." Among other things, section 1848 dealt with creating a fee schedule for the payment of provider services, the rate of increases in Medicare expenditures, and limits on the amounts that nonparticipating providers can charge Medicare beneficiaries. The establishment of the fee schedule replaced the "reasonable charge system" used to pay Medicare fees until January 1, 1992. OBRA 89 required that payments under the new fee schedule be based on nationally uniform "relative value units" (RVUs), which are related to the resources used in providing the service. Section 1848(c) of OBRA 89 established RVUs for physician work, practice (overhead) expense, and malpractice (liability insurance) costs.

To account for geographical differences in the cost of providing services (rent is higher in New York City than in Saint Paul, for example), the act implemented Geographic Practice Cost Indices (GPCIs), pronounced "gypsies" and sometimes called "geographic adjustment factors" (GAFs). Each state is divided into one or more geographical regions and assigned a work, practice, and malpractice GPCI value for each region. Each RVU value is then adjusted by its corresponding GPCI value, resulting in a resource-based relative value (RBRV). When this number is multiplied by a federally determined "converter," the result is the actual dollar amount the provider is paid for providing the service to the Medicare patient. This federal converter, called a "conversion factor" (CF) by the feds, is different for surgical services, nonsurgical services, anesthesia, and primary care services. Pub. L. No. 101-239, 103 Stat. 2106 (1989).

Omnibus Budget Reconciliation Act of 1990 (OBRA 90) Federal legislation that created the *Medicare Select* program, and included the *Patient Self-Determination Act (PSDA)*. See also *social HMO* under *health maintenance organization*. Pub. L. No. 101-508, 104 Stat. 1388 (1990).

Omnibus Budget Reconciliation Act of 1993 (OBRA 93) Federal legislation that included a provision, amending the *Employee Retirement Income Security Act (ERISA)*, that established health insurance equity between the adopted children of parents and their "biological" children. See also *Stark II*. Pub. L. No. 103-66, 107 Stat. 312 (1993).

OMP *Ophthalmic medical personnel*. See *ophthalmic medical assistant*, *ophthalmic medical technologist*, and *ophthalmic technician*.

OMR See *online medical record* under *electronic health record*.

OMS Online medical services; see *telemedicine*.

OMT See *osteopathic manipulative treatment* and *ophthalmic medical technologist*.

ONC See *Office of the National Coordinator for Health Information Technology*, and *Orthopaedic Nurse Certified* (under *orthopaedic nursing*).

on call Available during a specified period of time to respond to emergencies or other needs. For example, an obstetrician may be "on call" at a hospital maternity unit on Tuesday nights, so if a birth is imminent (or a problem arises) on a Tuesday night, the hospital would contact that physician to come in and handle it. If a physician is on "emergency room call" (ER call), she would be contacted if a patient needing her special services (for example, psychiatry) arrived at the ER during that time period. A physician may or may not be compensated for being on call, depending upon the agreement with the hospital.

ONCHIT See *Office of the National Coordinator for Health Information Technology*.

ONCHIT Framework See *Strategic Framework*.

ONCHIT1 A Request for Proposal (RFP) issued by the Department of Health and Human Services (HHS) in 2005, with the aim of bringing together organizations with a stake in health data standards to develop a healthcare information technology (HIT) standards harmonization process. The contract was awarded to ANSI, which established the **Healthcare Information Technology Standards Panel (HITSP)**. The term "ONCHIT1" sometimes is used to refer to the harmonization effort in general, or to HITSP. The formal name of ONCHIT1 was "The Evaluation of Standards Harmonization Process for Health Information Technology Program."

oncogene A gene that contributes to cancer formation when mutated or inappropriately expressed.

oncologist A physician specializing in oncology.

oncology The science of the diagnosis and treatment of tumors. See also **cancer**.

oncology nursing The area of nursing focusing on the needs of cancer patients

Advanced Oncology Certified Clinical Nurse Specialist (AOCNS) A registered nurse with a master's degree or higher, with experience in oncology nursing, who has passed an advanced examination of the Oncology Nursing Certification Corporation (ONCC). **www.oncc.org**

Advanced Oncology Certified Nurse (AOCN) A specialist in oncology nursing who has passed an advanced examination of the Oncology Nursing Certification Corporation (ONCC). This credential is no longer being offered, but is being renewed. **www.oncc.org**

Advanced Oncology Certified Nurse Practitioner (AOCNP) A nurse practitioner with a master's degree or higher, with experience in oncology nursing, who has passed an advanced examination of the Oncology Nursing Certification Corporation (ONCC). **www.oncc.org**

Certified Pediatric Oncology Nurse (CPON) A registered nurse with experience in pediatric oncology nursing who has passed an examination of the Oncology Nursing Certification Corporation (ONCC). **www.oncc.org**

Oncology Certified Nurse (OCN) A registered nurse with experience in oncology nursing who has passed an examination of the Oncology Nursing Certification Corporation (ONCC). **www.oncc.org**

100,000 Lives Campaign An effort, organized by the Institute for Healthcare Improvement (IHI), to help reduce medical errors and improve quality at participating hospitals (over 3,000), thus saving (a goal of) 100,000 patient lives. IHI estimated that after the first eighteen months, as of June 2006, 122,300 avoidable deaths had been prevented. Hospitals that participated committed to implementing some or all of the following changes:

- Activate a rapid response team at the first sign that a patient's condition is worsening and may lead to a more serious medical emergency.
- Prevent patients from dying of heart attacks by delivering evidence-based care, such as appropriate administration of aspirin and beta-blockers to prevent further heart muscle damage.
- Prevent medication errors by ensuring that accurate and continually updated lists of patients' medications are reviewed and reconciled during their hospital stay, particularly at transition points.
- Prevent patients who are receiving medicines and fluids through central lines from developing infections by following five steps, including proper hand washing and cleaning the patient's skin with chlorhexidine (a type of antiseptic).
- Prevent patients undergoing surgery from developing infections by following a series of steps, including the timely administration of antibiotics.
- Prevent patients on ventilators from developing pneumonia by following four steps, including raising the head of the patient's bed between 30 and 45 degrees.

This initiative was followed by the **5 Million Lives Campaign**.

Online Analytical Processing (OLAP) Computer software that uses *multi-dimensional* data bases and thus provides more detailed analyses and greater analytical speed than formerly possible. OLAP is distinguished from **Online Transaction Processing (OLTP)**, which typically uses relational databases that are characterized as being *two-dimensional* (rows and columns).

OLTP software supports many users who are adding, editing, and removing individual records in a database, one record at a time. To do a query in this context involves searching many individual records, which could bring even a powerful computer to a standstill if it involved many millions of records. OLAP, on the other hand, tends to deal with data that are already summarized in such a way as to support what is known as "multidimensional data analysis." By predigesting or "consolidating" the values contained in many separate records and storing the results back into the database, there is now a third dimension (time, or "trend") to the database that allows a much faster response time, no matter how large the database has become. Although the standard database language for two-dimensional, relational databases is SQL, OLAP databases will require a new language, possibly called MDSQL, for multi-dimensional structured query language. See also *database management system*.

online healthcare services (OHS) See *telehealth*.

online medical record (OMR) See under *electronic health record*.

online medical services (OMS) See *telemedicine*.

Online Survey Certification and Reporting System (OSCAR) A data network maintained by CMS containing information on the quality of long-term care facilities. OSCAR compiles all the data elements collected by state surveyors during the inspection conducted at nursing facilities for the purpose of certification for participation in Medicare and Medicaid. OSCAR includes information on the operations, patient census, and regulatory compliance of long-term care facilities.

Online Transaction Processing (OLTP) See *Online Analytical Processing*.

On Lok Short for On Lok Senior Health Services, a program in San Francisco's Chinatown that enables severely disabled and frail older persons to remain at home rather than be placed in nursing homes. (On Lok means "happy home.") **www.onlok.org**

ONTR Order not to resuscitate. See *do not resuscitate*.

OP See *outpatient*.

OPA See *organ procurement agency*.

OPCS-4 *Office of Population Censuses and Surveys Classification of Surgical Operations and Procedures, 4th Revision.* An "intervention classification" devised for translating or classifying all operations and surgical procedures that may be carried out on a patient during an episode of health care. Used by the National Health Service (NHS) in the United Kingdom.

open access A descriptive term for a managed care plan (MCP) or a health maintenance organization (HMO) in which the beneficiary or subscriber can go directly to a healthcare specialist without going through a gatekeeper. See also *managed care*.

open account See under *account*.

open-ended health maintenance organization (open-ended HMO) See *point-of-service*.

open enrollment A limited time period, usually occurring annually, during which individuals are given the opportunity to enroll in a healthcare insurance plan without medical screening, and without regard to their health status. Open enrollment is a characteristic of some Blue Cross and Blue Shield plans and some health maintenance organizations (HMOs). The time period is limited in order to minimize the potential for *adverse selection*. Open enrollment is an effort to approach *community rating* (see under *rating*).

OpenGALEN See *GALEN*.

open medical staff See under *medical staff*.

Open Source A reference to computer software that has been developed and distributed in conformance with the certification requirements of the **Open Source Initiative (OSI)** (**www.opensource.org**). OSI consists of a group of individuals, tied together through the Internet, who believe that when programmers have free access to a software's *source code*, the software can evolve and improve much more quickly than "closed source" (proprietary) software.

It is also argued that Open Source software is more secure and reliable, largely due to the fact that it undergoes more peer review. Probably the best known single example of Open

Source software is the Linux operating system. Also, much of the Internet's foundation consists of Open Source software, including the Apache web server and the TCP/IP, SMTP, HTTP, POP3, IMAP, NFS, and other open standard protocols.

The term "open source" (typically lower case) is increasingly used in a *generic* context to mean software that is a product of world-wide collaboration and is made freely available, for "the good of the community." However, Open Source software has a very precise definition, and is in fact licensed and restricted; see the **Open Source Definition** at **www.opensource.org/docs/definition.php**. Software that meets the OSI requirements receives the **OSI Certified** mark. It should not be confused with "shareware" or "freeware," which have significantly different licensing schemes, or with software that is in the public domain.

open staff See *open medical staff* under *medical staff*.

open standard A standard (norm) that is not proprietary. Notable examples of open standards in the healthcare industry include HL7, DICOM, and XML. An "open standard" shouldn't be confused with *Open Source*, in spite of their sharing related ideas.

Open Systems Interconnection See *OSI*.

OpenVistA See *Hui OpenVistA* under *VistA*.

operating room (OR) A room specially equipped for the performance of surgical *operations*. The OR is staffed by a specialized team of health professionals, commonly including the *operating surgeon* (see under *surgeon*), the *surgical assistant*, the *anesthesiologist* or *anesthetist*, the *circulator*, and the *scrub*. ORs may be general or specialized, such as for neurological or orthopaedic surgery.

operating room nurse See *perioperative nursing*.

operating room procedure See under *procedure*.

operating room technician (ORT) See *surgical technologist*.

operating statement See *income and expense statement*.

operation Sometimes an operation is defined as identical with a "surgical procedure" (see *procedure*). In general usage, however, the term "operation" is rarely used for a single procedure; the term suggests an event of sufficient magnitude that it requires special preparation of the patient, use of an operating room (OR), assistance to the operator by nurses and often other surgeons, sometimes anesthesia, and postoperative care. The term "procedure," on the other hand, usually refers to something that is discrete, and for which a relatively short time is required for execution.

An operation often actually consists of a number of procedures, and the array of procedures that make up a given operation will vary from patient to patient. For example, cholecystectomy (gallbladder removal) for one patient may include "exploration of the common bile duct," whereas for another, this procedure may be omitted. For this reason, a proper description of an operation requires that its procedures be listed.

operative In the context of a surgical operation. The word "operative" is usually encountered modified by pre-, intra-, post-, or peri-. **Preoperative** refers to events preceding a surgical operation, whereas **postoperative** refers to events following the operation. Events occurring during the operation itself are **intraoperative**, whereas **perioperative** describes all events surrounding the operation—before, during, and after.

OPHS See *Office of Public Health and Science*.

ophthalmic Having to do with the eye.

ophthalmic assistant See *ophthalmic medical assistant*.

ophthalmic dispenser A health professional trained in dispensing optical products and services. See *contact lens technician* and *dispensing optician*.

ophthalmic laboratory technician (OLT) A health professional who fulfills the prescriptions of optometrists and ophthalmologists by cutting, grinding, and finishing the lenses. Most learn on the job, although there are formal training programs.

ophthalmic medical assistant (OMA) A health professional trained to assist in an ophthalmologist's office by taking patient histories, making eye measurements, administering tests, and performing other tasks as directed by the ophthalmologist.

Certified Ophthalmic Assistant (COA) An ophthalmic medical assistant who has completed an accredited postsecondary program in ophthalmic medical assisting and met other requirements for certification by the Joint Commission on Allied Health Personnel in Ophthalmology (JCAHPO). **www.jcahpo.org/newsite**

Corporate Certified Ophthalmic Assistant (CCOA) An ophthalmic medical assistant who works for a company that supplies products and services to the field of ophthalmology, who has qualified for and obtained certification from the Joint Commission on Allied Health Personnel in Ophthalmology (JCAHPO). **www.jcahpo.org/newsite**

ophthalmic medical personnel (OMP) See *ophthalmic medical assistant*, *ophthalmic medical technologist*, and *ophthalmic technician*.

ophthalmic medical technologist (OMT) An ophthalmic medical assistant who has all of the skills of the ophthalmic technician, plus advanced training in microbiology, general medical knowledge, photography, pharmacology, and other areas.

Certified Ophthalmic Medical Technologist (COMT) An ophthalmic medical technologist who has passed an examination and met other requirements for certification by the Joint Commission on Allied Health Personnel in Ophthalmology (JCAHPO). **www.jcahpo.org/newsite**

ophthalmic nursing The area of nursing focusing on the needs of ophthalmic patients.

Certified Ophthalmic Registered Nurse (CRNO) A specialist in ophthalmic nursing who has passed an examination of the National Certifying Board for Ophthalmic Registered Nurses. **webeye.ophth.uiowa.edu/ASORN**

ophthalmic photography A specialized form of medical imaging dedicated to the study and treatment of disorders of the eye. See also *retinal angiography*.

ophthalmic surgical assistant (OSA) A health professional trained to assist in ophthalmic surgical procedures.

Certified Ophthalmic Surgical Assistant (COSA) An ophthalmic surgical assistant who has met the requirements for certification by the Joint Commission on Allied Health Personnel in Ophthalmology (JCAHPO). **www.jcahpo.org/newsite**

ophthalmic technician (OT) An ophthalmic medical assistant with additional training in the areas of clinical optics, visual fields, and other technical areas.

Certified Ophthalmic Technician (COT) An ophthalmic technician who has passed an examination and met other requirements for certification by the Joint Commission on Allied Health Personnel in Ophthalmology (JCAHPO). **www.jcahpo.org/newsite**

ophthalmic ultrasound biometrist (OUB) A health professional who uses sonography and biometrics to make assessments of patients under the supervision of an ophthalmologist.

Registered Ophthalmic Ultrasound Biometrist (ROUB) An ophthalmic ultrasound biometrist who has met the requirements for certification of the Joint Commission on Allied Health Personnel in Ophthalmology (JCAHPO). **www.jcahpo.org/newsite**

ophthalmologist A physician who specializes in the field of ophthalmology.

ophthalmology The study of the eye, its physiology, anatomy, and diseases. Subspecialty areas include vitreo-retinal surgery, cataract surgery, cornea surgery, glaucoma, lasik/refractive surgery, neuro-ophthalmology, ocular pathology, oculoplastic surgery, pediatric ophthalmology, and strabismus surgery.

opiaphobia A somewhat pejorative term, coined by some healthcare providers to describe other providers who, for a variety of reasons, are believed to be too hesitant in prescribing pain killing drugs to their patients. Typical reasons given for not prescribing these drugs include the fear of patient addiction, societal and regulatory censure, and diversion of drugs to unauthorized users.

OPO Organ procurement organization. See *organ procurement agency*.

opportunistic infection See under *infection*.

OPPS See *outpatient prospective payment system* under *prospective payment system*.

OP service See *outpatient service*.

optician See *dispensing optician*.

opticianry The profession of filling prescriptions for glasses and contact lenses, fitting glasses, and dispensing glasses and other ophthalmic devices.

optimal coding See under *coding (billing)*.

optionality When used in medical informatics, optionality refers to the amount of freedom a communication standard allows in requiring the presence of certain segments, or fields within those segments. In a standard with no optionality, each message conforming to that standard will contain all segments and fields, whether or not they happen to be needed in that particular message. In a standard with a high degree of optionality, messages being exchanged may vary greatly in their content. As one might guess, higher degrees of optionality can cause problems when information is exchanged between different environments because there is less certainty as to the format. The benefits of greater optionality include the ability to extend the standard to meet more varied needs, to tailor messages for specific purposes, as well as to reduce unnecessary overhead. See *HL7* for more discussion about communication standards.

optometrist A health professional who examines eyes for health, visual acuity, depth and color perception, and ability to coordinate and focus. An optometrist may prescribe corrective lenses and some drugs, assist eye surgery patients before and after surgery, and diagnose certain systemic diseases such as diabetes and high blood pressure. All states require licensure, for which a candidate must possess a doctor of optometry (OD) degree and pass a state or national examination.

optometry The branch of science that deals with measurement of vision and the effects of lenses and prisms on vision. Optometry is not a branch of medicine.

OR See *operating room*.

oral surgeon A dentist who specializes in surgical treatment of disorders, diseases, and injuries of the jaws and adjacent structures.

Orange Book The common name for *Approved Drug Products with Therapeutic Equivalence Evaluations*, a book published by the Food and Drug Administration (FDA). See *therapeutic equivalent*.

order (judge) A command of a court (judge) that a certain action be taken or not taken. A court order may be made before or during a lawsuit; a final order is issued once the case has been formally decided.

order (nurse) See *nursing order*.

order (physician) Doctor's order. A directive from a physician to a nurse or other individual as to drugs, treatments, examinations, and other care to be given to a patient.

orderly A hospital attendant, without professional qualifications, who does heavy or routine work, such as transporting patients.

order not to resuscitate (ONTR) See *do not resuscitate*.

Oregon Better Health Act (OBHA) Legislation proposed in Oregon in 2007 to reform the system of health care in the state so that all individuals are insured. OBHA proposes to reallocate the public dollars currently being spent on health care, including both state and federal funding (for example, Medicaid and Medicare) to optimize the health of Oregon citizens and maximize the value of healthcare expenditures. Financial incentives would be realigned to ensure fair and reasonable payment to providers, value-based cost-sharing for consumers, and the transition to a more efficient delivery system.

All state citizens would equitably contribute to a "pool" to fund basic health insurance for everyone, regardless of income or status. Each individual would be entitled to a defined set of essential health services (the "core benefit"), which would be determined according to a process and set of criteria similar to that used in the **Oregon Health Plan**. This benefit would be fully portable, because it would not be tied to employment. Everyone (including employers) would be free to offer and purchase secondary insurance for additional services (beyond the core benefit). OBHA would authorize the state to seek the necessary permission from Congress to reallocate the public funds. Also, a process would be created whereby everyone—the general public, employers, employees, senior citizens, and healthcare providers—would have an opportunity to compare the new system with the current system before a new system is implemented.

Oregon Death with Dignity Act A statute enacted by the Oregon legislature in 1997 under which physician-assisted suicide became a legal medical option. The act allows terminally ill Oregon residents to obtain from their physicians, and use, prescriptions for self-administered, lethal medications. The act states that ending one's life in accordance with the law does not constitute suicide. However, the term "physician-assisted suicide" is commonly used (even in Oregon) to describe the provisions of this law because this is the term used by the public, and by the medical literature, to describe ending life through the voluntary self-administration of lethal medications, expressly prescribed by a physician for that purpose. The Death with Dignity Act specifically prohibits euthanasia, where a physician or other person directly administers a medication to end another's life. Or. Rev. Stat. § 127.800 et seq.

Oregon Health Plan (OHP) A state health plan initiated in 1989 when Oregon passed the Oregon Basic Health Services Act (OBHSA), designed to ensure that all citizens would receive at least basic health care.

One part of the OHP expanded Medicaid coverage to all residents below the federal poverty level. This was done by prioritizing services offered on the basis of the cost-benefits of each of some 750 "diagnosis-treatment (or condition-treatment) pairs," which were carefully developed by physicians, other providers, and with significant community input. The Oregon Health Services Commission included most conditions that are encountered in caring for the Oregon population. The diagnosis-treatment pairs were ranked from highest priority (pairs expected to have full recovery from established treatments, such as acute appendicitis with appendectomy) to lowest priority (pairs such as minor cosmetic surgery). Actuarial analysis then determined how far down the list of pairs the available funds would go in providing the services to all the population. Those pairs above the line are funded, those below are not. The Prioritized List of Health Services is evaluated and modified every two years. In the mid 1990s, mental health and chemical dependency services were added.

In October 2006 the list had 710 pairs, and was funded through line 530. As an example of priorities, the first pair funded (at the top of the list) is "severe/moderate head injury: hematoma/edema with loss of consciousness" with the treatment "medical and surgical treatment." The last funded pair is "chronic otitis media" with "PE tubes/adenoidectomy/tympanoplasty, medical therapy." The very last pair on the list (number 710) is "disorders of refraction and accommodation" with "radial keratotomy." The full list can be seen at **egov.oregon.gov/DAS/ OHPPR/HSC/current_prior.shtml**.

A second part of the Oregon Health Plan required employers to cover employees and their dependents (this mandate never went into effect). A third required the small insurance market to form an all-payers' high risk pool (see **risk pool**). **egov.oregon.gov/DHS/healthplan**

organ A part of the body that carries out a specific activity or function, for example, digestion.

organizational liability See **enterprise liability** under **liability (legal)**.

organizational responsibility officer See **corporate integrity agreement**.

Organization for the Advancement of Structured Information Standards (OASIS) An international, nonprofit consortium that creates interoperable industry specifications based on public standards such as XML and SGML, and others related to structured information processing. **www.oasis-open.org**

Organized Health Care Arrangement (OHCA) An arrangement that allows, under HIPAA, legally separate covered entities to use and disclose a patient's protected health information (PHI) for the joint operation of the arrangement. For example, a hospital and a physician on its medical staff are separate covered entities for HIPAA's purposes; they can form an OHCA so that they can share PHI in treating patients. To create an OHCA, all of the covered entities to the arrangement must self-designate that they are participating in an OHCA. They would then prepare a joint Notice of Privacy Practice (NPP) to give patients.

organized medical staff See *medical staff.*

organized professional staff See under *staff (group).*

organized staff See *organized professional staff* under *staff (group).*

organ procurement The obtaining of human organs from donors for transplantation into other humans who need them.

organ procurement agency (OPA) An organization set up to keep records of persons needing organ transplants and donor organs available, and to match the two with such speed that the surgery can be performed. Also, an organization designated by CMS as qualified to obtain and supply organs for transplantation in the Medicare program. An OPA may also be referred to as an organ procurement organization (OPO). See *United Network for Organ Sharing.*

Oriental medicine See under *medicine (system).*

   Diplomate in Oriental Medicine (Dipl. O.M.) A practitioner of Oriental medicine who has met the requirements for eligibility and passed an examination of the National Certification Commission for Acupuncture and Oriental Medicine (NCCAOM). **www.nccaom.org**

orientation and mobility (O&M) specialist A health professional who teaches people who are blind or visually impaired how to travel independently and safely. This involves using the person's remaining senses to determine where they are and techniques to move from one place to another. Such techniques include use of a cane, soliciting (and declining) assistance, route planning, use of traffic control devices, use of public transportation, and so forth.

   Certified Orientation and Mobility Specialist (COMS) An orientation and mobility specialist who has passed a certification examination of the Academy for Certification of Vision Rehabilitation and Education Professionals (ACVREP). **www.acvrep.org**

Original Medicare Plan See under *Medicare.*

originating site The place where the patient and/or the patient's physician is located in the context of *telemedicine* services. The other end of the encounter is called the *distant site.* Synonyms: spoke site, patient site, remote site, rural site.

ORMH Office of Research on Minority Health; see *National Center on Minority Health and Health Disparities* under *National Institutes of Health.*

orphan drug A category of the Food and Drug Administration describing a drug used to treat a rare disease or condition. There is usually no financial incentive for pharmaceutical companies to research and develop these drugs, because the market is so small. The federal Orphan Drug Act (ODA) provides funding for research on rare diseases, and financial incentives for manufacturers to develop orphan drugs.

ORT Operating room technician. See *surgical technologist.*

orthodontics The branch of dentistry that deals with prevention and treatment of misalignment of the teeth and the jaws.

orthognathic surgery Surgical intervention to correct misalignment of the jaws or dentofacial deformity.

orthomolecular therapy The use of chemicals, such as magnesium, melatonin, and megadoses of vitamins, to restore health.

orthopedic Having to do with the musculoskeletal system. Alternative spelling is orthopaedic.

orthopaedic nursing The area of nursing focusing on the needs of orthopaedic patients.

   Orthopaedic Nurse Certified (ONC) A specialist in orthopaedic nursing who has passed an examination of the Orthopaedic Nurses Certification Board (ONCB). **www.oncb.org**

orthopedics The medical discipline pertaining to the bones and joints and the musculoskeletal system (the spine, extremities, and related structures). Also spelled orthopaedics.

orthopedic surgery Surgical specialty that focuses on bones, joints, and the musculoskeletal system. Also spelled orthopaedic.

orthopedic technologist (OT) A health professional trained to assist an orthopedist by applying and removing casts and splints, setting up traction apparatus, fitting and adjusting crutches, assisting in surgery, and other tasks as directed by the physician. Also spelled orthopaedic.

> **Certified Orthopaedic Technologist (OTC)** An orthopaedic technologist who has met the requirements and passed an examination of the National Board for Certification of Orthopaedic Technologists (NBCOT). **naot.org**

orthopedist A physician who specializes in orthopaedics. Also spelled orthopaedist.

orthoptics The study of eye movements, from the Greek "ortho" (meaning straight) and "optikos" (vision).

orthoptist A health professional who specializes in the diagnosis and treatment of eye muscle problems, such as misalignments, defects in eye movement, and binocular vision. An orthoptist has a bachelor's degree and has completed a two-year training program.

> **Certified Orthoptist (CO)** An orthoptist who has passed an examination of the American Orthoptic Council (AOC). **www.orthoptics.org**

orthosis The use of a mechanical device to correct or straighten a deformity, especially those affecting walking. Also means the device itself. Synonym: orthotic.

orthotic See *orthosis*.

orthotics The science of using mechanical devices to help correct or straighten a deformity or disability.

orthotist A health professional who designs, produces, and fits orthoses.

> **Certified Orthotist (CO)** An orthotist who has met the requirements of the American Board for Certification in Orthotics and Prosthetics (ABC). **www.abcop.org**
>
> **Certified Prosthetist-Orthotist (CPO)** See under *prosthetist*.
>
> **Orthotist, BOC-Certified (BOCO)** An orthotist who has met the requirements of the Board for Orthotist/Prosthetist Certification (BOC). **www.bocusa.org**

ORYX An initiative of the Joint Commission on Accreditation of Healthcare Organizations (JCAHO), introduced in 1997, to integrate outcome and other performance measurement data into the accreditation process. ORYX is not an acronym. (It also is not related to oryx, a type of antelope.) See *performance measure* and *National Patient Safety Goals*.

OS See *Office of Science* (under *Department of Energy*) and *Office of the Secretary of Health and Human Services*.

OSA See *ophthalmic surgical assistant*.

OSCAR See *Online Survey Certification and Reporting System*.

OSHA See *Occupational Safety and Health Administration*.

OSI Open Systems Interconnection. A set of standards for the electronic interchange of information among differing computer systems and applications. Developed by ISO.

osteopath A physician (Doctor of Osteopathic Medicine (DO)) who has been trained in and practices *osteopathy* (see under *medicine (system)*). By contrast, a Doctor of Medicine (MD) practices *allopathy* (see under *medicine (system)*). The majority of osteopaths are primary care physicians, but there are a number of osteopathic specialties; see *medical specialty*.

A few decades ago, the distinction in theory and procedures permitted the two (osteopathy and allopathy) under licensing acts was marked; today, the distinctions are in matters of detail, and licensure gives DOs and MDs equal permission for the practice of medicine.

osteopathic manipulative treatment (OMT) A hands-on treatment modality utilized by osteopaths.

osteopathic specialty See *medical specialty*.

osteopathy See under *medicine (system)*.

Oswestry score A disability measure obtained from the use of the Oswestry Low-Back Pain Disability Questionnaire, which the patient completes. The sections of the questionnaire pertain to (1) pain intensity, (2) personal care (washing, dressing, etc.), (3) lifting, (4) walking, (5) sitting, (6) standing, (7) sleeping, (8) sex life, (9) social life, and (10) traveling. Each section has a scoring range from 1 to 6, with the higher scores indicating greater disability. The score was developed at The Institute of Orthopaedics in Oswestry, U.K., and published in 1980.

OT See *occupational therapist*, *occupational therapy*, *ophthalmic technician*, and *orthopedic technologist*.

OTA See *occupational therapy assistant* and *Office of Technology Assessment*.

OTC Over-the-counter drug; see *nonprescription drug* under *drug*. See also *Certified Orthopaedic Technologist* under *orthopedic technologist*.

OTJ On the job.

otolaryngology The study of the ear and larynx and other elements of the upper respiratory system.

otology The study of the ear.

otoneurology See *neurotology*.

otorhinolaryngology (ENT) The study of the ears (-oto), nose (-rhino), and throat (-laryngo), hence the acronym "ENT."

otorhinolaryngology and head-neck nursing The area of nursing focusing on the needs of otorhinolaryngology patients, including those undergoing and recovering from surgical procedures.

    Certified Otorhinolaryngology and Head-Neck Nurse (CORLN) A specialist in otorhinolaryngology and head-neck nursing who has passed an examination of the National Certifying Board of Otorhinolaryngology and Head-Neck Nurses (NCBOHN). **www.sohnnurse.com**

OTPER See *Office of Terrorism Preparedness and Emergency Response*.

OTR See *Occupational Therapist Registered* under *occupational therapist*.

OUB See *ophthalmic ultrasound biometrist*.

outcome A term used very loosely, particularly in evaluating patient care and the healthcare system and its components. When used for populations or the healthcare system, it typically refers to changes in birth or death rates, or some similar global measure. In contrast, it may refer to the "outcome" (finding) of a given diagnostic procedure. It may also refer to cure of the patient, restoration of function, or extension of life, sometimes with an attempt to introduce into the calculation some quantification of the quality of life. For its use in quality management, see *process*. See also *nursing outcome* and *patient-reported outcome*.

    unanticipated outcome The outcome of a medical treatment or procedure that differs from the expected result. It may or may not be due to medical or other error. The Joint Commission on Accreditation of Healthcare Organizations (JCAHO) requires hospitals to inform patients (and their families, when appropriate) of treatment outcomes, including unanticipated outcomes. See also *adverse patient occurrence* and *sentinel event*.

Outcome and Assessment Information Set (OASIS) See under *data set*.

outcome based quality improvement (OBQI) A systematic approach used by home health agencies to improve quality of care, using the Outcome and Assessment Information Set (OASIS).

outcomes assessment See *quality of life scale*.

outcomes research Research attempting to evaluate the relative benefits of various kinds of treatment, medical care, delivery of health services, public health measures, and so forth, by measuring and evaluating the results. One basic question asked is, "Does treatment A or treatment B give the better outcome?" This is, of course, followed by "How much better is the one than the other?" and "How costly is the treatment with the better outcome?" And finally, there follows an evaluation of the cost/benefit relationship.

outercourse Sex without penetration (as opposed to intercourse); a way to have "safe sex." The term was invented in the late 1980s to describe activities that would not involve exchange of bodily fluids.

outlier A patient who requires an unusually long stay or whose stay generates unusually great cost. The term is used in the prospective payment system (PPS). About 5–6% of the budgets for regional and national rates have been set aside for payments for outliers. Outliers provide an escape hatch for the hospital, because they allow the hospital to negotiate for a fee higher than the DRG price that would otherwise apply to the patient. Outliers are of two kinds:

cost outlier An unusually costly case.

stay outlier An unusually long stay. Also called "day outlier."

out-of-area Beyond the geographical service area of a managed care plan (MCP). Out-of-area medical care requires providers who are not participating with the plan. Thus, it is not ordinarily covered by the plan unless it is emergency or urgent care.

out-of-area insurance See under *insurance*.

out-of-network See *out-of-plan*.

out-of-network provider See *out-of-plan provider*.

out-of-plan An adjective applied to either a healthcare provider or a provided service when the provider is not a part of the enrollee's health plan, system, or network. Also refers to a service that is not available within the plan, and thus the cost has not been the subject of prior agreement. Synonym: out-of-network. Antonyms: in-plan or in-network.

out-of-plan provider A provider who is not under contract with or a member of a managed care organization (MCO) or managed care plan (MCP). Under some healthcare financing arrangements, the MCO must permit beneficiaries to use out-of-plan providers, for whose performance (services provided, cost, quality) the MCO is then held responsible. There is at present no legal method by which the MCO can carry out this responsibility. Synonym: out-of-network provider.

out-of-pocket cap See under *cap*.

outpatient (OP) A person who receives care without taking up lodging in a care institution.

outpatient bundling See under *bundling*.

outpatient clinic A facility for the diagnosis and treatment of ambulatory patients. The term is usually applied to a unit of a hospital.

Outpatient Code Editor (OCE) Software published by CMS to assist providers in processing claims under the outpatient prospective payment system (OPPS), using *Ambulatory Payment Classifications (APCs)*. The OCE has been used by fiscal intermediaries (FIs) (now Medicare Administrative Contractors (MACs)) in Medicare since 1987. Originally OCE had about a dozen edits, such as verifying that a given procedure was consistent with the patient's sex (removal of an ovary was not permitted for a male). The edits cover four general functions: (1) accuracy of data, (2) actions to be taken by the MAC based on the content of the claim, (3) decision as to APCs to be assigned to the claim, and (4) making decisions on the effects of other factors on the payment to be allowed. OCE is subject to updating on a quarterly basis by CMS; it is distributed by the National Technical Information Service (NTIS).

outpatient commitment See *assisted outpatient treatment*.

outpatient facility A healthcare facility to provide services for patients who do not need lodging.

outpatient prospective payment system (OPPS) See under *prospective payment system*.

outpatient service (OP service) Service provided to patients who do not require lodging in a care institution.

outrage See *intentional infliction of emotional distress* under *emotional distress*.

overcoding See under *coding (billing)*.

over-the-counter (OTC) drug See *nonprescription drug* under *drug*.

overweight See *obesity*.

OWH See *Office of Women's Health* and *Office on Women's Health*.

P

PA See *pathologist's assistant*, *physician advisor*, and *physician assistant*. Also stands for *product administration* (see under *administration (management)*), professional associa-tion (see *professional corporation* under *corporation*), and *public accountant* (see under *accountant*).

PA-C See *Physician Assistant—Certified* under *physician assistant*.

PAC See *post-acute care*, *preadmission certification*, and *products of ambulatory care*.

PACE See *Program of All-Inclusive Care for the Elderly*.

pacemaker An electrical, battery operated system for increasing the heart rate in patients with an abnormally slow rate (a condition called bradycardia).

The pacemaker has a tiny computer that senses the heart rate electronically and sends elec-trical impulses to the heart at the proper rate. The system has three parts. Two are inside the body: a small metal case containing the pacemaker itself, which is implanted under the skin, and an insulated wire ("pacing lead"), which connects the pacemaker with the heart. The third part, which is external, is the programmer, a special computer that communicates wire-lessly with the pacemaker, and is used by the physician periodically to make sure the battery is properly charged and to adjust the pacemaker if needed. A pacemaker does not cure heart disease or prevent heart attacks; rather, it treats symptoms—shortness of breath and lack of energy—by enabling the heart to pump more blood. The first pacemaker was implanted in then-forty-three-year-old Arne Larsson in 1958. His heart—with the help of an additional twenty-six or so pacemakers—worked well until he died of skin cancer in 2001.

breathing pacemaker An implantable electronic device that periodically stimulates the phrenic nerves in the chest so that the diaphragm contracts and the patient inhales. When the electrical pulse stops, the diaphragm relaxes and the patient exhales. The device is useful for quadriplegic patients and patients with sleep apnea.

PACS See *picture archiving and communication system*.

PACT See *post-acute care transfer policy*.

PAD See *public access defibrillation*.

PADE Potential adverse drug event. See *adverse drug event*.

PAHPA See *Pandemic and All-Hazards Preparedness Act*.

PAI See *Inpatient Rehabilitation Facility Patient Assessment Instrument*.

pain and suffering The noneconomic injury that accompanies the physical injury a malprac-tice victim suffers as a result of professional negligence, for which the law allows an amount of money to be paid to the victim as compensation. Some states limit the amount that can be awarded for pain and suffering in malpractice lawsuits.

pain management The study of pain and ways to reduce it, using methods from various dis-ciplines. See also *pain medicine*.

Certified Pain Management Nurse A registered nurse with an associate degree or diploma, or a Bachelor of Science in Nursing or higher degree, who is qualified in pain man-agement nursing and has passed an examination of the American Nurses Credentialing Cen-ter (ANCC) (**nursingworld.org/ancc**). The credential is RN,C (Registered Nurse, Certified).

Credentialed Pain Practitioner (CPP) A multidisciplinary credential in pain management. The American Academy of Pain Management offers three levels of credentials for experi-enced practitioners: **diplomate** for those with doctoral degrees, **fellow** for master's level applicants, and **clinical associate** for those with bachelor's degrees. **www.aapainmanage.org**

pain medicine The medical discipline involving the study and prevention of pain, and the evaluation, treatment, and rehabilitation of people in pain. Physicians may obtain specialty certification from the American Board of Pain Medicine (ABPM). Subspecialty certification is jointly offered by the American Board of Physical Medicine and Rehabilitation (ABPMR), the American Board of Psychiatry and Neurology (ABPN), and the American Board of Anesthesiology (ABA). See also *pain management*.

palliative care Treatment to relieve or reduce pain, discomfort, or other symptoms of disease, but not to cure. In late 1996, HCFA (now CMS) added a code for palliative care to ICD-9-CM, which means such care may be reimbursed under Medicare. See also *comfort care*.

PALS See *Pediatric Advanced Life Support* under *life support*.

pandemic A disease outbreak affecting a large population or area, or crossing international boundaries; a global epidemic.

Pandemic and All-Hazards Preparedness Act (PAHPA) Federal legislation enacted in 2006 aimed at bolstering national preparedness for public health emergencies such as pandemics, terrorism, mass disasters—"all hazards." Among its many provisions, it established the *Biomedical Advanced Research and Development Authority (BARDA)* within the Department of Health and Human Services (HHS), required a vaccine tracking system, and centralized federal control for preparing for and responding to public health emergencies by placing the Secretary of HHS in charge. Pub. L. No. 109-417 (2006).

P&L Profit and loss statement. See *income and expense statement*.

P&T See *pharmacy and therapeutics*.

panel A group of individuals who are given a specific task. The term is used for groups such as the physicians who form a preferred provider organization (PPO) or those who are convened to review a grant application. In law, a panel is a group of people given the duty to review information, receive evidence, and make a decision.

In a court of law, a panel may be composed of judges; in other contexts, it may be made up of experts or laypersons. Also, the group of potential jurors from which a jury will be selected is called a "panel."

pretrial screening panel In malpractice cases, a group of physicians who review the case before trial and make a recommendation as to whether there was malpractice and, if so, the dollar amount of damages the plaintiff suffered as a result of it. The purpose is to encourage settlement; if one party turns down a settlement based on the recommendation, that party may be penalized if she or he loses at trial.

paradigm One's view of "the way things are"; an implicit framework within which "everything" fits or is understood. In science, for example, one's "world view" restricts what problems are considered legitimate for study and what methods are acceptable to pursue them. Sir Isaac Newton's "laws" of gravity and motion, developed in the seventeenth and eighteenth centuries, governed much of scientific thought for nearly two centuries. Einstein's paradigm not only explained the same phenomena, but also opened the way for new thought. When people thought the earth was flat, this paradigm governed thinking about stars, oceans, and travel. Proof that the earth was a sphere released entirely new thinking. See *paradigm shift*.

paradigm shift The change in one's "world view" in moving from one *paradigm* to another: replacing an old paradigm with a new one. Such a change may take a lot of energy, and usually has far-reaching consequences.

Among the paradigm shifts emerging today in health are: (1) from the view that knowledge processing is limited to the human mind, plus "paper and pencil," to the view that knowledge processing can be successfully extended through use of computer technology; (2) from the view that the physician should assume a "paternal" role of caring and making decisions for the patient, to the view that empowered patients are competent to collaborate in their own health care and that, in fact, many wish to and can *direct* their own care; (3) from the view that the government is responsible for the health of the community, to the view that the community itself is responsible; and (4) from the view that healthcare providers are there to provide "health care," to the view that "health" rather than "health care" is their goal.

paramedical personnel A term derived from "para-," meaning "beside." Generally refers to health professionals other than physicians, nurses, dentists, and pharmacists. See *allied health professional* and *health science discipline*.

parameter Any defining or characteristic factor, especially one that can be measured or quantified. See also *guidelines*, *indicator*, *performance measure*, and *standard (threshold)*.
    practice parameter A parameter relating to clinical practice. See *clinical practice guidelines* under *guidelines*.

parens patriae "Parent of his country." A legal term referring to the power of the state to protect its people—specifically, those unable to care for themselves, such as minors (children) and the mentally incompetent.

parent A term applied to both the father and mother of a child. With the advent of noncoital reproduction, it has become necessary to distinguish among the genetic parents, the gestational mother, and the rearing parents:
    genetic parent The parent who furnished the sperm (the genetic father) or the ovum (the genetic mother).
    gestational parent The woman who bore the child. (The father, who cannot bear a child, cannot be a gestational parent.) The gestational mother may also be the genetic parent, the rearing parent, or neither.
    rearing parent The parent who actually rears the child. This term would apply to both father and mother, and is used in connection with both noncoital reproduction and adoption.

parenteral Given other than via the alimentary tract or lungs ("*para*" = outside and "*enteron*" = intestine). Refers to giving a substance by intravenous, subcutaneous, intramuscular, or other injection. See also *enteral* and *nutrition support*.

Pareto principle A principle that states that in any series of steps in a process, such as the diagnosis of a patient's problem, there are a "vital few" steps and a "trivial many." The procedure for identifying the vital few and the trivial many is called a **Pareto analysis**. The Pareto analysis makes feasible productive efforts at quality improvement because once the "vital few" steps where efforts pay off can be identified, appropriate action can be taken. The Pareto principle is also the key to optimizing the care possible under a condition of limited resources. The principle was developed by J.M. Juran, an authority on quality, and named after an Italian economist named Pareto. See also *Juran Institute*.

parish nursing Providing nursing and other healthcare services to and through a church or other religious congregation.

parity Equalizing benefits for mental health care, to bring them in line with benefits for other kinds of healthcare needs. Historically, there have been significant differences in the way that healthcare services have been provided for behavioral and physical health needs. Many insurers and health plans exclude or minimize benefits for psychiatric, behavioral, and substance abuse treatment. By the late 1990s, strong legislative efforts were underway seeking to establish "parity" between the two, spurred on at least in part by the federal *Mental Health Parity Act* that took effect on January 1, 1998.

parochial and unconventional medicine (PUM) One of the two main categories of *unconventional healing practices (UHP)*. PUM is divided into three classes:
    Ethno-medicine: For example, Puerto-Rican spiritism and Hmong practices
    Religious healing: Includes Pentecostal churches and Christian Science
    Folk medicine practices: Include copper bracelets for arthritis and red string for nosebleeds
    See also *complementary and alternative medicine*.

parse analysis A tongue-in-cheek method described in 1969 by Paul Davis, MD, and Robert Gregerman, MD, in response to the burgeoning problems of multiauthorship of papers and perceived logarithmic differences (PLDs) in the quality of published papers. The parse analysis assigned decimal values to the real contributions of investigators to a multiauthored paper—e.g., 0.04 or 0.37. The rationale was that embarrassingly low parse values assigned to negligibly contributory authors would defeat the trend toward multiauthorship that emerged in the 1960s. When parse values and levels of statistical significance were regrettably confused in the subsequent scientific literature, many authors came to associate really low parse values with significant achievement.

In 1995, the authors submitted an update, concluding that the original concept had failed, and offering a new approach. They contended that there were not enough periodicals to go around, and that more journals would promote a reduction in multiauthorship. Multi-authored papers could be converted into shorter manuscripts, called **fractional pieces of work (FPWs)**, with smaller numbers of authors. Although the authors' combined contribution to the original work may have totaled only 5%, for example, in the FPW it expanded to 100% for purposes of distributing among the authors. This the authors call **parse inflation**, which was described by one enthusiast as "Wow, what a fractional piece of work that was."

Davis, P.J., & Gregerman, R.I. "Parse Analysis: A New Method for the Evaluation of Investigators' Bibliographies." *New England Journal of Medicine*, 1969;281:989–990. Davis, P.J., & Gregerman, R.I. "Parse Analysis II: A Revised Model That Accounts for Phi." *New England Journal of Medicine*, 1995;332:965–966.

Part D See *Medicare Part D* under *Medicare*.

partial hospitalization See under *hospitalization*.

partnership Two or more people (or organizations) carrying on a business for profit (for the purpose of making money). The law recognizes such an enterprise as a legal partnership, whether or not the partners have a verbal or written partnership agreement. In a general partnership, the partners share profits, losses, and management of the business, and are all equally liable should the partnership be sued. In a limited partnership, there is at least one general partner who manages the business, and one or more limited partners who put in money and share profits and losses, but who are liable only to the extent of their investments, and who do not have management control. To be recognized as a limited partnership, however, the business must comply with legal formalities.

Partnership for Long Term Care (PLTC) A program to pay for long-term care that provides an alternative to spending down or transferring assets by forming a partnership between Medicaid and private long-term care insurers. Participating states (in 2007, these were California, Connecticut, Indiana, and New York) work with insurers to create insurance policies that are more affordable and provide better protection against impoverishment than those commonly offered. Once private insurance benefits are exhausted, special Medicaid eligibility rules are applied if additional coverage is necessary. The authority for the program resides in state plan amendments rather than CMS waivers. A provision in Medicaid law allows a state to alter the asset eligibility criteria dependent on a state-specified requirement. In this case, it is the purchase of a state-certified long-term care insurance policy. The program, started in 1988, is sponsored by the Robert Wood Johnson Foundation.
www.gmu.edu/departments/chpre/research/PLTC

PAS See *physician-assisted suicide* (under *suicide*), *preadmission screening*, and *Professional Activity Study*.

passive smoking See *involuntary smoking*.

PAT See *preadmission testing*.

patch See *electrotransport*.

PATCH See *Planned Approach to Community Health* and *Psychogeriatric Assessment and Treatment in City Housing*.

patent A legal right to manufacture or produce a thing or substance, and to prevent anyone else from also manufacturing or producing the same or substantially similar thing or substance. This legal right can be enforced against others, even if the other party independently discovered or invented the same subject matter of the patent. This point is one of the distinguishing characteristics of a patent, as opposed to other intellectual property rights, such as *copyright* or *trade secret*. Administered by the U.S. government's Patent and Trademark Office (**www.uspto.gov**), the U.S. patent system is of the "first to invent" type, as opposed to the "first to file" standard found in most other countries. This means that in the event of a dispute over a patent in the United States, the patent would be granted to the party who could prove to have invented it first, regardless of the filing date.

design patent This type of patent protects the "ornamental" design (rather than functional) aspects of a product. A design patent may protect much of what can be covered under copyright protection, but the significant legal differences between patents and copyrights may afford the holder of a design patent greater or additional advantages. See also *utility patent*, below, and *copyright*.

medical procedure patent See *method or process patent*, below.

medical-process patent See *method or process patent*, below.

method or process patent A type of *utility patent* (see below) for a method or process, comparable to a patent for a product or device. Under patent law it is possible for a "pure medical or surgical procedure" (method or process) to be patented, and for the patent holder to require the payment of royalties for use of the method. The "pure" in this context means that the procedure for which the patent is sought is independent of the use of a medical device or drug. Such procedures were not considered patentable prior to 1952, but the U.S. Patent and Trademark Office (PTO) has granted many such patents since then. These are called **medical-process patents** or medical procedure patents. Examples of procedures for which patents have been obtained include using ultrasound methods for determining the gender of a fetus and injections of vasodilators to treat male impotence.

A famous case involved a surgeon in Arizona who obtained a patent on a "stitchless" technique used in cataract surgery and sued to collect royalties ($3–5 per procedure) from an ophthalmologist using and teaching the procedure. (A consent decree was entered that prohibited the surgeon from enforcing his patent; *Pallin v. Singer*, 36 USPQ 2d 1050 (1995).) This case attracted much attention and public debate ensued.

In 1995, the American Medical Association (AMA) took a stand against this patenting practice as unethical, and many other professional organizations adopted their own strictures against such patents. In 1996, federal legislation was passed that, although still allowing medical procedure patents, deprived patent holders of remedies against "medical practitioners" using the process during the course of "medical activity." Under the law, a court can find that a physician has infringed a patent, but cannot order that physician to pay damages or stop using the process. Remedies are available for other types of infringement, however (35 U.S.C. § 287(c) (2005)). More than eighty countries around the world expressly prohibit such patents, including most European countries.

plant patent A patent for a plant that has been invented or discovered, and asexually reproduced, which is distinct and new. It includes cultivated sports, mutants, hybrids, and certain types of newly found seedlings. A "sport" is a plant with abnormal or striking variation from the parent type as a result of spontaneous mutation.

utility patent A specific type of patent designed to protect invented functions, methods, or systems. Also included are algorithms and applied mathematical formulas. This type of patent protects much of the software used in health care, as well as the medical devices one normally would expect to be patented. Patent protection has a limited term, typically lasting twenty years for patents filed on or after June 8, 1995.

patent medicine See *nonprescription drug* under *drug*.

pathogen A microorganism or substance that can produce disease. Examples of pathogens include bacteria, viruses, fungi, and chemicals.

pathography The retrospective study of the possible influence and effects of disease on the life and work of a historical individual or group. A "contemporary pathography" is the story of an illness written by the patient.

Also, a biography that overemphasizes the negative aspects of a person's life and work, such as failure, illness, and tragedy. "[It] falls into pathography's technique of emphasizing the sensational underside of its subject's life" (Joyce Carol Oates).

pathological Abnormal. When the body structure or function is not normal, it may be called "pathological." When function or structure is normal, it is called "physiological."

pathologist A physician whose specialty is *pathology*. Sometimes referred to as "the doctor's doctor," because of the pathologist's role as a consultant to the physician.

pathologist's assistant (PA) A health professional with advanced training who provides anatomic pathology services under the direction and supervision of a pathologist. Tasks include gross examination of surgical pathology specimens and performance of autopsies. Many PAs have a bachelor's degree or have completed a two-year post-graduate pathology assistant program.

Pathologist's Assistant (PA(ASCP)) A pathologist's assistant with at least a bachelor's degree who has been certified as a specialist by the American Society for Clinical Pathology (ASCP) (**www.ascp.org/bor**) through a joint program with the American Association of Pathologists' Assistants (AAPA) (**www.pathologistsassistants.org**).

pathology The study of the structures of the body and their physiology (vital processes), and in particular the changes in both structure and physiological function that occur in disease. Pathology is sometimes referred to as "laboratory medicine" because of the use of laboratory tests to diagnose and treat disease. Pathology was recognized as the practice of medicine by the American Medical Association (AMA) in 1943. Physicians certified to practice this specialty are called pathologists. Their primary professional organization is the College of American Pathologists (CAP). See also *pathology laboratory* (under *laboratory*) and *telepathology*.

anatomic pathology The study of tissues removed at surgery, of biopsy specimens (specimens of tissue removed purely for examination by the pathologist), and of autopsy material. Anatomic pathology may be either gross (the study of an entire tissue, typically as visible to the naked eye) or microscopic.

clinical pathology The study of body tissues and fluids, with particular attention to changes in physiology (function) and biochemistry in disease. The site of the clinical pathology services in the hospital is the *clinical laboratory* (see under *laboratory*), where biochemical and other examinations are made of materials obtained from the body and body fluids.

forensic pathology The branch of pathology that deals with legal issues, particularly crime, and the cause of violent or mysterious death. Estimation of the time of death is also a forensic matter. A growing concern in forensic pathology is toxicology, the study of poisonous substances, their effects, and their detection in the body.

molecular pathology The study of body tissues and fluids, with particular attention to genomes.

neuropathology The branch of pathology that deals with the nervous system.

surgical pathology The study of tissues removed in surgical operations. It includes the examination of tissue during operation (often by frozen section) in order to help the surgeon determine the appropriate procedure for the remainder of the operation; it also includes the examination of tissue after surgery. During the operation, a determination as to whether the tissue is cancerous (malignant) may greatly influence the extent and type of surgery.

pathology laboratory See under *laboratory*.

patient A person who is receiving services from a healthcare provider. In a legal sense, a patient is a person who has established a contractual relationship with a healthcare provider for that provider to care for that person. A patient may or may not be ill or injured. A patient who is ill or injured, or who otherwise presents a health problem, is often referred to as a *case (health care)*. See also *client*.

patient advocacy See *health advocacy*.

patient advocate A person who helps patients with their complaints and problems with medical care and hospital and healthcare services and with the protection of their rights. The field is called "patient advocacy," one area of *health advocacy*. Synonyms: ombudsperson, patient representative, health advocate.

Patient Assessment Instrument (PAI) See *Inpatient Rehabilitation Facility Patient Assessment Instrument*.

patient assistance services Things done by volunteers for patients, such as reading to them and providing library services and toiletries.

patient card See *smart card*.

patient care The totality of things done for a patient to determine the cause of the patient's problem(s), plan for treatment of the causes, carry out the plan, and provide comfort and support. Patient care includes that provided by allied health professionals and their helpers as well as that given by nurses, physicians, and other health professionals. The care is for the whole patient, including social and spiritual needs, not just for the patient's diagnoses or the procedures involved in diagnosis and treatment. See also *medical care*.

progressive patient care A system of organizing patient care in the hospital in which the hospital establishes patient care units ready to provide different intensities of care (for example, intensive, intermediate, and self-care), and moves patients from unit to unit as they progress in their illnesses.

patient care audit (PCA) See under *audit*.

patient care committee A hospital committee, typically composed of medical, nursing, and other disciplines involved in direct patient care, along with hospital administration. The purpose of the committee is to monitor patient care practices, evaluate them against standards, and improve care through better liaison among the departments involved.

patient care coordinator (long-term care) An individual assigned the responsibility for coordinating all care given to a patient in a long-term care facility.

patient care coordinator (nurse) A registered nurse who manages, coordinates, or directs a nursing service, such as obstetrics, among two or more patient care units.

Patient Care Data Set (PCDS) See under *data set*.

patient-caregiver collaboration (PCC) A culture of health care in which the patient is enabled to collaborate with the physician in decisions about diagnostic, therapeutic, and other health matters. The knowledge asymmetry between the physician and the patient must be substantially reduced if there is to be meaningful PCC. Information sources, especially electronic, are increasingly available to close this knowledge gap. See also *informed shared decision making* and *patient empowerment*.

patient care management See *care management*.

patient care manager (PCM) See *gatekeeper (health care)* and *case management*.

Patient Care Partnership (PCP) A readable and up-to-date replacement of the American Hospital Association's former Patient's Bill of Rights. The AHA's "Patient Care Partnership" brochure is to be provided to patients upon their admission to the hospital. It describes not only what the patient should expect from the hospital, but also the patient's responsibilities in his or her care. Subtitled "Understanding Expectations, Rights and Responsibilities," the booklet's topics include High Quality Hospital Care, A Clean and Safe Environment, Involvement in Your Care, Protection of Your Privacy, Help When Leaving the Hospital, and Help with Your Billing Claims. It is available in eight languages: English, Arabic, Simplified Chinese, Traditional Chinese, Russian, Spanish, Tagalog, and Vietnamese.

patient care plan See *interdisciplinary patient care plan*.

patient care referral data set (PCRDS) See *Continuity of Care Record* under *data set*.

patient care unit (PCU) An organizational part of the hospital where inpatients are lodged during their hospitalization. Synonyms: nursing unit, unit, ward.

patient-carried record (PCR) See under *electronic health record*.

patient-centered care Health care that takes into account the patient's preferences, values, lifestyle, family, expressed needs, and fears; care approached from the patient's point of view. Such care includes education, physical comfort, emotional support, coordination of care, involvement of family and friends, and help with transitions. The Institute of Medicine's Health Care Quality Initiative names "patient-centered care" as one of six domains of quality. Synonym: patient-focused care. See also *Picker Institute* and *Planetree*.

patient-centric See *consumer-centric*.

patient condition A brief statement of "how ill" the patient is. Patient condition is described to relatives, other professionals, and in public information releases. It may be described in terms of progression of the illness, for example, as "improving" or "stable." It may also be described in terms of likelihood of favorable outcome, for example, "good," "fair," "poor," "serious," or "critical." In general, this latter series progresses from high likelihood of recovery (good) to low (critical). Although health professionals often use these terms in communicating with each other about patients, terms describing patient condition may also reflect specific patient needs, and may use measurements that translate the condition into requirements for nursing service in order to provide better the necessary hours of skilled or other nursing care. See also *severity of illness* and *staging (diseases)*.

patient-controlled analgesia (PCA) Pain-relief medication administered by the patient him- or herself, rather than by a caregiver. A computerized, medication-dispensing unit equipped with a pump is attached to an intravenous line, which is inserted into a blood vessel in the patient's hand or arm. The patient pushes a button whenever pain medication is needed. This is typically used by patients after surgery. It has been found that most patients use less medication overall than when a nurse administers the pain-killers, are more comfortable, and recover more quickly.

patient days The total number of inpatient service days, for all patients, during a specified period of time (for example, a month). Ordinarily this number will be expressed in three segments—adult days, pediatric days, and newborn days—because there almost certainly will be a desire to relate the usage in these three segments to the "adult inpatient bed count," the "newborn bed count," and the "pediatric inpatient bed count." Each bed count multiplied by the number of days in the period gives the "available bed days," the denominator in computing the *occupancy rate* (see under *rate (ratio)*). See also *bed count*.

patient-directed care Health care guided by the recipient of the care. A trend in medical practice stemming from the concept that patients should be empowered to make decisions as to their own health and health care. In patient-directed care, the physician advises and collaborates with the patient in determining the steps to be taken to discover the causes of problems and in treating those problems. See *patient empowerment*.

patient-driven health care See *healthcare consumerism* and *patient-directed care*.

patient dumping See *dumping*.

patient education See under *education*.

patient empowerment Enabling individuals to control their own health and healthcare decisions. "Empowerment" means granting power or authority; it also means enablement. Granting authority may mean simply giving permission, but enablement may also require the provision of information not ordinarily available and/or additional education. "Patient empowerment" requires using empowerment in both senses.

Patients have been given legal power at both the state and federal level. Many states have enacted a Patient's Bill of Rights, providing patients with rights to both consumer and healthcare protection. The federal Patient Self-Determination Act supports the implementation of an individual's right to make decisions concerning extraordinary treatment.

Enabling individuals to make intelligent, informed decisions concerning their health care, however, involves more than merely giving them the "right." They need tools—mostly information—and the cooperation and assistance of their health professionals. Patient empowerment requires a relationship between patient and physician (or other caregiver) in which both patient and physician understand that the patient has the authority to make (or share substantially in) the decisions concerning his or her medical care, with regard to both the diagnostic efforts to be employed and the treatment to be given. This collaborative relationship between patient and physician is called one of *informed shared decision making (ISDM)*.

Many physicians have become convinced that ISDM is desirable—the care is based on the patient's values; patients comply better with the care process when they understand it and have helped select it; most patients are pleased to be treated as responsible individuals; and the outcome is often superior. But employment of ISDM has been slow, in large part because of the *knowledge asymmetry* between the patient and the physician; that is, the professional not only knows a great deal more about medicine than does the patient, but has been brought up to respect that fact. This problem is diminishing with the development of decision-support software (DSS) systems, which provide current biomedical knowledge to guide both the physician and the patient at the time that the decisions need to be made. (See *Problem-Knowledge Couplers* as an example of one such guidance tool.) With these tools, the patient can become thoroughly informed as to the nature of the various options available, and their risks and benefits. The patient can then make truly informed decisions and can give truly informed consent.

The first widely distributed book advocating patient empowerment was *Primitive Physic*, published by John Wesley, founder of the Methodist religion, in 1747.

patient-focused care See *patient-centered care.*

Patient Management Category (PMC) Severity Scale A method of quantifying severity of illness based on the perceived needs of the patient for diagnostic and therapeutic services. The system assesses the overall severity of a hospitalized patient's illnesses based on the patient's unique clinical conditions, his or her interaction, and the resultant, combined risk of morbidity and mortality.

Patient Medical Record Information (PMRI) HIPAA required that the National Committee on Vital and Health Statistics (NCVHS) study issues related to the adoption of uniform data standards for Patient Medical Record Information and for the electronic exchange of such information, and to make recommendations to the Secretary of the Department of Health and Human Services (HHS). PMRI may refer, depending on who is using the term and the context, to the information (content) of the patient's medical record, the standards for that information, and/or the standards for the electronic exchange of that information. Some use it as a synonym for electronic health record (EHR) in its broadest sense.

In its 2000 report to the secretary, the NCVHS proposed the following definition of PMRI:

Patient medical record information (PMRI) is information about a single patient. Healthcare professionals generate this information as a direct result of interaction with the patient, or with individuals who have personal knowledge of the patient, or with both. PMRI documents the course of a patient's illness and treatment, communicates between care providers, assists in evaluating the adequacy and appropriateness of care, substantiates claims for payment, protects the legal interests of all concerned parties to the information, and provides case studies for education and data to expand the body of medical knowledge. PMRI includes patient demographics, health history, details of present illness or injury, orders for care and treatment, observations, records of medication administration, diagnoses/problems, allergies, and other healthcare information. PMRI facilitates the creation of a lifetime health record for individuals. PMRI of many individuals may be aggregated to provide the basis for continuous quality improvement, outcomes analysis, and population-based care management.

NCVHS recommended that the uniform standards for PMRI specifically address *data quality*, *interoperability*, and *data comparability*. Data quality standards involve issues of data capture, encoding, translation, transformation, communication, decoding, presentation, accountability, and integrity. The NCVHS proposed the following criteria for data quality:

- *Accessibility:* Data items should be easily obtainable and legal to collect.
- *Accuracy:* Data are the correct values and are valid.
- *Comprehensiveness:* All required data items are included.
- *Consistency:* The value of the data should be reliable and the same across applications.
- *Currency:* The data should be up-to-date (i.e., current for a specific point in time).
- *Definition:* Each data element should have clear meaning and acceptable values.
- *Granularity:* The attributes and values of data should be defined at the correct level of detail.
- *Precision:* Data values should be just large enough to support the application or process.
- *Relevancy:* The data are meaningful to the performance of the process or application for which they are collected.
- *Timeliness:* This is determined by how the data are being used and their context.

For interoperability, the NCVHS recommended in 2002 that *HL7* be recognized as the core message format standard and that *DICOM*, *NCPDP SCRIPT*, and *IEEE 1073* be recognized as standards for specific PMRI market segments; these were adopted for federal use by HHS, along with the Departments of Defense and Veterans Affairs, in 2003.

To assist with data comparability, NCVHS recommended the following as the "core set" of PMRI terminology standards:

- *SNOMED Clinical Terms (SNOMED CT)* (as licensed by the National Library of Medicine)
- *Logical Observation Identifiers Names and Codes (LOINC)* (laboratory subset)
- Federal Drug Terminologies: *RxNorm*; the representations of the mechanism of action and physiologic effect of drugs from *NDF-RT*; and ingredient name, manufactured dosage form, and package type from the FDA.

This core set was reviewed and modified by the *Consolidated Health Informatics (CHI)* initiative. The standards were adopted by 2004 for electronic exchange of clinical information across the federal government. Also adopted were the:

- HIPAA *Transactions and Code Sets*
- *Human Gene Nomenclature (HUGN)*
- Environmental Protection Agency's *Substance Registry System*

PMRI standards were still under development in 2007. These standards are one component of the broader national health information infrastructure; see *Nationwide Health Information Network*.

Patient Outcomes Research Team (PORT) A research group supported by the *Agency for Healthcare Research and Quality (AHRQ)* to conduct a specific study on a topic such as the values of various options for the treatment of prostate cancer and benign prostatic hyperplasia (BPH), the use of serum prostatic specific antigen (PSA) in screening for prostatic cancer, values of knee replacement surgery, and the treatment of back pain. PORTs were established in 1990 as a part of the agency's Medical Treatment Effectiveness Program (MEDTEP).

patient presenter See *presenter*.

patient privacy See under *privacy*.

Patient Protection Act See *Patient's Bill of Rights*.

patient record See *medical record*.

Patient Record Architecture (PRA) A framework being developed by *HL7* to use XML, a subset of SGML, to facilitate the exchange of documents among healthcare providers and their information systems. A key element of PRA documents is that they will be capable of sending and receiving HL7 messages. This framework was initially referred to as the "Kona Architecture" before being renamed in the late 1990s.

patient-reported outcome (PRO) The results of healthcare services from the patient's point of view. This is monitored chiefly by use of health outcomes assessment instruments—surveys that are completed by the patient or by interviewing the patient. See *quality of life* and *quality of life scale*.

patient representative See *patient advocate*.

patient safety The protection of patients from injury and illness caused by or during the provision of health care. Always a concern of hospitals, much attention was focused on this area with the 1999 publication of the Institute of Medicine (IOM) report, *To Err Is Human: Building a Safer Health System*. The IOM found that medical errors result in the deaths of between 44,000 and 98,000 people each year in U.S. hospitals. In addition, more than 7,000 people die each year in the United States due to medication errors (see *adverse drug event*), which exceeds the number of deaths due to workplace injuries. To reduce these errors, the IOM report specifically recommended: (1) building leadership and knowledge for patient safety, (2) developing a nationwide public mandatory reporting system and encouraging healthcare organizations and practitioners to participate in voluntary reporting systems, (3) raising performance standards for patient safety, and (4) creating safety systems in healthcare organizations. See also *adverse patient occurrence*, *Leapfrog Group*, *medical harm*, *National Patient Safety Goals*, *100,000 Lives Campaign*, and *Patient Safety and Quality Improvement Act of 2005*.

Another issue gaining attention in the context of patient safety is the number of nonstop hours worked by interns, residents, and other healthcare providers. A number of studies have linked long work shifts to increased medical errors, including one study that claimed staying awake for just twenty-four hours straight can impair performance as much as a 0.10% blood-alcohol level. In 2002, the Accreditation Council for Graduate Medical Education (ACGME) adopted rules that require hospitals to limit their residents' work week to eighty hours and no more than thirty consecutive hours per shift, to provide at least ten hours of rest between shifts, and to give residents at least one day off per week. See also *chronobiology*, *chronohygiene*, and *Libby Zion case*.

Patient Safety and Quality Improvement Act of 2005 (PSQIA) Federal legislation to create a voluntary, confidential reporting system for "medical errors" as recommended in the Institute of Medicine's 1999 report, *To Err Is Human: Building a Safer Health System* (see *patient safety*). The PSQIA calls for the creation of public and private **Patient Safety Organizations (PSOs)**, to be certified by the Agency for Healthcare Research and Quality (AHRQ). A PSO must have patient safety as its primary activity and must have contracts with more than one healthcare provider to receive patient safety data. (What constitutes "patient safety data" is not defined in the act.) The PSO collects and analyzes the data in a standardized way so that comparisons can be made, and feeds back to the providers recommendations on improving patient safety. (Note that useful comparisons will depend on the adoption of a standard classification of the medical errors to be considered.) The AHRQ is authorized to create a nationwide network of patient safety databases for use in analyzing regional and national statistics, including trends and patterns of healthcare errors.

The provider establishes a **Patient Safety Evaluation System (PSES)** to collect information on patient safety, which it then reports to the PSO. A PSES is defined as the collection, management, or analysis of information for reporting to or by a PSO. **Patient Safety Work Product (PSWP)** is defined as any information gathered for, and actually reported to, the PSO, and also any information prepared by the PSO for patient safety activities. PSWP is privileged and confidential, and can be released only under narrow circumstances specified in the act. In addition, an individual who in good faith reports patient safety information to a provider or PSO is protected from retaliatory action by his or her employer. Pub. L. No. 109-41, 119 Stat. 424 (2005).

Patient Safety Evaluation System (PSES) See *Patient Safety and Quality Improvement Act of 2005*.

Patient Safety Goals See *National Patient Safety Goals*.

Patient Safety Institute (PSI) A nonprofit membership organization governed by consumer, physician, and hospital advocates who work together to improve healthcare safety and quality while lowering the cost of health care. PSI was formed to provide the healthcare industry with a commonly owned, inclusive network utility to support communities (through Regional Health Information Organizations (RHIOs)) in delivering real-time health information at the point of care. The aim of PSI is to ensure that patients receive care from a provider who has access (with permission) to their personal health record (regardless of the source). **www.ptsafety.org**

Patient Safety Organization (PSO) See *Patient Safety and Quality Improvement Act of 2005*.

Patient Safety Work Product (PSWP) See *Patient Safety and Quality Improvement Act of 2005*.

Patient's Bill of Rights This phrase was first widely used in a statement by the American Hospital Association (AHA) in 1973 giving some twelve "rights" to which it felt that hospital patients were entitled. These include the right of the patient to be included in making treatment decisions, to be treated with dignity, to have privacy, and so forth. In several states, legislation has been passed codifying and augmenting these rights; some states extend these rights to nonhospitalized patients. The AHA's *Patient's Bill of Rights* has since been superceded by the *Patient Care Partnership*.

Over the years, the idea of patient's rights has grown to include legal rights concerning treatment decisions, insurance, and payment for care. Prompted by alleged abuses of managed care plans saving money by denying necessary treatment, many states have enacted or are considering legislation governing these issues. A federal patient's bill of rights, the Bipartisan Patient Protection Act, was proposed (but not enacted) in 2001 and addressed such issues as access to emergency care, specialty care, nonformulary drugs, clinical trials, direct access to pediatricians and obstetricians/gynecologists, continuity of care for those with ongoing healthcare needs, and access to important health plan information. Other issues included methods of dispute resolution (patients vs. health plans) and whether patients may sue their health plans over medical decisions and benefits. "Anti-gagging" provisions sought to prohibit plans from restricting their physicians' freedom to inform patients about treatment options. The federal law would have provided a minimum standard; state laws already in place that give patients similar or more protection would continue to govern.

patient's chart See *medical record*.

patients' compensation See under *compensation*.

Patient Self-Determination Act (PSDA) A federal law that requires most hospitals, nursing homes, and other patient care institutions to ask all admitted patients whether they have made *advance directives* as to their wishes concerning the use of medical interventions for themselves in case of the loss of their own decision-making capacity. The institution is required to furnish each patient with written information about advance directives. The act was passed as an amendment to the Omnibus Budget Reconciliation Act of 1990. 42 U.S.C. § 1395cc(a) (2004).

patient site See *originating site*.

patients' rights See *Patient's Bill of Rights*.

payback period The period of time it will take a new item of equipment to produce revenues or result in savings equal to its cost.

payer An organization or person who furnishes the money to pay for the provision of healthcare services.

  primary payer A payer who has the primary responsibility of paying for the healthcare services. This might be an individual or an insurance company, or workers' compensation, for example. The funds available for primary payment will be used up first, before any other party pays. See also *secondary payer* (below).

secondary payer A payer who is only obligated to pay on any balance remaining, after the primary payer has fulfilled its obligation to pay for the healthcare services. See *Medicare Secondary Payer Rules*.

third-party payer (TPP) A payer other than the patient. When healthcare services are provided, the first and second parties are the patient and the provider. A patient who pays for his or her own (or family's) care directly is called a "self-pay." If anyone else pays, that payer is a third party. Examples of third-party payers are the government (for example, Medicare), a nonprofit organization (such as Blue Cross and Blue Shield), commercial insurance, or some other entity. Increasingly, employers are paying directly for health care to save money paid to insurance companies or other third parties.

fourth-party payer Sometimes used to designate employers who buy health care for their employees, with or without the services of a third-party payer.

PAYERID See *National Payer ID*.

pay-for-performance (P4P) A model of payment for healthcare services designed to provide incentives for the improvement of quality and control of costs; sometimes called pay-for-quality. In a contractual arrangement between payer and provider, specific targets are set for achieving quality and/or containing costs. Two basic payment models are used: reward and punishment. In a reward-based (positive incentive) pay-for-performance program, the provider receives a bonus for meeting the target. In a "punishment" (negative incentive) system, money is withheld for failure to meet a target.

The quality targets, for example, may be based upon performance measures such as the National Hospital Quality Measures or the AQA physician performance measures. Cost containment may be based upon utilization targets, or upon standards of care that have proven to offer higher quality while reducing costs. For example, evidence-based programs of care have been developed for asthma, congestive heart failure, hypertension, and diabetes mellitus, which result in lower costs, improved quality of life, and better outcomes. Targets will typically be measured statistically (patterns of care) rather than by individual patients. See also *Bridges to Excellence*.

payment The act of paying or the amount paid for healthcare services.

Payment Error Prevention Program (PEPP) See *Hospital Payment Monitoring Program*.

payment error rate The ratio of the number of dollars paid in error divided by the total number of dollars paid for services under the prospective payment system (PPS) for a given period of time, typically a year. "Paid in error" basically means Medicare payments made for which the providers do not have proper documentation or do not meet the reimbursement requirements in some other way. The national error rate is calculated using a combination of data from the *Comprehensive Error Rate Testing (CERT)* program and *Hospital Payment Monitoring Program (HPMP)* with each component representing about 60% and 40% of the total Medicare fee-for-service dollars paid, respectively.

Payment Error Rate Measurement (PERM) A program of CMS to measure improper payments in the Medicaid program and the State Children's Health Insurance Program (SCHIP). See also *payment error rate*.

payment update An annual adjustment to the rates that hospitals and other providers are paid by Medicare.

payor See *payer*.

pay or play See *play or pay* under *mandate*.

PBM See *pharmacy benefit manager*.

PBT See *Phlebotomy Technician* under *clinical laboratory technician*.

PC See *professional component*, and *professional corporation* under *corporation*.

PCA See *patient care audit*, under *audit*, and *patient-controlled analgesia*. Also personal care account; see *health reimbursement account*.

PCC See *patient-caregiver collaboration*, *primary care center*, and *HCMA Professional Certified Chaplain* (under *chaplain*).

PCCN See *Progressive Care Certified Nurse* under *progressive care nursing*.

PCD(DONA) See *Postpartum Certified Doula* under *doula*.

PCDS See *Patient Care Data Set* under *data set*.

PCHRG See *Public Citizen Health Research Group*.

PCM Patient care manager or primary care manager; see *gatekeeper (health care)*.

PCN See *progressive care nursing*.

PCP See *Patient Care Partnership*.

PCPI See *Physician Consortium for Performance Improvement*.

PCR See *patient-carried record* under *electronic health record*.

PCRDS Patient care referral data set. See *Continuity of Care Record* under *data set*.

PCS See *Pediatric Certified Specialist* under *physical therapist*.

PC-stager See *stager*.

PCU See *patient care unit*.

PDP See *prescription drug plan*.

PDR *Physicians' Desk Reference*. A compendium of information on **prescription drugs** (see under **drug**) and diagnostic products. Sections include listings of drugs by manufacturer, type (action) of drug, and brand name. Detailed information as furnished by the manufacturer is the same as that found in the "package inserts" required by law. One section shows color photographs of products as an aid in identification in poison control, and for use with patients who are not sure of the prescriptions they are taking. Published on paper annually (with periodic supplements) and online by Thomson PDR, which also publishes a companion volume, *PDR for Nonprescription Drugs, Dietary Supplements and Herbs: The Definitive Guide to OTC Medications*. **www.pdr.net**

PE See *physician executive*.

PECOS See *Provider Enrollment Chain and Ownership System*.

pediatric Pertaining to children.

pediatric nursing The area of nursing focusing on the needs of children.

> **Board Certified Pediatric Nurse** A registered nurse with a Bachelor of Science in Nursing (BSN) degree who is qualified in pediatric nursing and has passed an examination of the American Nurses Credentialing Center (ANCC) (**nursingworld.org/ancc**). The credential is RN,BC (Registered Nurse, Board Certified).

> **Certified Pediatric Nurse** A registered nurse with an associate degree or diploma who is qualified in pediatric nursing and has passed an examination of the American Nurses Credentialing Center (ANCC) (**nursingworld.org/ancc**). The credential is RN,C (Registered Nurse, Certified).

> **Certified Pediatric Nurse (CPN)** A registered nurse with pediatric nursing experience who has passed an examination of the Pediatric Nursing Certification Board (PNCB). **www.pncb.org**

> **Certified Pediatric Nurse Practitioner (CPNP)** A nurse practitioner with pediatric nursing experience who has passed an examination of the Pediatric Nursing Certification Board (PNCB). There are exams for primary care and acute care. **www.pncb.org**

> **Clinical Specialist in Pediatric Nursing** A clinical nurse specialist with a graduate degree who is qualified in pediatric nursing and has passed an examination of the American Nurses Credentialing Center (ANCC) (**nursingworld.org/ancc**). The credential is APRN,BC (Advanced Practice Registered Nurse, Board Certified).

> **Pediatric Nurse Practitioner (PNP)** A nurse practitioner who is qualified in pediatric nursing and has passed an examination of the American Nurses Credentialing Center (ANCC) (**nursingworld.org/ancc**). The credential is APRN,BC (Advanced Practice Registered Nurse, Board Certified).

Pediatric Nursing Certification Board (PNCB) A certification organization for pediatric nurses and nurse practitioners. Formerly the National Certification Board of Pediatric Nurse Practitioners and Nurses (NCBPNP/N). **www.pncb.org**

pediatric rule A reference to a 1998 requirement by the Food and Drug Administration (FDA) that requires drug manufacturers to make sure that all drugs intended for pediatric use are properly labeled, based on scientific studies.

pediatrics The study of medicine as it applies to infants, children, and adolescents. The American Academy of Pediatrics definition includes young adults. The upper age limit for pediatrics varies with the region of the country and the hospital. In 1938, most hospitals were only admitting children up to age fourteen in their pediatric units. In 2007, U.S. pediatricians considered the age range up to twenty-one. For pediatric subspecialties, see *medical specialty*. Also spelled paediatrics.

pedigree A term used in genetics, referring to a diagram mapping the genetic history of a particular family.

pedorthics The design, manufacture, modification, and fit of footwear to prevent or alleviate foot problems caused by disease, congenital defect, overuse, or injury.

pedorthist A health professional who practices orthotics. A few states require licensure.

> **Certified Pedorthist (C.Ped)** A pedorthist who has been certified by the Board for Certification in Pedorthics (BCP). **www.cpeds.org**

peer review Review by individuals from the same discipline and with essentially equal qualifications (peers). "Peer review" in a hospital context usually means review of the performance of a physician, done by other physicians, although it applies to such activity within any discipline. Peer review sometimes leads to reduction or denial of privileges of a physician (or other professional) whose performance is reviewed. It is therefore especially important that the process be done fairly and in good faith to avoid legal liability.

"Peer review" sometimes has a narrower meaning, which can be determined only after careful listening and asking questions. Some use the term only for review conducted by a group of physicians appointed by a medical society, some use it as a synonym for a patient care audit, and some use it only when the reviewers are physicians.

Peer review also refers to the process that academic or scientific articles go through prior to publication, where the article is reviewed by experts in the relevant area.

peer review committee A committee of physicians, charged with review of the performance of other physicians. The committee may be that of a medical society, hospital department, medical staff, or other entity. See *peer review*.

peer review organization (PRO) The former name for a *quality improvement organization (QIO)*.

pen-based system A computer that accepts its instructions via a penlike device instead of a keyboard. Starting in the mid 1990s these computers became successful in small specialty niches where a high degree of portability was of critical importance and a relatively narrow set of tasks needed to be accomplished (such as package delivery services). As late as the year 2007, continuing problems with the computer's ability to recognize general handwriting successfully has kept pen-based systems from relegating the keyboard to obsolescence.

People's Medical Society, The A nonprofit medical consumer advocacy organization, founded in 1983, that sees itself as being at the forefront of the "medical consumerism movement," which holds that the most appropriate and best medical care goes to consumers who have the right tools and information. Among its many publications are *Medicine on Trial* (Charles B. Inlander, Lowel S. Levin, and Ed Weiner) and *Take This Book to the Hospital with You* (Inlander and Weiner). **www.peoplesmed.org**

PEPP Payment Error Prevention Program. See *Hospital Payment Monitoring Program*.

Pepper Commission An advisory body that in 1990 made recommendations as to universal health insurance coverage for both acute care and long-term care, and recommended the *play or pay* (see under *mandate*) method of financing. Most of the members of the commission were congressional leaders. The official name of the commission was the U.S. Bipartisan Commission on Comprehensive Health Reform.

per capita Per head (per person); see *capitation*.

percentile The size or magnitude of that element, in a series of elements that are arranged in order of magnitude, whose location in the series is at the designated percentage of the way from the small end of the series to the large end. For example, the fiftieth percentile is the magnitude of the element that is 50% of the way through the series—namely, the magnitude of the middle element, if the series has an odd number of elements. (Thus the fiftieth percentile is the same as the median.)

Algorithms (sets of rules) for calculating percentiles vary, and so their results for a given series may also vary somewhat. This is because the concept of "percentile" is not precise.

Grading of students is a familiar use of the percentile. All the test scores (either percentages or raw scores) are placed in order from lowest to highest. If there are eighty students in the class, the fortieth test score (from either end) is the fiftieth percentile (also known as the median). The sixtieth test score (from the low end) is the seventy-fifth percentile, the seventy-second (again from the low end) is the ninetieth percentile (90% of 80 students (scores) is 72).

percutaneous Through the skin.

per diem rate See under *rate (charge)*.

PERF See *perfusionist*.

performance The actual carrying out of an activity. The term occurs especially in connection with physicians' privileges, where the trend is to attempt to grant privileges, and to continue or terminate them, not only on the basis of the individual's credentials, but also on her or his performance, that is, the skill with which she or he carries out the activities under review. To be able to evaluate performance accurately requires considerable sophistication in the collection and analysis of data about the performance demonstrated. See *performance measure*.

performance data Data that are developed from the activities of an individual or institution. Traditional hospital statistics such as admissions and discharges, lengths of stay, and mortality are performance data. More sophisticated performance data can be developed from ongoing information systems, such as those for billing and medical records. These can describe patterns of medical and surgical management of cases, adherence to critical clinical practice guidelines, use of generic versus proprietary medications and conformance to recommended medication schedules, and similar information. See *performance measure*.

performance improvement (PI) The process of analyzing workers' capabilities—including skills, knowledge, and attitudes—and the organizational environment in which they work, and finding and implementing ways to improve their performance. In health care, some use this synonymously with *quality improvement* or *quality management*. In this context, the organization would collect data on *performance measures* and work to improve the measured performance.

performance measure Something used to gather data on and evaluate activities and/or outcomes; a synonym for *indicator*. The Joint Commission on Accreditation of Healthcare Organizations (JCAHO) uses the term in its *ORYX* initiative to describe things that must be monitored by hospitals and other healthcare organizations as part of the accreditation process. JCAHO defines a performance measure as "[a] quantitative tool (for example, rate, ratio, index, percentage) that provides an indication of an organization's performance in relation to a specified process or outcome."

JCAHO has developed five **core measure** sets for hospitals: for acute myocardial infarction (AMI), heart failure, pneumonia, pregnancy and related conditions, and surgical infection prevention. Performance measures for ICU, pain management, children's asthma care, and hospital-based inpatient-psychiatric services measures are planned. Hospitals must monitor and report on at least three core measure sets. Data are submitted to the JCAHO for accreditation purposes, and JCAHO reports back to the hospital its performance in relation to other hospitals. JCAHO also publishes the results online, for the public, as part of its *Quality Reports*; in this context, the core measures are called **National Quality Improvement Goals (NQIGs)**.

JCAHO performance measures are standardized, with technical specifications and defined data elements and values. To date, all JCAHO core measures have been endorsed by the National Quality Forum (NQF). Some of the core measures for AMI, heart failure, pneumonia, and surgical infection have been adopted by the Hospital Quality Alliance as *National Hospital Quality Measures*. See also *National Patient Safety Goals*.

Performance measures are not just for hospitals; physicians have been developing them, as well. See, for example, *AQA* and *Physician Consortium for Performance Improvement*.

physician performance measure See *AQA and Physician Consortium for Performance Improvement*.

performance measurement system (PMS) A system supplied by a vendor, and approved by the Joint Commission on Accreditation of Healthcare Organizations (JCAHO), for collecting and disseminating data on *performance measures*. The PMS must meet technical specifications so that data can be compared among different systems. In 2007 there were over fifty such systems providing services to hospitals and other healthcare organizations.

performance panel An information device for presenting key information, rapidly and graphically, primarily for the governing body of an institution. The term is replacing "dashboard" for this purpose. See *dashboard*.

performing arts medicine An area of health specialty that focuses on the etiology, prevention, and treatment of health problems common to performing artists. For more information, go to the Performing Arts Medicine Association (PAMA) web site. **www.artsmed.org**

perfusion Pouring through, especially the circulating of blood or other liquid through an organ or tissue. In certain cardiovascular surgery, this flow is assisted by mechanical pumping devices, such as a heart-lung machine.

perfusionist (PERF) A health professional trained to operate and monitor the machines that breathe and circulate blood for patients during surgery. Synonyms: extracorporeal technologist, perfusion technologist.

Certified Clinical Perfusionist (CCP) A perfusionist who has completed an accredited perfusion training program and passed an examination of the American Board of Cardiovascular Perfusion (ABCP). **www.abcp.org**

perfusion technologist See *perfusionist*.

perianesthesia nursing The area of nursing focusing on the needs of patients undergoing anesthesia, including pre- and postanesthesia care. See also *post anesthesia nursing*.

Certified Ambulatory Perianesthesia Nurse (CAPA) A specialist in perianesthesia nursing of ambulatory patients who has passed an examination of the American Board of Perianesthesia Nursing Certification (ABPANC). **www.cpancapa.org**

perinatal Pertaining to the infant in the period shortly before and after birth. It is often (but not always) defined as beginning with the completion of the twenty-eighth week of gestation (pregnancy) and ending one to four weeks after delivery.

perinatal nursing The area of nursing focusing on the needs of women and their babies during the perinatal period.

Board Certified Perinatal Nurse A registered nurse with a Bachelor of Science in Nursing (BSN) degree who is qualified in perinatal nursing and has passed an examination of the American Nurses Credentialing Center (ANCC) (**nursingworld.org/ancc**). The credential is RN,BC (Registered Nurse, Board Certified).

Certified Perinatal Nurse A registered nurse with an associate degree or diploma who is qualified in perinatal nursing and has passed an examination of the American Nurses Credentialing Center (ANCC) (**nursingworld.org/ancc**). The credential is RN,C (Registered Nurse, Certified).

periodic interim payment (PIP) A system of providing Medicare funds to providers on a regular basis. Periodic payments may be made monthly or semi-monthly to a hospital, home health agency, or skilled nursing facility in the Medicare program, based on the institution's estimated annual Medicare revenue. Adjustments are made later when actual revenue figures become available. Such a system of payment is also sometimes employed by other payers.

periodic payments A payment arrangement that allows money due to be paid in installments, over time, instead of in a lump sum. The term is used in regard to settlements (or judgments) in malpractice cases, which allow the defendant to pay for the patient's health care and other needs as those expenses accrue, or to pay a fixed sum in even portions over a given number of years.

perioperative See *operative*.

perioperative nursing The area of nursing concerned with the needs of patients before, during, and after surgery. Formerly called operating room nurse.

> **Certified Perioperative Nurse (CNOR)** A specialist in perioperative nursing who has passed an examination of the Competency and Credentialing Institute (CCI) (formerly Certification Board Perioperative Nursing). A retired Certified Perioperative Nurse may use the credential CNOR(E) (emeritus). **www.cc-institute.org**

Perioperative Nursing Data Set (PNDS) See under *data set*.

peripheral worker See *contingent worker*.

peritoneal dialysis See under *dialysis*.

peritoneal dialysis nurse See *Certified Peritoneal Dialysis Nurse* under *dialysis nursing*.

PERM See *Payment Error Rate Measurement*.

per member per month (PMPM) Refers to the cost (or charge) for a healthcare premium for an individual for one month.

per se "By itself." In antitrust law, where it is frequently referred to as the "per se rule," it refers to activities that, by themselves, are violations of the antitrust laws. No proof of intent, negative effect on competition, and so forth are required. *Price-fixing* is a "per se" violation of the Sherman Act. This rule is distinguished from the less strict test used in the *Rule of Reason*. See *antitrust*.

persistent organic pollutants (POP) Chemical substances—such as DDT, PCBs, and dioxins—that remain in the environment, accumulate through the food chain, and pose a continuing health risk to humans and animals. POPs travel throughout the globe, and are causing international concern.

personal care account (PCA) See *health reimbursement account*.

personal care aide See under *aide*.

personal care services Those services required to take care of the *activities of daily living (ADL)*. Synonym: personal care.

personal computer stager (PC-stager) See under *stager*.

personal health record (PHR) See under *electronic health record*.

personal information carrier (PIC) See under *electronic health record*.

Personal Membership Group (PMG) Groups within the American Hospital Association (AHA) made up of personal members (individuals, as opposed to hospitals) representing various disciplines in health care. In 2007 AHA had the following PMGs:

> American Society for Healthcare Central Service Professionals (ASHCSP)
> American Society for Healthcare Engineering (ASHE)
> American Society for Healthcare Environmental Services (ASHES)
> American Society for Healthcare Food Service Administrators (ASHFSA)
> American Society for Healthcare Human Resources Administration (ASHHRA)
> Association for Healthcare Resource & Materials Management (AHRMM)
> American Society for Healthcare Risk Management (ASHRM)
> American Society of Directors of Volunteer Services (ASDVS)

Association of Healthcare Administrative Professionals (AHAP)

Hospitals for a Healthy Environment—An AHA/EPA Partnership

Medical Fitness Association (MFA)

National Association of Healthcare Transport Management (NAHTM)

Society for Healthcare Consumer Advocacy (SHCA)

Society for Healthcare Strategy and Market Development (SHSMD)

Society for Social Work Leadership in Health Care (SSWLHC)

personal responsibility contribution (PRC) See *Healthy Americans Act*.

personal services Usually, services that are provided simply because the recipient wants them, rather than because they are essential to his or her medical or other care. Examples include beauty parlor services, catered meals, and the like. Such services are not included in the benefits of a health plan. See also *personal care services*.

personal trainer A health professional who provides fitness and health counseling and advice to individual clients on a one-to-one basis. The personal trainer may evaluate fitness, design an individualized fitness program, supervise the exercises, and generally provide support and encouragement for the client to meet his or her fitness goals. As a minimum, most personal trainers have at least a high school diploma and CPR certification. See also *athletic trainer*.

ACE Certified Personal Trainer (ACE-CPT) A personal trainer who has met the certification requirements of the American Council on Exercise (ACE). **www.acefitness.org**

ACSM Certified Personal Trainer A personal trainer who has met the certification requirements of the American College of Sports Medicine (ACSM). **www.acsm.org**

Certified Personal Trainer (NASM-CPT) A personal trainer who has met the certification requirements of the National Academy of Sports Medicine (NASM). **www.nasm.org**

NCSF Certified Personal Trainer (NCSF-CPT) A personal trainer who has met the certification requirements of the National Council on Strength and Fitness (NCSF). **www.ncsf.org**

NFPT Certified Personal Trainer (NFPT-CPT) A personal trainer who has met the certification requirements of the National Federation of Professional Trainers (NFPT). **www.nfpt.com**

NSCA-Certified Personal Trainer (NSCA-CPT) A personal trainer who has met the certification requirements of the National Strength and Conditioning Association (NSCA). **www.nsca-cc.org**

persons with AIDS (PWAs) Persons who are HIV-positive and have developed clinical symptoms of AIDS.

PERT See *program evaluation and review technique*.

PET Positron emission tomography; see *nuclear medicine*.

PETO A method for qualifying and quantifying workload requirements of pediatric patients, developed in the Eugene Talmadge Memorial Hospital in Augusta, Georgia, in 1970. The name was created from the first initials of the surnames of the three pediatric nurse researchers and a pediatrician who worked out the system: Poland, English, Thorton, and Owens. This workload management system has since evolved; see *GRASP*.

pet therapy Treatment provided to animals; sometimes used as a misnomer for *animal-assisted therapy*.

PFFS See *private fee-for-service* under *fee-for-service*.

PFGE Pulsed-field gel electrophoresis. See *PulseNet*.

P4P See *pay-for-performance*.

PFQI Physician Focused Quality Initiative. See *Quality Initiative*.

PFSH Past, family, and social history. The part of the medical record in which the caregiver records the patient's background information.

PFT See *pulmonary function technologist*.

PGx See *pharmacogenomics*.

phacoemulsification The liquidizing of cataracts and their removal by suction, using ultrasound.

phage A virus that affects a bacterium, sometimes destroying the bacterium but, in some cases, increasing the bacterium's virulence. Early in the twentieth century phages were increasingly used to treat bacterial diseases, but with the advent of antibiotics, they went into disuse except in certain areas of the former Soviet Union. With the increasing antibiotic resistance of bacteria throughout the world at the end of the twentieth century, interest in phages revived. Research methods have improved and phages are being identified and grown that destroy specific bacteria. Phages are able to mutate along with their counterpart bacteria, thus counteracting phage resistance on the part of the bacteria. Genetic engineering is being employed to design phages for specific purposes, and commercial ventures are appearing. Synonym: bacteriophage.

pharmaceutical An adjective pertaining to the manufacture, dispensing, and use of drugs used in health care. Also frequently used as a noun meaning a "pharmaceutical product."

  radiopharmaceutical Shorthand for "radiopharmaceutical product," a drug having radio-active properties, used in diagnosis or treatment.

pharmaceutical medicine The medical specialty devoted to the discovery, development, clinical trials, and monitoring of drugs.

pharmacist A person who is licensed to prepare, dispense, and control prescription drugs. A pharmacist need not be a pharmacologist.

  nuclear pharmacist A pharmacist who specializes in radiopharmaceuticals.

  Board Certified Nuclear Pharmacist (BCNP) A nuclear pharmacist certified by the Board of Pharmaceutical Specialties (BPS). **www.bpsweb.org**

  nutrition support pharmacist A pharmacist trained in treating patients who are receiving specialized nutrition support, including parenteral and enteral nutrition.

  Board Certified Nutrition Support Pharmacist (BCNSP) A nutrition support pharma-cist certified by the Board of Pharmaceutical Specialties (BPS). **www.bpsweb.org**

  oncology pharmacist A pharmacist who specializes in the pharmaceutical needs of patients with cancer.

  Board Certified Oncology Pharmacist (BCOP) An oncology pharmacist certified by the Board of Pharmaceutical Specialties (BPS). **www.bpsweb.org**

  pharmacotherapy specialist A pharmacist focusing on the safe, appropriate, and eco-nomical use of drugs in patient care. Often serves as a source of drug information for other health professionals.

  Board Certified Pharmacotherapy Specialist (BCPS) A pharmacotherapy specialist certified by the Board of Pharmaceutical Specialties (BPS). Added qualifications are avail-able in Cardiology and Infectious Diseases. **www.bpsweb.org**

  psychiatric pharmacist A pharmacist specializing in the pharmaceutical care of patients with psychiatric illnesses.

  Board Certified Psychiatric Pharmacist (BCPP) A psychiatric pharmacist certified by the Board of Pharmaceutical Specialties (BPS). **www.bpsweb.org**

pharmacoeconomics The study of the cost-effectiveness of health-related interventions. Applying the principles of economics to alternative drug therapies, pharmacoeconomics can include *quality of life (QOL)* considerations as part of its cost-benefit analysis. The initial attention was given to drugs, but these evaluations also include other health services, such as medical and surgical techniques and procedures, both diagnostic and therapeutic, and the use of technological tools. See also *International Society for Pharmacoeconomics and Outcomes Research*.

pharmacoepidemiology The study of the use and effects of drugs in a given population. Investigators using the methods of this discipline provide information used by, among oth-ers, agencies concerned with the regulation of medicines.

pharmacogenetics The study of how the genetic makeup of individuals (their "genotype") affects their response to drugs. Scientists are studying how to tailor drugs to the genes of specific individuals. In deciding on treatment, a patient would first be given genetic tests to determine his or her drug-response profile. Depending on the profile, only drugs that would be effective would be prescribed; drugs forecast to be ineffective or harmful would be avoided—one size does not fit all. The term comes from the words "pharmacology" and "genetics." See also *designer drug* (under *drug*) and *pharmacogenomics*.

pharmacogenomics (PGx) The general study of how genes affect the behavior of drugs. The term comes from the words "pharmacology" and "genomics." Sometimes the term is used interchangeably with *pharmacogenetics*.

pharmacokinetics The action of a drug (or other substance) within the body: time required to be absorbed, distribution throughout the body, duration of action, and how and when it is excreted.

pharmacologist A person trained in the science of drugs—their properties and reactions, and their therapeutic effects and drug interactions. A pharmacologist need not be licensed, and is not necessarily a pharmacist.

pharmacology The science dealing with drugs, their composition, preparation, chemical properties, actions, and uses.

pharmacopeia A document containing recipes for the preparation (compounding) of medicinal drugs and also standards for their strengths and purities. Many nations adopt official pharmacopeias. See also *formulary (pharmaceutical)* and *United States Pharmacopeia—National Formulary*.

Pharmacopeia of the United States See *United States Pharmacopeia—National Formulary*.

pharmacotherapy The treatment of disease through the use of drugs.

pharmacovigilance (PV) Attention to drug safety, especially monitoring *adverse drug events*.

pharmacy (discipline) The art and science of preparing and dispensing medicine (substance).

pharmacy (facility) A place where medicine is prepared and dispensed. A retail drug store is one type of pharmacy. In a hospital, the pharmacy is a department where medicine is prepared to be administered to inpatients, and to be kept in areas where drugs are administered; for example, the emergency department.

pharmacy and therapeutics (P&T) Usually, a committee of the medical staff, or of the hospital, that concerns itself with drugs to be stocked by the hospital pharmacy (facility) and their correct use. It ordinarily has physician, pharmacist, and nurse members.

pharmacy benefit manager (PBM) A company used by managed care providers and health insurers to increase the efficiency of providing drugs to their subscribers or members. These providers contract with PBMs to process claims for drugs or medications. To control the costs of providing these pharmacy benefits, the PBM might use generic (cheaper) drugs in place of brand names where possible, or gain financial benefits for the clients from rebates or other discount programs offered by some drug manufacturing companies. A software program or online service providing similar services might also be called a PBM. Synonym: prescription benefit manager.

pharmacy technician A health professional who assists a pharmacist in the various tasks related to the pharmacy, including administrative functions and many other duties that do not require a licensed pharmacist to perform, or that may be done under the direct supervision of the pharmacist. A pharmacy technician may work in a hospital or other facility, managed care organization, or free-standing pharmacy.

Certified Pharmacy Technician (CPhT) A pharmacy technician who has been certified by the Pharmacy Technician Certification Board (PTCB). **www.ptcb.org**

PHDSC See *Public Health Data Standards Consortium*.

phenotype The physical appearance of an organism, as contrasted with its genetic makeup, which is called its genotype.

pheromone A hormone-like substance that is released into the environment by certain animals, and perceived only by animals of the same species, which results in changes in social or sexual behavior.

PHI See *protected health information*.

PHIN See *Public Health Information Network*.

phlebology The study of veins.

phlebotomist See *Phlebotomy Technician* under *clinical laboratory technician*.

phlebotomy The procedure of opening a vein to draw blood.

Phlebotomy Technician (PBT) See under *clinical laboratory technician*.

PHN See *public health nurse* under *public health nursing*.

PHO See *physician-hospital organization*.

PHP Partial hospitalization program. See *partial hospitalization* under *hospitalization*.

PHPC See *Public Housing Primary Care*.

PHR See *personal health record* under *electronic health record*.

PHS See *Public Health Service*.

PHSA See *Public Health Service Act*.

PHSCC See *Public Health Service Commissioned Corps*.

PHS Pricing See *340B Drug Pricing Program*.

PhyloCode A method of classification of biological entities according to their genetic ancestry rather than their physical similarity. The PhyloCode grew out of a workshop at Harvard University in August 1998. It is being developed by the International Society for Phylogenetic Nomenclature (**www.phylonames.org**). Synonym: phylogenetic nomenclature. See also *Linnaean System*.

phylogenetic nomenclature See *PhyloCode*.

physiatrist A physician specializing in *physical medicine and rehabilitation*.

physiatry See *physical medicine and rehabilitation*.

physical Having to do with physics, that is, mechanics, heat, radiation, sound, electricity, and similar phenomena. It is contrasted with "chemical," which refers to the properties of substances. Also used as shorthand for *physical examination*.

physical examination The portion of the examination of an individual that the physician carries out by using his or her own senses—looking, touching, and listening—with or without the aid of devices to assist these senses. When the term is used in the context of a "complete physical" (examination), it may also include examination of the blood or body fluids and the use of special procedures such as x-ray and electrocardiography.

physical medicine and rehabilitation (PM&R) The branch of medicine concerned with the prevention, diagnosis, and treatment of disorders that cause impairment. Emphasis is on the musculoskeletal, cardiovascular, neurologic, and pulmonary systems, with the goal being restoration of function. Synonym: physiatry.

physical status classification (PS classification) See *ASA Physical Status Classification*.

physical therapist (PT) A health professional who provides physical therapy services to those with injuries or disease. The PT evaluates the patient's joint motion, muscle strength and endurance, function of heart and lungs, and performance of the activities of daily living (ADL). Treatment then includes therapeutic exercise, cardiovascular endurance training, and ADL training. Sometimes called a physiotherapist. PTs must be licensed by the state and, to do this, pass a national examination created by the Federation of State Boards of Physical Therapy (FSBPT). **www.fsbpt.org**

Cardiovascular and Pulmonary Certified Specialist (CCS) A licensed physical therapist who has met the certification requirements for cardiovascular and pulmonary physical therapy of the American Board of Physical Therapy Specialties (ABPTS). **www.apta.org**

Clinical Electrophysiologic Certified Specialist (ECS) A licensed physical therapist who has met the certification requirements for clinical electrophysiologic physical therapy of the American Board of Physical Therapy Specialties (ABPTS). **www.apta.org**

Geriatric Certified Specialist (GCS) A licensed physical therapist who has met the certification requirements for geriatric physical therapy of the American Board of Physical Therapy Specialties (ABPTS). **www.apta.org**

Neurologic Certified Specialist (NCS) A licensed physical therapist who has met the certification requirements for neurologic physical therapy of the American Board of Physical Therapy Specialties (ABPTS). **www.apta.org**

Orthopaedic Certified Specialist (OCS) A licensed physical therapist who has met the certification requirements for orthopaedic physical therapy of the American Board of Physical Therapy Specialties (ABPTS). **www.apta.org**

Pediatric Certified Specialist (PCS) A licensed physical therapist who has met the certification requirements for pediatric physical therapy of the American Board of Physical Therapy Specialties (ABPTS). **www.apta.org**

Sports Certified Specialist (SCS) A licensed physical therapist who has met the certification requirements for sports physical therapy of the American Board of Physical Therapy Specialties (ABPTS). **www.apta.org**

physical therapist assistant (PTA) A health professional skilled in using physical therapy to treat patients, who works under the supervision of a physical therapist. More than half of the states require PTAs to be licensed, certified, or registered.

physical therapy (PT) The use of physical means such as exercise, massage, light, cold, heat, and electricity, as well as mechanical devices, in the prevention, diagnosis, and treatment of diseases, injuries, and other physical disorders. Physical therapy does not include the use of x-rays or other types of radiation. Synonym: physiotherapy.

physician A person qualified by a doctor's degree in medicine (Doctor of Medicine (MD)) or osteopathy (Doctor of Osteopathic Medicine (DO)). To practice, a physician must also be licensed by the state in which she or he practices. Note that "physician" is the generic term; a surgeon is also a physician, but a physician is not necessarily a surgeon. For specialists, see *medical specialty*.

admitting physician The physician who orders the admission of a given patient to a hospital or other healthcare institution.

alternate physician In a long-term care facility (LTCF), the physician assigned responsibility for medical care to patients in the absence of the attending physician.

attending physician The physician legally responsible, at a given time, for the care of a given patient in an institution. May or may not be the operating surgeon (see *surgeon*).

board certified physician See *board certified*.

board eligible physician See *board eligible*.

contract physician A physician who provides care under a contract. A hospital, for example, may contract with a physician (directly or through a corporation) to provide emergency care. The contract sets out the physician's duties as well as the hospital's. The contract physician is an independent contractor, rather than an employee of the hospital.

first year resident physician A physician who has already had formal training in medicine, who is now obtaining his or her first year of supervised practical training. The term "graduate year 1" (GY-1) is now being applied to any residency program for the individual in the first year out of medical school. The term "intern" was formerly given to this person, but "intern" is no longer restricted to physicians; the term is applied in many disciplines.

full-time physician A physician who spends the major part of her or his time within one or more specific hospitals, as, for example, a pathologist, radiologist, or emergency department physician. Synonym: hospital-based physician.

geographic full-time physician A physician whose primary income is derived from a salary for services to a hospital, but who also engages in private clinical practice at that hospital.

graduate physician A physician who has completed the education leading to the Doctor of Medicine (MD) or Doctor of Osteopathic Medicine (DO) degree, and who has obtained that degree.

hospital-based physician See *full-time physician*, above. See also *hospitalist*.

locum tenens physician A substitute physician, hired temporarily to fill in for another. From the Latin for "holding the place."

marginal physician A physician whose performance is just at (or below) the standards of performance for such physicians, either in terms of quality of care or cost.

nonparticipating physician Under Medicare, a physician who has not signed a contract agreeing to refrain from charging a Medicare patient the difference between the physician's usual charge and the Medicare payment allowance.

participating physician Under Medicare, a physician who has signed a contract agreeing not to charge a Medicare patient for the balance between the physician's usual charge and the Medicare payment allowance for the service rendered.

primary care physician (PCP) A physician who specializes in primary care (family medicine, general internal medicine, general pediatrics, or obstetrics and gynecology). He or she provides the initial care for a patient, and refers the patient, when appropriate, for secondary (specialist) care. See also *primary care*.

referring physician A physician who has asked another physician to give a consultation or to take over the care of a given patient, or who has sent a patient to another institution.

resident physician A graduate physician who is in an approved hospital training program in graduate medical education (a residency). Upon successful completion of the program, the resident is granted a certificate of that fact. A resident physician may be called simply a "resident," a "medical resident," a "surgical resident," or something similar.

salaried physician A physician employed on a salary. Ordinarily such a physician does not also bill for services on a fee-for-service basis.

secondary care physician (SCP) A specialist; one who treats patients on referral from another physician, most often a primary care physician.

specialty care physician (SPC) A physician who practices any medical or surgical specialty other than a primary care specialty. The term is used to distinguish them from primary care physicians. Sometimes the term used is "secondary care physician."

physician advisor (PA) A physician who is involved with utilization review and/or quality management to advise on medical necessity and other medical issues, for example in the context of preadmission authorizations or concurrent review. The physician is normally contacted only if the case falls outside specific predetermined criteria. Synonym: physician reviewer.

physician assistant (PA) A health professional with advanced training who is licensed to practice medicine under the supervision of a physician. PAs take patient histories, perform examinations, order tests and x-rays, suture wounds, set casts, do other minor procedures, and make preliminary diagnoses. Most states permit PAs to prescribe drugs.

Physician Assistant—Certified (PA-C) A physician assistant who has completed an accredited PA program and passed a national examination administered by the National Commission on Certification of Physician Assistants (NCCPA). **www.nccpa.net**

Physician Consortium for Performance Improvement (PCPI) A group convened by the American Medical Association (AMA) to develop, test, and maintain evidence-based clinical *performance measures* and measurement resources for physicians. The consortium is composed of over 100 national medical specialty and state medical societies, the Council of Medical Specialty Societies (CMSS), the American Board of Medical Specialties (ABMS) and its member boards, experts in methodology and data collection, the Agency for Healthcare Research and Quality (AHRQ), and CMS. By the end of 2006, complete clinical and technical specifications were available for asthma, chronic stable coronary artery disease, heart failure, hypertension, major depressive disorder, osteoarthritis, pediatric acute gastroenteritis, and preventive care and screening (also five measurement sets including adult influenza immunization, colorectal cancer screening, problem drinking, screening mammography, and tobacco use). See also *AQA*.

physician contingency reserve (PCR) See *withhold*.

physician executive (PE) An executive in a healthcare organization who is a physician. See also *medical management*.

> **Certified Physician Executive (CPE)** A physician who has passed an examination of the Certifying Commission in Medical Management (CCMM) (**www.ccmm.org**). Prior to about 1997, PEs were certified by the American Board of Medical Management (ABMM).

physician extender A health professional who, usually under the supervision of a physician, provides services formerly given by physicians themselves. Nurse practitioners (NPs), advanced practice nurses, certified nurse midwives, and physician assistants are among those who serve as physician extenders. The use of physician extenders in private practice was still relatively new in the late 1990s, but large managed care providers, such as Kaiser-Permanente, have made extensive use of NPs since the 1970s.

physician-hospital-community organization (PHCO) Same as a *physician-hospital organization (PHO)*, except that the community is also represented on the governing board along with the hospital and physicians.

physician-hospital organization (PHO) A legal entity formed by a hospital and a group of physicians, often categorized as a "multiprovider network." The PHO serves as a negotiating and contracting unit to obtain managed care contracts directly with employers, or other payers (such as managed care companies). The physicians usually maintain their own practices, and contract with the PHO to provide services. If the provider members in the network comprise a significant percentage (typically 30% or more) of all available providers in an area, they must be careful to avoid actions that run counter to antitrust laws, such as *collectively* negotiating fee schedules. See also *provider-sponsored network* and *independent practice association*.

physician office laboratory (POL) The *Clinical Laboratory Improvement Amendments (CLIA)* subjected the physician office laboratory to the same regulations as independent laboratories. The amendments require, among other things, certification for all physician office labs except those performing only simple procedures (as defined by the FDA). The amendments also subjected the POLs to unannounced laboratory inspections. Synonym: physician-owned laboratory.

physician order entry (POE) See *computerized physician order entry*.

physician-owned laboratory (POL) See *physician office laboratory*.

physician-patient collaboration See *patient-caregiver collaboration*.

physician-patient relationship See *doctor-patient relationship*.

physician payment reform (PPR) A basic change in the way physicians were paid for services for Medicare patients, mandated by the Omnibus Budget Reconciliation Act of 1989 (OBRA 89), effective January 1, 1992. Prior to that date, payment had been based on *customary, prevailing, reasonable charges (CPR)*. Replacing that method, the new method was based on a *resource-based relative value scale (RBRVS)* (see under *relative value scale*).

One intent of the change was to reduce the premium (high fees) put on procedures, typically done by specialists, and increase the reimbursement for *cognitive services*, such as evaluation and diagnosis and patient management, services provided mainly by primary care physicians. A second component of the reform was application of Medicare Volume Performance Standards (MVPS), targets against which a physician's spending is measured. If a physician's standard is exceeded, the next year his or her rate of fee increase is reduced. A third component of the reform is a cap on the out-of-pocket charges that may be made to beneficiaries.

Physician Payment Review Commission (PPRC) A federal advisory body set up under the Consolidated Omnibus Budget Reconciliation Act of 1985 (COBRA 1985) to provide input to HCFA (now CMS) regarding methods of saving money in the payment of physicians for services to Medicare patients. Its recommendations helped form the basis of the Omnibus

Budget Reconciliation Act of 1989 that created the *resource-based relative value scale (RBRVS)* (see under *relative value scale*).

physician practice guidelines See *clinical practice guidelines*.

physician query form A type of paper form used by many healthcare facilities as a substitute for (or addition to) a physician's documentation that is required in the medical record to support Medicare reimbursement. It is the responsibility of the medical record department in these facilities to obtain the necessary documentation from the physicians, and they have traditionally had a hard time getting the physicians to comply.

Although the physician query form is seen as a labor saving device by the providers, the Medicare payer (CMS) and the Office of Inspector General (OIG) have seen the use of this form as increasing the likelihood of fraud and abuse. Their concern, justified by some past discoveries of DRG upcoding, centers primarily on the possibility of the forms' use of "leading questions" to encourage certain responses by physicians. In 2001, CMS stated that a query form would be considered acceptable to the extent it provides clarification and is consistent with other medical record documentation. The query form should not be leading, and it should not introduce new information not otherwise contained in the medical record. Synonym: coding summary form.

physician recruitment Finding, soliciting, and attracting physicians to a particular hospital or area. Hospitals devote resources to the search, and provide incentives, for physicians in specialties that are needed by the hospital and community. Such incentives may include relocation reimbursement and either initial employment of the physician or provision of a loan (with favorable terms) to enable the physician to start and build a practice in the area. See also *inurement*.

physician reviewer (PR) See *physician advisor*.

physician's assistant See *physician assistant*.

Physician Scarcity Area (PSA) A county with a low ratio of primary care or specialty care physicians to Medicare beneficiaries; the designation is made by CMS. The Medicare Modernization Act (MMA) established a payment incentive program for primary physicians in a primary care PSA, and for specialty physicians in a specialty PSA. Medicare pays these physicians a 5% bonus for Medicare services. See also *Health Professional Shortage Area*.

Physicians' Current Procedural Terminology (CPT) See *CPT*.

Physicians' Desk Reference (PDR) See *PDR*.

Physicians for Social Responsibility (PSR) The U.S. affiliate of the *International Physicians for the Prevention of Nuclear War (IPPNW)*. **www.psr.org**

Physician Shortage Area (PSA) A *Medically Underserved Area* that is particularly short of physicians. The term is defined in the Public Health Service Act and used to determine which areas have priority for assistance.

physician's information assistant (PIA) A proposed new type of physician assistant, who is specially trained in the electronic medical record (EMR) and other information systems.

physician site See *distant site*.

physicist A specialist in the science of physics.

>**health physicist** A physicist specializing in the prevention and control of radiation hazards. He or she may work in industry, government, defense, or the environment, as well as health care.

>>**Certified Health Physicist (CHP)** A health physicist with at least a bachelor's degree and six years of experience, who has passed an examination of the American Board of Health Physics (ABHP) (**www.hps1.org/aahp/abhp/abhp.htm**). Holders of ABHP certification may also identify themselves as Diplomates of the American Board of Health Physics (DABHP).

>**medical health physicist** A health physicist who specializes in the diagnostic and therapeutic uses of radiation. Usually works in the radiologic department of a hospital or clinic. May serve as the *radiation safety officer*.

medical physicist A physicist specializing in the uses and safety of radiation within the field of medicine. A *medical health physicist* (see above) is one kind of medical physicist. See also *nuclear medicine scientist*.

    Certified Medical Physicist (CMP) A medical physicist who has at least a graduate degree and has passed both a general examination and additional examinations in either Magnetic Resonance Imaging (MRI) Physics or Medical Health Physics given by the American Board of Medical Physics (ABMP) (**www.abmpexam.com**). A person with this credential may also be called a Diplomate of the American Board of Medical Physics (DABMP).

radiologic physicist A medical physicist specializing in *radiologic physics* (see under *physics*). The American Board of Radiology (ABR) offers Board Certification in three areas: *Diagnostic Radiologic Physics*, *Medical Nuclear Physics*, and *Therapeutic Radiologic Physics* (see below). **www.theabr.org**

physics The science of the properties of matter and energy and their interactions.

    health physics The science of promoting the safe use of radiation, while minimizing its dangers. It involves protecting people and the environment from hazards related to use of the atom.

        medical health physics The science of the safe use of x-rays, gamma rays, and electron and other charged particle beams of neutrons or radionuclides and of radiation from sealed radionuclide sources for diagnostic and therapeutic purposes.

    medical physics The application of the science of physics to medicine. See also *nuclear medicine*.

    radiologic physics A term encompassing diagnostic radiologic physics, medical nuclear physics, and therapeutic radiologic physics (see below).

        diagnostic radiologic physics The science of the diagnostic applications of x-rays, gamma rays from sealed sources, ultrasonic radiation, and radio frequency radiation.

        medical nuclear physics The science of the therapeutic and diagnostic applications of radionuclides (except those used in sealed sources for therapeutic purposes).

        therapeutic radiologic physics The science of the therapeutic applications of x-rays, gamma rays, electron and charged particle beams, neutrons, and radiations from sealed radionuclide sources.

physiological Normal. When the body is functioning normally, its processes and activities are said to be physiological; when the function is not normal, it is *pathological* (abnormal).

physiological chemist See *biochemist*.

physiology The science dealing with the life processes of living things, the chemical and physical activity of body organs and tissues. It is contrasted with "anatomy," which deals with the structures of the organs and tissues rather than their activities.

physiotherapy See *physical therapy*.

PhysPRC See *Physician Payment Review Commission*.

PI See *performance improvement*.

PIA See *physician's information assistant*.

PIC See *personal information carrier* under *electronic health record*.

Picker Institute An independent, nonprofit organization dedicated to the advancement of the principles of *patient-centered care* and the global patient-centered care movement. The institute was an outgrowth of the Picker/Commonwealth Program for Patient-Centered Care (see *Commonwealth Fund*), established in 1987 to investigate the discrepancies between routine investigations of patients' satisfaction and patients' own accounts of their healthcare experiences. Its aim is to promote healthcare quality assessment and improvement strategies in order to address patients' needs as patients themselves define them, and to work toward models of care that make the experience of illness and health care more humane. The institute has developed a group of tested patient survey instruments and videotapes, including the prize-winning *Through the Patient's Eyes*. There are also Picker Institutes in Europe, Switzerland, and Germany. **pickerinstitute.org**

picture archiving and communication system (PACS) A system to provide efficient archival, retrieval, communication, and display of digital medical images. Originally developed for use in radiology departments for x-ray pictures and other diagnostic images, their use has expanded to accommodate any kind of pictures (graphics) used in health care. A PACS system will depend on other standards for images, such as *DICOM*, to allow interoperability with other systems.

PICU See *pediatric intensive care unit* under *intensive care unit*.

PIE charting A charting system designed to provide an ongoing plan of care. It begins with the nursing assessment; some hospitals add checklists and flow sheets. A separate care plan is not written; instead, interventions are recorded in the nursing notes. After initial assessment, the nurse identifies actual problems or nursing diagnoses that arise during the shift. Problems and diagnoses are listed and numbered consecutively on a problem list during each twenty-four-hour period. In the narrative nursing notes, problems, interventions, and evaluations (PIE) are described, with reference to each problem by number. Problems are evaluated at least once every eight hours, and after twenty-four hours the problem list is rewritten, with resolved problems dropped and new ones added. The system was developed in 1984 at Craven County Hospital in New Bern, North Carolina.

pill mill A source of controlled substances (drugs) that are not medically indicated or legitimately prescribed, in violation of federal law. A doctor who prescribes pain medication, such as OxyContin, for patients who don't "need" it may be considered a pill mill. Also, a web site, for example, where one can get prescription medications (not just controlled substances) without a prescription is a pill mill. Collusion among doctors, clinic owners, and pharmacists to defraud Medicare or Medicaid by prescribing and distributing drugs mainly to obtain reimbursement also is called a pill mill.

PIP See *periodic interim payment*.

PKC See *Problem Knowledge Couplers*.

PKI See *public key infrastructure*.

placebo A sugar pill or other fake medication or treatment, used for comparison with a real drug or treatment in clinical studies. Physicians also sometimes prescribe a placebo for a patient demanding medication, but for whom no drug is indicated. There is a well-known "placebo effect," where the patient experiences real improvement, apparently from belief in the placebo. From the Latin meaning "I shall please." See also *nocebo effect*.

plaintiff The person (or organization) who brings a lawsuit against another person or entity, called the defendant. Commonly, the plaintiff in a lawsuit is someone who alleges she or he was injured by the acts of the defendant.

Planetree A nonprofit consumer healthcare organization dedicated to promoting *patient-centered care*. Its philosophy is based on consumer access to health and medical information, involvement of family and friends, and encouraging consumers to become active participants in improving, maintaining, and restoring their health. Planetree was founded in 1978 to humanize, personalize, and demystify the healthcare system for patients and their families.

The **Planetree Alliance** is a group of hospitals and healthcare institutions with shared values, goals, and experiences that are dedicated to implementing Planetree programs and developing more effective programs. Planetree has also developed a number of "Health Resource Centers" at hospitals and health centers to give consumers easy access to health and medical information. **www.planetree.org**

Plan ID See *National Payer ID*.

Planned Approach to Community Health (PATCH) A model for planning, conducting, and evaluating community health promotion and disease prevention programs, developed by the Centers for Disease Control and Prevention (CDC).

planner A person whose profession is planning.

planning The analysis of needs, demands, and resources, followed by the proposal of steps to meet the demands and needs by use of the current resources and obtaining other resources as necessary. See also *strategic planning*.

> **community-based planning** Planning in which the attempt is made to have the planning initiative within the local community rather than external to the community.

> **comprehensive health planning (CHP)** Attempts to coordinate environmental measures, health education, health care, and occupational and other health efforts to achieve the greatest results in a community.

> **corporate planning** The establishment of goals for a corporation, along with the policies and procedures to be used to attain those goals.

> **health planning** Planning (a formal activity directed at determining goals, policies, and procedures) for a healthcare facility, a health program, a defined geographic area, or a population. Health planning may be carried out by the organization itself or by a planning agency. When it is carried out for an area, and the people in the area itself furnish the initiative, it is called "community-based planning."

> **joint planning** Planning carried out jointly by two or more institutions, which may or may not envision sharing of services and facilities.

plan sponsor An entity that sponsors an employee benefit plan, with or without healthcare benefits. It is defined at length in the Employee Retirement Income Security Act (ERISA) (29 U.S.C. § 1002(16)(B) (2005)). The HIPAA Privacy Rule includes by reference the definition provided by ERISA.

plant engineer See *administrative engineer*.

plastic surgery This surgical specialty has two components: reconstructive and cosmetic surgery. Reconstructive surgery involves the repair, reconstruction, or replacement of abnormal structures in the face or body caused by trauma, burns, disease, or birth defects—for example, repair of a cleft palate and breast reconstruction after a mastectomy. Cosmetic (aesthetic) surgery is performed on normal body structures to enhance appearance—for example, facelift, rhinoplasty (nose surgery), breast augmentation, and liposuction. "Plastic" comes from the Greek word plastikos, meaning "to mold or shape."

plastic surgical nursing The area of nursing focusing on the needs of patients undergoing plastic surgery.

> **Certified Plastic Surgical Nurse (CPSN)** A specialist in plastic surgical nursing who has passed an examination of the Plastic Surgical Nursing Certification Board (PSNCB).
> **www.aspsn.org**

play or else See *employer mandate* under *mandate*.

play or pay See under *mandate*.

pledging of accounts receivable Short-term financing where accounts receivable are used to secure the financing. The lender does not buy the accounts receivable, but simply accepts them as collateral for the loan. Synonym: discounting of accounts receivable.

PLM See *product line management* under *management (organization)*.

PLTC See *Partnership for Long Term Care*.

plunge An educational visit to an unfamiliar environment. The term is being used in health care for a visit to a community in order to begin to learn about its population, organizations, resources, problems, needs, and interests.

pluralistic system A system that provides alternatives. The United States is described as favoring pluralism, as illustrated by the fact that medical care, for example, can be obtained from solo practitioners, group practices, or prepaid health plans.

PM See *post mortem*, *practice management system*, and *psychosomatic medicine*.

PM&R See *physical medicine and rehabilitation*.

PMC See *Patient Management Category Severity Scale*.

PM-DRG See *Pediatric-Modified Diagnosis Related Group* under *DRG*.

PMHNP See *Adult Psychiatric and Mental Health Nurse Practitioner* and *Family Psychiatric and Mental Health Nurse Practitioner*, both under *psychiatric and mental health nursing*.

PMPM Per member per month. Describes the basis for determining a capitation amount.

PMRI See *Patient Medical Record Information*.

PMS See *performance measurement system* and *practice management system*.

PNCB See *Pediatric Nursing Certification Board*.

PNDS See *Perioperative Nursing Data Set* under *data set*.

PNP See *Pediatric Nurse Practitioner* under *pediatric nursing*.

POA See *present on admission*.

POC See *point-of-care*.

POCTE See *Point of Care Testing Evaluator Program* under *clinical laboratory qualification*.

podiatrist A practitioner of podiatry. The podiatrist has the degree "doctor of podiatric medicine" (DPM), and must be licensed by the state to practice. A podiatrist may or may not be considered a physician. This distinction is often significant when the issue of *clinical privileges* comes up (see under *privileges*).

The American Board of Multiple Specialties in Podiatry (ABMSP) (**www.abmsp.org**) offers certification in three podiatric specialties: primary care in podiatric medicine, podiatric surgery, and prevention and treatment of diabetic foot wounds and in diabetic footwear. Certification in podiatric medicine and orthopaedics is offered by the American Board of Podiatric Orthopedics and Primary Podiatric Medicine (ABPOPPM) (**www.abpoppm.org**).

podiatry The diagnosis and treatment of foot disorders, diseases, injuries, and anatomic defects. Medical, surgical, and physical means may be employed. Formerly called chiropody.

POE See *computerized physician order entry* and *point-of-enrollment*.

point-of-care (POC) Clinical testing that is done near the patient—bedside, emergency room, intensive care unit, health fair—rather than in a laboratory. Tests most commonly performed at POC include glucose, urinalysis, and occult blood. Synonym: near-patient testing.

Point of Care Testing Evaluator Program (POCTE) See under *clinical laboratory qualification*.

point-of-enrollment (POE) A managed care plan in which the enrollee selects, at the time of enrollment, either (1) a lower-priced option, but one that requires the enrollee to use only providers within the plan, or (2) a higher-priced option that allows the enrollee a continuing option to choose providers of her or his choice, whether in-plan or out-of-plan. There are many variations on these options. See also *point-of-service*.

point-of-sale (POS) An information system in which the details about a transaction are picked up electronically, coincidentally with the transaction, and are used as input to an integrated computer system that transmits the details of the transaction to the places in the organization where they are needed and automatically records them.

The supermarket provides an illustration. Items for sale often carry "bar codes," which tell exactly what the item is, the quantity being purchased, and the price. At the checkout counter, an optical reader scans the bar code and picks up this information, which is "simultaneously" shown to the customer on the cash register display, is used in producing the customer's receipt (often showing the item and quantity as well as the charge made for it), adding the dollar amount to the day's sales total, and subtracting the amount of goods sold from the inventory for the item, so that reordering is systematized.

Similar applications are appearing in hospitals, which increase efficiency, decrease cost, and protect patients. For example, in the hospital pharmacy, as a medication order is dispensed for a given patient, the transaction is transmitted to an electronic medication file, where all drugs being given that patient are recorded. Here the newest medication order is checked (1) to see that the dosage is within the normal range for the drug (this is primarily a safeguard against clerical errors in the medication order) and (2) to see that the new drug is not incompatible with other drugs the patient is already receiving. A warning is issued automatically if there is a problem in either regard. At the same time, a charge for the medication order is made to the patient's bill, a notation is made for the medical record, the nursing station is informed, and the inventory of the pharmacy is adjusted. See also *medication error* and *drug utilization review*.

point-of-service (POS) Selection of a provider by a managed care plan enrollee at the time (and *each* time) the care is needed. The entire plan may be designed as point-of-service, or the *option* may be offered to enrollees, usually for a higher premium and/or copay amount. Most managed care plans require the enrollee to use only in-plan physicians and other providers, except in emergencies or when out of the service area. With POS, the provider need not be a participant with the plan; an enrollee may select in-plan or out-of-plan providers. A plan not allowing the POS option is sometimes referred to as a *point-of-enrollment (POE)* plan. POS plans are also known as "open-ended HMOs."

point-of-surgery (POS) Clinical testing that is done at the patient's bedside, at the same time the patient is undergoing surgery.

POL See *physician office laboratory*.

police power The authority of government to restrict the rights of individuals to protect the health and welfare of the public. In the healthcare context, police power may be invoked by public health officials, for example, to quarantine infected individuals in order to control an epidemic, or to carry out an unannounced inspection of a restaurant, housing, or an institution to ensure compliance with health and safety codes.

policy maker's paradox A dilemma concerning research into public health interventions. The paradox arises when there is a relatively small group of high-risk individuals who are tested for the efficacy of an intervention, when it may be that lower-risk individuals would have a greater benefit from the intervention. The concept is discussed in Brown, E., Viscoli, C., & Horwitz, R. "Preventive Health Strategies and the Policy Makers' Paradox." *Annals of Internal Medicine*, 1992;116:593–597.

polypharmacy A condition in which a person may be taking too many or conflicting medications. Some drugs should not be taken with each other because they have opposing effects. For example, diuretics lower blood pressure, whereas steroids raise it. Other drugs may have the same effects as each other, and their combined effect may be too much. For example, Valium and Tegritol are both tranquilizers; taking both at once may make a person confused and helpless. Other adverse effects can occur, or some of the medications may simply be useless. Polypharmacy arises when the prescribing physician is unaware (or does not take into account) what other medications the patient is already taking. It can also occur when a person is taking over-the-counter (OTC) remedies (cold medicine, vitamins, herbal supplements, etc.) that interact with each other and/or prescription medications. See also *brown bag program*.

polysomnogram (PSG) An electroneurodiagnostic procedure that uses polysomnography to monitor heart rate, eye movement, brain activity, blood oxygen levels, and other functions.

polysomnographic technologist (PSGT) An electroneurodiagnostic technologist who is specially trained in polysomnography procedures.

Registered Polysomnographic Technologist (RPSGT) An electroneurodiagnostic technologist who is registered in polysomnography by the Board of Registered Polysomnographic Technologists (BRPT). **www.brpt.org**

polysomnography The science of using EEG and other physiologic measures to evaluate sleep and sleep disorders.

POMR See *problem-oriented medical record* under *medical record*.

POP See *persistent organic pollutants*.

population A group of individuals occupying a specified area at the same time.

population genetics See under *genetics*.

population management A *disease management* program for an entire population (for example, all members of a health plan or a community) rather than a single individual.

population medicine Health care in which the goal is the improvement of the health of a population, such as a reduction in teenage pregnancies, lowered obesity rates, or an increase in cardiovascular fitness; this is in contrast with individual medicine, which concerns the health of an individual.

POR Problem-oriented record. See *problem-oriented medical record* under *medical record*.

PORT See *Patient Outcomes Research Team*.

portability An attribute of a healthcare payment system in which the beneficiary can move from one employer to another without loss of benefits or having to go through a waiting period. Without portable coverage, individuals often are unwilling to change employment because benefits will be lost. This condition is known as "job lock."

portal On the Internet, a portal is a "gateway" web site from which you link to information of the type that particular portal specializes in, such as a "healthcare portal." A healthcare provider such as a hospital may provide a portal for all of its patients that contains general health information, ways to locate a doctor, and also a way to make appointments with that doctor. A portal is typically distinguished from a normal web site by having some level of access control. These are sometimes known as "corporate" portals or "enterprise" portals. See also *vortal*.

Citizens Health Portal (myNDMA) A personal health record (PHR) portal, linked directly to the *National Digital Medical Archive (NDMA)*. Registrants at myNDMA can establish a secure, private electronic medical "locker" that includes personal medical history, medical records, and digital medical images. **www.myndma.com**

Medicare Beneficiary Portal A secure web site where Medicare beneficiaries can access personalized information about their Medicare benefits and services. At MyMedicare.gov, the beneficiary can check claim status; view eligibility, entitlement, and preventive services information; access online forms and publications; and so forth. **my.medicare.gov**

vertical portal See *vortal*.

portfolio The aggregate of the investments (stocks, real estate, and other assets) of an investor. Unless there is more than one kind of investment, a portfolio does not exist.

POS See *point-of-sale*, *point-of-service*, and *point-of-surgery*.

positioning A term used in public relations (marketing) indicating the place occupied by an institution or product in the minds of its constituency. For example, Microsoft is "positioned" in the number one spot with respect to software in most peoples' minds. Hertz has the same position in car rentals. See also *strategic positioning*.

positron emission tomography (PET) See *nuclear medicine*.

positron tomography See *nuclear medicine*.

post-acute care (PAC) Care provided to patients after discharge or transfer from an acute care hospital. Post-acute care may be provided in inpatient facilities (e.g., skilled nursing facilities (SNFs), rehabilitation hospitals, long-term care hospitals) or by home health care agencies or outpatient programs.

post-acute care transfer (PACT) policy A Medicare payment policy for acute care hospital patients with certain DRGs (CMS issues a list—in 2007 there were 182 such "transfer" DRGs) who are discharged or transferred to certain post-acute care settings rather than completing their care in the acute facility or being discharged (dying or being sent home). Receiving facilities triggering the PACT policy include skilled nursing facilities (SNFs), home health care, and prospective payment system (PPS)-excluded facilities (rehabilitation, long-term care, cancer, and psychiatric facilities). To comply with the policy, the acute-care hospital must report the transfer, and is then paid under a per-diem formula for the care it has provided rather than receiving the usual single-amount DRG payment. The total payment cannot exceed the DRG payment for the condition. Acute-care hospitals generally receive less reimbursement under this policy than under the regular DRG payment system.

postal medicine A term applied to the use of mail-order pharmacies, which are under some attack because of certain problems, such as the failure to protect certain sensitive medications from temperature extremes in transit and the possibility of children accessing the medications from unprotected mailboxes.

post anesthesia nursing The area of nursing focusing on the needs of patients coming out of anesthesia. See also *perianesthesia nursing*.

Certified Post Anesthesia Nurse (CPAN) A specialist in post anesthesia nursing who has passed an examination of the American Board of Perianesthesia Nursing Certification, Inc. (ABPANC). www.cpancapa.org

post mortem (PM) After death. The term also is used as an abbreviation for a postmortem (after death) examination of a body. See *autopsy*.

postnatal The period immediately after birth or delivery. The term refers to both mother and baby.

postoperative See *operative*.

postoperative recovery room See *recovery room*.

postpartum Following delivery.

potential adverse drug event (PADE) See *adverse drug event*.

potentially compensable event (PCE) An adverse event that is likely to require compensation (see *adverse drug event* and *adverse patient occurrence*).

potentially ineffective care (PIC) A measure developed at Stanford University for predicting which patients are unlikely to benefit from critical care. It is derived from a special use of *APACHE III* model information.

potential years of life lost (PYLL) The sum of the years that a group of individuals would have lived, had they not died early deaths. PYLL is a measurement of the loss to a society due to disease, war, auto accidents, or other causes. Synonym: years of potential life lost (YPLL).

POTS Plain old telephone system. Used to differentiate from all the "newer" telecommunications technologies. See also *telehealth*.

power of attorney A written agreement under which one person (the "principal") authorizes another (the "agent") to act on her behalf. The agent need not be a lawyer. An ordinary power of attorney automatically terminates if the principal becomes incompetent. The theory behind this is that the agent's power derives from the power of the principal herself, and when she is no longer legally competent (able to make decisions), the agent correspondingly loses authority to act.

durable power of attorney A power of attorney that remains (or becomes) effective when the principal becomes incompetent to act for herself. It should be noted that in most states, even an agent with a durable power of attorney cannot make medical treatment decisions for an incompetent patient, unless state law provides that she can or a court has given her specific authority.

PPA Preferred provider arrangement. See *preferred provider organization*.

PPO See *preferred provider option* and *preferred provider organization*.

PPR See *physician payment reform*.

PPRCS Perinatal/Pediatric Respiratory Care Specialist; see *Neonatal/Pediatric Respiratory Care Specialist* under *respiratory therapist*.

PPS See *prospective payment system* and *prospective pricing system*.

PRA See *Patient Record Architecture*.

practice (action) Verb. To carry on a profession, such as medicine.

delegated practice The medical activities of nonphysician providers performed under the authority and direction of a licensed physician.

practice (business) Noun. A business in which a profession, such as medicine, is carried out.

group practice A medical practice consisting of three or more physicians or dentists, associated to share offices, expenses, and income.

group practice without walls (GPWW) See *clinic without walls*.

multi-specialty group practice A group practice offering more than one medical specialty.

prepaid group practice A group practice providing care for a defined population under a prepayment plan.

single-specialty group practice A group practice in which all members of the group practice the same specialty.

solo practice A practice in which the physician (or other professional) is alone, that is, not a member of a group or associated with other physicians. Solo practitioners may, however, arrange with others to provide care for their patients when the practitioner is absent or ill.

practice guidelines See *clinical practice guidelines* under *guidelines*.

practice management system (PMS) A computer system (software) that carries out clerical functions for a clinic or physician's office. The following functions typically are included:

- Patient demographics and insurances
- Scheduling of appointments and use of resources
- Accounting, billing, and collection
- Communication, written and electronic, among physicians and with patients, including ticklers and reminders
- Patient referrals
- Prescription writing and recording
- Personnel time management, including hospital rounds
- Education
- Generation of management reports

Patient medical information must include the minimum clinical information and evidence of evaluation and management required for billing. Additional detail on medications, diagnoses, problems, progress notes, laboratory and other investigative detail, images, and documents may be sufficient to qualify the system as containing a full-fledged electronic medical record (EMR), but this is not essential to a PMS. Sometimes an EMR from a different vendor is associated with a PMS, and shares content. Similar systems are offered for other professionals such as lawyers and dentists. Also called simply PM.

practice parameters See *clinical practice guidelines* under *guidelines*.

practitioner An individual entitled by training and experience to practice a profession. Often such practice requires licensure, and the boundaries of the practice are prescribed by law. See also *allied health professional*, *general practitioner*, *independent practitioner*, *midlevel practitioner*, and *nurse practitioner*.

PRC Personal responsibility contribution; see *Healthy Americans Act*.

preadmission certification (PAC) A process by which elective care that is proposed for a patient is reviewed and approved by the payer before the patient is admitted to the hospital. When a PAC program is in effect, the care will not be paid for unless the certification is obtained.

preadmission process for admission A formal admission process (namely, initiating the paperwork) carried out by a hospital prior to doing preadmission testing (PAT) for an elective admission patient.

preadmission screening (PAS) A program of evaluation of applicants for admission to nursing homes under Medicare. Some states also require preadmission screening for private pay applicants.

preadmission testing (PAT) The carrying out of laboratory and other diagnostic work on an outpatient basis within a few days of hospital admission for the patient scheduled for elective hospitalization. It is less costly to have the tests performed in this manner and, in some instances, the test results will be such that hospitalization will be avoided or postponed. The hospital usually goes through a formal acceptance of the patient, called the preadmission process for admission, prior to carrying out the tests.

precautions Actions taken to prevent an undesired effect or outcome. In the healthcare context, the term "precautions" usually refers to measures taken to prevent the transmission of disease to a patient who is particularly vulnerable to infection because his or her immune system has broken down (such a patient is called a "compromised host"), or from a patient with an especially communicable disease.

special precautions "Extra" precautions that must be taken for a particular patient for whom special precautions are ordered, such as a patient vulnerable to infection or one with a highly contagious, airborne disease. For example, gowns, masks, and gloves must be worn in the patient's room, and visitors strictly limited. Special precautions may include the use of *quarantine*.

universal precautions (UP) A set of policies and procedures recommended by the Centers for Disease Control and Prevention (CDC), and required by the Occupational Safety and Health Administration (OSHA), for protecting patients, hospital staff, and physicians from the risk of contracting diseases, such as AIDS and hepatitis B, which are transmitted by blood and body fluids. "Universal" means that the precautions are to be taken with respect to *every* patient, not just those who are known to be particularly vulnerable or contagious. Recommended precautions include the use of gloves and special disposal of hypodermic needles to reduce accidental needlesticks.

predatory pricing A practice by insurers of giving a low rate on health insurance to a low-risk small group or individual, then raising the rates when the insured start filing claims. See also *cherry picking*. Synonyms: churning the books, price churning.

preexisting condition A physical or mental condition that has been discovered before an individual applies for health insurance. Insurers often deny insurance to individuals with certain preexisting conditions, invoke a waiting period, or reject a group unless such individuals are excluded. Some healthcare reform efforts insist that there be no exclusion of individuals for such conditions.

preferred provider arrangement (PPA) See *preferred provider organization*.

preferred provider option (PPO) A form of health plan in which certain physicians with whom the payer has contracted (usually called a "panel") are designated as preferred providers. When a beneficiary elects to receive care from these physicians, the physicians' charges are paid in full—there is no additional charge to the beneficiary. The beneficiary may elect to obtain care from other physicians, but if she does, there is a financial penalty to the beneficiary—she must pay part of the charges.

preferred provider organization (PPO) An alternative delivery system (ADS) designed to compete with health maintenance organizations (HMOs) and other delivery systems. A PPO is stated to be an arrangement involving a contract between healthcare providers (both professional and institutional) and organizations such as employers and third-party administrators (TPAs), under which the PPO agrees to provide healthcare services to a defined population for predetermined fixed fees. There is little uniformity among the organization of various PPOs. In fact, there are some who contend that there are as many organizational structures as there are PPOs. Max Fine, a leading PPO consultant, testified at a 1985 congressional hearing, "If you've seen one PPO, you've seen one PPO."

PPOs are distinguished from HMOs and other alternative delivery systems in that: (1) PPO physicians are paid on a fee-for-service basis, whereas in other delivery systems payment is usually by capitation or salary; (2) PPO physicians are not at risk—the purchaser of the service retains the risk—whereas HMOs are at risk; and (3) consumers are not locked in to using the PPO providers. The term "contract provider organization (CPO)" is preferred by the American Medical Association (AMA) for the arrangements discussed here. The term "CPO" might be preferable as a method of distinguishing a preferred provider organization from the other "PPO"—the preferred provider option. Synonym: preferred provider arrangement (PPA). See also *exclusive provider organization*.

preferred term See the diagram at *natural language*.

prelitigation screening panel Some jurisdictions require that plaintiffs submit all medical malpractice cases to a screening panel before bringing them to the courts. The panel usually contains at least a physician with expertise in the relevant area, and may include a judge, an attorney, and/or a layperson. The purpose of the panel is to identify claims that have merit and encourage their settlement. Further, they attempt to identify claims without merit and encourage dismissal or withdrawal of the claim. The panel's determinations are usually not binding, so that regardless of the determination, the plaintiff can still go to trial.

premature Before it should happen. In the case of birth, "premature" means before the thirty-seventh week of pregnancy, regardless of the birth weight of the infant. A baby born after forty-two weeks is called "post term." In between is called "full term."

premium A payment required for an insurance policy for a given period of time.

prenatal The fetus (baby) before birth; also the period of pregnancy before delivery, as in "the prenatal period" or "prenatal care" of the mother.

prenatal care Care for a pregnant woman in an effort to keep the woman healthy and to maximize the likelihood that the pregnancy will result in a full-term, full-birthweight, healthy infant.

preoperative See *operative*.

prepaid health plan See *health plan*.

prepayment Payment in advance. Under a prepayment system, a fee is paid to a third-party payer, such as a health maintenance organization (HMO), Blue Cross and Blue Shield plans, or commercial insurance, and the third party agrees to pay for stipulated care when it is provided.

prepayment plan A contractual arrangement for health care in which a prenegotiated payment is made in advance, covering a certain time period, and the provider agrees, for this payment, to furnish certain services to the beneficiary, member, or enrollee.

prescription A written direction for the preparation and use of anything for the treatment of a patient. The term "prescription" is most often thought of in connection with a drug (see *drug prescription*), but it is also used for eyeglasses, treatment such as physical therapy, and artificial limbs and other devices.

prescription benefit manager (PBM) See *pharmacy benefit manager*.

prescription drug See under *drug*.

prescription drug plan (PDP) Insurance or plan that meets the requirements for Medicare Part D prescription drug coverage. This is a stand-alone plan, purchased and paid for separately from Medicare Part A and Part B, or from a Medicare Advantage plan that does not include drug coverage. PDPs are offered by private companies; Medicare pays the companies a subsidy of approximately 75% of the cost of the plans, with beneficiaries paying the other 25% in premiums. People with limited incomes can get extra help paying the premiums. PDPs are required to use e-prescribing. See also *formulary (health plan)*.

    Medicare Advantage—Prescription Drug Plan (MA-PD) A *Medicare Advantage* plan that includes prescription drug coverage. Synonym: Medicare Advantage Drug Plan.

presenter In the context of telehealth and telemedicine, the presenter is the person on-site (the originating site), next to the patient, who is responsible for collecting information about the patient and transmitting it to the physician, specialist, or other provider at the distant site. The presenter is trained in the use of the telecommunications equipment, manages the camera, and performs any hands-on activities required to perform the examination of the patient. For example, a neurological exam would require a nurse (or other practitioner) capable of testing the patient's reflexes and other manipulative activities. However, some telehealth encounters may only require use of a camera, in which case the presenter need not be a healthcare professional. Synonym: patient presenter.

present on admission (POA) An indicator on the *UB-04* form that tells whether a coded "diagnosis" (condition, disease, or cause of injury) was present at the time of the patient's admission to the hospital. It is applied to both principal and secondary diagnosis codes.

president of the medical staff See *chief of staff*.

prevailing When used in conjunction with physicians' fees, "prevailing" refers to the charges made for the service in question in the area, provided by physicians of similar specialty qualifications. See *customary, prevailing, reasonable charge (or fee)*.

prevalence The number of events or cases of disease *present* in a given population at a given time. "Prevalence" is often confused with **incidence**, which is the number of new events taking place in a *defined period of time* in a specified area or population. Usually both incidence and prevalence refer to cases of disease or injury. Both are numerators in the calculation of an incidence rate or a prevalence rate, respectively, for the event in question. The denominator is, for both, the population at risk (the given population).

prevention paradox See *policy maker's paradox*.

preventive health services Services designed to (1) prevent disease or injury from occurring, (2) detect it early, (3) minimize its progression, and/or (4) control resulting disability.

preventive medicine The study of the prevention of disease.

PRI See *program-related investment*.

price The amount of money to be paid for something. Each DRG, for example, carries a price—the amount of money to be paid for the hospital care of a patient classified to that DRG.

price blending A method of adjusting a hospital's price for a given DRG under the prospective payment system (PPS) after comparing the hospital's cost per case for that DRG with the national average for the same DRG. Synonym: DRG-specific price blending.

price churning See *predatory pricing*.

price-elasticity A condition in which a seller can increase revenue by *reducing* prices (achieved, of course, by increased volume of sales). Elasticity means that the demand for a product will go up if the price goes down (and vice versa). Under *managed competition*, price-elasticity is a specific goal. See also *price-inelasticity*.

price-fixing Two or more competitors agreeing on prices (charges). Price-fixing is a per se violation of the Sherman Act, an antitrust law.

price-inelasticity A condition in which a seller can increase revenue only by *raising* prices. Inelasticity means that the demand for a product will not be influenced by the price. *Managed competition* seeks to avoid price-inelasticity. See also *price-elasticity*.

prima facie tort See under *tort*.

primary care The Institute of Medicine (IOM) defines primary care as "the provision of integrated, accessible healthcare services by clinicians who are accountable for addressing a large majority of personal health care needs, developing a sustained partnership with patients, and practicing in the context of family and community." It may be provided by physicians (typically family practitioners, internists, pediatricians, and obstetrician-gynecologists) or by other health professionals such as physician assistants (PAs) and nurse practitioners. Primary care often describes the care given at the initial contact of the patient with the healthcare system or with a healthcare provider, usually in an office or other outpatient setting. Primary care usually precedes referral to or consultation with a specialist (secondary care physician).

primary care center (PCC) An institution for furnishing primary care. A PCC may be freestanding or part of another institution.

Primary Care Evaluation of Mental Disorders (PRIME-MD) A diagnostic questionnaire designed to be used by primary care physicians (PCPs) to detect common mental and eating disorders. PRIME-MD evaluates four groups of disorders—mood, anxiety, somatoform, and alcohol—by use of a two-part procedure. First, before seeing the physician, the patient completes a one-page questionnaire (PQ) as an initial symptom screen. Second, if appropriate, the physician interviews the patient with one of five diagnostic modules (which one depends on the patient's responses) contained in a clinician evaluation guide (CEG). The results assist the physician in assessment of the patient.

primary care manager (PCM) See *gatekeeper (health care)*.

primary care network A group of primary care physicians who have formed a network in order to share the risk of providing services to enrollees in a prepaid plan.

primary care physician See under *physician*.

primary cell In genetics, refers to a cell taken directly from a living organism. See also *immortalized cell*.

primary nursing See under *nursing*.

principal (finance) An amount of money upon which interest is earned or owed.

principal (law) A person (or entity, such as a corporation) who authorizes another to act on his or her behalf as an agent.

prion A class of infectious agents that consist of protein and nothing else (i.e., they do not contain genetic material (nucleic acid (DNA or RNA)), material previously thought necessary to establish an infection in a host). Prion diseases typically are fatal, destroying portions of the brain. They occur quite frequently in animals; examples are scrapie in sheep and goats, and *mad cow disease*. In humans, prions have been shown to cause kuru (in New Guinea), Creutzfeldt-Jakob disease (CJD), Gerstmann-Straussler-Scheinker disease, and fatal familial insomnia. Pronounced "preeon."

privacy As a legal term, "privacy" is discussed in various contexts:

invasion of privacy A *tort* in which the wrongdoing is the subjecting of a person to unreasonable, unwanted publicity. For example, a physician was successfully sued by a patient for publishing "before" and "after" pictures of the patient's cosmetic surgery without her permission. It can also involve disclosure of private facts or intrusion into private areas (eavesdropping into someone's home, for example).

patient privacy Generally having less to do with whether or not a patient has a private room in a hospital than with the level of privacy and security with which that patient's health information (such as the medical record) is treated. Although a person's health information has traditionally been seen as basically confidential (see *confidentiality*), policies regarding this have been far from universal. Recent federal legislation (HIPAA) seeks to remedy this; see *Privacy Rule*.

right of privacy The right of the individual to be left alone, free from unwarranted intrusion. The U.S. Supreme Court has recognized this as a constitutional right, and used it as the basis upon which to restrict governmental intrusion in such matters as birth control, sterilization, abortion, and the right to refuse medical treatment (sometimes called the "right to die").

Privacy Act of 1974 See *Freedom of Information Act*.

privacy and security professionals Health professionals specializing in the protection of health information and information systems.

Certified in Healthcare Privacy (CHP) A health information professional who has demonstrated "advanced competency in designing, implementing, and administering comprehensive privacy protection programs in all types of healthcare organizations" by meeting specified requirements of the American Health Information Management Association (AHIMA). **www.ahima.org**

Certified in Healthcare Privacy and Security (CHPS) A credential sponsored jointly by the American Health Information Management Association (AHIMA) and the Healthcare Information and Management Systems Society (HIMSS).

Certified in Healthcare Security (CHS) A health information professional who has demonstrated "advanced competency in designing, implementing, and administering comprehensive security protection programs in all types of healthcare organizations" by meeting specified requirements of the Healthcare Information and Management Systems Society (HIMSS). **www.himss.org**

privacy officer A generic job title or description being increasingly used in business early in the twenty-first century for the person responsible for ensuring that the company's "privacy policy" is being correctly administered and enforced. This job is becoming more common due in large part to the popularity of the Internet, which allows massive amounts of information to be globally exposed—including information that many people would prefer to be kept private. The privacy officer takes steps to reduce the company's liability to others for wrongfully releasing "private" information. What is and isn't private isn't always clear (see *confidentiality* and *Privacy Rule*, for example). A privacy officer may also be referred to as a "chief privacy officer (CPO)." A privacy officer working for a healthcare company may also be assigned the duties of the *privacy official*, created under HIPAA. See also *privacy and security professionals* and *security*.

privacy official A position or duty mandated by the *Privacy Rule*. A privacy official, who may also be designated a "contact person," is responsible for the implementation and development of the *covered entity's* privacy policies and procedures under the rule. 45 C.F.R. § 164.530(a)(1)(i) (October 1, 2006).

privacy, patient See under *privacy*.

Privacy Rule A rule issued (under the administrative simplification provisions of HIPAA) by the Department of Health and Human Services (HHS), which calls it "the first comprehensive federal protection for the privacy of health information." The rule creates national standards to protect medical records and other personal *health information*. Among its provisions:

- Gives patients more control over their health information, including the right to examine and obtain a copy of their own health records and request corrections
- Sets limits on the use and release of health records
- Requires healthcare providers to protect the privacy of health information
- Imposes civil and criminal penalties for violations
- Balances privacy interests with public health interests

The rules apply to healthcare providers, health plans, and others defined as *covered entities*. Although it appears that the intent of the HIPAA legislation was to protect the privacy of health information when electronically transmitted, the actual effect of the final Privacy Rule is that most "*individually identifiable health information*" (see also *designated record set* and *protected health information*) is subject to its requirements. Healthcare providers who themselves may not be a covered entity will still likely be subject to the Privacy Rule if they have a business associate who is a covered entity (see *business associate agreement*). Some have advised to simply treat all healthcare information as covered by this rule, because proving exceptions is likely to cost more than compliance.

To help meet the demands of the rule, covered entities are required to designate an individual as their "privacy official." The full name of the rule is "Standards for Privacy of Individually Identifiable Health Information." Links to the text are available at **www.hhs.gov/ocr/hipaa/finalreg.html**. The Privacy Rule is codified at 45 C.F.R. §§ 160–164 (October 1, 2006). See also *audit trail* and *release of information*.

private contract See under *contract*.

private key See *public key* and *public key infrastructure*.

private room See under *room*.

privilege A special right, benefit, or advantage granted to one person or a group or entity, but not to everyone.

privileged communication Information that is legally protected from discovery in a lawsuit or use as evidence in a trial. Communications between a physician and patient are privileged communications, and cannot be revealed without the permission of the patient or a court order; most of the contents of a medical record are protected by this privilege. It should be noted that the privilege "belongs" to the person protected and can only be waived by that person; in this instance, the patient is the one whose rights are protected, so the privilege cannot be waived by the physician (or hospital), nor can the physician invoke the privilege if the patient waives it.

privileges Permission granted by the governing body of a healthcare organization to *physicians* and *allied health professionals (AHPs)* to carry out specified diagnostic and therapeutic procedures within the hospital (and/or other areas) and, in some cases, to admit patients. Medical staff membership may or may not be required; see *medical staff member*.

Privileges are usually granted upon recommendation of the medical staff, typically working through its credentials committee, which reviews the person's credentials and performance in determining the privileges to be recommended. Some hospitals have an allied health review committee (AHRC), which may or may not be associated with the medical staff, to review AHPs. Privileges may be withheld, increased, diminished, or withdrawn by the governing body at its discretion (subject, of course, to due process requirements).

Privileges granted by an institution are a kind of credential in themselves (e.g., the hospital has given the practitioner a "seal of approval" with the granting of privileges). See also *credentialing* and *recredentialing*.

admitting privileges Authority, granted by the governing body, to admit patients to the hospital. Generally, admitting privileges are restricted to physicians (MD and DO) who are active medical staff members. The privileges ordinarily are limited in relation to the qualifications of the physician; for example, a specialist in obstetrics and gynecology would not likely be granted privileges to admit psychiatric patients. Podiatrists and dentists may also be authorized to admit patients for their specialized care, but only under the supervision of a physician with "full" care privileges.

clinical privileges Privileges to perform designated diagnostic and therapeutic procedures and to treat specific types of patients. Privileges granted are based upon the professional's credentials (education, training, and licensure) and performance.

Privileges are determined upon initial appointment to the medical staff, and are subject to formal review periodically (usually no less frequently than every two years, or more frequently if required by law), and also ad hoc upon the practitioner's request or on the basis of allegations of performance problems. Privileges are expanded as the physician (or other professional) acquires additional credentials and/or experience and demonstrates proficiency; and should be reduced if warranted by the physician's performance (subject, of course, to due process requirements).

Initial privileges are typically provisional, with performance being observed by peers (other physicians or peer professionals on the medical staff) and periodically reviewed with the assistance of hospital personnel who collect data and provide them to a review body (usually the medical staff member's clinical department), which makes recommendations to the credentials committee regarding lifting or continuing the provisional status. Such periodic review continues for all medical staff members, even after the "provisional" requirements are dropped; it is a necessary part of quality management and of the process of reappointment of medical staff members. When used in the statement that a certain physician "has clinical privileges" in a given hospital, the term indicates that the physician has been appointed to the medical staff of that hospital, and has been granted specific privileges in a clinical category that permits her or him to treat patients there.

core privileges The basic set of *clinical privileges* (see above) granted to qualified practitioners of a specific specialty. These will be the treatments and procedures that are routinely covered in the residency training (or other standard training) for that specialty. The hospital delineates which privileges are "core" for each specialty. For example, core privileges in anesthesiology may include general anesthesia, regional anesthesia, acute pain management, endotracheal intubation, ventilator management, pulmonary artery catheterization, central venous cannulation, and arterial line placement. See also *special privileges*, below.

setting-specific privileges *Clinical privileges* (see above) that are restricted to a particular area or facility of the healthcare organization. The Joint Commission on Accreditation of Healthcare Organizations (JCAHO) requires that privileges be setting-specific, at least to delineate whether the privileges pertain to ambulatory care, long-term care, behavioral health, or a hospital-owned physician office practice setting. If the types of care and treatment are different in these settings than in the acute-care setting, because of available equipment, qualified personnel, and resources, then the clinical privileges must be altered to be specific to what can be done in each setting. The hospital defines what each "setting" is, and is free to define specific settings that may be smaller than the broad categories; for example, the emergency department, intensive care, endoscopy laboratory, and so forth.

special privileges *Clinical privileges* (see above) to do treatments or procedures that are not included on the list of *core privileges* (see above). These require additional training and qualifications. For example, in anesthesiology, management of chronic pain and transesophageal echocardiogram (TEE) may require special privileges.

privileging The process of granting and monitoring *privileges*. See also *credentialing*.

PRM Pediatric rehabilitation medicine.

prn As (often as) or if necessary.

PRO See *patient-reported outcome* and *peer review organization*.

probe A short segment of single-stranded DNA that is tagged with a reporter molecule, such as a radioactive atom, that is used in genetic studies to detect a matching DNA sequence.

probiotics Live microorganisms, such as bacteria and yeast, that can benefit human health by improving the balance of intestinal microflora.

problem A question to which an answer is desired, or a situation for which a remedy is desired. In health care, a problem is a disease, injury, or any other condition or situation that brings an individual into contact with the healthcare system. Certain conditions, such as alcoholism, are not admitted by all to be diseases, but they do bring individuals to health care, as do ill-defined symptoms, behavioral problems, the need for well-person examinations, and the like. This is the usage of the term "problem" in the "problem-oriented medical record (POMR)."

Chapter XXI of the *International Statistical Classification of Diseases and Related Health Problems* (see *ICD-10*), entitled "Factors Influencing Health Status and Contact with Health Services," lists among others the following "factors": loss of love relationship (code number Z61), removal from home (Z61), failed exams in school (Z55), stressful work schedule (Z56), and extreme poverty (Z59.5). Each of these could be said to be a problem in the healthcare context.

problem centered charting A charting method developed to follow a patient's problems, needs, and nursing diagnoses throughout the hospital stay. In the nursing assessment, a patient's needs are identified and a care plan is written, with numbers assigned to each problem. Problems are numbered in the order they occur, not in priority order. Documentation of routine care is reduced by reference to protocols instead of writing out each action. Nursing notes follow the patient's problems by number, with narrative notes supplemented by flow sheets or checklists. Notes document ongoing evaluation of the care plan, in addition to actions taken and patient responses. Resolution of a problem is noted and dated.

Problem Knowledge Couplers (PKCouplers) Interactive computer software for PC computers that elicits (profiles) the significant attributes of a patient and that patient's problem and then matches (couples) this profile of the patient with the existing juried literature that has a bearing on the understanding of or solution to that problem.

The concept was conceived by Lawrence L. Weed, MD, who developed the problem-oriented medical record (POMR). The purpose of PKCouplers is to assist the physician and other providers in accessing the medical knowledge available in the literature as to diagnosis and management of patients, and to do it instantly on demand, while patient and physician are together. Four kinds of PKCouplers are available: (1) baseline, (2) diagnostic, (3) management, and (4) triage.

PKCouplers not only prove invaluable in coping with the information explosion in health care, but also in providing the patient with knowledge, making the patient a true collaborator in reaching decisions about lifestyle, diagnostic efforts to be expended, and treatments to be undertaken. Furthermore, couplers, computerized and cumulative, are important building blocks toward an electronic health record (EHR), which not only keeps a record, but also assists and guides the caregiver and patient.

baseline problem knowledge coupler A class of PKCouplers that is typically used at the patient's first visit to provide a baseline of data about the patient. Under the heading of wellness, it collects information about the patient's lifestyle, habits, and health risks. It also develops a thorough medical and health history, and records baseline physical and laboratory findings. If any of the inventories detect lifestyle modifications or risk avoidance that would be beneficial, these are suggested to the physician and patient by the software. If medical problems are noted, the problem-specific diagnosis or management PKCouplers for them may be used to guide further investigation and management. Printouts are available for the patient and for the paper-based medical record.

diagnostic problem knowledge coupler A class of PKCoupler that uses, as do all PKCouplers, a two-step process. First it has a questionnaire that, when completed, constructs a patient's personal profile (database) for a given problem. This is done within a computer program that then, as step two, couples (matches) that profile with the medical literature's knowledge for the same problem.

The diagnostic PKCoupler for a given problem is structured to elicit data known to be helpful in discriminating among possible causes of the problem. Sources of the data are the patient's history, physical examination, investigative findings, response to therapy, and other factors. The knowledge database for that problem contains information on these same data items, maintained to reflect the current medical literature. Once the diagnostic coupler's patient profile is in the computer, where it is placed as a part of acquiring the data, coupling, on the physician's command, instantly matches the profile with the stored knowledge. The computer display (and printout) indicates which findings of the specific patient match each of the diagnoses (possible causes of the problem) in the knowledge database stored in the computer. The physician is given invaluable guidance from a thorough review of the possibilities.

Diagnostic couplers, as well as baseline and management couplers, are annotated with comments that provide the published background, competing theories, and the rationale for alternatives presented.

management problem knowledge coupler A class of PKCouplers used when the cause of the patient's complaint is known and the problem becomes one of treatment. The management PKCoupler gives guidance as to alternative treatment paths. It takes into account any other problems the patient may have, and other treatments that may complicate the picture, giving the pros and cons of the alternatives, such as contraindications, relative probability of success, side effects, and cost. Management PKCouplers use the same technique of collecting information from the patient (a structured questionnaire) and coupling it with the relevant literature as do the diagnostic and baseline couplers.

triage problem knowledge coupler A PKCoupler used at the door to route a patient, as quickly as possible, to the most appropriate care. With a triage coupler, the physician's triage assistant first elicits information about the patient's reasons (problems) for seeking health or medical care, including the problem's onset, history, severity, and other relevant factors.

Instead of the literature as the source of knowledge against which to couple the patient's profile, however, a triage coupler must be custom-tailored to the situation where it is to be employed. Its knowledge base for an office practice, for example, includes such information as the physician's kind of practice, the office's resources (such as laboratory and x-ray, and health professionals available), office hours, alternate physicians, and so on. Decision options might be, for example, direct hospitalization; referral to the emergency department; an office appointment immediately; an office appointment after indicated laboratory, x-ray, or other procedures; or an elective office visit.

Plans are under way to expand this triage concept to one-stop shopping for health care for an entire community.

problem-oriented information Information organized in such a fashion that it bears directly on a specific question asked or on a specific problem for which a solution is sought, in contrast with **subject-oriented information**, which is typically oriented around a field or branch of knowledge. A dictionary and a telephone book provide problem-oriented information, answers to the specific question, "What does this word mean?" or "What is John Doe's phone number?" A more complex example of problem-oriented information is found in a "how to" book. A standard textbook or a descriptive book provides subject-oriented information, such as "all about physics" or "all about Hawaii."

A chief distinction between the two classes of information is that a problem-oriented source will draw from as many sources or fields of knowledge as necessary to deal with the problem, whereas a subject-oriented source deals, in the main, with a single discipline. A strong movement toward providing information in the problem-oriented mode has come with the computer, which brings a number of attributes: virtually unlimited memory, high-speed access to information, hypertext linkage, multimedia (sound and visual images, both still and in motion), and interactivity. One of the best examples of a problem-oriented information source is found in medicine in *Problem Knowledge Couplers*.

problem-oriented medical record (POMR) See under *medical record*.

problem-oriented record (POR) See *problem-oriented medical record* under *medical record*.

proceduralist A physician in whose specialty the performance of procedures, diagnostic or therapeutic, such as endoscopies and surgical operations, is a significant element. See also *cognitive services*.

procedure In medicine, something that is "done" or "carried out" for a patient by a physician or other person. A procedure is usually discrete, and a relatively short time is required for its execution. Procedures are generally either diagnostic or therapeutic (treatment). A diagnostic procedure would be the taking of an x-ray or blood pressure, for example, whereas a therapeutic procedure might be anything from removing a splinter from a finger to an extensive operation such as repair of a hernia.

For the purposes of healthcare financing (charges and payments for procedures), a hernia repair "procedure" might also include both preoperative and postoperative care. For more information about procedures in financing terminology, see *service*. See also *cognitive services*, *operation*, and *surgery (treatment)*.

advanced emergency medical procedure A term sometimes applied to a procedure that the highest level of *emergency medical technician*—EMT-Paramedic—may perform, but that lower levels of EMTs may not. Such procedures may include, for example, insertion of a tube into the patient's airway for assistance in breathing, and administration of certain drugs. State statutes typically govern the designation of levels of EMTs, and the procedures authorized for each.

operating room procedure A term that, on its face, describes a surgical treatment of a patient, performed in the hospital's operating room. However, the term has a special function under the prospective payment system (PPS): If a patient has an "operating room procedure," that patient is placed in a different payment category than a patient in the same Major Diagnostic Category (MDC) who does not have an operating room procedure. For the purpose of making this allocation of patients, an arbitrary list of procedures (actually, a list of procedure codes) has been established by CMS. If the patient's data set submitted for payment has a code shown on the CMS list as an operating room procedure, that patient is considered to have had an operating room procedure, no matter where the procedure was actually done.

special procedure An umbrella term to cover examinations, tests, and therapies that require advanced training and/or technology. Examples are x-rays, magnetic resonance imaging, radiation therapy, and sonography (ultrasound).

surgical procedure A procedure that utilizes *surgery (treatment)*.

procedure capture The mechanisms by which one healthcare facility (a hospital, laboratory, or imaging service, for example) or specialist physician is selected in preference to another. Such "procedure services" are the results of referral, primarily from physicians, so "procedure capture" really is the sum of the efforts to persuade the referring person to make the referral to the institution or specialist seeking more business.

process The things done (for a patient, for example). It is commonly stated in quality management that three things can be measured: structure, process, and outcome. *Structure* refers to resources and organization. *Outcome* refers to the results of the process (see *outcome*). There is a tendency on the part of some individuals to take an "either-or" position, to the effect that one need only be concerned with one of the three dimensions, but this is not logical; all three must be considered. Clearly, certain structure is needed; and equally clearly, there is no way to change outcome except through changing process, because "outcome 'tells on' process."

proctor A person, typically a physician or surgeon, appointed to supervise (or simply observe) the work of another individual healthcare provider. The observed individual is typically applying for membership on a hospital medical staff or for certain clinical privileges. The use of a proctor, also referred to as proctoring, is one method used to maintain quality control among physician providers. See also *privileges*.

product Something that is made (or grown). Often used in a marketing context to refer to whatever is sold to the consumer; in this context, "product" may mean either a tangible item or a service. See also *biotechnology product*.

product administration (PA) See under *administration (management)*.

productivity The relationship between the number of units of service provided or products produced per unit of labor (or other cost) required, per unit of time. Productivity is said to increase in a hospital, for example, when patient stay can be reduced for a given illness with no sacrifice in quality and no increase in labor. On a larger scale, a hospital is sometimes considered more productive than another when it uses fewer employees, or has a lower cost per day.

product liability See under *liability (legal)*.

product line A term sometimes used in health care to denote the kinds of services offered by a healthcare institution, including, for example, the kinds of patients (defined by their diagnoses, procedures required, and age limitations accepted for care). For example, a hospital's product line might include three "products"—acute care, hospice care, and home health care—and might specifically exclude another product, obstetric care. See also *strategic business unit*.

product line management (PLM) See under *management (organization)*.

products of ambulatory care (PACs) A classification developed by the New York State Ambulatory Care Reimbursement Demonstration Project in 1985 as a "sophisticated ambulatory care product definition." There are twenty-four PAC categories, into which patient visits are allocated by computer depending on "who the patient is" (type of problem presented) and what is done (resources received).

Pro-DUR Prospective *drug utilization review*.

professional See *health professional*.

Professional Activity Study (PAS) The prototype hospital discharge abstract system, originating about 1950 and continuing into the 1990s. PAS was a program offered to hospitals first by the Southwestern Michigan Hospital Council and then by the Commission on Professional and Hospital Activities (CPHA). PAS used abstracts of hospital medical records from enrolled hospitals as input to a database, and provided hospitals with indexes of their medical records and statistics on hospital performance. The database was also available for computer research on hospital activities, epidemiology, and healthcare studies. PAS offered case mix management information and other services to member hospitals. The University of North Carolina at Chapel Hill in 1998 established the Vergil N. Slee Distinguished Professorship in Health Care Quality Management, and cited his work with PAS as "forming the principal foundation of what is now called health outcomes research."

professional association (PA) See *professional corporation* under *corporation*.

professional component (PC) The portion of healthcare services for which the physician gets paid. See also *technical component*.

professional review organization (PRO) Synonym for peer review organization; see q*uality improvement organization*.

professional service corporation (PSC) See *professional corporation* under *corporation*.

professional staff, organized See *organized professional staff* under *staff (group)*.

professional standards review organization (PSRO) An organization established under federal law to review medical necessity, appropriateness, and quality of services provided to beneficiaries of the Medicare, Medicaid, and maternal and child health (MCH) programs. These organizations were physician-sponsored. In 1982, the Tax Equity and Fiscal Responsibility Act (TEFRA) replaced PSROs in function by peer review organizations (PROs), also known as professional review organizations (PROs), which in 2002 changed to quality improvement organizations (QIOs).

profile A statistical report showing certain predefined information about a given subject. Physician profiles, for example, may display such information as the number of patients cared for, their average length of stay in the hospital, the physician's use of various drugs and other treatments, and other factors. When there are enough cases, the profiles may be refined by considering specific diagnoses and procedures. Physicians are compared with each other on these attributes in an effort to encourage efficiency and frugality.

Controversial and irritating to doctors is **economic profiling**, which seeks to find out which ones treat a given condition or carry out a given procedure with the least use of resources (i.e., which doctors give care at the lowest cost). Many of the profiles have been criticized because, among other things, they do not factor in such things as severity of illness and outcomes. Hospitals are also profiled to permit comparisons among hospitals on such matters as clinical services, mortality rates, and costs. See also *report card*.

profit Excess of income over expense. Actually means an increase in assets. The word "**gain**" is often used in nonprofit corporations as a substitute for the word "profit." See also *gainsharing*.

profit and loss statement (P&L) See *income and expense statement*.

profit sharing See *gainsharing*.

prognosis The physician's forecast as to the patient's future course. The prognosis is based on the usual course of progression of or recovery from a given disease or injury, modified by the physician's estimation of the patient's condition and other factors and their effects. A patient will have several prognoses covering length of illness, survival, recovery of function, and so on.

program evaluation and review technique (PERT) A process to identify the accomplishments of programs and the time and resources required to move from one accomplishment to the next. The PERT diagram shows the sequence and interrelationship of activities from the beginning to the end of a project.

Program of All-Inclusive Care for the Elderly (PACE) A Medicare service-delivery model designed to help frail elderly individuals remain in the community through intensive care management. Originally modeled on *On Lok*.

program-related investment (PRI) A short-term (from one- to ten-year) loan from a foundation or other philanthropic organization to a nonprofit organization that is eligible for grants or charitable contributions. Nonprofit organizations often have difficulty obtaining loans through normal channels because such organizations typically do not show profit margins, which the usual lending institutions see as essential in eligible borrowers. Recipients of PRIs may use the PRIs as collateral for obtaining loans through banks, as flexible lines of credit, or for other purposes. PRIs are only available for purposes that fall within the lending foundation's granting policy.

Program Safeguard Contractor (PSC) A private entity that has contracted with CMS to provide services under the Medicare Integrity Program. PSC functions, all designed to protect the Medicare Trust Fund, include prepay and postpay medical review of claims, data analysis, fraud and abuse investigation, provider cost report audits, and provider and beneficiary education. Many of these functions were previously carried out by Medicare carriers and fiscal intermediaries.

Program Support Center (PSC) A division within the Department of Health and Human Services (HHS) that provides administrative, financial management, and human resources services to agencies and departments both within and outside the HHS. **www.psc.gov**

progressive care nursing (PCN) *Critical care nursing* provided to patients "whose needs fall along the less acute end of the critical care continuum" (American Association of Critical-Care Nurses (AACN)).

> **Progressive Care Certified Nurse (PCCN)** A registered nurse with experience in progressive care nursing who has passed an examination of the American Association of Critical-Care Nurses (AACN). **www.aacn.org**

progressive patient care See under *patient care.*

Project Bioshield A federal program designed to guard the United States against a chemical, biological, radiological, or nuclear (CBRN) attack—weapons of mass destruction (WMD). The project provides funding and authorization to develop, acquire, stockpile, and make available critical *medical countermeasures (MCMs)*. It also established *Emergency Use Authorization (EUA)* to provide access to the countermeasures in an emergency. See also *Biomedical Advanced Research and Development Authority* and *Strategic National Stockpile.*

projection In statistics, a calculated estimate for a whole calculated from data for a part of the whole, or an estimate of a future situation based on information currently available. The term "projection" is often used when sampling has given information from a part of a whole (for example, a population), and a projection is made as to the actual situation in the whole population. For example, a candidate's actual performance in opinion polls is "projected" from the response of a sample of voters.

ProMED-mail An Internet-based reporting system dedicated to rapid global dissemination of information on outbreaks of infectious diseases and acute exposures to toxins that affect human health, including those in animals and in plants grown for food or animal feed. Sources of information include media reports, official reports, online summaries, local observers, reports by subscribers, and others. A team of expert human, plant, and animal disease moderators screens, reviews, and investigates reports before posting them to the network. Reports are distributed by email to direct subscribers and posted immediately on the ProMED-mail web site. This facilitates timely dissemination of essential information; for example, ProMED-mail was the first active surveillance system to notify the world of the outbreak that would later be known as SARS.

In 2007 ProMED-mail reached over 30,000 subscribers in at least 150 countries (there are no subscription fees). The program was established in 1994 with the support and encouragement of the Federation of American Scientists and SatelLife. Since 1999, ProMED-mail has been administered by the International Society for Infectious Diseases (ISID), with servers and software furnished by Oracle, Inc. The email service provider is located in the Harvard School of Public Health. **www.promedmail.org**

ProPaC See *Prospective Payment Assessment Commission.*

proportion A specific type of *ratio* in which the numerator is a part of the denominator. Proportions are always between 0 and 1 (inclusive). They are often expressed as rates such as percentages.

proprietary Privately owned and managed and, usually, for-profit.

prospective Pertaining to the future. When used to refer to prospectively collected data in a research study, "prospective" means that special care is taken that the desired data are obtained from all individuals starting as of a given date.

prospective payment A term often used as a misnomer for *prospective pricing*. Under some circumstances, prospective payment for goods or services is made in advance (prepayment), either in whole or in partial payments, with adjustments made to the total when the actual amount due is determined. Payment in advance provides cash flow for the payee.

Prospective Payment Assessment Commission (ProPAC) An advisory body established under Medicare legislation to give advice and assistance to CMS on matters pertaining to the prospective payment system (PPS) under which Medicare operates. Advice from ProPAC is not binding on CMS.

prospective payment system (PPS) A system used for paying for services for Medicare patients. Patients are classified into categories for which prices are negotiated or imposed on the hospital or other provider in advance (thus it is actually "prospective pricing" rather than "prospective payment"). This is in contrast to fee-for-service, where the provider is paid a fee for each service provided. PPS, although not mandated by federal law for payers other than Medicare, is being applied to patients under other health plans. PPS is sometimes referred to as the "DRG system." (The letters "PPS" are sometimes translated, incorrectly, to mean a prospective reimbursement system.) Synonym: health insurance prospective payment system (HIPPS). See also *DRG*.

home health prospective payment system (HH-PPS) The reimbursement program used by CMS to pay for home health care for Medicare patients. A nurse or therapist from the home health agency uses the *Outcome and Assessment Information Set (OASIS)* (see under *data set*) instrument to assess the patient's condition. OASIS items describing the patient's condition, as well as the expected therapy needs (physical, speech-language pathology, or occupational) are used to determine the case-mix adjustment to the standard payment rate. Eighty case-mix groups, called Home Health Resource Groups (HHRGs), are available for patient classification. On Medicare claims these HHRGs are represented as *HIPPS codes*. Grouper software run at a home health agency site uses specific data elements from the OASIS data set to assign beneficiaries to a HIPPS code, which is used on Medicare claims.

inpatient prospective payment system (IPPS) The system for payment for acute care hospital inpatient stays under Medicare Part A (hospital insurance). See *DRG*.

inpatient psychiatric facility prospective payment system (IPF-PPS) The payment system used by CMS to pay for Medicare patients in inpatient psychiatric facilities (IPFs). The basis is a per diem base rate, which is then adjusted by all applicable characteristics, including age, DRG assignment, certain comorbidities, electroconvulsive therapy, length of stay, presence or absence of a dedicated emergency department, outlier eligibility, transition year, teaching status, cost-of-living adjustment for Alaska and Hawaii, rural location, and wage index.

inpatient rehabilitation facility prospective payment system (IRF-PPS) The payment system used by CMS to pay for rehabilitation services provided by inpatient rehabilitation facilities (IRFs). As with DRGs, the goal is to group patients with similar uses of resources and lengths of stay. Each patient is assigned to a **Case-Mix Group (CMG)** (similar to a *Function Related Group (FRG)*) that, along with comorbid conditions and/or complications, determines payment. On Medicare claims these CMGs are represented as *HIPPS codes*, which are determined based on assessments made using the *Inpatient Rehabilitation Facility Patient Assessment Instrument (IRF-PAI)*. Grouper software run at an IRF uses specific data elements from the IRF-PAI data set to assign a patient to a HIPPS code. The Grouper outputs the HIPPS code, which is used on Medicare claims.

long-term care hospital prospective payment system (LTCH-PPS) The payment system used by CMS to pay for Medicare patients in long-term care hospitals (LTCHs). Like the ***inpatient prospective payment system*** (see above), it is discharge based (payment is made per discharge, rather than per diem). Patients are classified into DRGs that have been weighted to reflect the resources required to treat the medically complex patients cared for at LTCHs. The system provides for an adjustment for differences in area wages and a cost-of-living adjustment for LTCHs located in Alaska and Hawaii.

outpatient prospective payment system (OPPS) The system used by CMS for payment for outpatient care for Medicare patients. The OPPS applies to hospital outpatient departments, community mental health centers (CMHCs), and some services provided by comprehensive outpatient rehabilitation facilities (CORFs), home health agencies (HHAs), and services provided to hospice patients for the treatment of a nonterminal illness. See ***Ambulatory Payment Classification***.

skilled nursing facility prospective payment system (SNF-PPS) The payment system used by CMS to pay for Medicare patients in skilled nursing facilities (SNFs). The basis is a per diem base rate, adjusted by case mix according to a classification system (Resource Utilization Groups (RUGs)) based on data from the ***Resident Assessment Instrument (RAI)***. Grouper software run at the SNF uses specific data elements from the Minimum Data Set (MDS) in the RAI to assign beneficiaries to a RUG III code. The Grouper outputs the RUG III code, which is combined with the Assessment Indicator to create a ***HIPPS code***, which is used on Medicare claims. The labor portion of the federal rates is adjusted for geographic variation in wages using the hospital wage index. The base rate is increased each federal fiscal year using an SNF market basket index.

prospective pricing Setting (or agreeing upon) prices in advance for the furnishing of a product or service. This is in direct contrast with the concept of reimbursement, in which the service or product is provided first, and then the provider is paid whatever it cost. The ***prospective payment system (PPS)*** adopted for Medicare, and applied also for other payers, is the most widespread example of prospective pricing.

The first step in prospective pricing is the definition of the product or service for which the price is to be set. Thus the DRG system of classification of patients, used in the PPS, is the first step in that prospective pricing application. The definition of procedures in CPT could be a first step toward prospective pricing for physician services. Prospective pricing facilitates budgeting on the part of payers, because only the units of service or product likely to be needed have to be estimated or predicted; the cost of each unit is fixed in advance. On the other hand, prospective pricing increases the budgeting problems of the provider, because the provider is now at risk and must plan much more carefully or else lose on the prospectively priced "transaction." (Of course, the provider may also gain on the transaction.)

prospective pricing system (PPS) A sometimes translation of "PPS," which is generally translated to mean "prospective payment system." "Prospective pricing system" is, however, a more appropriate description of this payment system. See ***prospective pricing***.

prospective reimbursement See under ***reimbursement***.

prospectus A formal written statement addressed to a prospective investor (usually in securities), containing information needed for the investor to make an informed decision as to whether to invest.

prosthesis A manufactured substitute for a part of the body, such as an arm, a leg, a heart valve, or a tooth.

prosthetics The science of using artificial, manufactured parts to replace or augment body parts.

prosthetist A health professional who designs, produces, and fits prostheses. Requires at least a bachelor's degree.

Certified Prosthetist (CP) A prosthetist who has met the requirements of the American Board for Certification in Orthotics and Prosthetics, Inc. (ABC). **www.abcop.org**

Certified Prosthetist-Orthotist (CPO) A person who is certified in both orthotics and prosthetics by the American Board for Certification in Orthotics and Prosthetics (ABC). **www.abcop.org**

Prosthetist, BOC-Certified (BOCP) A prosthetist who has met the requirements of the Board for Orthotist/Prosthetist Certification (BOC). **www.bocusa.org**

protected health information (PHI) Under the *Privacy Rule*, this term means *individually identifiable health information* that is (1) transmitted by electronic media, (2) maintained in any medium described in the definition of electronic media (in the statute), or (3) transmitted or maintained in any other form or medium (certain educational and other records are excluded) (45 C.F.R. § 160.103 (October 1, 2006)). In other words, essentially all individually identifiable health information maintained or transmitted by a healthcare provider is protected health information. The Department of Health and Human Services (HHS) maintains a web site for this topic at **aspe.os.dhhs.gov/admnsimp**. See also *designated record set* and *health information*.

protected person A person for whom a guardian has been appointed, or who is otherwise "protected" by the law; for example, a minor or a legally incompetent person.

proteome See under *DNA*.

proteomics A branch of genetics involving the study of the proteins produced in cells and of how they are produced. Genes encode (give instructions for) the construction of the proteins, providing these instructions by the use of substances called *messenger RNA (mRNA)* (see under *ribonucleic acid*, under *DNA*). Proteomics is gaining increasing attention because the resulting proteins are the targets of much of current drug research. Synonym: study of protein expression.

protocol A plan of treatment or management. As used currently in hospital finance and quality management, a "protocol" typically means that, for a patient with a given problem, certain diagnostic and treatment procedures and length of stay (LOS) are expected. See also *clinical practice guidelines* under *guidelines*.

reverse protocol A term coined for the proposition that a given diagnostic or therapeutic procedure implies that a certain kind of diagnosis or problem must have been presented by the patient. For example, administration of a certain drug should have been explained by a class of disease (or prophylaxis) for which the drug was an appropriate treatment. Failure to find such a disease in the record would indicate an error in documentation or inappropriate use of the drug.

provider A hospital or other healthcare institution or health professional that provides healthcare services to patients. A "provider" may be a single hospital, an individual, a group or organization, or even the government.

The Institute of Medicine (IOM) recommends restricting the use of the term "provider" to a system of health care, and using the term "clinician" for the individual health professional.

healthcare provider A term that can be generically used to mean any person or organization that provides health care. Under *HIPAA*, it is defined as including "a provider of services (as defined in section 1861(u)), a provider of medical or other health services (as defined in section 1861(s)), and any other person furnishing health care services or supplies." As such, a healthcare provider is a *covered entity* under HIPAA.

provider credentialing specialist A health professional who verifies and monitors the status of physicians and other clinical health professionals to practice legally. This involves checking education, training, licensure, and current competence, according to applicable laws and regulations. See also *credentialing* and *medical staff services professional*.

Certified Provider Credentialing Specialist (CPCS) A provider credentialing specialist who has passed an examination of the National Association Medical Staff Services (NAMSS). **www.namss.org**

provider-driven system See under *economic system*.

Provider Enrollment Chain and Ownership System (PECOS) A national database of Medicare provider, physician, and supplier enrollment information. One purpose is to combat Medicare fraud and abuse.

provider organizations This term covers a number of—often loosely defined—entities:
provider service network (PSN)
provider-sponsored network (PSN)
provider service organization (PSO)
provider-sponsored organization (PSO)

Although the above terms are defined separately elsewhere in this book, this entry was needed to help sort through the unavoidable confusion regarding the definition and usage of these similar sounding terms. The authors have made every effort to sort out all the variations, but none of the terms really can "stand alone"—one must know the context, including the date and geographical location. A continuous stream of new legislation by the federal and many state governments, along with marketing practices, proprietary forms, and (to be honest) simply inaccurate usage, all add to a very complex picture.

Nevertheless, these "provider organizations" almost always have some traits in common:
- Provider owned or controlled (unlike an insurance company or HMO)
- Formed for the purpose of contracting with other entities, such as health plans, to provide health care to a particular group of persons, such as the plan's subscribers
- Bear some level of financial risk (like an insurance company or HMO)
- Licensed by some governmental agency (like an insurance company or HMO)
- Likely to have programs in place for internal quality assurance, utilization review, and credentialing of providers

A typical brief definition encountered for any of the above entities might be "a provider-based managed care entity, organized for the purpose of providing, financing, and managing the risk of healthcare services for subscribers."

An example would be a hospital and a group of physicians who contract with a public (or private) employee health plan to provide care to all of the plan's members. (But to confuse matters further, note that this example is remarkably similar to a *physician-hospital organization (PHO)*.)

Proponents of these provider organizations, as opposed to HMO-type managed care entities, point out that they (1) do not contract directly with covered persons, (2) are not central to the design of the plan, (3) do not set the premiums, and (4) do not perform the benefit administration. In other words, they are primarily in the business of providing healthcare services rather than in the business of insurance. Because of this, legislation frequently attempts to give "provider organizations" some breaks relating to capitalization and antitrust requirements. See the individual listings for more detail.

Provider Reimbursement Review Board (PRRB) A panel of five members appointed by the Secretary of the Department of Health and Human Services (HHS) to which a provider may appeal a decision of a fiscal intermediary denying payment for services under Medicare.

provider service network (PSN) A term without formal definition. The first popular usage of "provider service network" can probably be linked to a type of healthcare organization proposed in the Medicare Preservation Act of 1995. There a PSN was defined as a group (network) of healthcare providers that may contract with a *provider-sponsored organization (PSO)* to provide services to Medicare beneficiaries. The PSN would essentially be a subcontractor to the PSO, which was itself a creation of the same 1995 reform proposal. The PSN would be operated by providers and funded in part by the capital contributions of its members. It would require all PSN members to provide health care to Medicare beneficiaries, and would receive compensation on the members' behalf and distribute it among them. A PSN was given some antitrust protection under the bill with regard to establishment of fee schedules and the conduct of the network. A PSN was designed to operate like an HMO, offering HMO services and assuming risk, but was to be exempt from being regulated as an insurance company, like an HMO.

In 2007, it appeared that the current usage of the term "provider service network" includes its use as a proper name for a Boston area healthcare company, and as a legislatively created alternative Medicaid option in the state of Florida. See *provider organizations* for an overview of this and related terms.

provider service organization (PSO) A term that does not really exist. Most likely a reference to a *provider service network (PSN)*. Also a common, but erroneous, reference to a *provider-sponsored organization (PSO)*. In fact, when the provider-sponsored organization was first proposed in the Medicare Preservation Act of 1995, one congressman referred to it in a PBS interview as a "provider service organization," noting further that "[n]o one knows what it is." See *provider organizations* for an overview of all of these terms.

provider site See *distant site*.

provider-sponsored network (PSN) There is no formal definition for a provider-sponsored network. The speaker probably is referring to a *provider-sponsored organization (PSO)*. See *provider organizations* for an overview of this and related terms. See also *provider service network*.

provider-sponsored organization (PSO) A legislatively defined provider-based managed care organization in which the provider (or affiliated group of providers) provides a "substantial proportion" of healthcare services (CMS has defined substantial proportion to mean at least 75%), shares some amount of financial risk, and owns a majority interest in the PSO. Created by the Balanced Budget Act of 1997, PSOs were first proposed in 1995 by the Republican Medicare reform proposal, known as the Medicare Preservation Act of 1995.

The incentive for PSOs to be formed arose from their legislated ability to enter into direct contracts to provide healthcare services under the Medicare+Choice program, also created by the Balanced Budget Act of 1997. A PSO could seek to be established and enter into business without the necessity of obtaining state licensure as an insurance company. (Such licensure is required for other types of health plans, such as HMOs.) The state could issue a certificate that the PSO meets federal requirements. The PSO would not be subject to any state law imposing capitalization, enrollment, or insolvency requirements that prevented it from doing business. Although the PSO would still need to meet the federal requirements, it was expected that these would likely be easier to meet.

By late 2000, however, it was obvious that this mechanism wasn't working. Other than the thirteen "demonstration" PSOs, there was reportedly only one PSO that ever earned an HCFA (now CMS) waiver of state licensure (St. Joseph Healthcare, Albuquerque, New Mexico), and it ceased operations in December 2000. See also *Balanced Budget Act of 1997*, *Medicare*, and *provider organizations*.

proxemics The study of how body language (nonverbal signals) is used to communicate in different cultures.

proximate cause See under *cause*.

proxy Someone who stands in for another person and is authorized to act on that person's behalf. See *healthcare proxy* under *advance directive*.

PRRB See *Provider Reimbursement Review Board*.

PSA See *Physician Scarcity Area* and *Physician Shortage Area*.

PSC See *Program Safeguard Contractor* and *Program Support Center*. Also means professional service corporation; see *professional corporation* under *corporation*.

PS classification See *ASA Physical Status Classification*.

PSDA See *Patient Self-Determination Act*.

PSES Patient Safety Evaluation System; see *Patient Safety and Quality Improvement Act of 2005*.

PSG See *polysomnogram*.

PSGT See *polysomnographic technologist*.

PSI See *Patient Safety Institute*.

PSN See *provider service network* and *provider sponsored network*.

PSO Patient Safety Organization; see *Patient Safety and Quality Improvement Act of 2005*. See also *provider service organization* and *provider-sponsored organization*.

PSQIA See *Patient Safety and Quality Improvement Act of 2005*.

PSR See *Physicians for Social Responsibility*.

PSRO See *professional standards review organization*.

PS score See *ASA Physical Status Classification*.

PSWP Patient Safety Work Product. See *Patient Safety and Quality Improvement Act of 2005*.

psychiatric and mental health nursing The area of nursing focusing on the needs of individuals and their families to stay mentally healthy and deal with psychiatric disorders.

Adult Psychiatric and Mental Health Nurse Practitioner (PMHNP) A registered nurse with a master's degree or higher who is qualified in adult psychiatric and mental health nursing and has passed an examination of the American Nurses Credentialing Center (ANCC) (**nursingworld.org/ancc**). The credential is APRN,BC (Advanced Practice Registered Nurse, Board Certified).

Board Certified Psychiatric and Mental Health Nurse A registered nurse with a Bachelor of Science in Nursing (BSN) degree who is qualified in psychiatric and mental health nursing and has passed an examination of the American Nurses Credentialing Center (ANCC) (**nursingworld.org/ancc**). The credential is RN,BC (Registered Nurse, Board Certified).

Certified Psychiatric and Mental Health Nurse A registered nurse with an associate degree or diploma who is qualified in psychiatric and mental health nursing and has passed an examination of the American Nurses Credentialing Center (ANCC) (**nursingworld.org/ancc**). The credential is RN,C (Registered Nurse, Certified).

Clinical Specialist in Adult Psychiatric and Mental Health Nursing A clinical nurse specialist with a graduate degree who is qualified in psychiatric and mental health nursing of adults and has passed an examination of the American Nurses Credentialing Center (ANCC) (**nursingworld.org/ancc**). The credential is APRN,BC (Advanced Practice Registered Nurse, Board Certified).

Clinical Specialist in Child and Adolescent Psychiatric and Mental Health Nursing A clinical nurse specialist with a graduate degree who is qualified in psychiatric and mental health nursing of children and adolescents and has passed an examination of the American Nurses Credentialing Center (ANCC) (**nursingworld.org/ancc**). The credential is APRN,BC (Advanced Practice Registered Nurse, Board Certified).

Family Psychiatric and Mental Health Nurse Practitioner (PMHNP) A registered nurse with a master's degree or higher who is qualified in family psychiatric and mental health nursing and has passed an examination of the American Nurses Credentialing Center (ANCC) (**nursingworld.org/ancc**). The credential is APRN,BC (Advanced Practice Registered Nurse, Board Certified).

psychiatry The study of mental, emotional, and behavioral disorders.

psychic Referring to the mind.

Psychogeriatric Assessment and Treatment in City Housing (PATCH) A program that seeks to identify and provide services for elderly public housing residents with mental healthcare needs. Operated by Johns Hopkins Medical Institutions in Baltimore, Maryland.

psychographics The analysis of populations on the basis of certain characteristics of individuals, specifically their attitudes, values, and lifestyles. The psychographic attributes of individuals are obtained by surveys or forms of psychometric testing. Such analyses are extensions of demographics. The attributes involved are not what are usually considered demographic; the analyses combine the psychographic data with demographic data. For example, it may be essential for some purposes to know the social consciousness (a psychographic item) of a population as it relates to various age and sex groups (demographic items).

psychologist A health professional specializing in mental health and trained in psychological analysis, therapy, and research. Psychologists in independent practice must be certified or licensed by the state, which usually requires a doctorate in psychology, completion of an approved internship, professional experience, and passing an examination. A psychologist is distinguished from a psychiatrist in that the latter holds a medical degree.

psychology The science pertaining to the mind and to behavior.

clinical psychology The application of psychology in the clinical setting, with especial emphasis on testing and counseling. The specialty is practiced by a clinical psychologist (a nonphysician) who must, in some states, be licensed.

psychometric The measurement of intelligence and of mental processes.

psychosomatic medicine (PM) A subspecialty of psychiatry that studies the effects of psychological and emotional factors on health, disease, and disability; the relationship of mind and body.

psychotherapy The type of therapy that treats mental, behavioral, and emotional disorders by psychological methods rather than by chemical or other physical means.

psychotropic A drug that acts on the patient's mental processes; a drug used in treating mental illness. Such drugs may also be used for recreation; some are addictive.

PT See *physical therapist* and *physical therapy*.

PTA See *physical therapist assistant*.

public access defibrillation (PAD) The placement of *automatic external defibrillators (AEDs)* (see under *external defibrillator*, under *defibrillator*) in strategic locations, such as sporting event venues, shopping malls, airports, and airplanes so that they are available for health professionals or laypersons to use in cases of cardiac arrest.

public accountant (PA) See under *accountant*.

Public Citizen Health Research Group (PCHRG) An independent, nonprofit consumer advocacy organization founded in 1971 by Sidney Wolfe, MD, and Ralph Nader (who was associated with PCHRG until 1982). PCHRG's purpose is to represent healthcare consumer interests in Congress, the executive branch, and the courts. It publishes a monthly newsletter, *Health Letter*. www.citizen.org/hrg

Public Company Accounting Reform and Investor Protection Act of 2002 See *Sarbanes-Oxley Act of 2002*.

public domain A legal term of art that means "open to all." Something that exists in the public domain may be used or appropriated by anyone. This term is often used to describe products whose patents have expired, or literature whose copyrights have expired. If the patent for a particular drug has expired, any pharmaceutical manufacturer may now produce this drug (the new manufacturer's product is referred to as a generic equivalent drug). Information and systems produced by the federal government are generally in the public domain. Sometimes something is made available "free" for anyone to use, but is still subject to some sort of license, in which case it is not in the public domain. See *Open Source* as an example of this.

public health The organized efforts on the part of society to reduce disease and premature death, and the disability and discomfort produced by disease and other factors, such as injury or environmental hazards. Public health is also a branch of preventive medicine, a medical specialty. Specialization in public health also occurs in engineering, nursing, nutrition, law, and other disciplines.

Public Health Data Standards Consortium (PHDSC) A nonprofit membership-based organization of federal, state, and local government agencies, professional associations, and public and private sector organizations established to develop, promote, and implement national standards for population health practice and research. PHDSC serves as a mechanism for ongoing representation of public health interests in the implementation of HIPAA and in other data standards-development processes. **www.phdsc.org**

public health genetics See under *genetics*.

Public Health Information Network (PHIN) An initiative within the Centers for Disease Control and Prevention (CDC) to advance fully capable and interoperable information systems in the many organizations that participate in public health, at the local, state, and federal levels. Goals include integrated systems for disease surveillance, national health status indicators, data analysis, public health decision support, information resources and knowledge management, alerting and communications, and the management of public health response. See also *National Electronic Disease Surveillance System*. **www.cdc.gov/phin**

public health nursing The area of nursing concerned with the health of the community as a whole. Public health nurses work with groups, families, and individuals. Primary prevention and health promotion are basic concerns. Synonyms: community health nursing, public/community health nursing.

> **Board Certified Public/Community Health Nurse** A registered nurse with a Bachelor of Science in Nursing (BSN) degree who is qualified in public/community health nursing and has passed an examination of the American Nurses Credentialing Center (ANCC) (**nursingworld.org/ancc**). The credential is RN,BC (Registered Nurse, Board Certified).

> **Clinical Specialist in Public/Community Health Nursing** A clinical nurse specialist with a graduate degree who is qualified in public/community health nursing and has passed an examination of the American Nurses Credentialing Center (ANCC) (**nursingworld.org/ancc**). The credential is APRN,BC (Advanced Practice Registered Nurse, Board Certified).

> **public health nurse (PHN)** A registered nurse with special education and training in public health nursing. Many states require certification or registration.

public health nutritionist A health professional specializing in assessment of community nutrition needs and in planning, organizing, implementing, and evaluating appropriate nutrition-related services. Public health nutritionists are often members of a publicly funded health agency such as city, county, and state health departments. They usually serve selected groups having special nutritional needs, such as mothers and children, pregnant teenagers, and the poor. See also *nutritionist*.

Public Health Security Act See *Bioterrorism Act*.

Public Health Service (PHS) The division of the federal government charged with protecting and advancing the health of the American people. The PHS originated from a 1798 law establishing a system of hospitals and health care for merchant seamen, called the Marine Hospital Service (MHS). Over the years the MHS was assigned more duties, including the quarantine and medical inspection of immigrants beginning in the late nineteenth century. The name was changed in 1902 to the Public Health and Marine Hospital Service and in 1912 to the Public Health Service. Activities of the PHS during the twentieth century included controlling the spread of contagious diseases such as smallpox and yellow fever, conducting biomedical research, regulating the food and drug supply, providing health care to underserved groups, supplying medical assistance in the aftermath of disasters, and many others.

Today the Public Health Service is a part of the Department of Health and Human Services and consists of the Office of Public Health and Science (headed by the Assistant Secretary for Health and including the Surgeon General), ten Regional Health Administrators, and eight operating divisions: Agency for Healthcare Research and Quality (AHRQ), Agency for Toxic Substances and Disease Registry (ATSDR), Centers for Disease Control and Prevention (CDC), Food and Drug Administration (FDA), Health Resources and Services Administration (HRSA), Indian Health Service (IHS), National Institutes of Health (NIH), and Substance Abuse and Mental Health Services Administration (SAMHSA). See also *Public Health*

Service Commissioned Corps. For more about the history, visit the Office of the Public Health Service Historian at **lhncbc.nlm.nih.gov/apdb/phsHistory**.

Public Health Service Act (PHSA) Important legislation first passed in 1944 that authorizes a number of federal health-related activities. There have been numerous amendments to the act since that time. Among other things, the act provides grants for community health services and the development of community health centers (see *Federally Qualified Health Center*). The act established the National Health Service Corps and provided for a Loan Repayment Program and scholarship opportunities. The act also authorizes, for example, federally regulated public health programs, biomedical research, health manpower training, family planning, emergency medical service systems, regulation of drinking water supplies, and health planning and resources development. Authority to enforce the act is delegated to the Secretary of the Department of Health and Human Services (HHS). The act is codified at 42 U.S.C. §§ 254–257 (2004). A compilation of the act as amended is published periodically by the Committee on Energy and Commerce. **energycommerce.house.gov**

Public Health Service Commissioned Corps (PHSCC) One of the seven uniformed services of the United States. The PHSCC is under the direction of the Surgeon General, within the Public Health Service. Its mission is to protect, promote, and advance the health and safety of the American people. The PHSCC has approximately 6,000 officers in the following professional categories: physician, nurse, dentist, pharmacist, dietitian, engineer, scientist, environmental health, therapist (occupational therapy, physical therapy, and speech-language pathology and audiology), health services (computer science/informational technology), dental hygiene, medical (health) record administration (or health information management), medical technology, physician assistant, biological sciences, biostatistics, chemistry, epidemiology, health education, health physics, health services administration, public health, social work, clinical psychology, optometry, podiatry, and veterinarian. **www.usphs.gov**

Public Housing Primary Care (PHPC) A federal program to provide preventive and primary healthcare services to residents of public housing. The program was created under the Disadvantaged Minority Health Improvement Act of 1990 and reauthorized under the Health Centers Consolidation Act of 1996. See *Federally Qualified Health Center*.

public key A *cryptography* component of the *public key infrastructure (PKI)* used for securing the exchange of information. A "public key" is a relatively small amount of digital data (typically a string of 1,024 digits) that you provide to someone else from whom you want to receive private digital data. Although this technology can be applied to virtually any form of digital data storage and transfer, the following example shows its use in an email exchange, one of its most common applications.

Let's say you want Dr. X to email your lab results to you, but you want the email message to be encrypted while it travels over the public and insecure Internet, and you even want it to be encrypted when it finally arrives in your computer's email inbox. You first provide Dr. X with your public key, which you can safely send via a simple email, unencrypted ("in the clear"). Or, Dr. X may even look up your public key in a public directory somewhere if you have listed it (as part of obtaining a *digital certificate*). You may have seen these public keys as standard parts of some people's email signature forms, included on every email they send. Dr. X (whom you obviously trust to read your lab results) then uses *your* public key to encrypt the message, leaving it completely unreadable by anyone, including Dr. X. At this point, as you might guess, even the public key itself cannot decrypt the encrypted message, because it wouldn't be a secure system if it could. We now have a series of digital codes traveling in public, and although they can be intercepted and copied, they can't be understood. There is only one practical way to decrypt your lab results message, and that is with your "private key."

The **private key** is technically very similar to the public key, and is mathematically related to it. The main difference between the two is that the private key must be kept absolutely secure and confidential. The private key allows the message that has been encrypted with the public key to be decrypted and read, and anyone who possesses the private key has access to the contents of that message. The private key can also be used to create an electronic signature, used for authentication.

A pair of public and private keys must be generated at the same time, using the same algorithm (a popular one is known as "RSA"). The keys will only work as a pair, as described above. They are part of the *public key infrastructure (PKI)*.

public key infrastructure (PKI) A system using *public key* (asymmetric) *cryptography* to protect the privacy of digital information that exists on a computer, or travels across a network, especially a public network such as the Internet. Now the most common system used for protected health information (PHI), PKI is likely to be used by many to meet the security requirements of HIPAA.

PKI uses a public and a private cryptographic key pair that is obtained and shared through a trusted authority, known as a *certificate authority (CA)*. The CA provides a *digital certificate* that can identify an individual or an organization, as well as directory services that can store and, if necessary, revoke the certificate. Additionally, a registration authority (RA) verifies the CA before a digital certificate is issued to a requestor. Although the cryptography used in PKI is fairly well established, standards for the use of PKI are still far from settled, including its use on the Internet and the regulation of CAs. Implicit in PKI is also a system to manage all of the digital certificates.

public relations The efforts to communicate with the hospital's (or other organization's or an individual's) audiences and constituencies and to enhance the hospital's image.

PubMed A free web-based literature retrieval system that contains citations and abstracts from thousands of medical and science journals, dating back to 1966. The system allows the public to follow web links between *MEDLINE* abstracts and the publishers of the full-text articles. PubMed was established in 1997 as a result of collaboration between the National Library of Medicine (NLM) and major science publishers such as the *New England Journal of Medicine (NEJM)*, *Science, Journal of Biological Chemistry*, and *The Proceedings of the National Academy of Sciences*. **www.ncbi.nlm.nih.gov/entrez/query.fcgi**.

PubMed Central (PMC) Begun in 2000, is an electronic archive for full text (as opposed to just citations or abstracts) life science journal articles, offering unrestricted access to its contents. Every full text article in PubMed Central has a corresponding entry in PubMed. PMC, which is not itself a publisher, is operated by the National Center for Biotechnology Information (NCBI), a division of the NLM. Access to PMC is free and unrestricted. **www.pubmedcentral.nih.gov**

pulmonary disease The study of diseases and disorders of the respiratory (breathing) system.

pulmonary function technologist (PFT) A health professional trained to conduct diagnostic tests to evaluate normal and abnormal lung conditions, under the supervision of a physician.

Certified Pulmonary Function Technologist (CPFT) A PFT who has met the requirements and passed an entry-level examination of the National Board for Respiratory Care (NBRC). **www.nbrc.org**

Registered Pulmonary Function Technologist (RPFT) A Certified Pulmonary Function Technologist (CPFT) who has passed an advanced-level examination of the National Board for Respiratory Care (NBRC). **www.nbrc.org**

PulseNet An electronic network administered by the Centers for Disease Control and Prevention (CDC) linking state and local public health departments together with the CDC, Department of Agriculture (USDA), and Food and Drug Administration (FDA). The purpose of PulseNet is to eliminate food-borne illnesses, such as infections from *E. coli* and *Salmonella* bacteria. PulseNet performs DNA "fingerprinting" on bacteria that may be foodborne. The network permits rapid comparison of these "fingerprint" patterns through an electronic database at CDC. The DNA fingerprinting method is called **pulsed-field gel**

electrophoresis (PFGE). The formal name of the project is the National Molecular Subtyping Network for Foodborne Disease Surveillance. **www.cdc.gov/pulsenet**

PUM See *parochial and unconventional medicine*.

purchasing The function of the hospital (or other facility) that procures necessary items, both durable (from beds to CAT scanners) and nondurable (dressings, needles, etc.).

    group purchasing A shared service that combines the purchasing power of individual hospitals in order to obtain lower prices for equipment and supplies. Also may refer to arrangements where several small employers purchase health insurance collectively.

purine See under *DNA*.

Push Package See *Strategic National Stockpile*.

PV See *pharmacovigilance*.

PVRP Physician Volunteer Reporting Program. See *Quality Initiative*.

PVS See *persistent vegetative state* under *vegetative state*.

PWAs See *persons with AIDS*.

PYLL See *potential years of life lost*.

pyrimidine See under *DNA*.

Q

QA See *quality assessment*. Also quality assurance (see *quality management*).

QALY See *quality-adjusted life-year*.

QAM See *Quality Assurance Monitor*.

QAP Quality assurance professional; see *quality management professional*.

QAPI See *Quality Assessment and Performance Improvement*.

QASC See *Quality Alliance Steering Committee*.

QC See *quality control*.

QCYM See *Qualification in Cytometry* under *clinical laboratory qualification*.

qi The vital energy of the body. A central concept in traditional Oriental medicine. Pronounced "chi."

QI See *quality improvement*, *quality indicator* (under *indicator*), and *Quality Initiative*.

qi gong Exercises to benefit health by improving energy. Qi gong (also represented as "chi kung") literally means "energy cultivation." There are thousands of such exercises, all containing common principles concerning mind, eyes, movement, and breath.

QIHC See *Qualification in Immunohistochemistry* under *clinical laboratory qualification*.

QIO See *quality improvement organization*.

QIOSC See *quality improvement organization support center*.

QIP See *quality improvement project*.

QLC See *Qualification in Laboratory Compliance* under *clinical laboratory qualification*.

QLI See *Qualification in Laboratory Informatics* under *clinical laboratory qualification*.

QM See *quality management*.

QMMP See *Quality Measurement and Management Project*.

QMT See *quality management technologist* and *quality management technology*.

Q-Net Exchange A secure, interactive web site approved by CMS for the confidential exchange of information between two or more organizations. It is designed for use by hospitals, quality improvement organizations (QIOs), end stage renal disease (ESRD) facilities, ESRD networks, performance measurement systems (PMS) vendors, and the Clinical Data Abstraction Center (CDAC). **www.qualitynet.org**

QOL See *quality of life*.

QRM See *quality and resource management*.

QSAP Qualified *Substance Abuse Professional*.

qualification See *advanced qualifications* and *clinical laboratory qualification*.

qualified Having met certain requirements; usually refers to a health professional. The specific requirements will vary according to the field of specialty and purpose of qualification. Requirements may relate to education, experience, training, competence, applicable professional licensure, regulation or certification, registration, and/or privileges.

qualitative data See under *data*.

quality-adjusted life-year (QALY) A measure used in economic and other analyses of the benefits of various healthcare procedures and programs, including drug therapies. It combines both the quantity and quality of life. One year of perfect health is 1 QALY (1 = "perfect" life quality). If the quality of life for a person with a life expectancy of one year is less than perfect—say, 0.6—the QALY would be 0.6 (1 year × 0.6 quality of life). If that person could gain two more years with a medical intervention, but the quality of life would be reduced to 0.2, there would be no net gain (3 years × 0.2 quality of life = 0.6). See also *quality of life* and *quality of life scale*.

quality alliance See *AQA* and *Hospital Quality Alliance*.

Quality Alliance Steering Committee (QASC) An effort of AQA and the Hospital Quality Alliance (HQA) to work together to better coordinate the promotion of hospital and physician performance measures, reporting on performance to consumers and other stakeholders, and quality improvement efforts. The steering committee works closely with CMS and the Agency for Healthcare Research and Quality (AHRQ), which are key members of both the AQA and HQA. Synonyms: AQA-HQA Steering Committee, National Quality Alliance Steering Committee (NQASC).

quality and resource management (QRM) A term used in some hospitals to indicate that quality management and the conservation of resources are seen as a single topic, or at least, topics that are closely interrelated. Such hospitals may have, for example, quality management, utilization review, risk management, and infection control under the "QRM department" headed by the "QRM Director."

quality assessment (QA) The former name for quality assurance. The name of the activity was changed to reflect that the intent was to maintain and improve the quality of care rather than merely measure it (assess it). Current terminology has, in turn, replaced "quality assurance" with "quality management." Also see *quality management*.

Quality Assessment and Performance Improvement (QAPI) A program to evaluate the quality of healthcare services provided, initiate change in performance if required, and monitor after the change to see if the quality has improved. All Rural Health Clinics (RHCs) are required to have such a program in place.

quality assurance (QA) See *quality management*.

quality assurance coordinator See *quality management professional*.

quality assurance function See *quality function*.

Quality Assurance Monitor (QAM) A part of the *Professional Activity Study (PAS)*. The care of patients, as reflected in their computerized discharge abstracts, was compared with standards established by clinical specialty societies, and the findings were displayed for use in hospital quality management.

quality assurance professional See *quality management professional*.

Quality Chasm Series See *Institute of Medicine's Health Care Quality Initiative*.

Quality Check An online directory of healthcare organizations and programs that have been accredited by the Joint Commission on Accreditation of Healthcare Organizations (JCAHO). See *Quality Reports*. **www.qualitycheck.org**

quality circle A group that deals with concerns that relate to the quality of performance or quality of work life. Six "non-negotiable" characteristics of a group must be present if it is to be called a quality circle: (1) the group must be small; and (2) composed of individuals in the same work area (of a hospital, for example); (3) it must be voluntary; (4) it must consider problems (or opportunities for improvement) that the group itself selects; (5) the problems must affect the quality of work life or the quality of performance; and (6) the circle must propose solutions to management.

A quality circle is not to be confused with a committee or task force, both of which are appointed (not voluntary) and work on assigned tasks rather than self-selected tasks. Morale, productivity, and quality of performance are typically improved by the activities of quality circles. The groups often carry locally determined titles rather than being named "quality circles." Synonym: quality control circle.

quality control (QC) The sum of all the activities that prevent unwanted change in quality. In the healthcare setting, quality control requires a repeated series of feedback loops that monitor and evaluate the care of the individual patient (and other systems in the healthcare process). These feedback loops involve checking the care being delivered against standards of care, the identification of any problems or opportunities for improvement, and prompt corrective action, so that the quality is maintained. See the illustration at *quality staircase*.

quality control circle See *quality circle*.

quality function The sum of all the activities, wherever performed, through which the hospital achieves the *quality of care* it provides. This usage is comparable to speaking of the "fiscal function," which is the sum of the activities, wherever performed, through which the hospital achieves fiscal soundness. Formerly "quality assurance function."

quality improvement (QI) The sum of all the activities that create a desired change in quality. In the healthcare setting, quality improvement requires a feedback loop that involves the identification of patterns of the care of patients (or of the performance of other systems involved in care), the analysis of those patterns in order to identify opportunities for improvement (or instances of departure from standards of care), and then action to improve the quality of care for future patients. An effective quality improvement system results in stepwise increases in quality of care. *Quality control*, with which quality improvement is sometimes confused, is the sum of all the activities that prevent unwanted change in quality. See the illustration at *quality staircase*. See also *performance improvement*.

continuous quality improvement (CQI) As used in health care today, CQI means the application of industrial quality management theory in the healthcare setting, based upon principles of quality "gurus" W. Edwards Deming and Joseph M. Juran. Whereas traditional *quality control* theories seek out "fault" and attempt improvement by exhorting people to change their behavior, continuous improvement seeks to understand processes and revise them on the basis of data about the processes themselves. CQI sees "problems" as opportunities for improvement. The CQI process involves a project-by-project approach to systematically improve quality, not just to maintain the status quo.

Quality Improvement Goals National Quality Improvement Goals; see *performance measure*.

quality improvement organization (QIO) An organization that contracts with CMS to provide certain mandated services. Fifty-three QIOs, one in each U.S. state, the District of Columbia, Puerto Rico, and the Virgin Islands, work with providers and Medicare beneficiaries to improve the quality and effectiveness of health care—to "make sure patients get the right care at the right time," particularly among underserved populations. QIOs also review cases to see that payment is made only for medically necessary services (thereby protecting the Medicare Trust Fund), and investigate beneficiary complaints about quality of care.

The QIO program uses four strategies: (1) measure and report performance, (2) adopt healthcare information technology and use it effectively, (3) redesign process, and (4) transform organizational culture.

QIOs, originally called peer review organizations (PROs), were set up by the 1982 Tax Equity and Fiscal Responsibility Act (TEFRA) as a part of the prospective payment system (PPS) to carry out certain review functions under contract from HCFA (now CMS). The duties of the early PROs were chiefly retrospective, and included such tasks as determining whether the medical records of Medicare patients supported the diagnoses and procedures stated in the claims submitted; determining whether a changing pattern of care in a hospital, as reflected in its claims submitted, represented an actual change in the kinds of patients or their treatment, or was a fictitious result of the claims submission and reporting system; reviewing the medical necessity of DRG outliers; reviewing cardiac pacemaker implantations; and attempting to achieve certain changes in performance in hospitals within the jurisdiction of the PRO.

Thus the PROs originally were largely "watchdogs," with emphasis on detecting individual problems in care and working toward their correction. Over the years, however, they adopted the philosophies and techniques of quality improvement (QI) and became "guidedogs," with an emphasis on reviewing patterns of care and taking positive measures to improve care generally. The name change in 2002 was intended to reflect this new role. However, most of the watchdog functions, including individual case review, still remain. See also *American Health Quality Association*, *Health Care Quality Improvement Program*, *Hospital Payment Monitoring Program*, and *MedQIC*.

quality improvement organization support center (QIOSC) A quality improvement organization (QIO) that has contracted with CMS to help administer the QIO program and share information with other QIOs. There are two types of QIOSCs, cross-cutting and task-specific. Task-specific QIOSCs are assigned to a particular Health Care Quality Improvement Program (HCQIP) effort, such as nursing homes or physician offices. Cross-cutting QIOSCs focus on more general support, such as communications or general quality improvement. QIOSC is pronounced "kiosk."

quality improvement project (QIP) One activity in the process of continuous quality improvement (CQI). Each project involves a process that has been identified as deserving improvement, and which has been given priority. (Prioritizing of effort is critical in CQI.) For each project, a team is assigned consisting of representatives from all departments involved in the process targeted for improvement, along with support from senior management. The team studies the process, comes up with theories for improvement, tests the theories, puts successful theories into place, and also puts into place measures to assure that the improved quality is maintained.

Examples of hospital QIPs conducted as part of the National Demonstration Project on Quality Improvement in Health Care were reduction in medication errors, reduction of unbilled drugs (thereby increasing revenues), and reduction of delays in surgery starting times (with a corresponding savings in hospital staff overtime expenses). See also *Health Care Quality Improvement Program*.

quality indicator (QI) See under *indicator*.

Quality Initiative (QI) A program launched by CMS in 2002 "to assure quality health care for all Americans through accountability and public disclosure." It consists of a number of multifaceted initiatives, each with specific focus, carried out by a variety of partnerships, including quality improvement organizations (QIOs) in collaboration with providers, researchers and academic experts, federal and state organizations, consumer organizations, and others. Initial programs included the Nursing Home Quality Initiative (NHQI); Home Health Quality Initiative (HHQI); Hospital Quality Initiative (HQI); Physician Focused Quality Initiative (PFQI), which includes the Doctor's Office Quality Project (DOQ); the End Stage Renal Disease (ESRD) Quality Initiative; and the Physician Voluntary Reporting Program (PVRP). See also *Hospital Quality Alliance*. www.cms.hhs.gov/QualityInitiativesGenInfo

quality management (QM) Efforts to determine the *quality of care*, to develop and maintain programs to keep it at an acceptable level (*quality control*), to institute improvements when the opportunity arises or the care does not meet standards (*quality improvement*), and to provide, to all concerned, the evidence required to establish confidence that quality is being managed and maintained at the desired level. (These are the same elements that are inherent in industrial quality management.)

QM used to be called **quality assurance (QA)**. However, the term "quality management" has become more popular because (1) there is no implication of a "guarantee," an idea that may be suggested by the use of the word "assurance," which is sometimes used as a synonym for "insurance"; and (2) "quality management" is more accurate, because the achievement of quality depends on people carrying out their responsibilities without error, and getting people to perform is the task of management. See also *performance improvement* and *process*.

Total Quality Management (TQM) Used to describe a philosophy (and actions) of an organization that is dedicated to *continuous quality improvement (CQI)* (see under *quality improvement*) throughout the organization. A hospital with Total Quality Management will, for example, set specific quality goals, choose a number of high priority *quality improvement projects (QIPs)*, make quality improvement part of job descriptions throughout the organization and legitimize time spent on quality improvement, provide necessary resources (financial and otherwise), provide essential training for staff involved, and formally recognize quality improvement efforts. Total Quality Management requires commitment and personal involvement of senior management. It should be emphasized that quality control (prevention of unwanted change in quality) must be maintained in parallel with quality improvement, and that quality control demands the same energy commitment as does quality improvement.

quality management audit See under *audit*.

quality management professional A health professional who specializes in quality management. Also called healthcare quality professional. Older terms for those involved in healthcare quality activities included quality assurance professional (QAP) and quality assurance coordinator. See also *utilization review coordinator*.

Certified Professional in Healthcare Quality (CPHQ) A multidisciplinary credential for health professionals available from the Healthcare Quality Certification Board (HQCB). **www.cphq.org**

Certified Professional in Quality Assurance (CPQA) The same as the Certified Professional in Healthcare Quality (CPHQ) credential, but granted before 1992, when the Healthcare Quality Certification Board was called the Quality Assurance Certification Board.

Fellow of the American Institute for Healthcare Quality (AIHQ Fellow) A quality management professional with Health Care Quality Management (HCQM) and Patient Safety Certification who has met the requirements to be a Fellow of the American Institute for Healthcare Quality (AIHQ), a division of the American Board of Quality Assurance and Utilization Review Physicians, Inc. (ABQAURP) (**www.abqaurp.org**). Quality management professionals without HCQM certification may become AIHQ Members.

Health Care Quality Management (HCQM) and Patient Safety Certification A credential offered to qualifying physicians, nurses, and other health professionals who pass an examination developed by the American Board of Quality Assurance and Utilization Review Physicians, Inc. (ABQAURP) (**www.abqaurp.org**) in association with the National Board of Medical Examiners (NBME) (**www.nbme.org**). Those certified are called diplomates.

quality management technologist (QMT) A health professional trained in quality management technology.

Registered Technologist—Quality Management (RT(QM)) A *Registered Technologist (RT)* (see under *radiologic technologist*) with advanced qualifications in quality management technology from the American Registry of Radiologic Technologists (ARRT). **www.arrt.org**

quality management technology (QMT) Procedures and techniques to assure that tests and therapies are of the highest possible quality, with the lowest risk to patients and health professionals. QMT assures that test results are accurate, amounts of radiation are carefully controlled, images do not degrade, and equipment and supplies are up to standards.

Quality Measurement and Management Project (QMMP) A project of the Hospital Research and Educational Trust (HRET) of the American Hospital Association (AHA) to develop quality monitoring and management tools for hospitals.

QualityNet A web site developed by CMS to provide healthcare quality improvement news, tools, and other resources. **www.qualitynet.org**

quality of care The degree of conformity with accepted principles and practices (standards), the degree of fitness for the patient's needs, and the degree of attainment of achievable outcomes (results), consonant with the appropriate allocation or use of resources. The phrase "quality of care" carries the concept that quality is not equivalent to "more" or "higher technology" or higher cost. The "degree of conformity" with standards focuses on the provider's performance, whereas the "degree of fitness" for the patient's needs indicates that the patient may present conditions that override strict conformity with otherwise prescribed procedures.

The Institute of Medicine (IOM) defines quality as "the degree to which health services for individuals and populations increase the likelihood of desired health outcomes and are consistent with current professional knowledge."

quality of life (QOL) A condition often given as one attribute or dimension of health. It is ill-defined, depending on the individual and his or her goals, the social setting and expectations (often of others), and other factors. The goal of much of health care is stated to be improved quality of life. The World Health Organization (WHO) defines "quality of life" as "an individual's perception of their position in life in the context of the culture and value systems in which they live and in relation to their goals, expectations, standards and concerns."

One of the most challenging problems in health care is to measure quality of life so that (1) improvement can be identified, and (2) it can be used as a factor in cost-benefit analysis. There is a real danger that inability to express quality of life in numerical terms will mean that much valuable care will not be available because quality of life cannot be given a value and therefore cannot be used to justify the expenditure (to end up with a positive cost-benefit ratio rather than a negative ratio); consequently, mere survival could be the measure.

An illustration is the debate over the "value" of some coronary bypass operations; patients in some studies have not shown significantly greater life expectancy with the operation than without it, but the patients operated on regularly testify to their pleasure with their relief from pain. In some instances (intractable pain or helplessness, for example), life itself is of such low quality to the individual that he or she may prefer not to live. See also *quality of life scale* and *quality-adjusted life-year*.

health-related quality of life (HRQOL) A number of aspects of quality of life (QOL) that are related to health, such as mental health, perceived physical health, and social and role functioning. The relevant aspects are sometimes developed under the headings of "physical well-being, perceived health, emotional well-being, home management, work functioning, recreation, social functioning, and sexual functioning."

quality of life scale A method designed to measure the quality of life of an individual, based upon one or more aspects of life and health. Well over a hundred assessment instruments have been developed, most of which are completed by the patient (or by interviewing the patient), rather than by observation. (Some combine the two methods.) Some investigators have developed weighting methods by which to consolidate the data from a number of scale measurements into a single score for an individual.

These instruments are also sometimes called "health outcomes assessment" or "health status assessment" tools. They may be used, for example, to assess the progress of rehabilitation of an individual, the effect of chronic disease on a person or group, or the effectiveness of health care in a population. A quality of life scale may be generic (applicable to any group) or disease specific (asthma, for example). Special scales are also used for children and adolescents. Some representative generic scales are listed below. See also *patient-reported outcome* and *quality-adjusted life-year*.

Duke Health Profile (DUKE) A seventeen-item generic questionnaire that measures patient-reported functional health status and health-related quality of life during a one-week time period. It has eleven scales, six of which measure functional health: physical, mental, social, general, perceived health, and self-esteem. The other five scales measure dysfunctional health: anxiety, depression, anxiety-depression, pain, and disability. The DUKE profile has been used primarily for research on health-related outcomes in the clinical setting. It is a refinement of the original Duke-UNC Health Profile (DUHP), a sixty-three-item generic measure that was developed by Duke University and the University of North Carolina School of Public Health.

London Handicap Scale (LHS) A six-item instrument that measures health status in patients with chronic, multiple, or progressive diseases. "Handicap" is defined as disadvantage in role performance due to impairment or disability. The scale generates a profile of handicaps on six different dimensions (mobility, physical independence, occupation, social integration, orientation, and economic self-sufficiency) and an overall handicap severity score. Each dimension has six levels, arranged in order of increasing disadvantage. Together this information forms a descriptive profile of the individual. The scale is particularly appropriate for the elderly.

Quality of Well-Being Scale (QWB) A general health-related quality of life questionnaire measuring symptoms, mobility, physical activity, and social activity. The scale first classifies patients into functional levels based on their answers to standardized questions. Each level is then assigned a "quality of well-being score" based on previous population studies. Then the score is adjusted to reflect the patient's prognosis to produce a "well-life expectancy" value. The QWB is used to measure and monitor the health status of individual patients and of groups over time, and also to evaluate the effectiveness of clinical interventions. The QWB requires a trained interviewer; however, a questionnaire has been developed for patients to take by themselves, the QWB-SA (self-administered).

SF-36 Health Survey A thirty-six-item instrument for measuring health status and outcomes from the patient's point of view. Administered by interview or self-administered, the SF-36 covers eight health concepts: limitations in physical activities because of health problems, limitations in usual role activities because of physical health problems, bodily pain, general health perceptions, vitality (energy and fatigue), limitations in social activities because of physical or emotional problems, limitations in usual role activities because of emotional problems, and mental health (psychological distress and well-being). The scoring system provides eight health scores and two summary scores, as well as a self-assessed change in health status. The SF-36 is widely used to measure health status and monitor health outcomes. A shorter form (SF-12) is also available. Also called *Medical Outcomes Study* Short-form Health Survey or MOS SF-36. **www.sf-36.org**

Sickness Impact Profile (SIP) A 136-item generic questionnaire used to evaluate the impact of disease on both physical and emotional functioning. The SIP measures everyday activities in twelve categories: sleep and rest, emotional behavior, body care and movement, home management, mobility, social interaction, ambulation, alertness behavior, communication, work, recreation and pastimes, and eating. Patients identify statements that describe their experience. In addition to scores in each area, a total score is tabulated, as well as summary scores for physical and psychosocial domains.

WHOQOL World Health Organization Quality of Life Assessment. A generic measure to assess individuals' perceptions of the quality of their lives (see *quality of life*). WHO developed two instruments (the WHOQOL-100 and a shorter version, the WHOQOL-BREF) to measure quality of life and well-being in a variety of cultural settings while allowing the results from different populations and countries to be compared.

Six domains are included in the WHOQOL-100: physical health (e.g., energy and fatigue, pain and discomfort), psychological (self-esteem, thinking and learning), level of independence (mobility, activities of daily living), social relations (personal relationships, social support), environment (financial resources, physical safety and security, healthcare access), and spirituality/religion/personal beliefs. There are a total of 100 questions. A version is being developed for older adults (WHOQOL-OLD) and for people living with HIV and AIDS (WHOQOL-HIV).

Quality of Well-Being Scale (QWB) See under *quality of life scale*.

Quality Reports Summaries of information on the quality of accredited healthcare organizations and programs, made available to the general public by the Joint Commission on Accreditation of Healthcare Organizations (JCAHO) on a web site called Quality Check. For each organization, the report includes the following information:

- JCAHO accreditation decision and the effective dates of the accreditation award. For Provisional, Conditional, and Preliminary Denial of Accreditation decisions, the reports list the standards cited for Requirements for Improvement.
- Programs accredited by JCAHO as well as programs or services accredited by other accrediting bodies.

- Compliance with JCAHO's **National Patient Safety Goals**, as applicable to the organization.
- Performance on **National Quality Improvement Goals** (see **performance measure**) (hospitals only).
- Special quality awards, including recognition such as Disease-Specific Care Certification, Codman Award, Eisenberg Patient Safety Award, Franklin Award, Magnet Status, Medal of Honor for Organ Donation, and others approved by the JCAHO Board of Commissioners.

See also **Hospital Compare**. **www.qualitycheck.org**

quality staircase A method, developed by Vergil Slee, of representing the results of quality improvement efforts. Joseph M. Juran in the industrial setting has represented quality improvement as an ever-rising spiral, an inclined plane. The processes involved in making the product or providing the service are constantly monitored and, as opportunities for improvement are identified, changes are made that result in breakthroughs to higher levels of quality. In certain respects, the concept of a staircase is more appropriate than that of a spiral, because breakthroughs actually improve quality in steps rather than in a continuous fashion. See the illustration below.

Quality Control

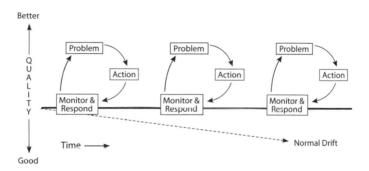

The Quality Floor: Preventing unwanted change for today's patients

Quality Improvement

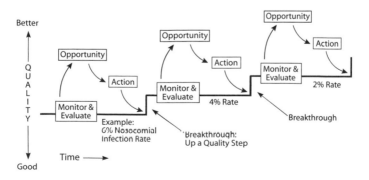

The Quality Staircase: Creating desired change for future patients

quantitative data See under *data*.

quarantine Isolation of a person or people to prevent the spread of an infectious disease. An individual may be quarantined (at home or in the hospital), or a quarantine may be imposed upon a population as a public health measure. Quarantinable diseases in the United States include cholera, diphtheria, infectious tuberculosis, plague, smallpox, yellow fever, viral hemorrhagic fevers (such as Ebola), and SARS (severe acute respiratory syndrome). Plants and animals may also be quarantined (for example, quarantine is usually required for animals being brought into the United States from other countries). See also *isolation*.

quick ratio See under *ratio*.

quill pen law A law that requires records to be maintained in written, rather than electronic, form.

qui tam claimant A person, usually a *whistleblower*, who brings an action under a statute that establishes a penalty for the omission or commission of a certain act. The person (claimant, or "relator") who is suing on behalf of him- or herself also sues on behalf of the state and consequently splits any recovery with the state. "Qui tam" is short for the Latin phrase "qui tam pro domino rege quam pro si ipso in hac parte sequitur," which means "Who sues on behalf of the King as well as for himself." See *False Claims Act*.

QWB See *Quality of Well-Being Scale* under *quality of life scale*.

R

RA See *Radiologist Assistant* under *radiologic technologist*.

Rabbi trust See *deferred compensation*.

RAC See *recovery audit contractor*.

Racketeer Influenced and Corrupt Organization Act (RICO) The federal racketeering statute. This and other state and federal laws were passed to control organized crime. Racketeering is a conspiracy to commit extortion or coercion. A person may be tried under RICO if he or she committed racketeering activity or merely had an interest in such activity. The Supreme Court has applied RICO to those who block access to family planning clinics that provide abortions. 18 U.S.C. § 1961 (2005).

radiant energy The energy of electromagnetic waves, including visible light, x-rays (see *x-ray (radiation)*), radio waves, and waves emitted by radioactive substances, such as radium.

radiation X-rays (see *x-ray (radiation)*) and other forms of radiant energy. The term "radiation" excludes visible light and radiation in the frequencies near the spectrum of visible light.

extremely low frequency (electromagnetic) radiation (ELF radiation) Radiation of 50 to 60 Hz from electric and magnetic fields. Such radiation comes from anything that produces electrical current, such as appliances, wall wiring, ground currents, and service distribution lines. Although both electric and magnetic radiation occur, the magnetic component is suspected of adverse effects such as leukemia (especially in children), brain cancer, and interference with cardiac pacemakers, according to the American Industrial Hygiene Association (AIHA) and the Environmental Protection Agency (EPA). Proper shielding and grounding of equipment and wiring, and siting of structures are possible ways to reduce the hazard.

radiation safety officer (RSO) A person in a hospital (or other facility utilizing radiation) who is responsible for making sure that radiation exposure of professionals and patients is within safe limits, that safety procedures are in place and working, and that the facility is in compliance with federal and state radiation safety regulations. See also *health physicist* under *physicist*.

radiation therapist A health professional trained to do radiation therapy.

Registered Technologist—Radiation Therapy (RT(T)) A *Registered Technologist (RT)* (see under *radiologic technologist*) who has been certified in radiation therapy by the American Registry of Radiologic Technologists (ARRT). **www.arrt.org**

radiation therapy Treatment by the use of x-rays and other forms of radiation.

radioactive A term applied to chemical elements that give off (or are capable of giving off) particles of radiant energy, such as alpha, beta, and gamma rays. Some chemical elements, such as plutonium, radium, and uranium, are radioactive as they are found in nature, whereas others can be made radioactive by special physical processes. Both natural and "artificial" radioactive chemical elements are used in nuclear medicine. See also *nuclide*.

radioactive isotope See *nuclide*.

radioactive nuclide See *nuclide*.

radioactivity See under *nuclide*.

radio frequency identification (RFID) A method of tracking a product by incorporating into the product a silicon chip and antenna that can transmit data to a receiver, so that it can be identified by a wireless reading device. Radio ID tags can be installed almost everywhere, even under the skin. "Passive" tags utilize power transmitted to the tag from the receiver (with a range of a few feet). "Active" tags have their own battery power (and can be read from much farther away). The Food and Drug Administration (FDA) is considering the use of RFID tags to track medical devices, such as external monitors and implanted devices such as pacemakers. Synonym: smart tag.

radiographer A health professional trained to take x-rays.

Registered Technologist—Radiology (RT(R)) A *Registered Technologist (RT)* (see under *radiologic technologist*) who has been certified in radiography by the American Registry of Radiologic Technologists (ARRT). **www.arrt.org**

radiography Examination of any part of the body by x-rays for the purpose of diagnosis. The result of the examination is usually recorded on photographic film. The use of x-rays and other radiation for treatment is radiotherapy.

contrast radiography Diagnostic examination of any part of the body by x-ray with the aid of a chemical that absorbs more or less of the x-rays than body tissues and thus in the x-ray image presents a contrast to the body tissues. The contrast material may be taken by mouth or injected. A barium enema and a "G-I series" use barium as the opaque contrast medium injected rectally or taken by mouth, respectively, which casts a darker shadow than the body tissues. Angiograms use an injected opaque substance as well. For some purposes, air, which is transparent to the x-rays, is the contrast medium.

radioisotope A radioactive form of a chemical element. Some radioisotopes are used in medical care for diagnostic and therapeutic purposes; this use is called *nuclear medicine*. See also *nuclide*.

Radiological Society of North America (RSNA) A national organization dedicated to promoting and developing the highest standards of radiology and related sciences through education and research. **www.rsna.org**

radiologic technologist A health professional who operates radiologic equipment, ordinarily under the supervision of a radiologist, and who assists in radiologic procedures. More than half the states require radiologic technologists (except sonographers) to be licensed. Synonym: radiological technologist.

Radiologist Assistant (RA) A health professional who has qualified and passed a certification examination of the American Registry of Radiologic Technologists (ARRT). **www.arrt.org**

Registered Technologist (RT) A radiologic technologist who has been certified by and registered with the American Registry of Radiologic Technologists (ARRT). Radiologic technologists become certified by completing an accredited program and passing a national examination in one of four primary areas:

(R): radiography (see *radiographer*)
(N): nuclear medicine technology (see *nuclear medicine technologist*)
(T): radiation therapy (see *radiation therapist*)
(S): sonography (see *diagnostic medical sonographer*)

They then are entitled to the credential RT(ARRT), and register annually with ARRT to verify continued qualification. RTs may obtain certificates of advanced qualifications ("postprimary" certifications) by passing examinations in the following areas:

(CV): see *cardiovascular-interventional radiography*
(M): mammography (see *mammographer*)
(CT): computed tomography (see *computed tomography technologist*)
(MR): magnetic resonance imaging (see *magnetic resonance imaging technologist*)
(QM): quality management (see *quality management technologist*)
(BD): bone densitometry (see *bone densitometrist*)
(S): sonography (advanced qualification) (see *diagnostic medical sonographer*)
(VS): vascular sonography (see *diagnostic medical sonographer*)
(BS): breast sonography (see *diagnostic medical sonographer*)
(CI): cardiac-interventional radiography (see *cardiovascular-interventional radiology*)
(VI): vascular-interventional radiography (see *cardiovascular-interventional radiology*)

An RT certified and registered in nuclear medicine technology and quality management, for example, would receive the designation RT(N)(QM)(ARRT). **www.arrt.org**

radiologist A physician specializing in radiology.

Radiologist Assistant (RA) See under *radiologic technologist*.

radiology The use of x-rays and other forms of radiation for diagnosis and treatment. Diagnostic radiology is a kind of imaging.

diagnostic nuclear radiology The branch of radiology that deals with making diagnoses with the use of radioactive materials.

diagnostic radiology The branch of radiology that deals with making diagnoses.

therapeutic radiology The branch of radiology that uses radiation in the treatment of disease.

radiology nursing The area of nursing focusing on the needs of patients undergoing diagnostic and therapeutic imaging procedures.

Certified Radiology Nurse (CRN) A specialist in radiology nursing who has passed an examination of the American Radiological Nurses Association (ARNA). **www.arna.net**

radiolucent A substance that is transparent to x-rays, and thus casts no shadow on an x-ray film. See also *radiopaque*.

radionuclide See under *nuclide*.

radiopaque Any material that blocks the passage of x-rays. Such materials are used in certain types of x-ray examinations; for example, in bowel examinations, the barium enema is radiopaque and will produce a contrast (shadow) on the film. See also *contrast radiography*, under *radiography*, and *radiolucent*.

radium therapy Radiation therapy through the use of radium.

RADTT Radiation therapy technologist. See *radiation therapist*.

RAI See *Resident Assessment Instrument*.

random A statistical term used in sampling that means every "element" or "event" in the whole "universe" being sampled has an equal chance of being "drawn." If a hospital wants to know how well patients like the food, for example, the universe could be all the patients who have been eating it; a random sample would mean that each eater had an equal likelihood of being questioned.

Rapid Estimate of Adult Literacy in Medicine (REALM) A test developed by Terry Davis and colleagues in 1991 to test the ability of an adult to pronounce a list of sixty six medical words of increasing complexity. It is used to assess *health literacy*. See also *Test of Functional Health Literacy in Adults*.

RAPs Radiologists, anesthesiologists, and pathologists. The acronym came into use with efforts in the 1987 federal budget to include payment for these three specialists in the DRG (prospective payment system (PPS)) payments to hospitals rather than paying the physicians directly, as was previously done.

rate (charge) A financial term referring to a hospital or other institution's charges. Typically rates are "fixed" in that they are for specified services, and the same rate is charged to all individuals or to purchasers of a given class (such as Medicare patients). For example, a hotel could have different rates for senior citizens, commercial travelers, and the general public.

blended rate A term used in the prospective payment system (PPS) of Medicare to designate a rate that is formed by combining the hospital-specific rate and the federal Medicare rate.

case rate A fixed charge covering a single procedure.

hospital-specific rate A term used in the Medicare prospective payment system (PPS) in the computation of the hospital's payment. This rate is "blended" with the federal Medicare rate in certain circumstances.

inclusive rate A prospectively established rate for a day of care that includes all hospital services that may be required, regardless of their nature or cost.

interim rate A temporary rate used in a reimbursement system that periodically makes payments to the hospital on the basis of an estimated figure. The rate is subsequently adjusted retrospectively to reflect actual expenses: additional payments are made to the hospital or the hospital refunds part of the payment it received, and corrections are made to future rates as appropriate. Using an interim rate provides operating cash for the hospital in a "retrospective reimbursement" payment system, where payment is based on actual costs as determined at the end of the fiscal period.

per diem rate A rate established by dividing total costs (plus a percentage for excess of income over expenses) by the total number of inpatient days of care for the same period. Thus the per diem rate is the same for each patient, regardless of the patient's illness, its severity, or the diagnostic or therapeutic measures required.

room rate Same as "daily service charge": the dollar amount the hospital charges for one day of inpatient care for "room and board" and basic nursing and hospital care. The term is not used when, for example, an inclusive rate system is employed because, in that case, the daily rate includes more than these items.

rural rate A type of rate computed by Medicare for hospitals it classifies as rural.

urban rate A type of rate computed by Medicare for hospitals it classifies as urban.

rate (ratio) A ratio or proportion, often expressed as a percentage (per 100), but which may also be expressed per 1,000, per 10,000, per 100,000, or even per million. These "per" numbers are called the "base." Thus a rate expressed per 100,000 is said to have 100,000 as the base. The base chosen is usually large enough to ensure that the rate will be expressed in whole numbers; the more rare the event, the larger the base chosen. A death rate of 7 per 10,000 is easier to understand than a rate of 0.07% (although both actually give the same information).

bed turnover rate The average number of times during a given period of time, ordinarily a year, that a change of occupants occurs in a hospital bed that is normally in use. For example, if the average stay were five days, the bed would have a bed turnover rate of 73 (365 divided by 5).

death rate See separate listing under "D."

infection rate The number of patients developing infections divided by the number of patients at risk (see *risk (health)*), usually expressed as a percentage (by multiplying by 100). Many different infection rates are used, depending on the group of patients at risk. For example, hospitals calculate postoperative infection rates, infection rates for various units of the hospital, and the like.

morbidity rate The number of occurrences of a particular disease, per year, within a certain population. See also *morbidity*.

mortality rate See *death rate* under "D."

occupancy rate The ratio between occupied and available beds, expressed as a percentage. The rate is calculated by dividing the average number of beds occupied for a given time period by the average number of beds available for that same time period (and multiplying by 100 to create the percentage). Sometimes the term "occupancy" alone is used.

readmission rate A statistic showing the proportion of a hospital's patients (or of a given class of patients) who enter the hospital a second (or subsequent) time within a given interval after discharge. This statistic is sometimes used to give, for example, an estimate as to whether the initial hospitalizations were of sufficient duration, on the theory that patients discharged prematurely will be readmitted more frequently than those with an adequately long initial stay.

There is no standard formula for this statistic. Therefore, the compiler of the statistic should (1) give the interval from the prior discharge in which a subsequent admission is to be classed as a "readmission," (2) state whether the readmission was for a condition related to the previous admission (for the purpose of the example above, only related readmissions should be included), and (3) give the time period over which the initial discharges took place. It usually is not feasible for one hospital to obtain information on admissions from other hospitals, so the readmission rate is likely to underestimate the frequency with which patients return to a hospital for further care (in other words, a patient discharged from one hospital may be soon thereafter admitted to another, rather than readmitted to the first hospital).

rate setting A process of regulation of hospital charges (see *rate (charge)*) by an external agency that sets the rates for the institution.

rating The determination, by an actuary, of the healthcare *risk (actuarial)* for a given group in order to establish the insurance premium to be charged.

community rating Establishment of insurance or health plan premiums on the basis of the average healthcare demands of an entire community (or enrolled population), so that all individuals in the community pay the same premium. A person's sex, age, or physical condition is not allowed to raise the premium, so there is no financial penalty for having a history of illness. Many states require HMOs to use community rating in setting their premiums. The alternative is *experience rating* (see below).

adjusted community rating (ACR) A way of setting group rates for the next year based on the actual experience of a group (enrolled population) during the past year. The average use of services for all members is used to predict the future use by the group. This adjustment factor is applied to the basic community rates, yielding the adjusted community rates. This method is used by many managed care plans to set premiums at a level predicted to be sufficient to cover the costs of the group's use of services the following year. However, after the rate is set, it may not be changed or adjusted retroactively.

community rating by class (CRC) A type of community rating in which prepaid premium rates may vary from group to group based on demographic "class" differences, such as age, sex, marital status, or the like. All enrollees in the same class, however, must receive the same rates, no matter which group they belong to. Using this method of rate setting preserves the feature of not penalizing those with a history of illness, but yet accounts for the fact that age, for instance, is related to the amount of health services required.

experience rating Establishment of insurance or health plan premiums on the basis of an actuarial analysis of the sex and age composition of the group, type of industry, and other factors, which are used to set the initial premiums. Experience rating calls for lower premiums for healthier subsets of the population and higher for subsets, such as the elderly, who require more care. In subsequent years, the actual record of the group may be used to modify the rating and the premiums. Often preexisting conditions are taken into the analysis and may be cause for rejection of enrollment of certain individuals. Actuarial analyses would, for example, give weights to sex and age: A preponderance of young males would point to a lower rate than females because of the lower obstetric exposure, but this would be countered by the higher accidental injury rates for males. Actuarial analysis is a complicated science. Experience rating is, of course, sought by employers of young, healthy individuals. The result is that the remainder of a given population, with poorer experience, pays more.

rating band The range of difference in insurance premiums for a specific class of individuals. Some healthcare reform proposals have required that such bands be eliminated, that is, all insurers must adopt the same rate for a given class of individuals.

ratio A value obtained by dividing one number (the numerator) by another (the denominator). See also *proportion*.

cost-benefit ratio See *cost-benefit analysis* under *cost-analysis*.

cost-to-charge ratio (CCR) A term used in finance, which shows whether a charge for a given product or service is set so that it covers the cost. A ratio of 1.0 means that the cost and charge are identical; a ratio greater than 1.0 means that the charge does not recover the cost, and a ratio less than 1.0 means that the charge exceeds the cost. See also *ratio of costs to charges*.

current ratio A financial term used to express liquidity. It is the ratio of *current assets* (see under *asset*) to *current liabilities* (see under *liability (financial)*). A ratio of 2:1 or higher is considered good.

debt ratio Total debt divided by total assets.

quick ratio The ratio of cash plus accounts receivable to current liabilities. This differs from the current ratio in that inventories are not included in the quick ratio (because they may not easily be convertible into cash in order to meet short-term obligations). A good ratio would be 1:1.

rationing A process of withholding goods or services when they are in short supply (see also *distributive justice*). Rationing of health care is, of course, in one sense always in effect, because it is not possible to provide all the care that has been proven effective to all the individuals who might benefit from it. In the climate of healthcare reform, discussion revolves around the problem of deciding the basis on which the limited financial and other resources will be allocated—on who will get what care there is. One method of rationing is financial: When the money runs out the care stops. This is "first-come first-served." Another rationing method is to identify certain groups of patients, such as Medicare and Medicaid patients, as eligible for the benefits. Other methods have been proposed, such as cutting benefits off on the basis of age. For an example of explicit rationing, see *Oregon Health Plan*.

ratio of costs to charges (RCC) A method of estimating costs in accounting. There is generally a desire that charges for health care reflect the costs of that care. This is fairly easy to achieve globally, that is, the total costs for a hospital, say, for a year can be ascertained and the charges or reimbursement can be matched to those costs. It is also easy to learn the total costs and the total charges for a revenue-producing department, such as radiology. Typically, the total charges exceed the total costs, and the ratio between these two figures is easily obtained.

Because it may be virtually impossible (or far more costly than can be justified) to find the actual costs of specific procedures and services, such as the cost of a chest x-ray, an approximation is made. Under the RCC approach, this is done by simply multiplying the charge for the procedure by the cost/charge ratio for the department, and using the resulting dollar amount as an estimate of the cost of the procedure. For example, if the total costs for the department are $100,000 and the total charges are $200,000, the ratio, $100,000/$200,000, is 0.5. Applying the RCC method, then, all charges would be multiplied by this ratio, and a chest x-ray, say, for which there is a $50 charge would be considered to have a $25 cost.

RBNI See *reported but not incurred*.

RBRVS See *resource-based relative value scale* under *relative value scale*.

RBRVU Resource-based relative value unit. See *Omnibus Budget Reconciliation Act of 1989* and *resource-based relative value scale* (under *relative value scale*).

RCB See *Recognized Certification Body*.

RCC See *Radiology Certified Coder*, under *coding specialist*, and *ratio of costs to charges*.

RCIS See *Registered Cardiovascular Invasive Specialist* under *cardiovascular technologist*.

RCS See *Registered Cardiac Sonographer* under *diagnostic medical sonographer*.

RCT See *Registered Care Technologist*.

RCVT Registered Cardiovascular Technologist. See *cardiovascular technologist*.

RD See *Registered Dietitian* under *dietitian*.

RDA See *Registered Dental Assistant* under *dental assistant*.

RD,BC-ADM Registered Dietitian, Board Certified—Advanced Diabetes Management. See *Advanced Diabetes Management Certification* under *diabetes management*.

RDCS See *Registered Diagnostic Cardiac Sonographer* under *diagnostic medical sonographer*.

RDH See *Registered Dental Hygienist* under *dental hygienist*.

RDMS See *Registered Diagnostic Medical Sonographer* under *diagnostic medical sonographer*.

RDRG See *Refined DRG* under *DRG*.

RDT See *Registered Drama Therapist* under *drama therapist*.

Read Codes See *Clinical Terms Version 3*.

readmission A second (or later) admission of a patient to a facility. Sometimes the term is used in a manner that implies that the readmission is for further treatment for the condition occasioning the previous admission, because of recurrence of the problem or failure of completion of care; however, this inference is not warranted. See *readmission rate* under *rate*.

REALM See *Rapid Estimate of Adult Literacy in Medicine*.

real time The time in which something is actually happening, rather than a delayed response. The term is frequently used in the computer context. A computer may analyze information and give back a report of what happened (last week, for instance), or it may tell what is happening exactly at this moment. If a computer can analyze and respond immediately to an event, it is said to be operating "in real time."

A real-time computer system, with the appropriate supporting software, can provide "instant" inventory control or give warning of immediate danger, as might be the case with a drug prescription error, thus preventing an adverse drug event (ADE). A physician typing in a prescription, for example, would receive an immediate warning if a patient had a contraindication for that drug. See also *computerized physician order entry* and *knowledge-based management*.

The implications of real-time computing are not limited to keyboarded entries, however. In fact, historically a computer operating in real time had direct inputs from sensors or measuring devices, or even other computers, rather than human input from a keyboard. All kinds of technological devices incorporate computers operating in real time. A pacemaker, which responds in real time to electronic signals from the heart, is an excellent example. Synonyms: real-time, realtime.

Realtime Outbreak and Disease Surveillance (RODS) A research laboratory at the University of Pittsburgh that investigates methods for real-time detection and assessment of disease outbreaks. RODS is home to four large projects that work with health departments to create surveillance systems: RODS software development (open source), the Public Health Data Center (a secure server facility used by public health personnel for surveillance projects), the National Retail Data Monitor (NRDM) (monitors sales of over-the-counter (OTC) healthcare products to identify disease outbreaks as early as possible), and the BioWatch Support Program (a Homeland Security program that guards thirty U.S. cities against possible biological attack). RODS, founded in 1999 by Drs. Rich Tsui, Jeremy Espino, and Michael Wagner, is a collaboration between researchers at the University of Pittsburgh and the Auton Laboratory in Carnegie Mellon University's School of Computer Science. Synonym: RODS Laboratory. **rods.health.pitt.edu**

reappointment The process of formally continuing the medical staff membership of a physician or other health professional, along with specific privileges. After the initial appointment to the staff, reappointment must take place at regular intervals (usually every year or two). During the reappointment process, the performance of the professional is evaluated, so that a proper determination can be made regarding renewal (or increase or decrease) of clinical privileges. If privileges are to be decreased or discontinued, certain due process procedures are required. See also *recredentialing*.

reasonable charge See *customary, prevailing, reasonable charge (or fee)*.

reasonable cost See under *cost*.

rebundling See *outpatient bundling* under *bundling*.

rebuttable presumption A fact that shifts the "burden of proof" from one party to the other in a lawsuit. It has been proposed that if a physician sued for malpractice has followed approved clinical practice guidelines, this would create a legal presumption that the physician was not negligent. Such a presumption may be rebutted by the plaintiff offering additional evidence, but it will be harder for the plaintiff to win in such a case.

receipt A document acknowledging that money or goods have been received.

recessive See *allele*.

reciprocity An agreement among specific states under which one state will grant a license to a physician or other health professional if that person produces evidence that she or he is licensed in any other state that is a party to the agreement. Usually the initial license must have been granted on the basis of an examination, either that of the National Board of Medical Examiners (NBME) or of the state of origin; in other words, a license granted on the basis of reciprocity cannot be used to gain another license by reciprocity. See also *board (credentialing)*.

recoding Placing data (cases, for example) from one classification (scheme) into categories of a second classification (when there is one-to-one correspondence) or by concatenating one or more categories from the first classification into the second, a sort of "compound grouping." Where the groups of the second classification are more specific than or different from those of the first classification, recoding should not be attempted, because no exact recoding is possible; data once coded to a category cannot be "split" without going back to more detailed sources. See *coding (process)*.

Recognized Certification Body (RCB) An organization that has been approved by the Department of Health and Human Services (HHS) to evaluate electronic health records (EHRs). See *Certification Commission for Health Information Technology*.

recombinant DNA (rDNA) See under *DNA*.

record See *database* and *medical record*.

record locator service (RLS) The "white pages" of a health information network, which is queried by authorized providers (and others) to find out what records are available on an individual patient and where they are located. The query includes demographic details on the patient (whatever is available), and the RLS uses a probability-weighted algorithm to identify the patient and locate the records. The RLS may return the query with a request for more data, with a zero response, or with the location(s) of any records found. There is always a risk that the wrong patient will be identified, which may result in a violation of the HIPAA *Privacy Rule*. See also *National Patient Identifier*.

recovery (get money) The money awarded by a court to the successful plaintiff in a lawsuit. The term can also mean the amount of money actually collected.

recovery (get well) Regaining of the condition of health or function that preceded the occurrence of a disease or disability. Used in the context of postoperative care, recovery refers to the period of time immediately following surgery, during which the patient is closely monitored in the recovery room until stabilized. Patients stay in the recovery room until they are ready to be returned to their hospital room (if inpatients) or to go home (if outpatients).

recovery audit contractor (RAC) A private auditing firm contracting with CMS to review Medicare claims of physicians, hospitals, nursing homes, and other providers to find instances in which the government paid too much or too little, and which were not found during the normal claims and review processes. The RAC seeks recovery of any overpayments. If an underpayment is found, the RAC notifies the Medicare Administrative Contractor (MAC) so that the provider can be paid. Required by the Medicare Modernization Act (MMA), this is a pilot project in three states—California, Florida, and New York—initiated in 2005, to run through 2008. The RAC gets paid only based on the amounts it recovers for Medicare; thus some have called these firms "bounty hunters."

recovery room A special patient care unit of the hospital used for the monitoring and care of postoperative patients until each patient's condition becomes stable after anesthesia. Synonym: postoperative recovery room.

recreation therapist See *therapeutic recreation specialist*.

recreation therapy See *therapeutic recreation therapy*.

recredentialing Determining and certifying as to the competency of a physician or other professional at some time after the initial determination of his or her qualification for licensure or hospital privileges. Recredentialing is required at periodic intervals in some hospitals and healthcare organizations. It is also under consideration by several states as a procedure to be followed at the time of renewal of licenses (most states simply require payment of a fee). As being discussed with regard to renewal of license, "recredentialing" does not rely on evidence of meeting continuing education requirements or written examination as to knowledge. The focus is on the physician's actual performance. Under consideration are computer-based "clinical" testing and the use of hospital-quality review records. In the case of physicians whose practice is entirely in their offices, an office audit system (now used in Canada) is under consideration. See also *credentialing*, *investigation*, and *reappointment*.

recruitment See *physician recruitment*.

recuse To reject or challenge an individual's qualification to serve in a given capacity, usually on the basis of conflict of interest or known bias. Usually used with respect to a judge or juror. Individuals may also recuse themselves voluntarily, to avoid the appearance of impropriety.

Red Cross See *American Red Cross*.

Redefining Progress A nonprofit public-policy and research organization in San Francisco committed to developing solutions that help people, protect the environment, and grow the economy, with a focus on sustainability. One of its efforts is an alternate way to measure the economic condition of the nation; see *genuine progress indicator*. www.rprogress.org

redlining See *blacklisting*.

R. EEG T. See *Registered Electroencephalographic Technologist* under *electroencephalographic technologist*.

reengineering healthcare A term sometimes used to describe the process of studying various aspects of health care and making changes in organization, procedures, or resources with the aim of increasing efficiency and/or effectiveness.

Reference Information Model (RIM) The definitive statement of *HL7* version 3 semantics, describing all aspects of the clinical care process, including administration, scheduling, and billing. The RIM is considered an improvement over the HL7 2.x standards, including the introduction of "conformance profiles," which require less custom programming. See also *Patient Record Architecture*.

reference point A measurement against which something can be compared to evaluate whether a desired performance or result has been achieved. Synonym: reference level. See *benchmark* and *indicator*.

referral The sending of a patient by one physician (the referring physician) to another physician (or some other resource) either for consultation or for care. Specialist care (secondary care) is ordinarily on referral from a primary care physician or another specialist. Care of the patient is given back to the referring physician if the referral was for consultation or where the specialist has completed the care required; otherwise the patient is transferred to the specialist, who takes over responsibility for the patient.

For example, if a primary care physician refers a patient suspected of having appendicitis to a surgeon (and the surgeon also diagnoses appendicitis), the surgeon customarily performs the appendectomy and returns the patient to the referring physician afterward. However, if a general internist refers a problem diabetic patient to an endocrinologist (specialist in diabetes and other endocrine diseases), the referral might result in the permanent transfer of the patient.

referral center A rural hospital classified as such by the federal government, for purposes of reimbursement under the Medicare prospective payment system (PPS).

referral site See *distant site*.

regimen A planned course of treatment or therapy (including such components as diet, drugs, and exercise) designed to achieve a specific result. The more complete phrase would be "therapeutic regimen"—the plan laid out for treatment of the patient.

regional health information network (RHIN) See r*egional health information organization*.

regional health information organization (RHIO) A term describing a joint effort among hospitals, physicians, other providers, health plans, pharmacies, public health entities, and others in a specific area to link together electronically to share patient information (electronic health records) in an effort to enhance patient care and increase economies. Some view RHIOs as the "building blocks" of the Nationwide Health Information Network (NHIN). The collaborative efforts span whole communities, states, and even multi-state regions. Unlike with earlier efforts (such as the community health information network (CHIN)), much of the needed technological infrastructure now exists (broadband Internet access, electronic medical records in more physicians' offices, wireless capability in hospitals to permit PDA (personal digital assistant) and laptop use), and there is increasing pressure to have the NHIN in place: Health information technology has been shown to reduce costs and promote patient safety and health. This means that there is more funding and support available for the regional efforts.

In the mid 2000s, there were over 100 RHIOs. One example is the California Regional Health Information Organization (CalRHIO), **www.calrhio.org**. Some RHIOs are funded by the federal government, whereas others are supported by private industry or state governments. RHIO has no "official" definition, but many of these efforts call themselves this. Synonyms: local health information infrastructure (LHII), health information exchange (HIE), regional health information network (RHIN). See also *community-wide health information system*.

registered A health professional who has met the requirements of a governmental or nongovernmental agency and is recorded on an official roster ("registry"). A qualified professional may be registered or certified, or both, depending upon the profession's requirements. Sometimes the registry is an organization rather than an agency, and the credential "registered" means the same as certified; see, for example, *Registered Health Information Technician* under *health information technician*.

Registered Care Technologist (RCT) A category of caregiver proposed by the American Medical Association (AMA) in 1988 in an effort to alleviate the nursing shortage. RCTs would have been required to have little education before entering a brief training program, after which they would have been "registered under an arm of the state medical board" (not the state nursing board) and would have given "technical" bedside care under the supervision of the physician.

registered nurse (RN) See under *nurse*.

registrar (admissions) See *admitting officer*.

registrar (government) A governmental official whose duty is to keep official records. There are a number of kinds of registrars keeping, for example, vital statistics such as births, deaths, marriages, and divorces, and legal documents such as deeds.

registration (credentials) A process established by a governmental or nongovernmental agency under which individuals meeting the agency's requirements can be recorded on an official roster ("registry") and can use "registered" ("registered nurse," for example) as a credential with the public and with their employment.

Registration is generally the least restrictive form of state regulation. As with *certification (credential)*, unregistered persons are usually permitted to practice the profession. Typically, exams are not given and enforcement of the registration requirement is minimal (registered nurse is a notable exception). See also *health professional* and *licensure*.

Registration is used in some contexts to denote that a health professional has met certain requirements and passed an examination to be credentialed in a specialty area. See, for example, *Registered Cardiac Sonographer* under *diagnostic medical sonographer*. In this sense, it essentially has the same purpose as certification.

registration (data) The recording of patient information in a *registry (data)*, such as a cancer, trauma, or tuberculosis registry.

registration (vital records) The official recording of births, deaths, marriages, and divorces, with maintenance of permanent records.

registry (credentials) An official roster, maintained by a governmental or nongovernmental agency, of individuals who have met the requirements set up by the agency as to qualifications (both initial, and, in some cases, continuing) that permit *registration (credentials)*. A person may use his or her listing on the registry as a credential to display to the public as, for example, in "Registered Dietitian."

registry (data) A central agency where data from an institution or specific geographic area can be collected and made available for study and, in the healthcare field, sometimes made available for assisting in patient care management. An illustration of the latter use is in sending reminders to patients when follow-up examinations are scheduled (for example, in the case of tumors).

cancer registry A repository of data on patients with cancers and other tumors. The cancer registry is used to develop statistics on the incidence and prevalence of cancer, relate data on the tumors to the characteristics of patients (such as age, sex, racial background, or other diseases), study relationships with patients' environment, attempt to evaluate therapy, and, in some instances, help keep the patients under treatment. The establishment and operation of tumor registries have been a special interest of the American College of Surgeons (ACS). Most states have cancer registries. Data from these are collected by the National Program of Cancer Registries (NPCR), administered by the Centers for Disease Control and Prevention (CDC), which maintains data on the occurrence of cancer; the type, extent, and location of the cancer; and the type of initial treatment. Synonym: tumor registry.

trauma registry A repository of data on trauma patients, including such information as the external causes of the trauma, diagnoses, treatment, and outcome, and demographic data about the patients.

tumor registry See *cancer registry*, above.

regression A statistical method used to measure and express the effect one variable, the "independent variable," has on another variable, the "dependent variable." A physician may want to increase the concentration of a drug in a patient's blood. The question: If the physician doubles the dose of a given drug (the dosage of the drug is the independent variable, because it can be controlled), will it double the concentration of the drug (the dependent variable) in the patient's blood, or will it less than double, and will the effects vary from patient to patient?

Regression is used to help answer this question. A collection of data on drug dosages (related to patients' weights, for example) and the same patients' blood concentrations of the drug is analyzed by an appropriate regression method. The analysis will tell the relationship between doses and blood levels—not only the probable increases (or decreases, which could happen) in proportion to dosage, but also the ranges of response that are likely to occur.

A common form of regression is a **linear regression**, in which the "model" chosen for the analysis is a linear equation.

regularly maintained beds See *bed capacity*.

regulation (corporate) A mandate adopted by a corporation or association as part of its internal *rules and regulations*. This type of regulation is seldom spoken of separate from the phrase "rules and regulations" of the corporation, and in fact is indistinguishable from a rule.

regulation (governmental) See *rule*.

rehabilitation Efforts to assist an individual to achieve and maintain her or his optimal level of function, self-care, and independence, after or in correction of a disability. The disability may be physical, mental, or emotional. See also *vision rehabilitation therapy*.

cognitive rehabilitation Therapy for brain-injured individuals to help restore cognitive functions—perception, memory, thinking, and problem solving—when possible, and to compensate for impaired functions that cannot be restored. Cognitive rehabilitation is provided by psychologists, neuropsychologists, speech/language pathologists, occupational therapists, and other healthcare professionals.

Rehabilitation Act of 1973 Federal legislation that prohibits discrimination against a qualified individual based solely on his or her disability. The act applies only to institutions that receive federal funds. This act was significantly expanded by the *Americans with Disabilities Act (ADA)*. 29 U.S.C. § 794 (2005).

rehabilitation counselor A health professional who advises disabled individuals and assists them to achieve and maintain an optimal level of self-care and independence.

    Certified Rehabilitation Counselor (CRC) A rehabilitation counselor who has met the requirements of the Commission on Rehabilitation Counselor Certification (CRCC). **www.crccertification.com**

    vocational rehabilitation counselor (VRC) A person who counsels disabled individuals with respect to vocations and vocational training in order to best fit together the individual and a vocation suitable to his or her physical, mental, and emotional abilities.

rehabilitation nursing The area of nursing focusing on the rehabilitation needs of individuals with disabling injuries or chronic illnesses.

    Certified Rehabilitation Registered Nurse (CRRN) A specialist in rehabilitation nursing who has passed an examination of the Rehabilitation Nursing Certification Board (RNCB). **www.rehabnurse.org**

rehabilitation potential Realistic goals for the individual patient with respect to (1) management of the patient's specific health problems and (2) achievement of self-care, independence, and emotional well-being. These goals are set and stated by the attending physician for each patient at the time of admission to a rehabilitation hospital or long-term care facility (LTCF).

rehabilitation teaching (RT) See *vision rehabilitation therapy*.

rehabilitative care Coordinated rehabilitation care, provided under the supervision of a physician.

rehabilitative nursing care A nursing care program directed at assisting each long-term care patient to achieve and maintain an optimal level of self-care and independence.

Reiki A method for relaxation, stress reduction, and healing by placing hands upon the person to be treated with the intent to direct energy to flow to and within the patient. The word "Reiki" means "life force energy."

reimbursement The payment to a hospital or other provider, after the fact, of an amount equal to the provider's expenses in providing a given service or product. The trend is away from such a "blank check" approach and toward *prospective pricing*, that is, toward agreement in advance as to the amount that will be paid for the service or product in question.

    cost-based reimbursement Payment of all allowable costs incurred in the provision of care. The term "allowable" refers to the terms of the contract under which care is furnished.

    prospective reimbursement A term sometimes used, incorrectly, instead of prospective pricing or prospective payment. See *prospective payment system*. Also, "prospective reimbursement" is sometimes used to describe the prospectively estimated amount to be paid a hospital on a current schedule so that it will have operating cash, with the understanding that adjustments will be made later in the light of actual operating cost data. The concept is similar to that of the *periodic interim payment (PIP)*.

    retroactive reimbursement Additional payment to a provider for costs not considered at the time of original reimbursement.

    retrospective reimbursement Payment based on actual costs as determined at the end of the fiscal period. See also *retrospective rate derivation*.

    third-party reimbursement (TPR) Payment for healthcare services by a third-party payer, such as an insurance company.

reimbursement specialist A person who is involved with working out the terms and details of reimbursement systems with third-party payers. Sometimes just refers to a person who prepares the statements and other materials needed to obtain reimbursement from third-party payers and insurers for services, and who maintains the related records. May also be called an insurance clerk.

reinsurance See under *insurance*.

relational database See *database management system*.

relative value scale (RVS) A numerical system (scale) designed to permit comparisons of the resources needed (or appropriate prices) for various units of service. The RVS is the compiled table of the relative value units (RVUs) for all the objects in the class for which it is developed.

An RVS takes into account labor, skill, supplies, equipment, space, and other costs to create an aggregate cost for each procedure or other unit of service. The aggregate cost is converted into the RVU of the procedure or service by relating it to the cost of a procedure or service selected as the "base unit." For example, the developer of the RVS for laboratory work might decide to use the cost of a red blood cell count as the base unit. Its actual cost might be $5, but, as the base, its RVU would arbitrarily be set at 1.0. If a blood sugar estimation, then, actually cost $25, it would have an RVU value of 5.0 ($25 divided by $5). If a urinalysis cost $3, it would have an RVU of 0.6.

resource-based relative value scale (RBRVS) A method of determining physicians' fees (for services provided under Medicare) based on the time, training, skill, and other factors required to deliver various services. The term came into use in 1988 upon release of the report of a study commissioned by the Department of Health and Human Services (HHS) and carried out under the direction of Harvard economist William Hsiao, PhD. It became law with the passage of the Omnibus Budget Reconciliation Act of 1989. Previously, physician payment for Medicare services had been based on *customary, prevailing, reasonable charges (CPR)*. See a full discussion of RBRVS in context under *Omnibus Budget Reconciliation Act of 1989*.

relative value unit (RVU) The numerical value given to each procedure or other unit of service in a *relative value scale*.

release A giving up of a legal claim or right, to the person against whom the claim could have been asserted. For example, when a malpractice case is settled, the injured patient signs a release freeing the physician and hospital from any further liability for the injury, in exchange for the money paid in the settlement.

release of information (ROI) Also known as "disclosure," an action by a healthcare provider or related party that causes any information about a patient to be given to another, whether a third party or not. Originally focused on making available copies of a patient's medical record, ROI now covers virtually any information known about the patient by anyone involved with the patient's care.

Typically no information about a patient may be released without the patient's authorization, unless it's immediately necessary for the patient's care (as in a medical emergency in which the patient is incapacitated). Legal rules pertaining to authorization and exceptions are often defined by state law, and may be similar to those applying to informed consent. HIPAA has specific rules governing the release of *protected health information (PHI)* (see *Privacy Rule*).

reliability The degree of accuracy of results over a period of time, a number of trials, or among different observers or investigators. Also, the probability that a system will perform its function properly for a given period of time.

interrater reliability The degree of agreement among different persons (raters) expressing judgments (ratings) on the same data or observations.

intrarater reliability The degree of agreement among judgments (ratings) by the same person (rater) made on the same data or on the same observations at different times.

relief What is sought by a plaintiff in a lawsuit; usually whatever it is that would make the plaintiff "whole" or at least compensate for the injury. For example, in a malpractice suit the plaintiff may ask for money; a physician suing a hospital for denial of privileges may ask that her or his privileges be reinstated. The term "relief" may also refer to that which has been granted by the court, or in general to the fact that the plaintiff won or lost the suit ("relief was denied"). See also *remedy*.

remediation The process of testing an organization's privacy and electronic transaction policies and systems to ensure compliance with *HIPAA* requirements.

remedy In law, something a court (or a statute) grants to redress a wrong or make an injured person whole. The most common remedy is money. Another, less common remedy is an injunction (ordering the defendant to do something or stop doing something). See also *relief*.

    exclusive remedy A remedy provided by law that precludes a person from trying to obtain any kind of compensation other than that provided by the law. An example is workers' compensation, which is the exclusive remedy for on-the-job injuries; an injured worker who is entitled to receive workers' compensation benefits may not sue his or her employer for damages. But see also *dual injury doctrine*.

remote medical diagnosis (RMD) See *telemedicine*.

remote site See *originating site*.

renal Having to do with the kidneys.

renal dialysis See under *dialysis*.

renal dialysis unit See *hemodialysis unit*.

reportable event See *serious reportable event*.

report card A generic term for statements pertaining to the performance of health professionals and providers. Report cards are being issued increasingly by healthcare institutions, regulatory agencies, insurers, managed care organizations, accrediting bodies, and others, giving information such as healthcare outcomes, costs, charges, severity of illness of patients, intensity of services, institution staffing, medical staff composition, patient satisfaction, provision of preventive services, and other data. Report cards may be designed for such purposes as internal information, for employers, or for release to the public. See *Hospital Compare* and *Quality Reports*.

reported but not incurred (RBNI) An obligation of a managed care plan under its benefit structure that is planned and perhaps scheduled, and that has been reported to the plan, but that has not been provided to the patient. An example would be surgery scheduled for a future date. Distinguish from *incurred but not reported*.

R. EP T. See *Registered Evoked Potential Technologist* under *evoked potential technologist*.

required request law A law that requires hospitals to develop programs for asking families of deceased patients to donate the organs of the deceased for transplantation. Synonym: routine inquiry law.

research study See *clinical trial*.

reserve accounts Earnings retained for a specific purpose.

reserved powers Generally, a reservation is a right that is both created and preserved (retained) by the grantor. In structuring a corporation, the bylaws may reserve certain corporate decisions or actions to be made by a shareholder, possibly the parent corporation. These reservations can be termed as the reserved powers of the parent corporation. These decisions are usually major, for example whether to sell large amounts of the corporate property or whether to merge with another corporation.

residency A program in a hospital or other healthcare institution or organization that has been approved for providing medical or other professional training by allowing the individual in training to perform actual duties under supervision. In medicine, a formal *Residency Review Committee* grants approval to *medical residencies* (see below) that meet established standards. *Administrative residencies* (see below) need only be acceptable to the institution in which the trainee (administrative resident) is enrolled.

administrative residency A position in a healthcare organization or institution where a student in a healthcare administration education program may obtain a practical training phase of his or her education. Upon completion of the administrative residency training, the student returns to the educational institution for further training. The student may be enrolled in the educational institution at the undergraduate or graduate level.

medical residency A generic term that may be used for a residency providing training for graduate physicians in any medical specialty. The term may also be used specifically for a residency in internal medicine. Residency programs are approved in the United States by the Accreditation Council for Graduate Medical Education (ACGME) and in Canada by the Royal College of Physicians and Surgeons of Canada.

Residency Review Committee (RRC) A national committee of experts that reviews individual clinical training programs in medical specialties (such as internal medicine, surgery, or psychiatry) for determination of quality. RRCs submit recommendations for accreditation of the programs to the Accreditation Council for Continuing Medical Education (ACCME).

resident (patient) A patient residing in a long-term care institution.

long-term resident A term sometimes applied to a patient who is not acutely ill, but who needs hospital care.

resident (trainee) An individual undergoing training by carrying out actual duties under supervision in a residency program in an institution or organization.

administrative resident A student in an *administrative residency* (see under *residency*) program.

medical resident A resident physician who is specializing in internal medicine.

medical specialty resident A resident physician in training in a medical specialty.

surgical resident A resident physician who is undergoing training in a surgical specialty.

Resident Assessment Instrument (RAI) A tool to evaluate the functional status and health of residents of skilled nursing facilities (SNFs), required for certification by CMS for Medicare and Medicaid patients. The **Minimum Data Set (MDS)** provides the core information about the patient for this assessment. The MDS includes such elements as demographics and patient history, cognitive status, communication/hearing, vision, mood/ behavior patterns, psychosocial well-being, physical functioning, continence, disease diagnoses, health conditions, medications, nutritional and dental status, skin condition, activity patterns, special treatments and procedures, and discharge potential. (The full name for MDS is Minimum Data Set for Nursing Facility Resident Assessment and Care Screening.)

An RAI must be completed for each resident and serves as the foundation for a plan to help the resident achieve optimal functioning and well-being. The RAI was initiated by the Nursing Home Reform Act (NHRA) in 1987. CMS also requires a similar assessment for inpatients of inpatient rehabilitation facilities (IRFs); this is called the IRF-RAI.

residential treatment center (RTC) A term generally used for residential centers that provide mental health treatment.

resident valet (RV) A person working in a long-term care facility (paid or volunteer) who assists residents with dining, housekeeping, laundry, and so forth.

res ipsa loquitur "The thing speaks for itself." A legal doctrine that states that a plaintiff (person filing suit) does not have to prove negligence in a specific factual situation; rather, negligence may be presumed from the facts that are proved, and it is up to the defendant to prove that she or he was not negligent. Res ipsa loquitur is applied when it is obvious that there was negligence (the injury could not have been caused without someone's negligence), but the knowledge regarding the negligent act is solely within the control of the defendant(s). An example is the leaving of a sponge in a surgical patient: The unconscious patient could not possibly know who left it there, but there is no doubt that the act was negligent.

It should be noted that the doctrine of res ipsa loquitur varies a great deal among legal jurisdictions, and that not all courts will permit its application. For example, some courts hold that the doctrine does not apply if more than one person could have committed the negligent act.

resistant bacteria See under *bacteria*.

Resource and Patient Management System (RPMS) An electronic health record (EHR) and practice management system (PMS) developed and used by the Indian Health Service (IHS). More than fifty software applications are incorporated; many components are based on *VistA*. The RPMS software is in the public domain.

resource-based relative value scale (RBRVS) See under *relative value scale*.

resource-based relative value unit (RBRVU) See *Omnibus Budget Reconciliation Act of 1989* and *resource-based relative value scale* (under *relative value scale*).

Resource Mothers Development Project (RMDP) Former name of *MotherNet*.

Resource Utilization Groups (RUGs) A patient classification system (similar to DRGs for inpatients) used for skilled nursing facility patients for reimbursement under the Medicare prospective payment system.

respirator A machine that performs or assists in the function of breathing for a patient.

respiratory arrest The cessation of breathing.

respiratory diseases unit A patient care unit of the hospital set aside for the care of inpatients with respiratory (breathing) problems.

respiratory therapist A health professional trained to provide respiratory therapy services. Requires an associate or bachelor's degree and, in most states, licensure.

    Certified Respiratory Therapist (CRT) A respiratory therapist who has passed the entry-level examination of the National Board for Respiratory Care (NBRC). **www.nbrc.org**

    Neonatal/Pediatric Respiratory Care Specialist (CRT-NPS or RRT-NPS) A respiratory therapist specially trained to work with newborns and children. Must be a CRT or RRT and pass a special examination of the National Board for Respiratory Care (NBRC). **www.nbrc.org**

    Registered Respiratory Therapist (RRT) An experienced Certified Respiratory Therapist (CRT) who meets additional requirements and has passed advanced examinations of the National Board for Respiratory Care (NBRC). **www.nbrc.org**

respiratory therapy (RT) Evaluation and treatment of respiratory (breathing) problems. Therapies may include administration of oxygen, treatments to drain the chest of mucus, and the use of breathing exercises.

respiratory therapy assistant (RTA) A health professional who helps a respiratory therapist by maintaining and transporting equipment, transporting patients, teaching, and so forth. Duties may or may not overlap those of the respiratory therapy technician, depending on knowledge and skills.

respiratory therapy technician (RTT) A health professional who assists the respiratory therapist by preparing and operating equipment; setting controls to regulate the flow of oxygen, gases, and so forth; monitoring patients during treatment; and teaching patients how to use the equipment at home if necessary.

respite care Short-term care (usually a few days) for a long-term care patient in order to provide a respite (rest and change) for those who have been caring for the patient, usually the patient's family. Respite care may involve hospitalization of the patient, or provision of round-the-clock care at home or in a nursing home as needed.

respondeat superior A legal doctrine that makes an employer liable for the negligent acts of its employees, even though the employer was itself not negligent. For the doctrine to apply, the employee must have been acting within the scope of his or her employment—a frequently complex legal determination all by itself. Similarly, a principal is liable for the acts of its agent. Note that this is only a way to also hold the employer liable; it does not necessarily absolve the employee from responsibility for his or her own actions. "Respondeat superior" is Latin for "Let the master answer." See also *captain of the ship doctrine*.

responsible party The individual or organization responsible for placing a patient in a healthcare facility and ensuring that adequate care is given to that patient there. For example, a parent is usually the responsible party in the case of a child; the parent is not only responsible for the child receiving care, but also for the payment for that care. In less formal usage in the hospital, the term "responsible party" is used to mean simply "responsible for payment." Legally, there can be more than one responsible party. For example, one person, such as a guardian, may be authorized to make treatment decisions, while another person may be responsible for payment.

rest home A free-standing facility set up to provide care for patients who are unable to live independently, that is, who need assistance with the activities of daily living (ADLs), and who may need occasional assistance from a professional nurse. Such nursing service is obtained from a visiting nurse. Regulations usually apply the designation of a rest home to a facility with over, say, six beds, but as a practical matter it is usually not economical to operate a rest home with fewer than thirty or forty beds. A facility providing similar service to a smaller number of persons may be called (and licensed as) a "family care home" (FCH) or "adult foster home." Rest home was formerly called "custodial care home."

rest home care See under *nursing care*.

restriction endonuclease An enzyme used to cut a DNA molecule. A number of these enzymes are available to cut at specific locations in the DNA molecule. Synonym: restriction enzyme.

restrictive covenant See *covenant not to compete*.

restructuring Reorganization of a corporation (a hospital, for example) in order better to handle new functions and enterprises. The restructuring may involve the creation of several corporations where there was only one, consolidation or merger of corporations, establishment of foundations, and the like. Restructuring is often essential to achieve effective diversification.

RESTT See *respiratory therapy technician*.

resuscitate To restore vital functions after the person is apparently dead, for example, to restart the heart. See also *life support*.

resuscitation See *cardiopulmonary resuscitation*.

retainer practice See *concierge physician practice*.

retinal angiography A procedure that involves injecting dye into a patient's arm, then photographing the retina using special cameras and colors of light as the dye travels through its vessels.

   Certified Retinal Angiographer (CRA) A health professional specializing in *ophthalmic photography*, who has been certified in retinal angiography and fundus (inner lining of the eye) photography by the Ophthalmic Photographers' Society (OPS). **www.opsweb.org**

retirement center A facility that provides social activities to senior citizens, usually retired persons, who do not require health care. The provision of housing is not required for an institution or organization to be called a retirement center. A retirement center may furnish housing and may also have acute hospital and long-term care facilities, or it may arrange for acute and long-term care through affiliated institutions.

retroactive date The date stipulated in a *claims-made coverage* policy (see under *insurance coverage*) as the earliest date an event may occur and be covered under that particular claims-made policy. For example, a policy for calendar year 1990 with a retroactive date of January 1, 1985, would cover an event occurring anytime on or after January 1, 1985, if the claim based on that event is made during 1990.

retrospective rate derivation A method of determining the cost for health insurance premiums that divides the risk between the insurance provider and the insurance purchaser.

The purchaser is typically an employer who purchases such coverage for its employees as a group. Although the two parties negotiate the percentages in advance, the actual amounts paid in premiums depend on the actual healthcare costs incurred by the group over a previous period, hence the "retrospective" aspect. Sometimes simply referred to as "retro," although it shouldn't be confused with going back to the 1970s when used in this way.

retrovirus A type of virus with certain unique genetic properties, specifically the ability to "reverse copy" its genome into a host cell's chromosome. The best known of this class of virus is the human immunodeficiency virus (HIV), which causes AIDS. (The family of viruses was named "retro" because they contain an enzyme called "reverse transcriptase.")

revenue An increase in an organization's assets or a decrease in its liabilities during an accounting period. This is in contrast with income, which refers to money earned during an accounting period.

marginal revenue The addition to or subtraction from total revenue resulting from the sale of one more or one less unit of service or product.

revenue-producing service A service of the institution for which charges are made directly on the patient's bill, such as use of the operating room.

reverse protocol See under *protocol*.

review The processes of examination and evaluation.

admissions review An evaluation of the appropriateness of the admission of the patient to the hospital. The admissions review determines whether the patient in question was in a condition that warranted use of the hospital, or could (or should) have been treated in some other setting (for example, at home or as an outpatient, or in a hospital more suited to managing his or her problem). Typically, the admissions review is carried out at or shortly after admission.

capital expenditure review (CER) A process carried out by a state agency prior to granting permission to the hospital to incur a capital expenditure.

claims review Retrospective review of hospital claims by a third-party payer in order to determine the: (1) liability of the payer (whether the benefit was included in the contract), (2) eligibility of the beneficiary and the provider, (3) appropriateness of the service, and (4) appropriateness of the amount claimed.

concurrent review Evaluation of medical necessity for admission and appropriateness of services, carried out while the patient is in the hospital (concurrent with the care). The advantage of concurrent review is that if any action (change in the care) is found to be necessary as a finding of the review, it can be taken while the patient is still in the hospital.

continued stay review Concurrent review (review while the patient is in the hospital), conducted at a specified time after admission, for the purpose of determining the appropriateness of continuation of hospital care for the individual patient.

drug utilization review (DUR) See separate listing for *drug utilization review*.

medical services review Retrospective review of the use of services (and failure to use services), for both inpatients and outpatients, with respect to the medical appropriateness of the services and, in some situations, review of whether the services are included in the patient's insurance benefits.

peer review See the separate listing for *peer review*.

preadmission review Evaluation, prior to admission, of the necessity for elective hospitalization for the individual patient in question.

preprocedure review Review of a case prior to the performance of a given procedure in order to determine (1) if the procedure is medically indicated, and (2) if the procedure could equally well be performed in an alternate setting.

private review Utilization review performed on patients whose care is paid for by private sources (sources other than government).

prospective review A term sometimes used to refer to evaluation of a patient's need for hospitalization prior to admission. "Preadmission review" is a better term for this meaning.

Prospective review is also a misnomer for what should be called concurrent review. A third use for the term is a review of the planning for a patient's future treatment, site of care (home, hospital, and so on), and other details.

rate review Review by a regulatory agency of a hospital's budget and financial picture in order to determine the reasonableness of the hospital's proposed rates and rate changes. Rate review is also applied to rates for certain prepayment plans, such as Blue Cross and Blue Shield, depending on state laws.

retrospective review Review after the fact. The term most often refers to a patient care audit (PCA) (see *audit*).

utilization review (UR) See the separate listing for *utilization review*.

RFID See *radio frequency identification*.

Rh See *Rhesus factor*.

RHC See *Rural Health Clinic*.

RHCP See *Rural Health Care Program*.

Rhesus factor (Rh factor) An attribute on the red blood cells of the rhesus monkey that has been found to occur on the red blood cells of certain humans. When it does occur, the person is Rh positive (RH^+); when it is absent, the person is Rh negative (RH^-). This factor provided one of the earliest tests for blood grouping.

rheumatologist A physician who specializes in the diagnosis and treatment of "rheumatism" or "rheumatic disorders," that is, disorders of the joints and related muscles and other structures.

rheumatology The study of rheumatic conditions—pain and other disorders of the joints or other parts of the musculoskeletal system.

RHIA See *Registered Health Information Administrator* under *health information administrator*.

RHIN Regional health information network. See *regional health information organization*.

RHIO See *regional health information organization*.

RHIT See *Registered Health Information Technician* under *health information technician*.

RHN See *rural health network*.

ribonucleic acid (RNA) See under *DNA*.

RICO See *Racketeer Influenced and Corrupt Organizations Act*.

right (legal) See *duty (legal)*.

right of privacy See under *privacy*.

right to die The legal right to refuse life-saving or life-sustaining treatment. A competent adult has the legal right to refuse medical treatment, even if that treatment is essential to sustain life. Some refer to this right as the "right to die." The issue of the right to die arises in the situation where a person has a condition in which the quality of life is so intolerable that death, at least in the belief of that individual (or those responsible for that person), is preferable. If the person is conscious (and mentally competent), he or she may exercise the right to refuse treatment for him- or herself; if he or she is unconscious or otherwise incompetent, others must make the decision for him or her. Serious legal and ethical issues are involved in the latter case. See also *advance directive*, *death with dignity*, *euthanasia*, and *suicide*.

RIM See *Reference Information Model*.

risk (actuarial) An actuary's statement of the risk presented by a group of individuals that is being considered for enrollment in healthcare insurance. This risk statement is the basis for rating the group (i.e., determining the insurance premium to be charged). For community rating, the risk statement is for the entire community; for experience rating, the statement is for a smaller group, such as the employees of a given corporation. See *rating*.

risk (financial) A chance of monetary loss; direct exposure. A health plan (for example, a health maintenance organization) is said to be at risk if it offers prepaid care for a given fee or premium. The plan is at risk because it must provide the care within the premium funds available, find the money elsewhere (the individual assets of the partners, for example), or suffer a loss.

risk (health) The likelihood of disease, injury, or death among various groups of individuals and from different causes. Individuals are said to be "at risk" if they are in a group in which a given causal factor is present. Patients who smoke are at risk from smoking; patients undergoing appendectomy are at risk from this operation. This definition is that employed in public health.

Risk may also refer to danger for individual patients. For example, a hemophiliac is a high-risk patient for any type of invasive surgery. A healthy, normal 22-year-old would ordinarily be a low-risk surgical patient.

risk (insurance) Chance of loss, the type of which can usually be covered by insurance. To a healthcare institution, the risk may arise through general liability (such as a visitor slipping and falling on hospital premises) or professional liability (harm to a patient from medical or hospital care). It may also arise because of other hospital liability (antitrust violations, for example) or physical property damage.

risk (software) As used in connection with computer software, the probability of failure and the consequences of that failure.

risk-adjusted capitation See *capitation*.

risk adjustment The use of severity of illness measures to estimate the risk to which a patient is subject.

risk contract See under *contract*.

risk factors Factors in the individual's genetic and physical makeup, lifestyle and behavior, and environment that are known (or thought) to increase the likelihood of physical or mental problems. Risk factors are typically specific for given kinds of problems. For example, obesity, high blood pressure, high cholesterol, high blood sugar, and smoking are all considered risk factors for coronary artery disease (blood vessel disease in the heart); several of these are also related to cerebrovascular disease (blood vessel disease in the brain). Risk factors for poisoning of children are such things as failure to properly store drugs and household chemicals.

There are also risk factors that contribute to *getting* a risk factor; for example, people who live sedentary lives are more likely to have high blood pressure than those who are physically active.

The term was coined by the ***Framingham Heart Study***.

risk management The process of minimizing risk (insurance) to an organization at a minimal cost in keeping with the organization's objectives. Risk management includes risk control and risk financing. *Risk control* involves: (1) developing systems to prevent accidents, injuries, and other adverse occurrences; and (2) attempting to handle events and incidents that do occur in such a manner that their cost is minimized. The latter might involve, for example, special attention to personal relations with the injured party, attempts to reach satisfactory settlement without lawsuit, and the like. *Risk financing* involves the procurement of adequate financial protection from loss, either through an outside insurance company or through some form of self-insurance. See also ***patient safety***.

risk management professional A health professional who specializes in risk management. **Certified Professional in Healthcare Risk Management (CPHRM)** A risk management professional who has met the certification requirements of the American Hospital Association (AHA) Certification Center. **www.aha.org/aha/Certification-Center**

risk manager A hospital (or other institution or organization) employee who coordinates the hospital's activities with respect to risk management.

risk pool A fund set up as a reserve for unexpected expenses in a prepaid health plan. Organizations that provide prepaid health care for a fixed fee typically set up such pools to cover, for example, unusually large demands for hospital care or specialist services.

high risk pool A fund set up to offer health insurance to small groups and individuals who have been denied coverage or whose medical history makes rates too high.

risk selection Action by a health plan or insurer that seeks to enroll only healthy persons (low risk), thus reducing the risk to the plan. Of course, adverse selection results in enrollment of a group of persons who are below the norm in health, and thus likely to be more costly for the plan. Many healthcare reform proposals would, along with requiring community rating, prevent risk selection.

risk sharing The division of financial risk among those furnishing the service. For example, if a hospital and group of physicians form a corporation to provide health care at a fixed price, they will ordinarily do it under an arrangement in which the hospital and physicians are both liable if the expenses exceed the revenue; that is, they share the risk.

RKT See *Registered Kinesiotherapist* under *kinesiotherapist*.

RLS See *record locator service*.

RMA See *Registered Medical Assistant* under *medical assistant*.

RMD Remote medical diagnosis; see *telemedicine*.

RMDP Resource Mothers Development Project. See *National Commission to Prevent Infant Mortality*.

RMT See *Registered Medical Transcriptionist* under *medical transcriptionist*.

RN See *registered nurse* under *nurse*.

RNA See *ribonucleic acid* under *DNA*.

RN,BC Board certified registered nurse, a credential offered by the American Nurses Credentialing Center (ANCC). Does not designate the specialty in which the nurse is certified. See *certified nurse*.

RNC Registered Nurse, Certified, a credential offered by the National Certification Corporation (NCC). Does not designate the specialty in which the nurse is certified. See *certified nurse*.

RN,C Certified Registered Nurse, a credential offered by the American Nurses Credentialing Center (ANCC). Does not designate the specialty in which the nurse is certified. See *certified nurse*.

RN,Cm Formerly a designation for a nurse with *modular certification*.

R.NCS.T. See *Registered Nerve Conduction Studies Technologist* under *nerve conduction technologist*.

Roadmap See *Connecting for Health (U.S.)*.

Robert Wood Johnson Foundation (RWJF) The nation's largest philanthropic organization devoted exclusively to health and healthcare issues. It concentrates its grantmaking in four areas: access to health care, delivery of care to the chronically ill, substance abuse, and healthy communities and lifestyles. The RWJF, which is based in Princeton, New Jersey, was created in 1972 by the late Robert Wood Johnson, who built the family firm, Johnson & Johnson, into a worldwide health- and medical care products company. He endowed the foundation with a $1.2-billion bequest from his personal fortune. See also *Alpha Center*, *Community Health Intervention Partnership*, and *Partnership for Long Term Care*. www.rwjf.org

Robinson-Patman Act A federal antitrust law that prohibits price discrimination. A seller cannot charge a buyer a discriminatory price and a buyer cannot knowingly benefit from such a price. The prohibition applies only to sales of goods. Discrimination may be justified in some cases if the seller can show a relationship between the discount and the cost of manufacture or delivery of the product (for example, in a volume discount), or if the discount is needed to meet the competition.

An important exemption from the Robinson-Patman Act is that granted to nonprofit hospitals (and certain other organizations) that purchase supplies for their own use. For example, "own use" has been interpreted to prohibit a hospital from selling prescription drugs (which it obtains at favorable prices) to the general public and outpatients coming in for refills, but to allow the hospital to sell or furnish drugs to inpatients, outpatients seen at the hospital, and physicians and employees and their families. The Robinson-Patman Act is an amendment to Section 2 of the Clayton Act. 15 U.S.C. §§ 13–13b.21(a) (2005).

RODS See *Realtime Outbreak and Disease Surveillance*.

Roentgen ray See *x-ray*.

Roe v. Wade The landmark U.S. Supreme Court case that liberalized abortion law in 1973. The Court struck down restrictive state abortion laws as unconstitutional, ruling that those laws violated the individual's right of privacy to make her own decisions concerning her body. *Roe v. Wade* held that the state could regulate abortions only where necessary to serve a compelling state interest. Those state interests were recognized to be protection of the life and health of pregnant women, and protecting the "potentiality of human life."

In *Roe v. Wade* the Court balanced the state interests against those of the individual. It found that during the first trimester of pregnancy, the risk to a woman's health from an abortion was less than the risk of childbirth; therefore, the state's interest in maternal health did not outweigh the right of privacy. Thus the state could regulate abortions during the first trimester only as it might restrict other surgical procedures (for example, requiring that they be performed only by licensed physicians). During the second trimester, the risk accompanying abortion was greater, and therefore greater restrictions could be placed to protect maternal health, as long as they did not unreasonably interfere with the woman's right to make her own abortion decision.

Once the fetus became viable, however (at about twenty-eight weeks in 1973), the Court ruled that the state's interest in protecting potential life became compelling, and therefore the state could prohibit third trimester abortions altogether except where abortion was necessary to protect the life or health of the mother. The Court did not address nor did it decide the question of when life began or when the fetus became a "person" as far as the law of abortion was concerned. 410 U.S. 113 (1973), rehearing denied, 410 U.S. 959 (1973).

ROI Return on investment. See also *release of information*.

room An enclosed area within a healthcare facility in which one or more patients are lodged, cared for, and/or treated.

private room A hospital room for only one patient.

semi-private room A hospital room set up to accommodate two to four patients.

treatment room A room in which procedures or other treatments are performed; usually the patient is not lodged in the room.

ward (room) A patient care room for more than four patients. See also *patient care unit*.

rooming-in An organization of the maternity and newborn services of a hospital that permits the newborn to share the room with the mother.

room rate See under *rate (charge)*.

ROUB See *Registered Ophthalmic Ultrasound Biometrist* under *ophthalmic ultrasound biometrist*.

routine inquiry law See *required request law*.

RPFT See *Registered Pulmonary Function Technologist* under *pulmonary function technologist*.

RPh Registered pharmacist.

RPh,BC-ADM Registered Pharmacist, Board Certified—Advanced Diabetes Management. See *Advanced Diabetes Management Certification* under *diabetes management*.

RPMS See *Resource and Patient Management System*.

RPSGT See *Registered Polysomnographic Technologist* under *polysomnographic technologist*.

RPT See *Registered Phlebotomy Technician* under *Phlebotomy Technician*, under *clinical laboratory technician*.

RPVI See *Registered Physician in Vascular Interpretation* under *diagnostic medical sonographer*.

RRA Registered Record Administrator. See *Registered Health Information Administrator* under *health information administrator*.

RRC See *Residency Review Committee*.

RRT See *Registered Respiratory Therapist* under *respiratory therapist*.

RSN Real soon now.

RSNA See *Radiological Society of North America*.

RSO See *radiation safety officer*.

RT See *respiratory therapy* and *Registered Technologist* (under *radiologic technologist*). Also means rehabilitation teaching; see *vision rehabilitation therapy*.

RTA See *respiratory therapy assistant*.

RTC See *residential treatment center*.

RTT See *respiratory therapy technician*.

rubric The title or label given to a category in a classification (scheme).

RUGs See *Resource Utilization Groups*.

rule Also frequently referred to as a regulation, the rule is the administrative agency (see *agency (administrative)*) equivalent of a statute (legislation). It has the force of law, as contrasted with an administrative guideline, which is merely advisory. The agency is typically given the power to create rules ("rulemaking") and regulations ("regulatory powers") by a particular statute. The rules and regulations implement the necessary details of that statute. A law passed in the healthcare field, for example, may require the Department of Health and Human Services (HHS) to issue rules and regulations spelling out in detail how the law's goals are to be achieved.

At the federal level, a rule or regulation is typically "adopted" by a federal agency as a result of being published in the *Federal Register* (FR) for a period of time. In this case, the regulation is typically referred to as a **Final Rule**, and it attains the force of law. To avoid confusion, federal law prohibits the agencies from making the contents of the regulations public until they have become "final." A proposed rule, on the other hand, is published in the *Federal Register* so as to invite review and comments from the public.

Rule of Reason A doctrine in antitrust law that states that only unreasonable restraints of trade are prohibited. Thus, in most cases of alleged anticompetitive behavior, the specific facts must be examined to decide whether an antitrust violation has occurred. For example, an exclusive contract between a hospital and a group of radiologists is anticompetitive on its face; that is, it precludes other radiologists from practicing in the hospital. However, courts have decided, by applying the Rule of Reason, that such arrangements may be upheld for reasons of quality of care, administrative efficiency, or other valid institutional goals. By contrast, if the per se standard were applied, the exclusive contract would be illegal regardless of its purpose. In healthcare cases, courts have been more likely to apply the Rule of Reason analysis than they have been in other industries.

Rule of Rescue The principle that saving a patient from imminent death has priority over any other medical duty. This "rule" is stated by some as a fact of the human psyche in connection with discussions of the rationing of health care.

rule out To eliminate (as a possible diagnosis or cause) by further investigation. See *rule out list*.

rule out list A list of *possible diagnoses* (see under *diagnosis*) that the physician typically places in the medical record at the beginning of the diagnostic investigation to determine the cause of the patient's symptoms. The list includes all the conditions that come to mind as possibly responsible for the patient's problem. Unless the final diagnosis is established before the elimination process is complete, every effort is made to eliminate (rule out) each diagnosis on the list, even when to do so requires use of diagnostic procedures not relevant to the diagnosis (or diagnoses) finally established. Such procedures may be challenged, in hindsight, as "unnecessary," because they don't "go with" the final diagnosis. It is of interest that in an early instruction for coding for Medicare, all diagnoses in the rule out list were to be coded as though actually present—a coding rule that was later rescinded. See also *differential diagnosis* (under *diagnosis*).

rules and regulations Official statements (statements authorized or commissioned by the governing body) as to the conduct of the organization's affairs in specific areas. In hospitals, the term often applies to statements that supplement the medical staff bylaws. Such rules and regulations have the force of the bylaws themselves, but contain more detail than would be appropriate in the bylaws; also, the process for their revision is less cumbersome than that for the revision of bylaws. For example, the bylaws could require the keeping of a medical record on each patient, whereas the rules and regulations could specify more detailed requirements concerning the content of medical records, promptness of completion, penalties for failure to comply, and so on.

rural area An area outside an urban, densely populated area. "Rural" may be defined differently for different purposes (in various laws and programs, for instance). The Oregon Office of Rural Health defines rural as "all geographic areas 10 or more miles from the centroid of a population center of 30,000 or more." To be designated by CMS as a *Rural Health Clinic (RHC)*, a facility must be located outside an *urbanized area*.

Rural Health Care Program (RHCP) A division of the *Universal Service Fund (USF)* that makes discounts available to eligible rural healthcare providers for telecommunication services and monthly Internet service charges, so that they pay no more for telecommunications than their urban counterparts.

Rural Health Clinic (RHC) A healthcare organization cert:fied to receive enhanced Medicare and Medicaid reimbursement. The purpose of the RHC program is to improve access to primary care in underserved rural areas. To qualify, a clinic must use a team of physicians and midlevel practitioners (nurse practitioners, physician assistants, and certified nurse midwives) to provide services. The clinic must be staffed at least 50% of the time with a midlevel practitioner. An RHC must be located in a "non-urbanized area" (see *urbanized area*) with a current healthcare shortage designation as either a Medically Underserved Area (MUA), Health Professional Shortage Area (HPSA), or Governor-Designated Shortage Area (GDSA). It must provide at least outpatient primary care services and basic laboratory services. In addition, an RHC must have a Quality Assessment and Performance Improvement (QAPI) program. RHCs may be public or private, for-profit or nonprofit. See also *Federally Qualified Health Center*. Further information may be obtained from the National Association of Rural Health Clinics (NARHC) at **www.narhc.org**.

rural health network (RHN) An organization with at least one Critical Access Hospital (CAH) and at least one full-service acute care hospital in which the participants have worked out agreements on such items as patient referral and transfer, use of communication systems (such as medical telemetry devices and electronic sharing of patient data), and transportation of emergency and nonemergency patients. See *Critical Access Hospital Program*.

rural hospital See under *hospital*.

rural site See *originating site*.

RV See *resident valet*.

RVS See *relative value scale*, and *Registered Vascular Specialist* under *cardiovascular technologist*.

RVT See *Registered Vascular Technologist* under *diagnostic medical sonographer*.

RVU See *relative value unit*.

RWJF See *Robert Wood Johnson Foundation*.

Rx See *prescription* and *treatment*.

RxNorm A standardized nomenclature for clinical drugs, produced by the National Library of Medicine (NLM). In this context, a clinical drug is "a pharmaceutical product given to (or taken by) a patient with a therapeutic or diagnostic intent." Both prescription and OTC drugs are included, both branded and generic. In RxNorm, the name of a clinical drug combines its active ingredient + strength + dose form (the physical form in which the drug is administered or is specified to be administered in a prescription or order). For example:

Acetaminophen 500 MG Oral Tablet: for a generic drug name

Acetaminophen 500 MG Oral Tablet [Tylenol]: for a branded drug name

RxNorm's standard names for clinical drugs are connected to the varying names of drugs present in many different controlled vocabularies within the UMLS Metathesaurus. These connections are intended to facilitate interoperability among the computerized systems that record or process data dealing with clinical drugs. **www.nlm.nih.gov/research/umls/rxnorm**

Ryan White CARE (Comprehensive AIDS Resources Emergency Care) Act A 1990 federal act, named for an Indiana boy with AIDS, that provides funding to states and other public or private nonprofit entities to develop, organize, coordinate, and operate more effective and cost-efficient systems for the delivery of essential health care and support services to medically underserved individuals and families affected by HIV/AIDS. The CARE Act was extended by the Ryan White HIV/AIDS Treatment Modernization Act of 2006 (Pub. L. No. 109-415). Pub. L. No. 101-381, 104 Stat. 576 (1990).

S

SA See *surgical assistant*.

SAE See *sexual assault examiner*.

safe harbor An assurance that a certain specified behavior or action will not result in civil or criminal penalties when done in a specified way. This is generally an effort made by lawmakers to avoid some law's having an unnecessarily chilling effect. Note, however, that behavior may fall outside a safe harbor and still not incur legal liabilities. See *safe harbor regulations*.

safe harbor regulations Regulations that describe certain acts or behaviors that will *not* be illegal under a specific law, even though they might otherwise be illegal. Typically this refers to federal regulations (42 C.F.R. § 1001.952) that specify conduct exempt from the fraud and abuse laws. As a result of the antikickback laws, providers were unsure of what conduct was prohibited and what was allowed. The Department of Health and Human Services (HHS) Office of Inspector General (OIG) promulgated a series of "safe harbors"; that is, conduct that is acceptable under the Medicare and Medicaid fraud and abuse laws. Generally, the safe harbors allow some discount arrangements, certain investment interests, space and equipment rentals, sales of practices by retiring physicians, warranties, and elaborate specific referral arrangements that are not prohibited. Further, there is a limited safe harbor for waivers of beneficiary coinsurance and deductible amounts in certain areas. Finally, a safe harbor exists for Medicare and Medicaid managed care organizations to offer certain incentives to enrollees. See also *Antikickback Statute* and *fraud and abuse*.

Safe Medical Devices Act of 1990 (SMDA) Federal legislation authorizing the Food and Drug Administration (FDA) to regulate companies that manufacture and distribute *medical devices* and equipment. The SMDA prescribed changes to the *Federal Food, Drug, and Cosmetic Act of 1938*, as amended, for the regulation of medical devices, and also modified the Medical Device Amendments of 1976, which established a comprehensive framework for the regulation of medical devices.

The SMDA also requires healthcare facilities (including hospitals and nursing homes) that use medical devices to report to the FDA all incidents involving a medical device that probably caused or contributed to the death, serious illness, or injury of a patient. Pub. L. No. 101-629, 104 Stat. 4511 (1990).

Safe Practices See *30 Safe Practices*.

safety See *patient safety*.

safety-critical See under *critical (essential)*.

safety net provider A provider obliged to provide health care to patients whether or not they are able to pay for it. A report published in 2000 by the Institute of Medicine (IOM) entitled *America's Health Care Safety Net: Intact but Endangered* distinguishes "core safety net providers" as having the following two characteristics:
1. Either by legal mandate or explicitly adopted mission they maintain an "open door," offering access to services for patients regardless of their ability to pay, and
2. A substantial share of their patient mix is uninsured, Medicaid, and other vulnerable patients.

See also *safety net hospital* and *disproportionate share hospital*, both under *hospital*, *Federally Qualified Health Center*, and *Emergency Medical Treatment and Labor Act*.

same-day surgery See *ambulatory surgery* under *surgery (treatment)*.

SAMHSA See *Substance Abuse and Mental Health Services Administration*.

sample A part of a population, intended to be in some way representative of the entire population.

sampling A technique used in statistics in which a part of a whole is examined with the intent that the results of the examination can be taken as representing the condition of the whole.

A large body of theory and experience has been developed as to various sampling methods (methods of drawing samples) and their reliability, that is, the trustworthiness of the projections made from them.

In general, the more random the sample, the better (i.e., the more likely the sample will accurately reflect the condition of the whole). One example of sampling involves coal, which is sometimes sold on the basis of its heating value. Small quantities thought to represent the whole are analyzed, and payment is based on these analyses. The same principle is used in polls as to a political candidate's popularity: A sample of people are questioned and their responses are projected as representative of the whole population from which they were selected (for example, a city). Most skepticism about sampling revolves around whether the sample was a correct one for the purpose.

SAMS See *Society for Advanced Medical Systems*.

sanction A term used with two, opposite meanings: (1) a kind of permission or support, and (2) discipline, punishment, or prohibition. Only by the context can one determine which meaning is intended.

SANE-A See *Sexual Assault Nurse Examiner—Adult/Adolescent* under *sexual assault examiner*.

SAP See *student affairs practitioner* and *Substance Abuse Professional*.

Sarbanes-Oxley Act of 2002 (SOX) A federal law enacted in response to high-profile financial scandals, such as Enron and WorldCom, to protect investors and the public from accounting errors and fraudulent practices. The law is wide-ranging and establishes new or enhanced standards for all U.S. public company boards, management, and public accounting firms. Among other requirements, companies must establish financial accounting systems that can generate financial reports that are readily verifiable with traceable source data. This source data must remain intact and cannot undergo undocumented revisions. In addition, any revisions to financial or accounting software must be fully documented as to what was changed, why, by whom, and when.

The act is administered by the Securities and Exchange Commission (SEC). SOX also created the Public Company Accounting Oversight Board (PCAOB), a private, nonprofit organization that oversees the auditors of public companies. Although SOX is limited to for-profit, publicly traded companies (with just a few exceptions), some states, either through their attorneys general or legislation, have applied principles from Sarbanes-Oxley to non-profit corporations.

Synonyms: the Public Company Accounting Reform and Investor Protection Act of 2002, SarbOx. Pub. L. No. 107-204, 116 Stat. 745 (2002).

SBB See *Specialist in Blood Banking* under *clinical laboratory specialist*.

SBU See *strategic business unit*.

SC Service corporation; see *professional corporation* under *corporation*. See also *Specialist in Chemistry* under *clinical laboratory specialist*.

scalability In the informatics world, the capability of a system to change from one size to another, typically from a small system to a bigger one, and then to a "humongous" one, without undue difficulty. An example would be a web site for the world Olympics, which works fine for 3.9 years with an average of three visitors a day. Then, during the actual games, it gets 300 million visitors a day. If it can handle that traffic without breaking, it is said to be very **scalable**.

SCAMC See *Symposium on Computer Applications in Medical Care*.

ScD Doctor of science (postgraduate degree).

SCH See *Sole Community Hospital* under *hospital*.

SCHIP See *State Children's Health Insurance Program*.

school counselor A counselor with special education and training in the needs of students. Synonym: guidance counselor.

National Certified School Counselor (NCSC) A credential for school counselors offered jointly by the American Counseling Association (ACA) (**www.counseling.org**), the American School Counselor Association (ASCA) (**www.schoolcounselor.org**), and the National Board for Certified Counselors (NBCC) (**www.nbcc.org**).

school nursing The area of nursing focusing on the health needs of elementary and secondary students.

National Certified School Nurse (NCSN) A registered nurse with at least a bachelor's degree who has passed an examination in school nursing given by the National Board for Certification of School Nurses (NBCSN). **www.nbcsn.com**

School Nurse Practitioner (SNP) A specialist in school nursing who has passed an advanced examination of the American Nurses Credentialing Center (ANCC). No longer offered.

school rule A legal doctrine that states that the ***standard of care (legal)*** in a malpractice lawsuit will be measured by the degree of care exercised by professionals within the same specialty or "school" of medicine. For example, under the school rule, osteopaths (DOs) would be measured by the practices of other osteopaths, not those of medical physicians (MDs). Some states use this rule; others do not. See also ***locality rule***.

SCI Spinal cord injury.

scintigraphy An imaging technique in which a camera sensitive to emissions from radioactive substances is used to photograph the distribution in the body of a radioactive drug administered internally.

SCIP See ***Surgical Care Improvement Project***.

SCM See ***Society for Computer Medicine***.

scoring A term used in connection with legislative budgeting in estimating the effects on revenue of tax policy changes, depending on their influence on behavior. **Static scoring** is used when no effect on behavior is expected from the change in tax policy; **dynamic scoring** is used when behavior is expected to change. An example of a behavioral change in response to tax policy has been the noticeable change to automobile leasing from purchasing as a response to the elimination of the deductibility of personal interest expense. The Congressional Budget Office (CBO) tends to use static scoring in its budget predictions. Synonym: cost estimating.

screening (diagnostic) Giving diagnostic tests to "normal" individuals or a population in order to detect diseases. The tests employed include examinations of the blood and urine, x-rays, blood pressure measurements, height and weight, questionnaires, and vision and hearing testing. Screening may be employed for detection of a single problem, such as hypertension (high blood pressure) or drug usage, or it may be a "broad spectrum" screening for "anything abnormal" that can be suspected by using a battery of tests. The latter approach is called ***multiphasic screening*** (see below).

Increasing attention is being given to the cost-benefit ratios of various screening approaches. In a population with very little tuberculosis, for example, the cost of finding new cases by chest x-ray screening is far higher than finding cases by examining contacts of known cases; consequently, chest x-rays are rarely included today in community screening programs. On the other hand, automation of blood chemical determinations has made it often cheaper to perform the standard battery of tests provided by the analyzer than to single out specific tests (which are included in the battery). The laboratory work done in routine examinations on admission to the hospital is primarily a screening process. For example, even though the physician may be most interested in the patient's blood sugar, the whole array of tests—which screens for other disorders—is done simultaneously. Furthermore, such screening on admission to the hospital provides a clinical database on the patient that often helps in timing the onset of abnormalities.

multiphasic screening Applying batteries of diagnostic tests, usually to persons "on the street" (primarily adults without symptoms) in such settings as shopping malls and county fairs. Often the tests include some blood chemistry determinations (such as for sugar and cholesterol levels), hearing, blood pressure, intra-eyeball pressure (for detection of glaucoma), and chest x-rays. The process has been criticized as to its value, on account of such problems as cost per case identified, false positive findings, false negative findings, and unnecessarily alarming the persons tested.

screening (quality) A method for separating some kinds of things or patients from others. The term is often employed in one method of assessing quality of care, in which medical records of patients are subjected to a "screen" that isolates for detailed review the records of those with unusually long stays, or those with complications of care, for example.

generic screening Screening in which the criteria used to "screen" cases apply to patients regardless of their diagnoses and procedures employed; thus the criteria are "generic" rather than diagnosis or procedure specific. Examples of generic screening criteria include injuries, incidents, documentation failures (including informed consent), failure to respond to abnormal laboratory or x-ray findings, and nosocomial (hospital-acquired) infections. Many of the criteria that define adverse patient occurrences (APOs) are generic.

occurrence screening The process of examining medical records and other data in the hospital (or other healthcare settings) in order to find cases in which there may have been adverse patient occurrences (APOs), cases that meet predefined criteria. The cases detected by the screening are reviewed by experienced personnel who make judgments as to whether each case should enter the occurrence reporting process for further review.

SCRIPT See *NCPDP SCRIPT*.

scrub A health professional who prepares the sterile field, scrubs and gowns the members of the surgical team, and prepares and sterilizes the instruments before and after a surgical procedure. May be a *surgical technologist*, a *first assistant*, or a *registered nurse (RN)* (see under *nurse*).

"To scrub" means to prepare to carry out or assist in a surgical operation. The term "scrub" is taken from the routine of thorough hand washing (scrubbing) prior to putting on sterile rubber gloves and operating garments.

SCS See *Sports Certified Specialist* under *physical therapist*.

SCT See *Specialist in Cytotechnology* under *clinical laboratory specialist*.

SCT-enabled application A software application designed to support the use of SNOMED CT.

SCU See *surge capacity unit*.

SDHP Self-directed health plan; see *consumer-driven health plan*.

SDM Shared decision making. See *informed shared decision making*.

SDO See *standards development organization*.

SDRG See *Severity DRG* under *DRG*.

SDTM See *Study Data Tabulation Model*.

secondary care Specialized care provided by a physician or hospital, usually on referral from a primary care physician. Synonym: specialized care.

second opinion A consultation that involves the examination of a patient by a surgeon, and the rendering of an opinion by that surgeon, with respect to the need for elective (nonemergency) surgery that has been recommended by another surgeon. Also known as a "second surgical opinion" (SSO). The SSO sometimes results in treating the medical problem with cheaper, nonsurgical alternatives. Either the patient, the provider, or the payer may suggest or require the second opinion.

second opinion program A mandatory or voluntary program calling for second opinions for elective (nonemergency) surgery prior to authorization of the performance of the surgery.

secretariat The base office of an organization, including its professional and clerical staffs, along with the essential technological and other resources necessary for carrying out the work of the organization.

Section 105 HRA plan See *health reimbursement account*.

Section 1122 A section of the Social Security Act that denies payment for certain capital expenditures not approved by state planning agencies.

Section 330 The original section of the Public Health Service Act that provided for funding of community health centers for medically underserved populations. Although the section has been renumbered (it is now Section 254b of the act, codified at 42 U.S.C. Chapter 6A (2004)), it is still referred to as Section 330, and funding pursuant to that section is called a "Section 330 grant." See *Federally Qualified Health Center*.

Section 330 Health Center See *Federally Qualified Health Center*.

security Traditionally, "security" has meant locked doors, lighted parking lots, and video cameras in remote areas of parking garages. It also was typified by the command to "call security" when someone needed to be thrown out of the building. However, since the passage of HIPAA, it is increasingly used to refer to patient privacy (see *Privacy Rule*). In this context, a healthcare provider's "security officer" may be a vice president, and not wear a uniform. See also *health security*.

security professional See *privacy and security professionals*.

sedation A process of calming the nervous system.

> **conscious sedation** A depressed level of consciousness in which a patient is able to independently maintain an airway and respond appropriately to physical stimulation, verbal command, and pain. Synonym: analgesic sedation.

> **deep sedation** A state induced by the use of medications, in which the patient does not respond appropriately to pain or to verbal or physical stimulation, and requires assistance in and monitoring of respiration.

self-care Care provided by the individual to her- or himself in order to maintain health and to carry out courses of treatment. Self-care is essential in chronic conditions such as diabetes and chronic cardiac conditions. Increasing attention is being given to educating patients as to details of the care required and to providing support for them, through individual instruction, classes, and Internet services. Internet "online self-care systems" offer support tools that include software that tracks adherence to diets and exercise routines; maintains both numerical and graphic records of such measurements as weight, blood sugar levels, and blood pressure; issues reminders as to medications and periodic examinations; facilitates filling of prescriptions; and schedules contacts with physicians and other healthcare providers.

self-directed health plan (SDHP) See *consumer-driven health plan*.

self-governance A term commonly used in connection with the medical staff, to which the hospital governing body delegates certain duties, for example, those connected with evaluation of care or the control of physician practices. It should be noted, however, that the governing body retains the ultimate responsibility for the care in the hospital, even where the medical staff is described as "self-governing."

self-insurance See under *insurance*.

self-pay patient A patient who pays either all or part of the hospital bill from his or her own resources, as opposed to a third-party payer. Synonym: self-responsible patient.

self-referral (patient) When a patient directly contacts a specialist to obtain secondary care. This is distinguished from a primary care physician (PCP) making the referral on behalf of the patient.

self-referral (physician) A physician referring a patient so as to create a conflict of interest. Physicians are prohibited by federal law from accepting payments from any provider resulting from the referral of Medicare or Medicaid patients. See also *Antikickback Statute*, *fraud and abuse*, and *safe harbor regulations*.

self-responsible patient See *self-pay patient*.

SEM See *somebody else's money*.

semi-private room See under *room*.

Senior Plan Network (SPN) An alliance of health maintenance organizations (HMOs) that offers enrollment in the SPN, and thus in its constituent HMOs. Medicare prepays part or all the cost of enrollment in an SPN as it does in an HMO under certain circumstances.

sentinel event In health care, an unexpected occurrence that results in, or poses a risk of, serious injury or harm. It is called sentinel because it may be symptomatic of a system problem. Thus its occurrence should always "raise a red flag" or sound a warning that requires immediate attention. Healthcare providers attempt to prevent the reoccurrence of sentinel events by correcting any system problems detected (i.e., by getting at the root cause). See also *adverse patient occurrence*, *medical harm*, and *unanticipated outcome* (under *outcome*).

separate billing See under *billing*.

separation A term used in Canada to mean the same as patient discharge in the United States. It is the formal release of a patient from a hospital (or other care).

serious adverse event Not synonymous with, but defined and discussed under, *adverse drug event*. See also *adverse patient occurrence*, *medical harm*, *sentinel event*, and *serious reportable event*.

serious reportable event (SRE) In 2002, the National Quality Forum (NQF) published "Serious Reportable Events in Healthcare," a list of twenty-seven adverse events in health care that should never happen. Examples are wrong-site surgery, stage 3 or 4 pressure ulcers acquired after admission, and leaving a foreign object inside a patient after surgery. NQF has since endorsed a set of definitions and measures to standardize data collection and reporting of these events, which are grouped into six categories: surgical, product or device, patient protection, care management, environmental, and criminal acts. The list is updated as necessary, to include events that are:

- Of concern to both the public and healthcare professionals and providers.
- Clearly identifiable and measurable, and thus feasible to include in a reporting system.
- Of a nature such that the risk of occurrence is significantly influenced by the policies and procedures of the healthcare facility.

Some states require the reporting of these events. This is also called the "never list." Synonyms: never event, reportable event. See also *adverse drug event*, *adverse patient occurrence*, *medical harm*, and *sentinel event*.

serology The study of serum. Serum is the liquid portion of a body fluid (for example, blood) that remains after clotting. Serum contains immune substances (antibodies) that represent the response of the body to exposure to certain disease-causing agents (see *agent (substance)*). For many diseases, these antibodies are highly specific (each disease tends to cause the production of a unique substance). Detection of the presence of disease-specific antibodies is helpful in making diagnoses and in keeping track of the progress of the diseases for which the antibodies develop.

Serology is also involved in preparation of serums used to protect persons against certain diseases. An example of such a serum is tetanus antitoxin, used to give *passive immunity* (see under *immunity*) against tetanus (a bacterial disease).

serostatus A term referring to the result of a test of blood serum to determine whether an individual has had previous exposure to a disease or other agent, such as an allergen. If there has been previous exposure, and the individual has developed an immune response, the test is positive; the person is seropositive. A seronegative individual either has had no previous exposure or has failed to respond to the exposure.

Determining serostatus is an important measure in finding and treating patients with HIV infection, for example, before symptoms appear. It is also important in carrying out public health measures to curb HIV epidemics, because HIV seropositive individuals are contagious (are "hidden cases") before illness is evident. Treatment at this stage of disease is usually desirable, suppressing or minimizing symptoms, often for a long period of time, and reducing the likelihood of transmission of the disease.

serum hepatitis See *hepatitis B*.

service The term "service" has many meanings in health care, and must always be interpreted in context.

In *healthcare financing*, a service (or a procedure) is a thing that the payer pays for. Service here means something "done" for a patient by a physician or other person. In medicine, the term "procedure" *also* means something done for a patient. In fact, it is sometimes difficult if not impossible to distinguish the two, because a specific act might equally well be called a "procedure" or a "service." There are some general guidelines: Procedures tend to be distinct actions, and carried out in a brief time as, for example, a surgical operation (a procedure or group of procedures); services (such as preoperative and postoperative care) are less distinct and are carried out over longer (and variable) periods of time. The real answer to what is a service or procedure in financing is whatever the system used by the payer says it is. For physician services, the guide is **CPT** *(Physicians' Current Procedural Terminology)*. In *CPT*, for example, the physician's "initial hospital care" of a patient is called a service, although it is largely limited (in billing for care) to what is done upon admission of the patient; each subsequent day's care is defined as another service. However, the "50-minute hour" in the psychiatrist's office for "medical psychotherapy" is listed as a procedure. For purposes of payment, a service (or procedure) might more accurately be defined as "the unit for which a charge is made." See also **procedure**.

Hospitals sometimes use the term "service" to refer to a division of the hospital organization, such as the nursing service, or of its medical staff, such as the oncology service. Hospitals also use it for major functions: nursing service, food service, pharmacy, medical records, laboratory, and diagnostic radiology. Hospitals as well as other healthcare institutions may mean support service when they say service (e.g., purchasing, maintenance, supplies). These services support the activities of other departments. Hospital services are typically directed by a specific individual who is responsible for their execution, but direction may be provided from one central point ("centralized service") or from a number of points in the organization ("decentralized service").

The *marketing* department will use the term "service" broadly to describe a variety of facilities, programs, and capabilities that provide for various needs of patients and the community. For example, a hospital may provide open heart surgery, genetic counseling, hemodialysis, organ transplants, psychiatric intensive care, weight loss programs, blood pressure screening, and so forth. Each of these might be described as a service.

The American Hospital Association uses "service" *to classify hospitals* as general or specialized and, if specialized, the nature of the specialty. For example, a hospital's classification according to service could be "children's general hospital" or "alcoholism and other chemical dependency" hospital. A given hospital can be put in only one class according to service.

In *economics*, "service" means the supplying or meeting of some public demand, as contrasted with producing goods. The healthcare industry is a "service" industry.

service animal The Americans with Disabilities Act (ADA) defines a service animal as "any guide dog, signal dog, or other animal individually trained to provide assistance to an individual with a disability." The animal need not be certified or licensed. A service animal is explicitly not a pet. Examples are "seeing-eye" dogs for the blind, dogs who alert their masters to sounds, animals who assist with mobility, and dogs trained to pick up things or pull wheelchairs. Some dogs have been trained to remind their owners when it's time to take medications. The ADA requires that service animals be accommodated in employment, housing, transportation, and so forth.

In 2003, the Department of Transportation (DOT) issued guidance on service animals for the airline industry. The DOT expanded the definition (which had required training for service animals) to include an "animal that has been shown to have the innate ability to assist a person with a disability" (such as a seizure-alert dog) or an **emotional support animal** (sometimes called "furry Prozac"). Airline personnel are to first ask the passenger whether the animal is a service animal or a pet. If necessary, they may require documentation for a trained animal or, for an emotional support animal, a letter from a mental health professional stating that the animal is necessary to assist the passenger with a mental health–related disability.

There has since been much controversy over the definition of a service animal, and some people have taken advantage of the DOT guidelines to claim their pets as emotional support animals. Airlines have accommodated any number of dogs, but also cats, rabbits, miniature horses, goats, and at least one duck. The issue also arises as to when animals must be permitted in housing, restaurants, hospitals, stores, theaters, workplaces, and so forth, because the DOT's guidelines only apply to air transportation.

Synonyms for "emotional support animal" include assistance animal, comfort animal, emotional-needs animal, emotional service animal, and psychological or psychiatric service animal. See also **therapy animal**.

service area The geographic area served by a hospital or other facility or, perhaps more accurately, the area from which the institution or organization draws its patients or clients. A "service area" is sometimes referred to as a "catchment area." The catchment areas of organizations with like services may overlap.

service benefits See under **benefits**.

service contract See under **contract**.

service mark See **trademark**.

settlement An agreement made by the parties to end a dispute or lawsuit before (or during) the hearing or trial, without a formal adjudication (decision by the arbitrator, judge, jury, or other decision-maker) of the merits of the dispute. The term "settlement" is also sometimes used to refer to the specific terms of the agreement (such as the amount of money to be paid).

structured settlement A settlement that provides for payment of money in a personal injury or workers' compensation case in other than one lump sum. A structured settlement often provides for payment of an agreed-upon amount in installments over a period of time. In some cases, a structured settlement might provide that medical and other expenses will be reimbursed as they occur, rather than by an advance estimate. Other variations are possible, because the terms of the structured settlement are negotiated by the parties.

severity of illness The gravity of a patient's condition. Patients with the same diagnosis often vary from being mildly ill to being extremely ill, or even dying. The original DRGs did not make allowance for the severity of a patient's illness; every patient with the same diagnosis (actually, every patient within a given DRG) was given the same "price tag." Alternative methods have been developed to take severity of illness into account; see **All Patient Refined DRG**, **All-Payer Severity-adjusted DRG**, and **Severity DRG**, all under **DRG**; also **Medical Illness Severity Grouping System (MedisGroups)** and **staging (diseases)**. See also **severity score**.

severity score A mathematical score that expresses the **severity of illness** of a patient according to one of several severity measurement methods. The goal is to use such scores in a formula for determining payment for care, and in quantifying the quality of care. See also **APACHE III**, **AS-SCORE index**, **Comprehensive Severity Index**, **Instrumental Activities of Daily Living scale**, and **Patient Management Category Severity Scale**.

sex chromosome See under **chromosome**.

sex-linked characteristic A genetic characteristic, such as color-blindness, that is determined by a gene on a sex chromosome and shows a different pattern of inheritance in males and females.

sexual assault examiner (SAE) A registered nurse or other qualified health professional specially trained to perform the forensic examination of sexual assault victims and alleged perpetrators. An SAE is immediately notified, usually by police or emergency room personnel, whenever there is a victim of sexual assault. The nurse interviews the patient and conducts the physical examination, including collection of evidence. He or she talks to the patient about risks of disease and pregnancy, and refers for follow-up care. The SAE also helps law enforcement officials and may testify in court. See also *forensic nursing*.

Sexual Assault Nurse Examiner—Adult/Adolescent (SANE-A) A registered nurse who has been Board Certified by the Forensic Nursing Certification Board (FNCB). **www.forensicnurse.org**

sexual harassment A form of discrimination in the workplace that violates the Civil Rights Act of 1964. "Sexual harassment" can be of two forms: (1) "quid pro quo" (the employee must submit to sexual advances to obtain tangible job benefits, or be penalized for refusing); or (2) "hostile environment" (the workplace is offensive, and seriously affects the employee's well-being). Offensive conduct may include unwelcome advances, comments, touching, questions about marital status, and so forth. Both men and women may be victims.

sexually transmitted disease (STD) A disease that may be transmitted by sexual contact. The "classical" sexually transmitted (venereal) diseases were syphilis and gonorrhea. Today, AIDS, genital herpes, chlamydia, hepatitis B, and others are included.

sexual misconduct (in medical practice) The American Medical Association (AMA) Code of Medical Ethics states that sexual contact between a physician and his or her patient is "sexual misconduct," and that the physician-patient relationship should be terminated before any romantic or sexual relationship is initiated.

SF-36 Health Survey See under *quality of life scale*.

SH See *Specialist in Hematology* under *clinical laboratory specialist*.

shadow pricing Setting the price for a product by matching the price for the same or similar product to that of a competitor. Some HMOs are said to have failed because they have used this method in establishing their premiums rather than actuarial analysis, in which the premium is set by defining a specific benefit package to be provided to a population whose demographic characteristics are carefully considered. See also *tailgate pricing*.

share See *stock*.

shared decision making (SDM) See *informed shared decision making*.

Shared Decision Making Programs (SDMP) Interactive computer programs that assist patients in medical decision making by providing them with general and specific information about their condition and the potential harms and benefits of the alternative medical and surgical treatments. SDMP are available for an increasing number of conditions, including benign prostatic hyperplasia, low back pain, mild hypertension, breast cancer surgery, and breast cancer adjuvant therapy. The system is designed to be used in the healthcare setting, where the physician refers the patient to the appropriate program on the basis of eligibility criteria. The system was developed by John E. Wennberg, MD, and his group at the *Foundation for Informed Medical Decision Making (FIMDM)*.

shared service organization An organization, external to the hospital, set up to provide shared services, such as group purchasing. Such an organization may or may not have been set up by the organizations receiving the services, and may or may not be under their joint control.

shared services Administrative, clinical, or other services provided by or for two or more institutions. The services are used jointly or under some arrangement that improves service, reduces cost, or both. A common type of shared service is group purchasing. Synonym: cooperative services.

Shared Visions—New Pathways An initiative of the Joint Commission on Accreditation of Healthcare Organizations (JCAHO) to "sharpen the focus of the accreditation process on operational systems critical to the safety and quality of patient care."

shareholder The owner of shares of stock in a corporation. Synonym: stockholder.

sharp In the context of biohazardous waste, a sharp is a hypodermic or suture needle, pipette, glass slide, blood vial, scalpel blade, or other object that can invade the skin. A sharp that has been in contact with an infectious agent, such as the HIV virus, poses a serious threat to the safety of health professionals and others. See also *needlestick*.

Sherman Act One of the primary federal *antitrust* laws. Section 1 of the Sherman Act prohibits contracts, combinations, and conspiracies in restraint of trade; Section 2 prohibits monopolies and attempts to monopolize. The Sherman Act has been interpreted by the courts to apply only to unreasonable restraints of trade, because every contract restrains commerce to some extent. 15 U.S.C. §§ 1–2 (2004). See also *Rule of Reason*.

SHM See *Society of Hospital Medicine*

S/HMO See *social HMO* under *health maintenance organization*.

Sickness Impact Profile (SIP) See under *quality of life scale*.

sick role A concept introduced by Talcott Parsons in the 1950s that pictures the role of a sick person as a temporary, medically sanctioned form of deviant behavior (as opposed to the normal, "social" role). The sick person has two rights: exemption from normal social role responsibilities and the privilege of not being held responsible for being sick. In exchange, there are two responsibilities: to try to get better, and to find proper help and follow the physician's advice.

side effect An effect of a drug that is other than the intended, desired effect. See also *adverse drug reaction*.

SIDS See *sudden infant death syndrome*.

SIG Special interest group.

sigma The Greek letter (σ) commonly used in statistics as a symbol for standard deviation (SD), which is a common measure of dispersion or variability in a distribution. (The uppercase Sigma (Σ) is used as the "summation" symbol.) See also *Six Sigma*.

sign See *diagnosis*.

signing out (the patient) Discharging the patient; the act of the attending physician that records her or his permission for the patient to leave the hospital. By this act, the physician in effect states that, in her or his opinion, the patient does not require further care in the institution. See also *discharge*.

sign oneself out The act of a patient to sign a document (release form) (1) refusing the recommendations of the physician, and (2) releasing the physician and the hospital from liability—"signing himself out" (discharging himself) rather than being "signed out" (discharged) by the physician, which is the normal procedure—and leaving the hospital. The act of leaving the hospital without permission and not returning is tantamount to signing oneself out. Synonyms: discharge against medical advice, AMA. See also *discharge*.

sign out See *discharge*.

silent PPO An insurance scam where a payer takes discounts it's not entitled to in paying claims. For example, say Dr. Jones has an agreement with a legitimate preferred provider organization ("Real PPO") to accept discounted fees (say a 30% discount) for all patients who are members of the PPO. Mrs. Smith is not a member of the PPO, having her indemnity insurance from "Acme Insurance," which has no connection with Real PPO. Mrs. Smith visits Dr. Jones and Acme is subsequently billed for the services (let's say $1,000). Acme finds out the Real PPO discount rate (sometimes via a contract with the PPO or a third party) and pays Dr. Jones according to that rate; in other words, Dr. Jones get $700 from Acme. Dr. Jones never had any agreement with Acme to accept discounted rates. There are variations on this scheme, but the result is that the physician is cheated. Synonyms: blind PPO, ghost PPO.

silo Something that is kept separate from others; compartmentalized. As a verb, silo means to keep separate. In information technology (IT), silo refers, for example, to a separate computer system supporting finance, another supporting human resources, and yet another for management—"system islands" (which don't necessarily talk to each other). This is in contrast to an integrated system. Synonym: silo effect.

single-diagnosis category See under *category*.

single-gene disorder A hereditary disorder caused by a single gene. Examples are Huntington's disease, Tay-Sachs disease, and sickle cell anemia.

single-payer plan A method of healthcare financing in which there is only one source of money for paying healthcare providers. The Canadian-style system is the prime example of a single-payer plan, but not all elements of the Canadian program need be included for a plan to be "single payer"; in fact, the single payer could be an insurance company. The scope of the plan also does not have to be national; it could be employed by a single state or community. Proponents of a single-payer plan emphasize the administrative simplicity for patients and providers, and the resulting significant savings in cost.

single photon emission computer tomography (SPECT) See *nuclear medicine*.

single strand One of the two strands of DNA that form the double helix carrying genetic information.

single-stream funding Consolidation of all sources of healthcare funding—particularly those for mental health services—to maximize their availability for the needs of patients.

sin tax A tax on products or activities that are allegedly harmful; for example, alcohol and cigarettes.

SIP See *Sickness Impact Profile* under *quality of life scale*.

site management organization (SMO) An independent organization that contracts with the sponsor or clinical investigator of a clinical trial. Federal regulations do not define an SMO or describe its responsibilities. See also *contract research organization*.

602 Pricing See *340B Drug Pricing Program*.

Six Sigma A quality improvement process, named and registered by Motorola during the 1980s, with the goal of keeping the quality of the product within Six Sigma (six standard deviations), rather than the "best" performance of three to four sigma of most companies. Three sigma means about 66,000 defects per million units or service operations. Six Sigma means only 3.4 defects per million.

  Six Sigma applies to repetitive processes. Leaders of the Six Sigma movement emphasize the need for top management to deploy the effort, which they define as personally participating, proactively, to demonstrate their commitment, rather than delegating, which assigns the effort and implies that it has low priority. Six Sigma results in a culture change in the organization.

  Healthcare organizations are increasingly using the Six Sigma process, which involves five steps: (1) defining the quality improvement project, (2) measuring the key product attributes, (3) analyzing to identify the key causes and process determinants, (4) improving by changing the process and optimizing performance, and (5) holding the gains.

skilled nursing care See under *nursing care*.

skilled nursing facility (SNF) A free-standing facility set up to provide *skilled nursing care* (see under *nursing care*). To qualify as an SNF, the facility must have an *organized professional staff* (see under *staff (group)*) including medical and nursing professionals, and meet the other social and health needs of patients who do not require acute hospital care, but who do need inpatient professional nursing care. An SNF typically must have on-site *registered nurse* (see under *nurse*) supervision for at least two nursing shifts each day. Patients may be discharged from an acute hospital and then admitted to an SNF. A portion of an SNF may be organized so as to provide *intermediate care* (see under *nursing care*), and called the *intermediate care unit* of the SNF. Skilled nursing care may be provided in a portion of an acute hospital, in which case that portion is called a "skilled nursing unit" (SNU). Formerly called extended care facility (ECF).

skilled nursing facility prospective payment system (SNF-PPS) See under *prospective payment system*.

skilled nursing services A Medicare term referring to nursing and to other rehabilitation services provided to Medicare beneficiaries under conditions set up by the Medicare program.

skilled nursing unit (SNU) A portion of a hospital devoted to providing *skilled nursing care* (see under *nursing care*), rather than acute care. To qualify as an SNU, the unit must have an *organized professional staff* (see *staff (group)*) including medical and nursing professionals, and meet the other social and health needs of patients who do not require acute hospital care, but who do need professional nursing care as inpatients. An SNU typically must have on-site registered nurse supervision for at least two nursing shifts each day. Patients may be discharged from an acute hospital and then admitted to its SNU. A free-standing facility offering the same skilled nursing care is called a *skilled nursing facility (SNF)*. Formerly called extended care unit (ECU).

skim A term that, in hospital usage, usually means to select patients who will be financially profitable (for example, because they have an illness for which the prospective payment system (PPS) favors the hospital, or because they have insurance and are not charity patients).

slander Spoken words that injure the reputation of another; oral defamation. Written defamation is called "libel." See *defamation*.

sleep medicine The medical discipline pertaining to sleep, circadian rhythm, and sleep disorders.

SLP See *speech-language pathologist*.

SLS See *Specialist in Laboratory Safety* under *clinical laboratory specialist*.

SM See *Specialist in Microbiology* under *clinical laboratory specialist*.

small employer The definition depends on the context in which the term is used, typically a particular statute or regulation. Generally, small employers are those that employ less than fifty people, although at least one health reform proposal put the limit at 100 employees. The distinction is important because the designation of "small employer" may exempt a business from having to comply with certain requirements, such as federal legislation dealing with the employment relationship (e.g., the Family Medical Leave Act). Some states have enacted Small Employer Insurance Reform to ease the hardship for the small employer in the healthcare market.

small employer pool The banding together of several small employers in order to compete in purchasing power with large employers. See *managed competition*.

small group market reform See *small group reform*

small group reform An approach to healthcare reform that would regulate insurers who sell policies to small businesses, to make insurance more available and affordable. Such regulations may, for example, outlaw cherry picking, predatory pricing, medical underwriting, and other questionable practices.

smart card A card that stores in magnetic or optical form information about a patient that can be read by an electronic device. The typical storage medium is a magnetic strip.

SMDEP See *Summer Medical and Dental Education Program*.

SME See *standard of medical expertise* under *divided standard of medical care*, under *standard of care (clinical)*.

SMO See *site management organization*.

SMSA Standard Metropolitan Statistical Area.

SNDO *Standard Nomenclature of Diseases and Operations.* A nomenclature and coding system for diseases and operations published by the American Medical Association (AMA), with its final, 5th, edition appearing in 1961. Until its replacement by the successive revisions of the *International Classification of Diseases (ICD)*, *SNDO* provided the coding system used most widely for indexing and retrieval of medical records in the United States. The 1st edition was published as *Standard Classified Nomenclature of Disease* in 1933, with a preliminary printing in 1932. The name changed with the 3rd edition in 1942 to *Standard Nomenclature of Disease* and *Standard Nomenclature of Operations*. At the 4th edition, 1952, the name was simplified to *Standard Nomenclature of Diseases and Operations*, with R.J. Plunkett, MD, and Adeline C. Hayden, RRL, editors. *SNDO* was the first major nomenclature using the principle of transforming the original language in which the diagnoses and operations were recorded into standardized, structured language, which was then coded, rather than the original language being coded.

SNF See *skilled nursing facility*.

SNF-PPS See *skilled nursing facility prospective payment system* under *prospective payment system*.

sniff Common pronunciation of the initialism SNF. See *skilled nursing facility*.

SNIP See *Strategic National Implementation Process*.

SNO See *subnetwork organization*.

SNODENT *Systematized Nomenclature of Dentistry*. Standardized terminology of dentistry, developed and maintained by the American Dental Association (ADA).

SNOMED *Systematized Nomenclature of Medicine*, developed by the College of American Pathologists (CAP). The system was first created and published by the SNOMED Division of the College of American Pathologists (CAP) in 1993 (with portions copyrighted by the American Veterinary Medical Association; it was originally called the *Systematized Nomenclature of Human and Veterinary Medicine*). It is the outgrowth of the *Systematized Nomenclature of Pathology* (SNOP) (CAP, 1965). See *SNOMED Clinical Terms*.

SNOMED Clinical Terms (SNOMED CT) A comprehensive clinical terminology covering diseases, clinical findings, and procedures. In 2007 SNOMED CT contained over 300,000 "concepts." A concept is defined as a "unit of meaning," described by:

- A unique numeric code
- A unique name ("fully specified name")
- A set of terms (descriptions)
- One "preferred term"
- One or more synonyms

There are more than 770,000 English language descriptions for expressing the clinical concepts. For example, for the "concept":

Pain in throat (fully specified name)

There are these associated "descriptions":

Sore throat
Throat pain
Pain in pharynx
Throat discomfort
Pharyngeal pain
Throat soreness

The concepts are organized into nineteen hierarchies (each with subhierarchies); these are listed below, with examples:

Clinical finding
   Finding (swelling of arm)
   Disease (pneumonia)
Procedure (biopsy of lung)
Observable entity (tumor stage)
Body structure (structure of thyroid)
   Morphologically abnormal structure (granuloma)
Organism (DNA virus)
Substance (gastric acid)
Pharmaceutical/biologic product (Tamoxifen)
Specimen (urine specimen)
Qualifier value (right)
Record artifact (death certificate)
Physical object (suture needle)

Physical force (friction)
Events (flash flood)
Environments/geographical locations (intensive care unit, Canada)
Social context (organ donor)
Situation with explicit content (no nausea)
Staging and scales (Barthel index)
Linkage concept
    Link assertion (has etiology)
    Attributes (finding site)
Special concept (inactive concept)

In addition, over 900,000 defining "relationships" serve to link concepts both within a hierarchy and across hierarchies.

Although comprehensive on its own, SNOMED CT cross-maps to other classifications already in use, avoiding duplicate data capture. In the July 2006 release, mappings were available for ICD-9-CM Epidemiological/Statistical Mapping, ICD-O-3, ICD-10 (U.K. edition), *OPCS-4* (U.K. edition), Nursing Interventions Classification (NIC), Nursing Outcomes Classification (NOC), NANDA International (NANDA-I), Perioperative Nursing Data Set (PNDS), Clinical Care Classification (CCC), and the Omaha System. In addition, SNOMED CT is aligned with key health information standards, including HL7, DICOM, ANSI, and ISO.

SNOMED CT, first published in 2002, was the result of a collaboration between *SNOMED International* and the United Kingdom National Health Service (NHS). It combines the content and structure of the SNOMED Reference Terminology (SNOMED RT) Version 1.0 with the United Kingdom's Clinical Terms Version 3 (CTV3) (formerly known as the Read Codes). SNOMED CT is available to U.S. users through the UMLS Metathesaurus. It is owned by the *International Health Terminology Standards Development Organisation*. See also *SNOMED*.

SNOMED CT See *SNOMED Clinical Terms*.

SNOMED International A division of the College of American Pathologists (CAP) that delivers SNOMED terminology and implementation support products and services. SNOMED International was responsible for *SNOMED Clinical Terms (SNOMED CT)* until April 2007, when CAP transferred ownership to the *International Health Terminology Standards Development Organisation*. www.snomed.org

SNOMED Reference Terminology (SNOMED RT) The last version of SNOMED issued (in 2000) prior to the publication of SNOMED Clinical Terms (SNOMED CT).

SNOP *Systematized Nomenclature of Pathology*; see *SNOMED*.

SNP See *special needs plan*. Previously also meant School Nurse Practitioner; see *school nursing*.

SNS See *Strategic National Stockpile*.

SNU See *skilled nursing unit*.

SOAP A common form of organization for a *problem-oriented medical record (POMR)* (see under *medical record*). "SOAP" stands for Subjective (complaints), Objective (observations, test results), Assessment, Plan.

SOAPIER See *charting by exception*.

social consciousness The awareness of an individual of the needs of society and of the impact of events on society. It is contrasted with what might be called "personal consciousness," an awareness of the needs of the individual and the relationship of events to the individual.

social health maintenance organization (S/HMO) See under *health maintenance organization*.

Social Security Act A major piece of legislation originally signed into law on August 14, 1935. It created an insurance program to pay retired workers age sixty-five or older a continuing income after retirement, as well as several other provisions related to the general welfare.

The act is available online at **www.ssa.gov/OP_Home/ssact/comp-ssa.htm**. See also *Social Security Administration*. Pub. L. No. 74-271, 49 Stat. 620 (1935), codified at 42 U.S.C. § 301 et seq. (2004).

Social Security Administration (SSA) The federal agency that administers the federal government's largest domestic program. The SSA was established as an independent agency in 1995. Originally triggered by the economic crisis in the United States known as the "Great Depression," the forerunners of the SSA began with President Franklin D. Roosevelt's 1934 message to Congress that he intended to provide a program for "social security." The resulting *Social Security Act* was signed into law on August 14, 1935. It created an insurance program to pay retired workers age sixty-five or older a continuing income after retirement, as well as several other provisions related to the general welfare.

The passage of the act required a massive organizational effort that resulted in the issuance of 35 million Social Security Numbers (SSNs) within the next two years. Beginning in January 1937, after the SSNs were assigned, the first Federal Insurance Contributions Act (FICA) taxes were collected. Since then, over $4 trillion have been paid out of the special Trust Funds set up for the purpose. There is currently quite a bit of concern that these Trust Funds are being depleted more quickly than they are being filled, due to a number of economic and demographic trends.

The Social Security Amendments of 1954 added a disability insurance program to the scope of the SSA's protection. In 1965 the Medicare bill's signature resulted in an additional 20 million beneficiaries for the SSA over the next three-year period. In the Social Security Amendments of 1972, a number of overlapping and inconsistent programs for the needy, largely administered by the states, were folded into the SSA under the Supplemental Security Income (SSI) program, adding another 3 million beneficiaries.

A serious financial crisis for the SSA in the early 1980s prompted a study by the Greenspan Commission, whose recommendations resulted in the 1983 Amendments that made many changes in both Social Security and Medicare programs, including the taxation of Social Security benefits. These 1983 Amendments also established the **prospective payment system** for hospital reimbursement, using DRGs. Both Medicare and Medicaid are now administered by CMS. **www.ssa.gov**

social services See *social work*.

social work Assistance to patients and their families in handling social, environmental, and emotional problems (in healthcare usage, primarily such problems associated with illness or injury). Synonym: social services.

social worker A person who does social work with patients and their families. Most social workers have at least a bachelor's degree in social work (BSW), psychology, sociology, or a related field.

> **forensic social worker** A social worker specializing in issues related to law and the legal system.

> **hospital social worker** A person designated as a social worker by the hospital.

> **medical social worker** A person qualified by a master's degree (MSW) to do social work in the hospital or other healthcare setting.

> **psychiatric social worker** A person qualified by a master's degree (MSW) to do social work in the psychiatric or mental health setting.

social worker designee A member of the staff of a long-term care facility (LTCF) responsible for identification of the emotional and social needs of a patient and for the services to meet these needs. Note that this term pertains to the duties assigned the employee, rather than the employee's qualifications.

Society for Advanced Medical Systems (SAMS) A national organization that merged with the Society for Computer Medicine (SCM) to form the *American Association for Medical Systems and Informatics (AAMSI)*.

Society for Computer Medicine (SCM) A national organization that merged with the Society for Advanced Medical Systems (SAMS) to form the ***American Association for Medical Systems and Informatics (AAMSI)***.

Society of Hospital Medicine (SHM) The professional association for the nation's ***hospitalists***. The association held its first meeting in 1998, and had nearly 5,000 members by 2007. Formerly called the National Association of Inpatient Physicians (NAIP). **www.hospitalmedicine.org**

software Computer programs and systems, as contrasted with "hardware," which refers to the physical (hard) components of the computer and its accessories. See also ***firmware***.

solo practice See under ***practice (business)***.

somatic gene therapy See under ***gene therapy***.

somatoform Physical symptoms that suggest a medical condition but that are not fully explained by such medical condition.

somebody else's money (SEM) Said to be a significant factor in the upward spiral of healthcare costs in the United States. The normal human inclination to be more willing to spend somebody else's money, rather than your own, results in reducing the incentive to shop more carefully for services and products, or forego them altogether. See also ***moral hazard***.

sonogram See ***sonography***.

sonographer See ***diagnostic medical sonographer***.

sonography The use of ultrasound to produce dynamic visual images of organs, tissues, or blood flow, by recording the reflection of the sound waves by the tissues. The imaging procedure (called a sonogram or ultrasound scan) is used to examine many parts of the body for diagnostic purposes, and is also being used to assist in other procedures—for example, to help guide a fine needle to take a tissue biopsy. No radiation is used. Miniaturized ultrasound devices are now available that allow bedside scanning. Synonym: ultrasonography.

SOP See ***standard operating procedure***.

source code The part of a computer program that exists in a form comprehensible to humans, as opposed to the part that is only "machine readable." Source code is typically written by humans for further processing ("compiling") into a binary form that the computer can execute directly. Source code always exists in some computer "language," such as Basic, Cobol, or C. Some source code languages can be executed directly by a computer, in which case they are known as "interpreted" languages (as opposed to "compiled").

Most people use computer programs successfully without ever looking at the source code for their programs, and in fact their license for proprietary programs typically forbids their doing so. Not having access to the source code prevents a user from making changes to the program itself, including the finding and fixing of "bugs" (which nearly any complex program will contain). Source code is available to users, however, for programs that are in the public domain or published under an ***Open Source*** license.

SOW Statement of Work. See ***Health Care Quality Improvement Program***.

SOX See ***Sarbanes-Oxley Act of 2002***.

SPD See ***sterile processing and distribution***.

SPE See ***standardized patient encounter*** under ***encounter***.

Speak Up An initiative of the Joint Commission on Accreditation of Healthcare Organizations (JCAHO) to prevent errors and increase patient safety by educating and encouraging patients to become involved in their own care—be informed about their care, ask questions, and speak up if something is not right.

special care unit An area of the hospital for critically ill or injured patients. Special care units include intensive care, burn, neonatal (newborn) intensive care, and cardiac care units.

special diet See under ***diet***.

specialist A person who has special experience and training in a portion of the field (discipline) of his or her major expertise. Although a person may simply claim to be a specialist, in most instances, there are specific credentials, such as being board certified in medicine, that can be obtained by qualified individuals to back up the claim. For example, a physician may be a specialist in internal medicine, with board certification to prove it. See *specialty*.

specialized care See *secondary care*.

special needs plan (SNP) A managed care plan available to Medicare beneficiaries who belong to a defined group with "special needs," for example, long-term care patients, those eligible for both Medicare and Medicaid ("dual eligibles"), or those with certain chronic or disabling conditions, such as diabetes. Established by the Medicare Modernization Act of 2003 and introduced in 2005, these plans are not available in all areas.

special procedure See under *procedure*.

specialty A particular branch of medicine, or a limited division of another profession, such as nursing. The practitioner of a specialty is a "specialist," usually qualified by added training, plus added experience, within the branch of the discipline. See *medical specialty* and *nursing specialty*.

specialty association See *specialty society*.

specialty board See under *board (credentialing)*.

specialty boards See under *boards*.

specialty site See *distant site*.

specialty society A society whose membership is made up of specialist physicians, such as surgeons or internists. Synonym: specialty association. See also *medical society*.

species A class of related organisms that can freely interbreed.

SPECT Single photon emission computer tomography; see *nuclear medicine*.

speech-language pathologist (SLP) A professional who examines, evaluates, and helps provide treatment for speech, language, cognitive-communication, and swallowing problems.

Board Recognized Specialist in Child Language (BRS-CL) A speech-language pathologist who has met the requirements for this advanced credential of the American Speech-Language-Hearing Association (ASHA). **www.asha.org**

Board Recognized Specialist in Fluency Disorders (BRS-FD) A speech-language pathologist who has met the requirements for this advanced credential of the American Speech-Language-Hearing Association (ASHA). **www.asha.org**

Board Recognized Specialist in Swallowing and Swallowing Disorders (BRS-S) A speech-language pathologist who has met the requirements for this advanced credential of the American Speech-Language-Hearing Association (ASHA). **www.asha.org**

Certificate of Clinical Competence in Speech-Language Pathology (CCC-SLP) A credential granted to speech-language pathologists who meet the requirements of the American Speech-Language-Hearing Association (ASHA). **www.asha.org**

speech pathology The science that concerns disorders of speech.

spell of illness A term, used in determining Medicare benefits, that is defined as a period of time starting when the patient enters the hospital and ending at the conclusion of a sixty-consecutive-day period during which the patient has not been an inpatient of any hospital or skilled nursing facility (SNF). (The patient's actual illness ordinarily would have started prior to the hospitalization, and might or might not have concluded within the sixty-day period outside the hospital.)

spend-down eligibility A method of determining eligibility for medical assistance that originated with Medicaid. A person may not have income above a certain level to qualify for the assistance (for example, $500 per month). However, a person with an income of $600 may "spend-down" $100 per month for health care, and qualify for assistance for monthly expenses over $100. This is similar to a deductible.

SPIN See *Standard Prescriber Identification Number*.

spinal cord injury medicine The medical discipline devoted to the prevention, diagnosis, treatment, and management of traumatic spinal cord injury (SCI) and nontraumatic spinal cord dysfunction.

spin density See *nuclear magnetic resonance imaging*.

SPI See *strategic planning*.

SPL See *Structured Product Labeling*.

SPMI Serious and persistent mental illness.

SPN See *Senior Plan Network*.

SPo See *strategic positioning*.

spoke site See *originating site*.

spoliation The intentional, reckless, or negligent destruction, loss, material alteration, or concealment of evidence that is relevant to litigation. This would include the failure of a hospital to produce a medical record necessary to a malpractice case, or the unauthorized or illegal alteration of the medical record.

sponsor (clinical trials) The organization (such as a pharmaceutical company or research institution) that initiates but does not actually conduct a clinical trial. The sponsor must ensure compliance with Food and Drug Administration (FDA) regulations.

sponsor (managed competition) The intermediary between the purchasers of health care and the provider(s). Large employers would usually serve as sponsors themselves, whereas a health alliance (HA) would be the sponsor for small employers (and people not covered by their employment). See *managed competition*.

sports medicine The study of sports injuries, including their treatment and prevention. Sports medicine has expanded to include all aspects of health related to sports and other similar physical activities, such as fitness programs, nutrition, and psychology. The subspecialty of sports medicine is available in the fields of emergency medicine, family medicine, internal medicine, and pediatrics.

squeal rule A law requiring a family planning agency to report to parents when family planning advice or services are provided to a minor.

SR See *USDA National Nutrient Database for Standard Reference*.

SRE See *serious reportable event*.

SRS See *Substance Registry System*. Also sexual reassignment surgery.

SRU See *standard of resource use* under *divided standard of medical care*, under *standard of care (clinical)*.

SSA See *Social Security Administration*.

SSDO See *SNOMED Standards Development Organization*.

SSI See *Supplemental Security Income*.

SSO Second surgical opinion (see *second opinion*) and *standard setting organization*.

ST See *surgical technologist*.

staff (group) A term that means either the body, or the individual members, of one of these hospital groups:

hospital staff The body of hospital employees. This term may easily be misused when the intent is to designate the medical staff. One must deduce the meaning of "hospital staff" from the context.

house staff The body of house officers, physicians, and dentists in residency training in an accredited graduate medical education (GME) (see *education*) program in a *teaching hospital* (see under *hospital*). The house officers may or may not need to be licensed.

medical staff Physicians, dentists, and other professionals who are officially members of the organized medical staff of the hospital. Members of this group are often referred to as "hospital staff" or merely "staff"; however, in better usage, "hospital staff" refers to hospital employees, and "staff" alone is ambiguous unless taken in context. See the separate listing for *medical staff*.

organized professional staff An ill-defined term, applied primarily to hospitals, that refers to the formal organization of the health professionals on its staff. Usually there must be one or more physicians on the staff, and the term may also imply delegation of certain responsibilities with respect to the quality of care of the organized professional staff. The term "organized medical staff" is, in contrast, well defined by the Joint Commission on Accreditation of Healthcare Organizations (JCAHO); see the separate listing for *medical staff*. Synonym: organized staff.

staff (structure) A term that, in the context of "line and staff," refers to positions (persons) in an organization who assist those with *line* authority. Those with line authority have responsibility, in an organizational hierarchy, to require those beneath them to perform tasks, and to set the standards for that performance. Staff persons have such authority only within the confines of the staff department in which they work.

staff development The in-service training of hospital employees. See *training*.

stage A point or period in the course of an illness. For example, many illnesses first have an acute stage, which is followed by a chronic stage. For some diseases, such as cancers, the stages are specifically identified and named by processes called "staging," with the stages important in both treatment and prognosis. See *staging (disease)* and *staging (tumors)*.

stager A method or device for performing staging of diseases.

personal computer stager (PC-stager) A method for quantifying the severity of illness using data specially abstracted from the medical record.

staging (diseases) One of the methods developed for taking into account a patient's *severity of illness*, in addition to simply the diagnosis and surgical procedures, in predicting and analyzing the length of stay, cost, and outcome. For a number of diagnoses, objective factors have been identified by which the patient's condition can be classified into several "stages" representing degrees of severity. For example, a diabetic person whose diabetes is under control could be in "stage 1," and not require hospitalization, whereas one in a diabetic coma (a life-threatening condition) could be in "stage 4," and require intensive care in the hospital. In this system, the severity score is specific to the disease. Synonym: disease staging.

staging (tumors) A term applied to various systems devised for describing the extent of tumors, both as to the tumor itself and its spread through the body, and with consequent implications as to the patient's likelihood of survival. Some of the staging systems for bowel cancer are, for example, the Dukes system, the Kirklin system, the Astler-Coller system, and the TNM (tumor, node, metastases) system. Synonym: tumor staging.

stakeholder An individual who has an interest in the activities of an organization and the ability to influence it. A hospital's stakeholders, for example, include its patients, employees, medical staff, government, insurers, industry, and the community.

standard (norm) An agreement reached via consensus that an object, method, or technology will always have certain attributes or properties. A "standard" credit card will always be the same size, no matter who has issued it. This type of standard is frequently spelled out somewhere and may be sponsored by an organization. In the case of the ubiquitous credit card, it must meet the relevant *ISO* standard so that it will physically fit into the slot of any cash machine in the world. As information processing has gotten increasingly important in the healthcare industry (healthcare informatics), standards (as norms) have also become increasingly important because without them it is extremely difficult to put the right information in the right place at the right time. See also *standards development organization* and *standard setting organization*.

standard (threshold) A measure of quality or quantity, established by an authority, by a profession, or by custom, that serves as a criterion for evaluation. It is in the nature of a "threshold," below which one should not fall. This type of standard is distinguished from a standard that is simply a "norm." See also *benchmark*.

standardization A statistical procedure for permitting valid comparisons among several populations. The procedure involves adjustments so that the rates of occurrence of some variable (a disease, for example, by age and sex) are applied to a "standard" distribution of persons by age and sex. Standardization is basically an application of weighting of averages.

standardized nomenclature See *nomenclature*, and the diagram at *natural language*.

standardized patient encounter (SPE) See under *encounter*.

Standard Nomenclature of Diseases and Operations (SNDO) See *SNDO*.

standard of care (clinical) The principles and practices that have been accepted by a healthcare profession as expected to be applied for a patient presenting a specific problem under ordinary circumstances. Standards of care are developed from a consensus of experts, based on specific research (where such is available) and expert experience. "Under ordinary circumstances" refers to the fact that a given patient may have individual conditions that are overriding; absent such considerations, a medical staff or nursing staff quality review committee will expect the generally accepted principles and practices to be carried out.

For example, the standard of care for a bedfast patient requires the nursing service to carry out certain procedures to minimize the patient's chances of developing bedsores. The standard of care for a patient with a suspected fracture is to x-ray the area; however, severe bleeding may override (for an extended period of time) the standard calling for the x-ray. In other words, the *first* standard of care is that the individual patient's needs come before the "general" standard. See also *guidelines*.

divided standard of medical care A proposal by E. Haavi Morreim and others that the "standard of medical care" should be divided into two components: the standard of medical expertise (SME) and the standard of resource use (SRU) (see below) in order to distinguish between that which physicians are expected to do for their patients and the resources, monetary and technological, that insurers and others owe to provide to their wards. This divided standard concept is based on the argument that, although physicians throughout the United States have essentially equal access to training and knowledge, and thus could, in general, be held to one SME, the availability of resources is quite a different matter, and the SRU depends on what insurance coverage the patient has, and what facilities and other resources are available.

standard of medical expertise (SME) The standard of care for physicians that measures performance against national norms of training, knowledge, and practice.

standard of resource use (SRU) A proposed standard of care for a healthcare provider that measures the resources used in the care of the patient against national norms of use of the same kind and amount of resources. For example, the treatment options available to one physician in an affluent area may not be available to another physician, due to lack of funding or payment, lack of technology, state laws, and so forth. The argument is that a physician should not be held liable for resource inadequacies for which the physician is not responsible.

standard of care (legal) The measure to be applied, in a malpractice suit, to the actions of the health professional in order to determine if the professional was negligent. The rule for determining the standard varies from state to state, but it can be generally stated that the standard of care for health professionals is to exercise that degree of care and skill practiced by other professionals of similar skill and training (and, in some states, in the same geographic locality) under similar circumstances.

The legal standard of care may or may not be the same as the medical standard of care (see *standard of care (clinical)*) in a particular case. The jury (or, in some cases, the judge) in a malpractice case decides what the appropriate "degree of care and skill" is in *that* case, based on the facts and upon the expert testimony offered by both the plaintiff and the defendant. Differences in juries' opinions on the relevant standard of care is one reason why two malpractice cases with similar facts can have different results.

On rare occasions, the legal standard of care may be higher than that of the healthcare profession. For example, a thirty-two-year-old woman developed glaucoma and suffered permanent eye damage, after her physicians failed to detect the condition while treating her from 1959 until 1968. Medical experts for both the plaintiff (the woman) and the defendant ophthalmologists testified that the standards of the ophthalmology profession did not require routine glaucoma testing for patients under forty years of age. However, the court concluded that because the test was simple, inexpensive, and painless, the standard itself was negligent. *Helling v. Carey*, 83 Wash.2d 514, 519 P.2d 981 (1974).

standard of medical expertise (SME) See under *divided standard of medical care* under *standard of care (clinical)*.

standard of resource use (SRU) See under *divided standard of medical care* under *standard of care (clinical)*.

standard operating procedure (SOP) An action (or series of actions) to be carried out in a given situation. An SOP may or may not be written. For example, it is "SOP" in most households to lock the doors at night.

Standard Prescriber Identification Number (SPIN) An early attempt by the *National Council for Prescription Drug Programs (NCPDP)* to establish a unique identifier for drug prescribers for use by retail pharmacies. By 1997 the NCPDP had changed the name of SPIN to the more catchy phrase "work group 3 standard identifiers" (WG3), under which label it continued its work. See *HCIdea*.

standards development organization (SDO) A formally accredited organization whose members work to create and refine standards (see *standard (norm)*) in an area where the lack of any standards hampers progress towards a universally desired goal. An SDO, most often a nonprofit organization, typically includes members from the relevant industries (stakeholders), interested individuals from academic institutions, and representatives from various governmental units.

A distinction should be made regarding organizations that take initiatives and promote the development of standards, such as CPRI-HOST, but which are not officially SDOs; see *standard setting organizations*. See also *ANSI*, *HL7*, and *ISO*.

standard setting organization (SSO) A general term for an organization that develops, maintains, promulgates, coordinates, revises, interprets, or endorses standards. A *standards development organization (SDO)* is one type of SSO, but not all SSOs are SDOs, which require accreditation.

standards manual See *accreditation manual*.

standards organization See *standards development organization* and *standard setting organization*.

standing orders A type of medical protocol that provides specific, written orders for care of patients under prescribed circumstances, such as in preparation for specific diagnostic procedures or surgery. Standing orders are to be followed for all such patients unless the physician or surgeon directs otherwise.

Stark I Legislation passed in 1989 as part of the federal Omnibus Budget Reconciliation Act of 1989 (OBRA 89). The bill was introduced by Representative Pete Stark and originally introduced as the "Ethics in Patient Referrals Act." The bill prohibited a physician to refer a patient to a clinical laboratory if the physician or an immediate family member of the physician had a financial interest in the laboratory. There were three exceptions: (1) if the physician services were provided by another physician in the same group, (2) for "in-office" ancillary services that were furnished by the referring physician or another physician in the same group, and (3) for services furnished by HMOs, CMPs, or other prepaid health plans. This bill differed from the *Antikickback Statute* because it prohibited self-referral as opposed to referral to another physician. The law was intended to save Medicare dollars by discouraging overuse of health services. The Stark legislation was amended substantially in 1993. See *Stark II* and *fraud and abuse*. 42 U.S.C. § 1395nn (2004).

Stark II The *Stark I* legislation was amended in this bill, Stark II, as part of the Omnibus Budget Reconciliation Act of 1993 (OBRA 93), codified at 42 U.S.C. § 1395nn(h)(6) (2004). This legislation prohibits a physician from referring a patient covered by Medicare or Medicaid to a facility in which the physician has a financial interest. Stark II extended the reach of Stark I to cover physical therapy services, occupational therapy services, radiology and other diagnostic services, radiation therapy services, durable medical equipment, parenteral and enteral nutrients, equipment and supplies, prosthetics and orthotics, home health services, outpatient prescription drugs, and inpatient and outpatient hospital services. Stark II also extended coverage to Medicaid-financed services (42 U.S.C. § 1396b(5) (2004)). The practical effect of this and other fraud and abuse laws was to encourage physicians to form groups and join health systems as employees. See also *Stark I* and *fraud and abuse*.

stat Medical shorthand for "do at once."

state approved A term that comes up especially often in nursing with regard to nursing education programs. To be eligible for registration (to be able to become a *registered nurse (RN)*; see under *nurse*), a nurse must be a graduate of a program approved by the State Board of Nursing. The program, however, may or may not have been accredited by the National League for Nursing (NLN), the voluntary body that accredits professional and vocational schools of nursing, because state approval may not require meeting the standards set by the NLN.

state board of medical examiners See *state medical board* under *board (credentialing)*. (Do not confuse this term with *medical examiner*.)

State Children's Health Insurance Program (SCHIP) A federal program that uses a block grant mechanism to help states set up healthcare programs for needy children and families not otherwise covered by health insurance (including Medicaid). Typical children in this target group have parents who earn too much to qualify for Medicaid, but not enough to afford private health insurance. A significant force in getting this legislation created and passed was Marian Wright Edelman, a person with a long-time commitment to the interests of children. Created by the *Balanced Budget Act of 1997*.

state mandate See under *mandate*.

state medical board See under *board (credentialing)*.

statement of work (SOW) See *Health Care Quality Improvement Program*.

State of the Science Statement See *National Institutes of Health Consensus Development Program*.

statute A law enacted (passed) by a legislative body. Distinguish from *rule*.

Statute of Frauds A law specifying which kinds of contracts must be evidenced by a written document to be enforceable. Examples are contracts concerning real estate (except short-term leases), sales of goods with a price of more than $500, and contracts that by their terms cannot be performed within a year. The entire agreement does not have to be written to satisfy the Statute of Frauds; all the law requires is a memorandum signed by the party against whom enforcement is sought.

statute of limitations A law requiring that certain types of lawsuits be initiated within a specific length of time. For example, if a patient wishes to sue for malpractice, state law may require that the suit be started within two years after the date of the alleged act of malpractice (the length of time varies from state to state). In some states, the time period begins when the patient discovers (or should have discovered) the injury, rather than on the date of the alleged act of malpractice; this is called the "discovery rule."

In certain circumstances, the law allows the statute of limitations to be suspended ("tolled"). For example, a minor is not legally competent to file suit. Therefore, the law allows that minor to reach majority before the time period begins to run. Thus, even though a statute of limitations for malpractice may be only two years, a suit could be initiated as long as twenty years after the birth of an injured infant (eighteen years to reach majority, plus the two-year limitations period).

STD See *sexually transmitted disease*.

STEEEP Safe, Timely, Effective, Efficient, Equitable, and Patient-centered. See *Institute of Medicine's Health Care Quality Initiative*.

steering committee A generic term for a committee set up to provide broad guidance for a program, project, or activity.

stem cell A cell whose daughter cells (descendent cells) may differentiate into cells of different types. Human stem cells are the first cells formed when a sperm fertilizes an egg. The single cell formed has the ability to split repeatedly and eventually form the entire human being. This cell is called a "totipotent" cell because it can form all other kinds of cells (i.e., it can form an entire embryo). After the first cell division, there are two totipotent cells that, if separated, can each go on to produce identical twins.

After the first few days of cell division, a cell mass called a blastocyte is formed, the outer layer of which produces the placenta and other tissues needed to permit the fetus to develop. The internal cells retain the ability to form various organs, but not the placenta and supporting tissues for the fetus. These internal cells are no longer totipotent; they are "pleuripotent," meaning that they can form the many other kinds of cells needed by the body. Because they are not totipotent, they are not embryos.

In the context of the current discussions of stem cell research, the "embryonic stem cells" most often discussed are, according to a fact sheet provided by the federal government, the *pleuripotent* stem cells. Pleuripotent stem cells, as they divide, produce more stem cells, which are further specialized, such as blood stem cells and skin stem cells—classes of cells that are called "multipotent." Blood stem cells, for example, persist throughout life and make possible the constant replenishing of the blood supply. The National Institutes of Health (NIH) has an "official resource" web page for stem cell research at **stemcells.nih.gov**.

step therapy A protocol that requires more simple or conservative measures to be tried first to control a disease or condition and then, if those fail, more complex therapies can be tried. In prescription drug usage, this approach usually means that the most cost-effective and safest drug must be prescribed first, and a new drug prescribed only if the first has failed to achieve the desired result. Drug plans may require an enrollee to try a cheaper drug before it will pay for a more expensive one. Synonyms: step-care therapy, step protocol, "fail first."

sterile (aseptic) Free from all living bacteria, viruses, and other living organisms and their spores (resistant forms of such life). Synonym: aseptic.

sterile (non-reproductive) Without capacity to produce offspring, a condition that may or may not be reversible. Sterile is a more definite term than "infertile," which is used when there is felt to be a greater possibility of correcting the condition. Sterility may be natural or the result of having undergone *sterilization (contraceptive)*, a procedure intended to remove the capacity to reproduce.

sterile processing and distribution (SPD) Cleaning, disinfection, sterilization, and inventory management activities in a healthcare setting.

CBSPD Certification Certification of an individual by the Certification Board for Sterile Processing and Distribution. Five levels are offered: Technician, Surgical Instrument Processor, Ambulatory Surgery Technician, Supervisor, and Manager. **www.sterileprocessing.org**

sterilization (antiseptic) The process of treating an object in such a manner that all living microorganisms are destroyed. Surgical instruments and dressings, for example, must be sterilized so that they do not transmit infections. Sterilization may be accomplished by heat, certain chemicals, radiation, ultraviolet light, or other means.

sterilization (contraceptive) Making a person unable to reproduce. Sterilization may be undertaken simply to prevent conception ("contraceptive sterilization"), to prevent inheritance of a mental or physical disability or disease ("eugenic sterilization"), or because bearing children would be harmful to the individual ("therapeutic sterilization"). To prevent inappropriate sterilizations, especially of those unable to give voluntary consent, there are often special laws concerning consent for sterilization. For example, federal regulations govern all sterilizations performed under federally financed programs. Those regulations require, among other things, that the person to be sterilized be at least twenty-one years old, not institutionalized, and fully informed about the procedure, and that he or she wait for thirty days after giving consent except in an emergency.

stigma Clinically, stigma means a mark on the skin, or the indicia of a disease. However, the term is also used to denote the use of negative labels or portrayals of those with a particular disease or condition—for example, AIDS or mental illness. Such labels show ignorance (and often fear) of the disease and disrespect for the individuals living with it. Stigmas can discourage people from getting needed health care for fear of discrimination and humiliation.

stock Evidence of ownership of a corporation, and of a claim against the company's assets and earnings. Synonym: share. Stocks are of two kinds:

common stock Evidence of ownership of a corporation, but with claims on assets and earnings having lower priority than preferred stock. Common stockholders have voting rights and dividend rights.

preferred stock A class of stock that has preference over common stock in the distribution of earnings or in the case of liquidation of the corporation. Preferred stockholders do not ordinarily have voting rights.

stockholder See *shareholder*.

stone center A *lithotripsy* facility.

stop-loss insurance See under *insurance*.

store and forward (S&F) A type of telehealth encounter that uses still digital images of a patient to assist in rendering a medical opinion or diagnosis, for example in providing radiology, pathology, dermatology, and wound care services. Data from the patient are stored and then forwarded to the consulting physician (for example, in an email attachment). The term also refers to the asynchronous (at different times) transmission of clinical data, such as blood glucose levels or electrocardiogram (ECG) measurements, from one site (such as the patient's home) to another site (for example, a home health agency, hospital, or clinic).

strategic business unit (SBU) A term applied to each *product line* of an organization employing *product line management (PLM)* (see under *management*). An SBU is a more or less distinct line of business (for example, in a hospital, knee replacement surgery or alcoholism rehabilitation) that has a specific market, resource requirements, and management demands. The hospital operating under PLM acts as though it were managing an array of more or less independent SBUs, rather than thinking of itself as a hospital. Thus it would, for example, advertise each product line separately, staff it more or less independently, and expect each product line to be profitable.

Strategic Framework A report issued by the U.S. Office of the National Coordinator for Health Information Technology (ONC) in July 2004 laying out a ten-year strategy to achieve the Nationwide Health Information Network (NHIN) and other national health information technology (HIT) goals. The full title is "The Decade of Health Information Technology: Delivering Consumer-Centric and Information-Rich Health Care—Framework for Strategic Action." The report lists seven "critical needs" for HIT: (1) avoid medical errors, (2) improve use of resources, (3) accelerate diffusion of knowledge, (4) reduce variability in access to care, (5) advance the role of the consumer, (6) strengthen privacy and data protection, and (7) promote public health and preparedness.

The Framework has four specific goals, with three strategies for each goal:

Goal 1: Inform Clinical Practice. Bring information tools to the point of care, especially by investing in EHR systems in physician offices and hospitals.

> *Strategy 1.* Incentivize EHR adoption.
> *Strategy 2.* Reduce risk of EHR investment.
> *Strategy 3.* Promote EHR diffusion in rural and underserved areas.

Goal 2: Interconnect Clinicians. Build an interoperable health information infrastructure, so that records follow the patient and clinicians have access to critical healthcare information when treatment decisions are being made.

Strategy 1. Foster regional collaborations.

Strategy 2. Develop a national health information network.

Strategy 3. Coordinate federal health information systems.

Goal 3: Personalize Care. Use health information technology to give consumers more access and involvement in health decisions.

Strategy 1. Encourage use of Personal Health Records.

Strategy 2. Enhance informed consumer choice.

Strategy 3. Promote use of telehealth systems.

Goal 4: Improve Population Health. Expand capacity for public health monitoring, quality of care measurement, and bringing research advances more quickly into medical practice.

Strategy 1. Unify public health surveillance architectures.

Strategy 2. Streamline quality and health status monitoring.

Strategy 3. Accelerate research and dissemination of evidence.

In addition, several "Key Actions" are described, including establishing standards for interoperability, supporting the Connecting Communities for Better Health (CCBH) program, launching a "portal" for Medicare beneficiaries (see **Medicare Beneficiary Portal** under **portal**), and requiring Medicare prescription drug plans (PDPs) to offer e-prescribing. Synonyms: Decade of Health Information Technology (DHIT), Framework for Strategic Action (FSA), ONCHIT Framework.

Strategic National Implementation Process (SNIP) A *Workgroup for Electronic Data Interchange (WEDI)* dedicated to a collaborative healthcare industry-wide process resulting in the implementation of standards and furthering the development and implementation of future standards, especially those required by HIPAA. **www.wedi.org/snip**

Strategic National Stockpile (SNS) Large quantities of medicine and medical supplies to protect the American public if there is a public health emergency (such as a terrorist attack, flu outbreak, or earthquake) severe enough to cause local supplies to run out. The stockpile includes such items as antibiotics, chemical antidotes, antitoxins, life-support medications, IV administration supplies, airway maintenance supplies, and medical/surgical items. One item is called a **Push Package**; this is a cache of a broad spectrum of pharmaceuticals, antidotes, and medical supplies to respond to an emergency as soon as possible, perhaps even before the exact threat is known. When needed, these supplies can be delivered to any state in the United States within twelve hours. If a disease agent is well defined, products will be sent specific to that agent. Each state has plans to receive and distribute SNS supplies to local communities as quickly as possible. In case the SNS runs out (or does not have an item), arrangements are in place with vendors to provide medicines and supplies directly; this is called **vendor managed inventory** (VMI). The SNS is managed by the Coordinating Office for Terrorism Preparedness and Emergency Response (COTPER), within the Centers for Disease Control and Prevention (CDC). **www.bt.cdc.gov/stockpile**

strategic planning (SPI) A term derived from "strategy" in the military sense; planning that is long range, and that is intended to lay out the nature and sequence of the steps to be taken to achieve the large goals of the organization. In traditional thinking, strategic planning should precede the development of the *tactics* with which it is implemented. A current insight is that a successful strategy can only be developed after the available tactics are assessed; then they can be used to their maximum. This is called **bottom-up planning**.

Strategic planning is based on the principle that, with goals and objectives specified, strategies can be developed for achieving them, resources can be generated to implement the strategies, and progress can be continually monitored. See discussion in *strategic positioning*.

strategic positioning (SPo) The concept behind strategic positioning is that it is often more important for an organization to expend its energy on being ready (positioned) to take whatever action is necessary in order to reach its visions of what it wants to happen, at the time such action is necessary, than to spend the energy on *strategic planning (SPI)*. Strategic planning works well in known markets, but strategic positioning has significant advantages in a market—health care, for instance—in which there is little predictable in the foreseeable future.

Strategic planning and strategic positioning may be contrasted in several ways:

In SPl, relatively few key decisions can be made, and actions can be held to them, whereas in SPo, decisions must be made continuously by many people who must keep the vision in focus (this is in line with the thinking of continuous quality improvement (CQI)).

In SPl, resources are considered as finite, whereas in SPo, resources are infinite and new sources can constantly be discovered.

In SPl, investment is heavy in plants, equipment, technology, and staffing, whereas in SPo, investment is heavy in training on how to seize opportunities and to leverage resources.

In SPl, effort is made to implement, monitor, and adjust to keep the plan on track, whereas in SPo, effort is made to experiment, learn, and change to keep moving toward the vision.

In SPl, the process is seen as a road to be travelled, whereas in SPo, the process is a compass—one is always looking for a better road.

In SPl, the plan often takes on a life of its own, whereas in SPo, the people are the life of the effort.

The term was coined by Michael Winer.

strategy A term derived from the military, and which concerns the long-range, large goals of the organization. In traditional thinking, strategy should precede the development of the **tactics** with which it is implemented. A current insight is that a successful strategy can only be developed after the available tactics are assessed and used to their maximum.

stroke The sudden stoppage of blood flow to the brain, typically caused by either blood clots or the bursting of defective arteries in a region of the brain. A stroke may be described as the brain's version of a heart attack (see **myocardial infarction** under **infarction**). Although the majority of strokes occur in older people, strokes ranked third as the cause of death for thirty-five- to forty-five-year-olds in the mid 1990s.

According to the American Heart Association, the warning signs for a stroke are the following: sudden and severe headache with no apparent cause, sudden trouble seeing in one or both eyes; sudden weakness or numbness of the face, arm, or leg, especially on one side of the body; sudden confusion; sudden trouble with talking or understanding speech; sudden dizziness, trouble walking, or loss of balance or coordination.

If you suspect someone is having a stroke, it is suggested that you "act F.A.S.T.":

1. *F*ace: Ask the person to smile; look to see if one side of the face droops.
2. *A*rms: Ask the person to raise both arms; look to see if one drifts downward.
3. *S*peech: Ask the person to repeat a simple sentence; see if the words are slurred or if the sentence is incorrect.
4. *T*ime: If any of the symptoms are present, time is of the essence; call 911 or rush to the emergency room.

(National Stroke Association, **www.stroke.org**)

Response to a stroke should be immediate emergency treatment, just as with a heart attack, because there is a three-hour window after the stroke occurs during which much permanent damage may be prevented.

About one third of all strokes are preceded by a "ministroke" known as a **transient ischemic attack (TIA)**, typically lasting no more than five minutes and otherwise displaying the usual stroke warning signs. TIAs should be treated as an emergency, like any other stroke. Risk of stroke may be minimized by avoiding excess fat and cholesterol in your diet, not smoking, not drinking alcohol excessively, maintaining a healthy weight, and not ignoring TIAs.

structure See *process*.

Structured Product Labeling (SPL) A pharmaceutical document XML standard to facilitate reliable communication of drug information among various groups needing access, such as the Food and Drug Administration (FDA), hospitals, doctors, and consumers. It has been approved by HL7 and adopted by the FDA.

student affairs practitioner (SAP) A counselor with special education and training in the needs of college and university students. Sometimes the phrase "student affairs in higher education" is used to describe this discipline.

Study Data Tabulation Model (SDTM) A standard for submitting clinical trial data tabulations to the Food and Drug Administration (FDA), developed by the FDA, Clinical Data Interchange Standards Consortium (CDISC), and National Institutes of Health (NIH).

subacute care A transitional level of care between acute care and traditional skilled nursing or home care. In some states, subacute care is provided in skilled nursing facility beds.

subcutaneous Beneath the skin, but outside the muscle. (Within the muscle is "intramuscular.") "Subcutaneous" refers to the administration of medication or nourishment.

subject-oriented information See *problem-oriented information*.

subnetwork organization (SNO) A network that supports data exchange subordinate to the larger nationwide network (*Nationwide Health Information Network (NHIN)*). A SNO is a building block of the NHIN. It is loosely defined as an affiliation of users who share health information and adhere to a common IT framework. A SNO encompasses the notion of a *regional health information organization (RHIO)* and expands it to include other types of organizational structures.

subpoena An order to appear in court (or at a deposition) to give testimony. "Subpoena" is Latin for "under penalty."

subpoena duces tecum An order to appear in court (or at a deposition) and to bring specific documents within the possession or control of the person being subpoenaed. The hospital does not permit medical records out of its custody without legal authority. Thus when medical records are required for a legal proceeding, a subpoena duces tecum requesting the records is sent to the health information administrator of the hospital, who personally (or by a delegee) takes the records to the court or deposition. The term is Latin for "under penalty" plus "bring with you."

subscriber As used in health insurance and with prepayment plans, the subscriber is the person (the eligible employee, for example) who signs up and pays the premiums. Dependents of the subscriber, as well as the subscriber her- or himself, are all *enrollees* (sometimes called members or "covered persons"), but not all enrollees are subscribers.

subspecialist A term often applied to a physician, nurse, or dentist whose field of special training, experience, and, usually, practice is a subdivision of a broader specialty. For example, a cardiologist is a physician who has narrowed her or his field from the specialty of all of internal medicine to the subspecialty concerned with just the diseases of the heart and circulatory system (cardiology). This development might perhaps more accurately have been termed "superspecialization" rather than "subspecialization." See *specialist* and *specialty*.

substance Matter or material. A generic word used for simplicity, as in "dangerous substance," to be inclusive of all chemicals, drugs, biological agents (see *agent (substance)*), and other materials that are dangerous. See also *controlled substance*.

substance abuse The excessive use of a drug or use of a drug for a purpose for which it was not medically intended. See also *substance dependence*.

Substance Abuse and Mental Health Services Administration (SAMHSA) An agency within the Department of Health and Human Services (HHS) that conducts and funds biomedical research designed to alleviate mental health problems as well as those related to drug and alcohol abuse. It includes the Center for Mental Health Services (CMHS), Center for Substance Abuse Treatment (CSAT), Center for Substance Abuse Prevention (CSAP), and Office of Applied Studies (OAS). **www.samhsa.gov**

Federal efforts to improve mental health and reduce the harm caused by drug and alcohol abuse are concentrated in SAMHSA, plus three institutes within the National Institutes of Health (NIH): (1) the National Institute on Alcohol Abuse and Alcoholism, (2) the National Institute on Drug Abuse, and (3) the National Institute of Mental Health.

substance abuse counselor A counselor specializing in the needs of individuals affected by substance abuse. Several states provide for certification of substance abuse counselors. Synonym: drug abuse counselor.

substance abuse facility A hospital or other facility specializing in the treatment of patients suffering from alcoholism or chemical dependency.

Substance Abuse Professional (SAP) A health professional specially qualified to evaluate airline pilots, truck drivers, and others who violate a U.S. Department of Transportation (DOT) drug and alcohol program regulation. The SAP makes recommendations concerning education, treatment, follow-up testing, and aftercare of the worker. SAPs include physicians, psychologists, social workers, employee assistance professionals, and drug and alcohol counselors who have met the requirements of the DOT.

substance dependence Compulsive use of a drug despite negative consequences. Physical dependence on a substance is not the same as addiction; a person can be dependent on blood pressure medication or insulin, for example. Cocaine, on the other hand, does not cause physical withdrawal symptoms but mainly depression. Of course, some substances cause both physical and psychological dependence. Synonym: addiction. See also *alcoholism*.

Substance Registry System (SRS) The central system of the Environmental Protection Agency (EPA) for information about regulated and monitored substances. The SRS provides a common basis for identification of chemicals, biological organisms, and other substances listed in EPA regulations and data systems, as well as substances of interest from other sources, such as publications. Examples of substances are mercuric acetate (chemical), *Agardhiella subulata* (biological organism), and bread crumbs (miscellaneous object). The Consolidated Health Informatics (CHI) initiative has adopted it as a standard. **www.epa.gov/srs**

substituted judgment doctrine A legal rule, applied by some courts, that requires a guardian or other person making treatment decisions on behalf of an incompetent person to base that decision on what the incompetent person him or herself would want under the circumstances, as distinguished from what the decision-maker believes would be in the best interests of the incompetent patient.

sudden infant death syndrome (SIDS) The sudden death of an infant younger than one year that remains unexplained after a complete postmortem investigation, including autopsy, examination of the death scene, and review of the clinical history. Synonym: crib death.

suicide Intentionally and voluntarily acting in a way that brings about one's own death.

assisted suicide A suicide involving someone other than the person dying. It is a crime in most jurisdictions to help someone to kill her- or himself. See also *euthanasia*.

physician-assisted suicide (PAS) A controversial practice in which a physician, on request of a patient with an incurable disease or an intolerable (to the patient) physical condition, helps the patient to commit suicide. The practice has gained public attention through the activities of Jack Kevorkian, MD (see *Doctor Death*) of Michigan and the *Oregon Death with Dignity Act* of 1997. See also *euthanasia*.

suicide contagion The exposure to suicide or suicidal behavior in a person's family, within his or her peer group, or in the media. Such exposure sometimes results in an increase in suicidal behavior by those at risk for suicide, especially adolescents and young adults.

Summer Medical and Dental Education Program (SMDEP) An intensive summer program to prepare eligible college students for medical and dental school, sponsored by the Robert Wood Johnson Foundation (RWJF) and the Association of American Medical Colleges (AAMC). Established in 1988, it was originally focused on minority groups that continue to be underrepresented in U.S. medicine—African Americans, Hispanics, and Native

Americans (American Indians, Alaskan Natives, and Native Hawaiians). Over the years the program has broadened to include students from rural areas, those who are economically disadvantaged, and students from groups that have historically received substandard health care regardless of their racial or ethnic background. Formerly (until 2003) called the Minority Medical Education Program (MMEP). **www.smdep.org**

superbill A paper or electronic form used by the physician to communicate with her or his office staff (and on to the payer) what services were rendered to the patient and why they were necessary by providing for the entry of diagnoses and their ICD-9-CM category codes, procedures and their HCPCS (CPT) codes, E&M billing codes, and preventive service "G" codes. Because of its use in communicating within the office, the superbill usually indicates when the patient should be seen again, special instructions, and desired referrals. Superbills may be custom-designed for a particular practice or specialty, and this is often reflected by offering "check-off" entry of the most common diagnoses and procedures for that office, a practice that encourages recording to "the nearest thing" when an exact match is not found. Provision is also made for linking the procedure(s) with the appropriate diagnosis(es).

Supplemental Security Income (SSI) A federal income support program for low-income aged, blind, and disabled individuals.

SUPPORT See *SUPPORT Prognostic Model.*

support group A group of individuals with the same or similar problems who meet periodically to share experiences, problems, and solutions, in order to support each other. For example, group members may themselves have, or have a family member or friend suffering from, a disease such as cancer, Alzheimer's, or alcoholism, or a behavioral problem such as gambling. The group may be sponsored by the individual members, a healthcare institution, a church, or another body.

SUPPORT Prognostic Model A system (model) for developing objective estimates of the probable survival over a 180-day period of seriously ill hospitalized adults. The acronym comes from the name of the study that developed the method, "Study to Understand Prognoses and Preferences for Outcomes and Risks of Treatment." The model uses each patient's diagnosis, age, number of days in the hospital before study entry, presence of cancer, neurologic function, and eleven physiologic variables recorded on day three after study entry. The study reports that this relatively small number of readily available items of information can provide as good estimates of the probability of survival for 180 days as could physicians' estimates. Somewhat better predictions resulted from combining both the objective predictions with physicians'.

support service A service that is necessary for the operation of the institution, but for which direct charges are inappropriate. Heating, for example, is essential, but is not itemized on the patient's bill. The cost of support services is recovered by allocating the costs to the revenue-producing services, using an appropriate accounting method.

surge capacity unit (SCU) An inflatable, portable hospital, similar to the mobile hospitals used by the military. An SCU can be used to provide extra beds, equipment, and supplies in case of emergency, mass disasters, epidemics—anytime the capacity of regular facilities is inadequate—and for quarantine when needed. Synonym: surge hospital. Sometimes called a MASH unit after the Mobile Army Surgical Hospital.

surgeon A physician specializing in surgery.

operating surgeon The surgeon responsible for a given surgical operation and the care directly associated with that operation. She may have other surgeons assisting, but the one surgeon has the prime responsibility. If the operating surgeon admits the patient herself, she is also the *attending physician* (see *physician*). But often a patient is admitted by another physician, who does not operate. If an operation is deemed necessary, this is performed by a surgeon (the operating surgeon) and, unless the patient is transferred to the surgeon's care, the first physician remains the attending physician.

surgeon assistant See *surgical assistant*.

surgeon general The head medical officer in the U.S. Air Force, Navy, Army, or Public Health Service, or any one of the states' public health services. Generally a commissioned (military) officer as well as a doctor.

Surgeon General of the United States The head of the Office of the Surgeon General, a division within the Office of Public Health and Science (OPHS) in the Department of Health and Human Services (HHS). The Surgeon General is responsible for administering the Public Health Service Commissioned Corps (PHSCC) and being a spokesperson for national health concerns. The position dates back to the 1870s when Congress wished to provide health care to American sailors, leading ultimately to the formal beginning of the Public Health Service in 1912.

Appointed by the president, subject to senate confirmation, the Surgeon General's office has become best known in recent years for lending authority to the position that the use of tobacco and certain other substances is unhealthy, resulting in governmental actions such as requiring warning labels on certain products and restrictions on advertising their sale in certain media. The office continues working to educate the nation on health concerns. Its public health priorities in 2007 included disease prevention, eliminating disparities in health, public health preparedness, improving health literacy, organ donation, children and healthy choices, and bone health and osteoporosis. **www.surgeongeneral.gov**

surgery (room) A term sometimes given to an operating room or a treatment room.

surgery (specialty) The medical discipline that utilizes surgery to diagnose and treat injury, disease, and deformity, or to enhance appearance.

surgery (treatment) The treatment of disease, injury, or deformity by means of operation, which usually involves the use of instruments and the removal of body tissues or the rearrangement, rebuilding, or replacement of body structures. Treatment by manipulation is also included under the term "surgery."

ambulatory surgery Surgery performed on an outpatient, with arrival and departure on the same day. If the patient has to be kept overnight, he or she is admitted and then discharged the next day. Synonyms: outpatient surgery, same-day surgery.

elective surgery Surgery that does not have to be done immediately in order to prevent death or serious disability. If surgery can be scheduled at some future date it is, by definition, elective. Thus, there is time for a second opinion to be obtained without hazard to the patient because of delay. Elective surgery may be performed for correction of medical problems, such as the repair of a hernia or the removal of a uterus, or it may be performed because of the wishes of the patient, as in the case of cosmetic surgery, face lifts, or hair transplants.

emergency surgery Surgery that the physician has determined should be performed without delay in order to prevent death or serious disability. Such surgery is not subject to second opinion programs.

incidental surgery A surgical procedure that is not the reason for the operation, but that is done because, during the course of the original operation, the surgeon finds a condition that can be corrected without additional trauma to the patient. A classic example is removing the appendix "en passant"—"in passing"—at the same time as gallbladder removal. The rationale is that the patient can no longer have appendicitis.

keyhole surgery See *laparascopic surgery*, below.

laparascopic surgery Abdominal surgery carried out by inserting instruments for seeing inside the abdomen and instruments for manipulation (such as cutting, application of lasers, sewing) through small incisions, often under local anesthesia. When surgery by this method is appropriate for a given patient, it is usually preferable, because the procedure usually becomes one for "same-day" (ambulatory) surgery. The technique is being used for gallbladder removal (laparascopic cholecystectomy), for example. Synonym: keyhole surgery.

laser surgery Surgery that employs a laser, instead of earlier methods, to cut, to coagulate blood and stop bleeding, or to vaporize tissue or other substances.

major surgery A term no longer in repute, which referred to surgery that was extensive or hazardous, in contrast with "minor surgery," which was neither extensive nor hazardous. However, both terms defied precise definition, and various tongue-in-cheek definitions were used. (One definition, offered by a surgeon, was "Surgery that I do or that is done on me is major surgery." Another definition considered surgery with a price tag above a certain point as "major," and surgery with one below that as "minor.") In light of the failure to develop an acceptable definition, the terms "major" and "minor" were dropped, and specific operations were studied and reviewed.

Nevertheless, there clearly remains a wide range of complexity to the procedures carried out as surgery. Currently the problem of such a distinction arises in the prospective payment system (PPS), where it is the general policy that care for a patient in a given DRG should have a higher price if the patient has "major" surgery than if she or he does not. The solution has been to devise the *operating room procedure* (see under *procedure*) as a surrogate for "major." Any procedure that the PPS has declared to be an "operating room procedure" as defined by its *ICD-9-CM* code—whether or not it was done in an operating room—is "major surgery."

minimally invasive surgery (MIS) Methods for operating on patients, using very small incisions. Such surgery carries decreased operative risk and quicker recoveries. It is being used in virtually every surgical specialty, including otolaryngologic, thoracic, urologic, neurologic, orthopaedic, cardiac, plastic, and general surgery. MIS techniques have cut recovery times for many operations from weeks to days, even permitting same-day surgery for many procedures.

A news story about the removal of a kidney described the procedure as . . . involving several very small incisions that admit tools that are only one-fourth to one-half inch wide and a similarly sized telescope called a laparascope, which is connected to a camera. The surgeon, working off the camera image displayed on a television screen, frees the kidney from attached blood vessels and places it into an impermeable pouch. The surgeon then passes the drawstrings [and mouth] of the pouch through one of the incisions. Once the neck of the sack has been delivered to the surface of the abdomen, the sack is carefully opened, and the kidney is fragmented into small pieces and removed . . . [thus removing] kidneys bearing tumors that weigh as much as two pounds through a one-half inch incision. (*Washington University Record*, August 10, 2001)

Apparently this technology is taking some inspiration from the lowly spider, who for several millennia has been using a similar technique. In the spider's case, however, the patient is known as a victim, and the surgery goes well beyond being minimally invasive, as substantially all of the body's contents are removed.

minor surgery A term no longer in repute, which referred to surgery that was neither extensive nor hazardous, in contrast with "major surgery," which was considered either extensive or dangerous; however, both terms defied precise definition. See *major surgery*, above.

operating room surgery Literally, surgery that should be or ordinarily is done in an operating room, in contrast with surgery that may be done in the patient's bed, physician's office, or a treatment room. At present, a more specific definition is used in the prospective payment system (PPS); see *operating room procedures* (under *procedure*).

outpatient surgery See *ambulatory surgery*, above.

same-day surgery See *ambulatory surgery*, above.

unjustified surgery Surgery that was, in the judgment of the surgeon's peers, not "justified" by the evidence presented by the patient prior to operation—his or her history, physical examination, laboratory, or other data available. Surgery may be "justified," that is to say, the surgeon's peers would have operated under the circumstances, but it may prove (in retrospect) to have been *unnecessary surgery* (see below). Sometimes the added evidence provided by the operation itself reveals that the case could have been treated without operation (or by a different operation).

unnecessary surgery Surgery that, at least in retrospect, was not required as treatment for the patient's condition. A distinction is made between "unnecessary surgery" and *unjustified surgery* (see above). Unnecessary surgery could have been justified, but the condition proved (often with the added information provided by the surgery itself) to be one that, in hindsight, could have been managed without the operation (or by some other operation). Some surgery is both unjustified and unnecessary.

surgical When used in reference to therapy, "surgical" means "by the use of surgical methods, operation and manipulation." It is contrasted with "medical," which means nonsurgical, the avoidance of surgical methods.

surgical assistant A health professional and member of the operating room team who directly assists the operating surgeon in such ways as holding retractors, tying and clamping blood vessels, and assisting in cutting and suturing tissue. May be a physician, registered nurse (RN), or other qualified professional. See also *first assistant*.

Certified Surgical Assistant (CSA) A surgical assistant who has met the qualifications of the National Surgical Assistant Association (NSAA). **www.nsaa.net**

Surgical Care Improvement Project (SCIP) A national partnership of organizations, initiated by CMS and the Centers for Disease Control and Prevention (CDC), committed to improving the safety of surgical care through the reduction of postoperative complications. SCIP's goal is to reduce the national incidence of surgical complications by 25% by the year 2010. About twenty surgical performance measures (for example, readmission within thirty days of surgery) have been developed to help achieve this goal.

surgical resident See under *resident*.

surgical specialty A *medical specialty* within the discipline of surgery; for example, thoracic surgery.

surgical technologist (ST) A health professional who is a member of the operating room (OR) team with a variety of functions, including presurgical preparation of the OR, the patient, and essential equipment; maintaining the "sterile field" during the surgery; assisting the surgeon in such ways as passing instruments, sponging and suctioning, preparing suture material, and preparing specimens for pathologic analysis; and afterwards applying dressings and preparing the OR for the next patient. The ST may also function in the nonsterile role of circulator. The earlier term for the ST was operating room technician (ORT). See also *first assistant*.

Certified Surgical Technologist (CST) A surgical technologist who has completed an accredited program and passed an examination of the Liaison Council on Certification for the Surgical Technologist (LCC-ST). **www.lcc-st.org**

surrogate A person designated to act in place of or substitute for another.

survey In the context of accreditation of a healthcare facility, a survey is an on-site inspection; for example, by a team from the Joint Commission on Accreditation of Healthcare Organizations (JCAHO). See also *health survey*.

surveyor A person who carries out an accreditation *survey* or a *health survey*.

survival analysis A type of statistical process that deals with analysis of a group of individuals with respect to the time intervals between the onset of a given disease and significant events in its progress, such as cure, recurrence, or death. It is used in evaluating the effectiveness of treatments, for example, and making prognostic statements.

SV See *Specialist in Virology* under *clinical laboratory specialist*.

Symposium on Computer Applications in Medical Care (SCAMC) An annual meeting under the auspices of the *American Medical Informatics Association (AMIA)*. Now called the AMIA Annual Symposium.

symptom See *diagnosis*.

symptom complex A group of symptoms that occur together, and that may or may not be characteristic of a specific disease. See also *syndrome*.

syndrome A pattern of signs and symptoms that occurs together and forms a picture of a given disease. See also *symptom complex*.

system (anatomical) One of the functional components of the body, for example, the respiratory (breathing) system or the circulatory (heart and blood vessels) system.

system (economic) See *economic system*.

system (process) A process by which a complex of people and machines (and other essential resources) works together in an orderly fashion to accomplish a given task.

Systematized Nomenclature of Dentistry See *SNODENT*.

Systematized Nomenclature of Human and Veterinary Medicine See *SNOMED*.

Systematized Nomenclature of Medicine See *SNOMED*.

Systematized Nomenclature of Pathology (SNOP) See *SNOMED*.

systemic A term that, in referring to a disease, means a disease that affects the body as a whole.

systems analysis An analysis of the resources (personnel, facilities, equipment, materials, funds, and other elements), organization, administration, procedures, and policies needed to carry out a given task. The analysis typically addresses alternatives in each category, and their relative efficiency and effectiveness.

systems review The traditional method of organizing the medical record under headings such as "respiratory," "past illnesses," or "cardiac." See also *problem-oriented medical record* under *medical record*.

systems theory The theoretical framework explaining how systems consisting of complexes of people and machines (and other essential resources) work together in an orderly fashion to accomplish a given task.

T

TA Technology assessment. See *health technology assessment*.

tactics A term derived from the military usage concerning actions that, although directed toward the large goal, are smaller in scale or scope than strategic actions. Tactics are those actions through which a "strategy" is carried out. See also *strategy*.

TAG Technical Advisory Group. See *U.S. TAG*.

tail coverage See under *insurance coverage*.

tailgate pricing A pejorative term used to describe pricing that the commentator feels simply responds to the demand of the market (competition) at the moment, that is, pricing that is not based on costs or a consistent pricing policy. See also *shadow pricing*.

tailored drug/catalyst therapy An approach to treating a specific disease, for example, a cancer, by attaching a "prodrug component" to the diseased tissue and then triggering its activation by administering a "catalytic component" that "turns on" the drug. The drug then treats only the specific tissue (disease) for which it has been designed, leaving the normal tissue unaffected.

target The desired performance, outcome, or result. See *quality indicator* under *indicator*.

TAS See *Tobacco Addiction Specialist* under *tobacco addiction counselor*.

task force A group of persons established to carry out a specific task. Its assignment is usually fact-finding or advisory. A time limit is typically given by the appointing authority for completion of the task, and upon its completion the task force is automatically disbanded. A task force is not to be confused with a committee, which is a standing body, or a quality circle, which selects its own tasks.

TAT See *turnaround time*.

tax credit An amount that can be subtracted from the tax owed by an individual. Some healthcare reform proposals include tax credits. These save the individual more money than would the same amount taken as a tax deduction. In some cases, the credit may only reduce the amount of tax owed; in other cases, the credit may actually be refunded to the taxpayer.

tax-deductible A contribution or other expense that may be taken as a *tax deduction*. For example, contributions to 501(c)(3) corporations are tax-deductible, so no tax is paid on the amount of the contribution. The tax deduction is taken by the donor; the term does not refer to the receiving corporation.

tax deduction An amount of money that can be subtracted from the income of an individual before the amount of taxable income is determined. Some healthcare reform proposals include tax deductions as a way to help the individual finance health care; for example, allowing taxpayers to deduct the cost of health insurance from their income. Tax deductions save the individual less money than would the same amount taken as a *tax credit*.

Tax Equity and Fiscal Responsibility Act (TEFRA) A 1982 federal act that, among other things, permitted HCFA (now CMS) to enter into risk contracts with health maintenance organizations (HMOs) and competitive medical plans (CMPs), to pay for hospice care, and to extend coverage for ancillary services. It also prohibited employers from keeping employees ages sixty-five to sixty-nine from participating in the employer's health plan and requiring them to use Medicare instead. See also *Medicare Secondary Payer Rules*. Pub. L. No. 97-248, 96 Stat. 324 (1982).

tax-exempt A nonprofit organization that is not required to pay certain federal (and/or state) taxes. A tax-exempt organization may also qualify to receive tax-deductible donations; see *501(c)(*)*.

tax incentive A method of encouraging behavior by providing favorable tax treatment (exemptions, deductions, or credits).

taxonomy A classification arranged according to the logical relationships of the terms with respect to a particular viewpoint; for example, diagnoses would have different taxonomies (e.g., relationships) from the point of view of their etiology (cause) as opposed to their physiological manifestations (symptoms, for example). See *Linnaean System* and *PhyloCode*.

Taxpayer Bill of Rights A federal law enacted in 1988 and officially entitled the "Omnibus Taxpayer Bill of Rights" (Pub. L. No. 100-647, 102 Stat. 3730). In 1996, legislation was enacted to extend this law, entitled the "Taxpayer Bill of Rights 2" (TBR2) (Pub. L. No. 104-168, 110 Stat. 1452). "Taxpayer Bill of Rights 3," the Internal Revenue Service Restructuring and Reform Act of 1998 (Pub. L. No. 105-206, 112 Stat. 726), made additional changes. Collectively, this legislation made substantial changes to the Internal Revenue Code (IRC) and the rights and duties of the Internal Revenue Service (IRS). See also *excess benefit transaction rule*.

Tax Relief and Health Care Improvement Act of 2006 Legislation that averted Medicare reimbursement cuts for physicians, raised the contribution limit for Health Savings Accounts (HSAs), and provided, among things, for physicians to be paid incentives for voluntarily reporting on performance measures and for hospital outpatient services and ambulatory surgical centers to report on specified performance measures or face reductions in Medicare payments. Public Law 109-432.

Taylorism A theory of management based on "science." Work behaviors are examined for effectiveness and efficiency, and tasks are standardized. Workers are scored and ranked. Introduced by Frederick W. Taylor (an engineer) in his 1911 book, *The Principles of Scientific Management*, "Taylorism" has had an enormous impact on manufacturing and business management practices in the United States. It has been taught for years in business schools as the "gospel of economics." Synonym: scientific management.

TB unit See *tuberculosis unit*.

TC See *technical component*.

TCGA See *The Cancer Genome Atlas*.

TCS See *Transactions and Code Sets*.

TC 215 See *ISO/TC 215*.

TC 251 See *CEN TC 251*.

TCU See *transitional care unit*.

TCWF See *California Wellness Foundation, The*.

Td vaccine Tetanus/diphtheria *vaccine*.

TE See *therapeutic equivalent*.

team nursing See under *nursing*.

Technical Advisory Group (TAG) See *U.S. TAG*.

technical committee (TC) See *CEN TC 251*.

technical component (TC) The portion of healthcare services for which the hospital (or other institution) gets paid. See also *professional component*.

technician A person qualified to carry out specific technical procedures.

technologist A scientist skilled in applying knowledge to solve problems; has more independence than a technician.

technology assessment (TA) See *health technology assessment*.

Technology Assessment Conference (TAC) A conference held as part of the *National Institutes of Health Consensus Development Program* that addresses a topic concerning *health technology*.

technology transfer (TT) Moving technology developed by one organization into another. It applies to the procedure by which an invention that has been developed (often under a federal grant or contract) by an investigator at a university or other nonprofit organization, or by the government (NASA, for example), may be put to commercial use and at the same time provide income to the organization. The invention must first be patented by the organization, after which it may be licensed by the organization to the commercial market, which, in return, pays "license income" to the organization. The procedure is the result of the **Bayh-Dole Act** (also known as the University and Small Business Patent Procedure Act of 1980, 35 U.S.C. § 200 et seq. (2004)), which was passed by Congress in 1980 in order to replace the previous arrangement under which such inventions became the property of the federal government. At that time there was no process either for rewarding the organization or for making sure the invention was put to use.

Many universities now have technology transfer programs that keep track of the science involved and the marketplace, and act as match-makers between the two. Examples of inventions resulting from these programs are Internet search engines, medical diagnostic technologies, and gene-splicing techniques. University income from licensing must be shared with the investigator and support specified activities within the university. For example, at one university the researcher gets 45% of the income after expenses, the university technology transfer program gets 15%, and the university's research and academic programs get the remaining 40%.

As an example of activity, in 1998 technology transfer resulted in $33.5 billion in economic activity, 280,000 jobs, 4,808 U.S. patents, 3,668 new licenses, and the formation of 364 companies in the United States. Prior to the Bayh-Dole Act's passage, only about 250 patents per year were issued for university research.

The Robert C. Byrd National Technology Transfer Center (NTTC) was established by Congress in 1989 to assist in the technology transfer process by linking U.S. industry with federal labs and universities that have technologies facilities and researchers. **www.nttc.edu**

TEFRA See *Tax Equity and Fiscal Responsibility Act*.

TEHRE Toward an Electronic Health Record Europe. An international conference that was sponsored by the Centre for the Advancement of Electronic Health Records (CAEHR).

telecommunications Pertaining to the technical aspects of telephones, computer wiring (intra- and inter-building), intercommunication, radio, paging, wireless, and other communications systems and networks (excluding computer networks). Includes both voice and data transmissions. Synonym: telecom.

teleconference A conference held via telecommunications equipment among individuals who are physically separated (perhaps by thousands of miles). Ordinarily the individuals all participate in the "conversation" interactively, that is, each in response to the input of the others. Telecommunication equipment includes computers, telephones, and television. In the healthcare field, one of the earliest applications of teleconferencing was in continuing medical (and other professional) education, usually with the educator at an education center and the students in their hospitals or other settings. Teleconferencing may also be used, for example, for official meetings, such as governing body meetings (provided the institution's bylaws and relevant statutes permit). See also *telehealth*.

teleconsultation A "face-to-face," real-time encounter between a patient or a patient's physician and another physician or practitioner by means of audio and video telecommunications. See *telehealth*.

telehealth The use of telecommunications, computers, and other information technology to deliver healthcare services and information over distances, both large and small. It may be used in clinical patient care, professional and patient education, and public health and health administration. The *tele-* prefix is sometimes added to specific disciplines; see, for example, *telemedicine* and *telenursing*. Synonyms: eHealth services, online healthcare services (OHS). See also *interactive health communication*.

CMS uses the terms "telehealth" and "telemedicine" interchangeably. It does, however, distinguish three types of telehealth services. The first is a remote, "face-to-face" encounter between provider and patient, utilizing audio and video technology. CMS calls this a "teleconsultation" and permits it to substitute for an in-person, "hands-on" encounter for consultation, office visit, individual psychotherapy, and pharmacologic management. Reimbursement is limited to certain providers (physicians, nurse practitioners, clinical psychologists, and others), facilities (physician or practitioner's office, hospital, Critical Access Hospital, Rural Health Clinic, or Federally Qualified Health Center), and only for services with CPT codes. The second type is remote, non-face-to-face services, delivered using telecommunications technology but not requiring the patient to be present during their implementation, such as interpretation of electrocardiograms and x-rays. These services, called **store and forward**, are not considered telemedicine or telehealth by CMS, but are covered just as if they were delivered on-site. The third type is home health services delivered by means of telecommunications; these are not covered by Medicare because they do not involve personal contact as required for a home health visit.

telehealth nursing See *telenursing*.

telemedicine Medical care provided through telecommunications when the patient and the caregiver are at separate physical locations or when the patient and the primary caregiver are at one location (the originating site), and a specialist or other consultant is at a separate location (distant site). May involve the use of interactive audio-visual technology, as well as remote patient monitoring.

Telemedicine is developing many specialties, such as telepathology, teleradiology, teledermatology, telepsychiatry, and so forth. Synonyms: remote medical diagnosis (RMD), online medical services (OMS). See also *presenter* and *telehealth*.

telementoring See *mentor*.

telemetry See *medical telemetry device*.

telenursing The practice of nursing utilizing *telehealth* modalities. Synonym: telehealth nursing. See also *telephone nursing practice*.

telepathology The use of technology to transmit microscopic images from a remote location to a pathologist for study. One technique is to scan or otherwise obtain a digital image of the slide and transmit it to the pathologist (the quality of the image will vary greatly depending upon the equipment used); this is called a "static image" system. In another technique, called "real-time" telepathology, a television camera records the image, which is then transmitted by wire or radio to a remote site where the pathologist can examine the image as though she or he were looking directly through the viewing microscope. The microscope is a special, robotically controlled device, so that the pathologist at the remote location can move the slide about and examine various areas, vary the magnification, change the brightness, introduce optical filters, and focus, just as though she or he were actually seated at an optical microscope.

These techniques make possible a number of advances in the quality of care, including providing pathology services to isolated areas, consultations, and instant second opinions. Further possibilities include the examination of entire organs as well as microscopic sections. See also *pathology* and *telemedicine*.

telephone nursing practice (TNP) The area of nursing focusing on serving patient needs by providing direct first contact by telephone. Synonym: call center nursing. See also *telenursing* and *teletriage*.

Telephone Nursing Practice Nurse (RNC) A registered nurse specializing in telephone nursing practice, who has passed an examination of the National Certification Corporation (NCC) and received the credential Registered Nurse Certified (RNC). **www.nccnet.org**

teleradiology The electronic transmission of radiologic images, such as x-rays, CTs, and MRIs, from one location to another for the purpose of interpretation and/or consultation.

teletriage Use of the telephone (usually by a nurse) to talk to a patient about a health problem, and then advise the patient on home treatment and whether to seek medical care; especially, whether to wait to make a doctor's appointment or go to the emergency room (or call 911) immediately. See also *telephone nursing practice*.

telomere The end of a *chromosome*.

Temporary Status by Qualification (TSQ) A credential offered by the National Credentialing Agency for Laboratory Personnel (NCA) (**www.nca-info.org**) to international clinical laboratory professionals who lack experience in U.S. clinics. It is granted to a clinical laboratory technician, technologist, or specialist who has passed an NCA examination. After four years of qualified experience, the TSQ may be converted into the appropriate NCA certification.

TEPR Toward an Electronic Patient Record. An annual conference, sponsored by the Medical Records Institute (MRI), that seeks to assist providers and other health professionals in moving towards electronic health records. **www.tepr.com**

term A word or phrase used for naming an entity (item) in a universe.

termcode The term used in *SNOMED* for the alphanumeric code for a given term in the nomenclature.

terminal Relating to or at the end. A terminal illness is one expected to cause death, and for which there is no known or available cure.

terminal care Care for a patient in the terminal stages of his or her illness; care for a dying patient. See also *hospice.*

terminal care document See *living will* under *advance directive.*

terminology The set of all the words (or groups of words—phrases) that have a special meaning within a given field of knowledge. The words and phrases are called terms. The reference work you are now reading, for example, defines the terms that are used in the *non-clinical* healthcare environment.

Some terms will be exclusive to the field; for example, one is not likely to encounter otorhinolaryngology outside of the medical world. On the other hand, common words may take on special meaning when used within a specific field. For example, typing commonly refers to a way of putting words on paper; in blood banks, it means determining certain characteristics of a blood sample. Risk to many people has to do with taking a chance—but a financial expert sees risk as a special kind of chance, that of losing money. An insurance adjuster will see risk as the odds of having to pay an insured for a loss (a hospital "risk management" department tries to minimize this type of risk). A physician will see the likelihood to a patient of disease, injury, or death—a person with high blood pressure, for example, is at risk for stroke or heart disease.

Terminology includes not only proper language, but also acronyms, eponyms, initialisms, abbreviations, and local jargon. Terminology varies regionally, and even varies within the same healthcare institution. It involves terminology from all of the disciplines that record information in the medical record—nursing, medicine, physical therapy, radiology, and so on. Because of all these characteristics, healthcare terminology is an uncontrolled (and uncontrollable) set of terms. The set for clinical records must include any term that is *actually* used, even if only locally and only for a few individuals, and whether everyone likes it or not. Distinguish *vocabulary*, and see the diagram at *natural language*.

terrorism The U.S. Federal Bureau of Investigation (FBI) defines terrorism as the "unlawful use of force or violence against persons or property to intimidate or coerce a government, the civilian population, or any segment thereof, in furtherance of political or social objectives." This definition is relevant in determining whether a death or injury was caused by terrorism; see *Classification of Death and Injury Resulting from Terrorism*. See also *agroterrorism* and *bioterrorism*.

tertiary care Care of a highly technical and specialized nature, provided in a medical center (usually one affiliated with a university), for patients with unusually severe, complex, or uncommon problems. Tertiary care is the highest level of care.

test A term without specific definition, which in health care generally refers to a laboratory procedure.

testing Evaluation of a product to see whether and how well it serves its intended purpose. The term is often used in referring to evaluation of questionnaires or software, for example.

Such products are usually subjected to two rounds of testing after their initial development:

alpha testing The first "round" of testing of a product by persons and institutions for which the product is ultimately intended to be used. The results of alpha testing are studied by the designers of the product, indicated changes are made in the product, and then it is tested again in many more settings in what is called beta testing.

beta testing The second "round" of testing of a product, after alpha testing, by persons and institutions for which the product is ultimately intended to be used. Problems uncovered in beta testing result in further changes, and then the product is usually ready for release for general use.

Test of Functional Health Literacy in Adults (TOFHLA) A test, published in 1995 by Parker et al., that measures an adult's ability to read and understand medical instructions and healthcare information when that information is presented in written form such as prescription drug bottle labels and appointment slips. It is used to assess *health literacy*. See also *Rapid Estimate of Adult Literacy in Medicine*.

TG See *transgender*.

thanadoula See under *doula*.

The Cancer Genome Atlas (TCGA) A collaboration of the National Cancer Institute (NCI) and National Human Genome Research Institute (NHGRI), both parts of the National Institutes of Health (NIH), to accelerate our understanding of the molecular basis of cancer through the application of genome analysis technologies, including large-scale genome sequencing. **cancergenome.nih.gov**

The Medical Directive See under *advance directive*.

therapeutic For the purpose of *therapy*.

therapeutic equivalent (TE) A drug classified by the Food and Drug Administration (FDA) as expected to produce the same clinical effect and safety profile as another drug, so that it may be substituted for that drug. To be TE, a drug must (1) be the pharmaceutical equivalent (contain the same active ingredient(s), dosage form and route of administration, and strength); (2) meet standards of strength, quality, purity, and identity; (3) be bioequivalent; (4) be adequately labeled; and (5) be manufactured in compliance with Current Good Manufacturing Practice regulations. Once classified, the TE drug receives a two-letter TE code providing information on the FDA's evaluations. Approved drugs and TEs are published by the FDA in *Approved Drug Products with Therapeutic Equivalence Evaluations*, commonly referred to as the "Orange Book." See also *generic equivalent*.

therapeutic recreation specialist A health professional who provides therapeutic recreation therapy services. Sometimes called activities therapist.

Certified Therapeutic Recreation Specialist (CTRS) A therapeutic recreation specialist who has been certified by the National Council for Therapeutic Recreation Certification (NCTRC). **www.nctrc.org**

therapeutic recreation therapy (TRT) Providing individual patients or patient populations with recreational activities to improve, restore, or maintain their physical and mental well-being. Activities may include arts and crafts, sports, outings, social gatherings, and so forth. Sometimes called activities therapy (see also *creative arts therapies*).

therapist A health professional who provides therapy. "Therapist" will almost always be modified by a term specifying the type of care, for example, physical therapist or radiation therapist. The term by itself is sometimes interchanged with *counselor*.

therapy Sometimes used interchangeably with *treatment* to refer to the care of a patient. For example, "the patient is undergoing therapy" means that the patient is being treated. However, it usually refers to a *specific type* of treatment method or technique. See, for example, *gene therapy*.

Some therapies are directed at the *cause* of a problem, designed to accomplish a specific result (kill cancer cells, for example). These include, among others, chemotherapy, electroconvulsive therapy (ECT), radiation therapy, and radium therapy.

Therapy may describe a group of techniques that address a specific *condition*. For example, respiratory therapy treats breathing difficulties by administration of gases, such as oxygen, and the use and teaching of breathing exercises.

Some therapies include a range of methods designed to result in improvement in a specific area, such as speech or movement, or a patient's social life or emotional well-being. These therapies often focus on the *result desired* rather than on the cause of the patient's problem. See, for example, **animal-assisted therapy**, **behavior therapy**, **creative arts therapies**, **occupational therapy**, **physical therapy**, and **therapeutic recreation therapy**.

therapy animal An animal, such as a dog, utilized in **animal-assisted therapy**. See also **service animal**.

thermogram An image made by thermography.

thermography A diagnostic technique that detects and records heat in tissues. Tissues in different states of chemical activity have different temperatures, and mapping the pattern of temperatures is used, for example, in efforts to find tumors in breasts.

third party administrator (TPA) An organization that administers healthcare benefits (and other employee benefits), primarily for corporations that are self-insured. The third party administrator's services include claims review and claims processing, primarily of medical claims but also dental, disability, workers' compensation, life insurance, and pension claims.

third party payer (TPP) See under **payer**.

third sector A term describing the nonprofit sector of the economy, to distinguish it from the public sector (government) and the private, for-profit sector.

30 Safe Practices A set of thirty practices recommended for healthcare providers that evidence shows can work to reduce or prevent adverse events and medical errors. These were identified by the National Quality Forum (NQF), with support from the Agency for Healthcare Research and Quality (AHRQ). Examples: "Use only standardized abbreviations and dose designations"; "Implement a computerized prescriber-order entry system"; "Upon admission, and regularly thereafter, evaluate each patient for the risk of aspiration." The complete report, entitled *Safe Practices for Better Healthcare: A Consensus Report*, is available from the National Quality Forum. Synonym: NQF-endorsed Safe Practices. See also **Leapfrog Group** and **patient safety**.

Thomson Medstat See **Medstat**.

thoracic Having to do with the chest and structures inside the rib cage.

340B Drug Pricing Program A law that limits the cost of covered outpatient drugs to specified federal grantees (including Federally Qualified Health Centers (FQHCs)), FQHC Look-Alikes, and disproportionate share hospitals (DSHs). The 340B price specified is a ceiling price, meaning that entities may negotiate with the drug companies for lower prices. 340B prices have been found to be about 50% of the average wholesale price. The program was established by Section 602 of the Veterans Health Care Act of 1992 (Public Law 102-585), which is codified as Section 340B of the Public Health Service Act. Synonyms: PHS Pricing, 340B Pricing, 602 Pricing.

thymine (T) See **DNA**.

TIA Transient ischemic attack. See **stroke**.

tie-in sale See **tying arrangement**.

tiered benefit plan A health plan with two or more levels (tiers) of benefits; subscribers choose a level and pay the corresponding premiums—higher levels of benefits will have higher premiums.

tiered formulary See **formulary (health plan)**.

tiered health plan See **tiered benefit plan**.

Time Banking The term used for local, tax-exempt barter currency in a concept initiated by Edgar Cahn. Individuals participating in a Time Banking program earn "Time Dollars" by helping others (tutoring, childcare, transportation, etc.). One Time Dollar is earned for each hour of volunteer service. A Time Bank account is maintained formally for each participant, and it may be drawn upon by the participant for services by other participants. Synonym: service credits. More information is available from TimeBanks USA, founded by Dr. Cahn. **www.timebanks.org**

tissue A collection of cells of the same type, along with the materials between them, which have a similar function. Muscle, bone, and blood are examples of tissues. An organ may be made up of several kinds of tissues.

tissue bank A facility for collecting, cataloging, storing, and distributing body tissues for use in surgery. Bone, for example, is a commonly stored tissue. Although the term "tissue" may cover entire organs, organs ordinarily are immediately transplanted rather than banked. The tissues stored in a tissue bank are primarily human. As implantation and transplantation technology advance, an increasing variety of tissues may be expected to be banked, rather than being available only by immediate transfer from donor to recipient. A concomitant development in health care has been the establishment of regional (and national and international) communications networks that help bring together available tissues (and organs) and people who need them.

tissue committee A committee of the medical staff whose purpose is to review the appropriateness of the surgery performed in the hospital. The "tissue committee" got its name because many surgical procedures result in the removal of tissue, which is then examined by a pathologist, who formally reports on her or his findings. The tissue committee does not confine itself to operations involving tissue removal, but rather considers the appropriateness of all surgery. See also *unjustified surgery* and *unnecessary surgery* under *surgery (treatment)*.

Title VI program A program established in a community under the federal Older Americans Act (OAA) to respond to the needs of older American Indians, Aleuts, Eskimos, and Hawaiians. See *area agency on aging*.

Title XIX See *Medicaid*.

Title XVIII See *Medicare*.

TLC Tender, loving care.

TMR See *translucent medical record*.

TNM system See *tumor, node, metastases system*.

TNP See *telephone nursing practice*.

tobacco addiction counselor A counselor specializing in helping people with tobacco addiction.

Tobacco Addiction Specialist (TAS) A person who has been trained and certified by NAADAC, the Association for Addiction Professionals (formerly the National Association of Alcohol and Drug Abuse Counselors) (**www.naadac.org**). Offered jointly with the University of Florida and Patient Support International (PSI). This credential is available to physicians, physician assistants, nurses, pharmacists, respiratory therapists, licensed or certified counselors, and other qualified health professionals.

To Err Is Human A landmark report published by the Institute of Medicine in 1999; see *patient safety*.

TOFHLA See *Test of Functional Health Literacy in Adults*.

tort A wrong for which the law provides a civil remedy, and which is not a breach of contract. (Contracts are covered by a separate body of laws.) A person who commits an act that is a tort is legally liable (responsible) to anyone injured by the act. "Civil remedy" means that the person doing the legal "wrong" must pay the victim money to make good his or her losses. (A few other civil remedies exist, which are less often used; for example, if A publishes a defamatory statement about B, A may be required to print a retraction.)

An act that is a tort may also be a crime. If someone steals a car, she can be prosecuted by the state (the public) for the crime of theft, and possibly pay a fine or go to jail. She can also, however, be sued by the car's owner for the tort of "conversion" (taking another's property without his permission).

There are three basic kinds of torts: *intentional torts* (see below), *negligence*, and *strict liability* (see under *liability*). Torts that are important for health professionals to know about include *malpractice*, *invasion of privacy* (see under *privacy*), *false imprisonment*, *intentional infliction of emotional distress* (see under *emotional distress*), *abuse of process*, *fraud*, *defamation*, and *tortious interference with business relationship*.

intentional tort A tort that is done intentionally, maliciously, or recklessly. (This is in contrast to negligence, which usually is done accidentally and without any intent to do harm.)

prima facie tort A tort "on the face of it." A legal term that describes a tort that has no legal classification, but that the law will recognize on the facts of a case because there should be a remedy. This is a cause of action that has been defined by Justice Holmes as "the intentional infliction of harm, resulting in damage, without excuse or justification, by an act or series of acts which would otherwise be lawful, and which acts do not fall within the categories of traditional tort." *Aikens v. Wisconsin*, 195 U.S. 194 (1904).

tortfeasor A person who commits a *tort*.

tortious interference with business relationship A *tort* in which someone wrongfully interferes with a business relationship and causes someone else an economic loss, such as a broken contract, loss of job or position, or suspension from the medical staff.

tort reform A change in the way in which individuals who are "harmed" by the healthcare system may be compensated. In the United States, patients injured through malpractice or otherwise generally file a lawsuit seeking damages; such suits themselves cost a great deal, take up a lot of time and resources, and may result in enormous sums to the patient. Some see tort reform as simply putting a "cap" on noneconomic damages or limiting attorneys' fees, but keeping the present system of litigation. Others believe the present system is broken, and that alternatives would be more fair, result in faster (and often more useful) settlements, and save money. Tort reform is sometimes, in the healthcare context, referred to as "malpractice reform," although it is not necessarily limited to malpractice cases. See also *alternative dispute resolution*, *early offer*, *enterprise liability* (under *liability (legal)*), *health court*, and *tort*.

Total Quality Management (TQM) See under *quality management*.

Toward an Electronic Patient Record (TEPR) See *TEPR* and *TEHRE*.

toxicity The degree to which a drug (or other substance) can be poisonous.

toxicogenomics The study of the effects of toxic substances on the human genome, and their relationship to disease.

toxicology The study of poisonous substances, their effects, their detection, and the treatment of poisoned individuals.

TPA See *third party administrator*.

TPP See *third party payer* under *payer*.

TPR Hospital jargon meaning "Temperature (reading), Pulse (rate), and Respiration (rate)." See also *third party reimbursement* under *reimbursement*.

TQM See *Total Quality Management* under *quality management*.

trademark A type of intellectual property right that affords protection for the name or special appearance of a product or service. (If it's a service, the trademark is called a **service mark**.) The purpose of the trademark is to identify the source of the product or service, chiefly for the protection of the consumer. Often there are significant resources invested in publicizing a product's name or appearance, which results in a measurable economic benefit referred to as "goodwill." Trademark protection is designed to prevent others from unfairly capitalizing on this goodwill by using an identical or "confusingly similar" name.

A person (or company) can obtain rights in a trademark only by actually using it in commerce (e.g., putting it on product labels and selling the product) before anyone else does. Owners of trademarks may use the trademark sign (™) at any time, even if they have not formally registered the trademark. (The ™ has no legal significance.) However, they cannot use the registered trademark sign (®) unless they have registered the mark with the U.S. Patent and Trademark Office (**www.uspto.gov**). The trademark must be used in commerce before it can be registered. Trademark protection will go on indefinitely as long as the mark is used in commerce; if it is abandoned, the rights are lost. Federal registration may be renewed every ten years. See also *patent* and *copyright*.

trade secret A type of intellectual property right that affords protection for an economically valuable product or process that cannot be readily known or ascertained by others. To be protected as a trade secret, it must also be shown to provide a competitive advantage. The owner of the trade secret must make reasonable efforts to protect the secrecy of the trade secret. These efforts typically include required "nondisclosure agreements" from all who may come near the trade secrets, as well as simply keeping trade secrets under lock and key. Even though an employee is under an implied legal duty not to disclose his or her employer's trade secrets without any written agreement, such an agreement provides numerous advantages for maintaining trade secret protection. Unlike patent and copyright protection, trade secret rights can theoretically last forever. However, unlike patent protection, trade secret protection does not protect against independent development by someone else. See also *patent* and *copyright*.

training A systematic process for achieving proficiency in a specialized area. Whereas "education" may focus on broad principles and the acquisition of knowledge, training focuses on action, on skills, and on the direct application of principles learned.

    in-service training Training carried out, usually within the institution, while employees carry out their regular duties. In-service training may take the form of "courses" integrated into the work schedule, or "coaching." Synonym: staff development.

training coordinator An individual in an institution who has responsibility for coordinating in-service training programs.

transaction See *Transactions and Code Sets*.

Transactions and Code Sets (TCS) Standards for Electronic Transactions and Code Sets, as required by HIPAA. Under HIPAA, a **transaction** is an activity involving the electronic transfer of healthcare information for a specific purpose. HIPAA requires that if a provider engages in one of the transactions identified below, it must comply with the electronic data interchange (EDI) standards for that transaction:

- Health Care Claims or Equivalent Encounter Information
- Eligibility for a Health Plan
- Referral Certification and Authorization
- Health Care Claim Status
- Enrollment and Disenrollment in a Health Plan
- Health Care Payment and Remittance Advice
- Health Plan Premium Payments
- Coordination of Benefits

Under HIPAA, a **code set** is any set of codes used for encoding data elements, such as tables of terms, medical concepts, medical diagnosis codes, or medical procedure codes. The following were adopted as the standard medical data code sets as of 2007:

- *International Classification of Diseases*, 9th Edition, Clinical Modification (ICD-9- CM), Volumes 1 and 2
- *International Classification of Diseases*, 9th Edition, Clinical Modification (ICD-9- CM), Volume 3 Procedures
- National Drug Code (NDC)
- Code on Dental Procedures and Nomenclature (CDT)
- Centers for Medicare & Medicaid Services (formerly known as Health Care Financing Administration) Common Procedure Coding System (HCPCS)
- *Current Procedural Terminology*, 4th Edition (CPT4)

transactions standards See *electronic transactions standards.*

transcription (genetics) The process of producing a ribonucleic acid (RNA) copy from DNA.

transcriptionist See *medical transcriptionist.*

transcriptome See under *DNA.*

transfer The formal shifting of responsibility for the care of a patient from one physician to another, from one institution to another, or from one unit of the hospital to another. There are specific Medicare payment implications depending on the type of transfer. In general, the following types of institutional transfer are recognized:

discharge transfer A transfer from one institution to another; the patient is discharged from one and admitted to the other.

intrahospital transfer A transfer within the same hospital (1) from one patient care unit to another, (2) from one clinical service to another, or (3) from the care of one physician to another.

transfer in A term used in Medicare for a patient admitted to the hospital by transfer from another short-term hospital, or "nonexempt distinct part unit" of the same hospital, for whose care the hospital is to receive a portion of the DRG "price" under the formula prescribed by the prospective payment system (PPS).

transfer out A term used in Medicare for a patient transferred from the hospital (or from a "nonexempt distinct part unit" of the same hospital) directly to another short-term hospital, or to another "nonexempt distinct part unit" of the same hospital, and for whose care the recipient hospital or unit is to receive a portion of the DRG "price" under the formula prescribed by the prospective payment system (PPS).

transfer agreement A formal agreement between two institutions regarding the conditions under which there can be transfer of patients between them and the exchange of clinical information on the patients.

transfer ribonucleic acid (tRNA) See under *ribonucleic acid*, under *DNA.*

transforming A term used in discussion of coding and classification for the process in which the meaning of a term is forced into a standardized, structured language (such as SNOMED Clinical Terms (SNOMED CT)) by dissecting the term into its components, each component having its own standard terminology (and codes).

transfusion hepatitis See *hepatitis B.*

transgender (TG) A very broad, umbrella term used to describe individuals who identify themselves with a different gender, or whose expression of gender varies in some way from the societal "norm." This includes, for example, cross-dressers, intersexed individuals, and transsexuals. Sometimes called "gender different."

transgene A gene in the genome of an organism that comes from a different organism.

transgenic Any organism, plant or animal, in which a foreign DNA gene (a transgene) has been incorporated into its genome early in embryonic development. Under these circumstances the transgene is in both somatic (body) and germ cells and is inherited by offspring. In agriculture, for example, a transgenic soybean was developed in which the transgene was taken from a Brazil nut in order to increase the nutritional value of the soybean. Patients known to be allergic to Brazil nuts were tested for allergy to the transgenic soybeans, and were found to react as though they were tested against the Brazil nuts themselves, indicating the ability of genetic engineering to transfer an allergen. Unless foods that have been "gene-altered" in this manner are labeled to reflect this, consumers are not likely to be able to distinguish them from the unaltered varieties.

transient ischemic attack (TIA) See *stroke.*

transitional care A term covering care that is not acute care and not long-term care. "Transitional care" includes care in postacute convalescence, rehabilitation, and psychiatric care, whether given within acute or long-term care facilities, or in separate programs or facilities.

transitional care unit (TCU) A patient care unit (PCU) to provide transitional care.

transitional year A type of medical residency with the purpose of providing a balanced experience in a variety of (two or more) clinical disciplines. The name is somewhat misleading because, rather than being used by physicians seeking to change from one specialty to another, most of the transitional year positions are occupied by physicians in their first year of graduate medical education. Transitional year programs are approved by the Accreditation Council for Graduate Medical Education (ACGME).

translational research Research that transforms scientific laboratory research into applications that benefit patient health and medical care. Synonym: bench-to-bedside.

translocation In genetics, the exchange or relocation of large chromosome segments, typically between two different chromosomes.

translucent database See *translucent medical record*.

translucent medical record (TMR) A proposed type of electronic medical record (EMR) that uses translucent database technology to prevent access to selected portions of the record by unauthorized viewers. The concept of the TMR is most easily understood if one thinks of the EMR as simply a specialized database—one that contains a single person's health information. Unlike traditional databases, to which access is either "all or nothing," a translucent database allows access to any, all, or none of the information stored in the database.

In a traditional online database, for example, if you enter a valid username and password, you are authorized to access the entire reference work—nothing is held back from your view. In a translucent database, however, one or more fields of the database (e.g., name, address, phone number) are further protected from view, in spite of the fact that you have already gained access to the database itself. The added security possible in this latter type of database holds great promise in the healthcare field, especially as a tool in implementing the HIPAA requirements relating to protected health information (PHI).

In the translucent medical record, those parts deemed to be PHI may be protected by the use of a software method known as a "one-way hash" (sometimes mistakenly described as "one-way encryption," which is a misnomer because encryption is by definition a two-way process). The hash process converts the readable information into a format that appears, to a human, to be gibberish. For example, the password "swordfish" might end up looking like "8c99b59fcc47392e3fe1b." People who are authorized to see the protected portions of the database will see the information in its original (unhashed) human-readable form. This approach results in information being both more accessible and more protected, at the same time.

The translucent database technology is not new, having been developed for (and in long-term use) guarding passwords in the Unix and Linux operating systems. However, it appears not to be currently used in health care, and the TMR remains hypothetical so far. See also *electronic health record*.

transparency initiative The effort by the Department of Health and Human Services (HHS) to collect, and make available (visible) to the public (consumers and purchasers), data on the quality and cost of healthcare services. The goal is to improve quality and reduce cost. One part of this effort is the requirement that hospitals report their performance in relation to the *National Hospital Quality Measures* to CMS in order to receive full Medicare payment. See also *AQA*, *pay-for-performance*, and *value-driven health care*. www.hhs.gov/transparency

transparent Free from deceit; readily understood; easily detected. In health care, this means that features of the system that used to be obscured, or at least unavailable to public view, are now visible—chiefly the price of healthcare services and the quality of care being provided. Some suggest that hospitals be transparent (open) about "everything"—executive compensation, charity care, community benefit, staffing numbers, billing, discounts, governance, financial data, and so forth. See also *accountability (governance)*.

transplant To move one living part of the body to another, or from one individual (the "donor") to another. The organ or tissue transplanted is called an "allograft" if from a donor, and an "autograft" (or "homograft") if from the same individual. The term "transplant" may also be used as a noun to indicate the tissue or organ that is transplanted. Synonym: graft. See also *implant*.

transplant hepatology The medical discipline pertaining to liver transplantation.

transport nursing The area of nursing concerned with the needs of individuals during air or ground medical transport. These include emergency patients and patients being transferred from one facility to another (for example, a critically ill infant might be transferred to a tertiary care center). Transport nursing involves not only standard nursing practices, but also special skills such as emergency and critical care, cardiac life support, neonatal resuscitation, and trauma care, and special knowledge about the effects of altitude on physiology. Synonym: air and surface transport nursing. See also *flight nursing*.

Certified Transport Registered Nurse (CTRN) A registered nurse specializing in critical care ground transport nursing who has met the certification requirements of the Board of Certification for Emergency Nursing (BCEN). **www.ena.org/bcen**

transposition In genetics, the movement of a chromosome segment within the same chromosome.

transposon A relatively small DNA segment that has the ability to move from one location to another in a chromosome.

trauma A wound or injury. Although one can speak, properly, of psychic trauma, the term in healthcare usage ordinarily refers to physical injury. Thus "trauma centers" are set up to care for victims of accidents and other violence.

trauma care system See *trauma system*.

trauma center A center for the emergency and specialized care of patients who are injured. A trauma center may also be used for patients who are critically ill. It may be within a hospital, where it may be called either a "trauma center" or a "trauma unit," or it may be free standing.

trauma system A multidisciplinary system to respond to the needs of severely injured patients from the time of injury through the provision of definitive care. Such systems call not only on the healthcare system, but also on public safety, communication, and other community resources. Several studies have published criteria for a trauma system, based on the recommendations of the American College of Surgeons (ACS). In general, a trauma system should have (1) a lead agency with authority to designate trauma centers; (2) a formal process for trauma center designation; (3) the use of ACS standards for trauma centers; (4) the use of a neutral, out-of-area team for making the trauma center designation; (5) a limitation on the number of trauma centers, in recognition of the superior care and lower cost provided by highly specialized and active centers; (6) the use of written patient categorization and triage criteria for bypassing non-trauma-center hospitals; (7) ongoing information and monitoring systems, including a trauma registry; and (8) state-wide availability. Trauma systems are cited as models that could well be followed in the design of regionalized systems for such conditions as cardiac surgery, organ transplantation, and high-risk neonatal care.

travel medicine See *emporiatrics*.

treadmill exercise score A method for giving a numeric value (ranging from −25 to +15) to the response of an individual's heart to exercise, based on the individual's performance on a *treadmill exercise test*, taking into account the duration of exercise, the electrocardiogram taken during the exercise, and the degree of angina (chest pain) that develops. An interesting use of the score is that it reportedly can discriminate between those patients for whom cardiac catheterization would give further useful information, and those for whom no added information could be expected from the further testing. Sometimes called the Bonow test.

treadmill exercise test A method of examining the ability of an individual's heart (cardiovascular system) to handle exercise. The individual is first examined at rest in order to determine the base electrocardiogram, heart rate, blood pressure, and symptoms, and then the individual walks on a treadmill while the same information is collected during the exercise.

The test was developed at Duke University. It is important that the exercise and observations be standardized, and a "protocol" for standardization (i.e., requirements as to degree of exercise, duration, and so on) has been developed. The most frequently used protocol is that developed by Robert A. Bruce. The result of the test is expressed as a ***treadmill exercise score***.

treatment Any or all elements of the care of the patient for the correction or relief of the patient's problem. Sometimes designated with the shorthand notation "Rx." See also ***therapy***.

    extraordinary treatment Medical treatment or care that does not offer a reasonable hope of benefit to the patient, or which cannot be accomplished without excessive pain, expense, or other great burden. The decision as to whether to provide extraordinary treatment is basically an ethical determination; also, whether treatment is "extraordinary" can only be determined in relation to the condition of the patient and the prognosis. See also ***futile care***.

    investigational treatment Treatment that is still being tested; "investigational" will be given a specific definition depending on the context. For example, a health plan may not cover investigational treatment defined as therapy not approved by the Food and Drug Administration (FDA).

treble damages See under ***damages***.

tree structure A term used by the U.S. National Library of Medicine (NLM) in its ***Medical Subject Headings (MeSH)***. Each document in the biomedical literature in the library has been classified to *all the subjects* to which it pertains according to a hierarchical list of subjects reviewed and revised annually by the NLM. The list is published in two forms, an alphabetical list of the subjects along with their reference code numbers (MeSH numbers), and a "tabular list," called the tree structure, in which the subjects are categorized and subdivided, often to several levels, according to the hierarchical arrangement of the classification. It is this branching structure of the hierarchies that gives the tree structure its name.

    The tree structure is the basis of searching for a given subject in the literature, because it groups together the documents pertaining to each subject. Each tree structure is itself a ***classification (scheme)*** of the subjects within its purview. Note that a given document usually will be found in more than one branch of the tree, that is, under more than one heading, having been classified to as many subjects as logically necessary.

triage Sorting or classification of patients according to the nature and urgency of their illnesses or injuries, and assigning priorities for treatment. There is a distinction between triage that takes place in an environment where healthcare resources are extremely limited, such as on the battlefield, and triage as performed in a modern medical facility. In the former, triage attempts to allocate resources in a manner that will save the most lives or return the most persons to duty quickly; in the latter environment, triage identifies the patients with the most serious conditions so they can be treated first or can best use the facilities offered. For example, an amputation would be given high priority in a facility where reattachment was an available option.

TRICARE The program that provides supplemental benefits to the Uniformed Services direct medical care system. It pays for health care for eligible persons, who include retired members of the uniformed services of the United States and their dependents, dependents of deceased members of the military services, and dependents of North Atlantic Treaty Organization (NATO) members if the NATO member is stationed in or passing through the United States on official business. TRICARE offers three options:

    TRICARE Prime is a voluntary "HMO-type" plan that emphasizes preventive care. All active duty service members are automatically enrolled in Prime, which uses a network of civilian and military providers.

    TRICARE Extra is a preferred provider organization (PPO) option, which also uses a network of civilian doctors and military providers.

    TRICARE Standard (same as the original CHAMPUS (Civilian Health and Medical Program of the Uniformed Services) program) pays a share of the cost of covered healthcare services obtained from a non-network civilian healthcare provider.

The programs are administered by the Military Benefit Association (MBA). TRICARE eligibility precludes coverage under **CHAMPVA**. **www.militarybenefit.org**

trigger An event that forces another event to happen. For example, a trigger could be written in legislation so that if healthcare costs increased beyond a specified rate of growth in a year, price controls would "automatically" be invoked, or a billing system could have the sales tax "automatically" computed at a rate triggered by the state or city in which the purchaser is located.

Computer programs also use triggers to either draw attention or cause some other event to happen, based on certain logic conditions becoming true. An example is a program that compares a drug prescription for a patient with that patient's medical record, and then triggers an immediate warning if an adverse drug event (ADE) is likely.

TRT See *therapeutic recreation therapy.*

trustee A member of the *governing body* when that body is called a board of trustees. When the governing body is called the board of directors, then each member is called a "director."

TSEs Transmissible spongiform encephalopathies. A specific group of generally fatal degenerative diseases of the nervous system in animals, including humans. TSEs are presumably caused by *prions*, have long incubation periods, and result in spongy holes in the brain. TSEs have gained much attention since the epidemic of *mad cow disease* in Great Britain and cases of scrapie in sheep. Human TSEs include traditional Creutzfeldt-Jakob disease (CJD), and a new variant of that disease (vCJD) described in 1996, thought to be caused by eating meat contaminated by mad cow disease.

TSQ See *Temporary Status by Qualification.*

TT See *technology transfer.*

tuberculosis unit (TB unit) A patient care unit for persons with tuberculosis.

tumor An abnormal growth of tissue that is not a temporary response to inflammation or injury, and that stems from tissue already in place. Certain kinds of tumors possess the potential for unlimited growth, and are called "malignant" or "cancers." Other kinds do not have this potential, and are called "benign."

tumor, node, metastases (TNM) system A method of staging tumors. See *staging (tumors).*

tumor staging See *staging (tumors).*

turnaround time (TAT) The time it takes to complete a certain process; for example, the time between discharge of the patient and the completion of that patient's medical record.

28th Amendment The constitutional right to health care. In a widely referenced editorial, Drs. Frank Davidoff and Robert Reinecke proposed that the right to health care should be as basic a human right as the right to legal counsel, for example, and that this be accomplished by an amendment to the U.S. Constitution stating, "All citizens and other residents of the United States shall have equal access to basic and essential health care." (There are now twenty-seven amendments; the next one would be the twenty-eighth.) *Annals of Internal Medicine*, 1999;130:692–694.

two-tier health care A pejorative description of a healthcare system in which those with more money presumably get better, faster care than those with less money. The term is often used to describe a system that provides "public" health care (the lower tier), available to all, and has "private" health care (the higher tier) available to those willing to pay more. Those with private insurance typically have shorter waiting times to get care, and a wider range of benefits. The care may or may not be "better."

tying arrangement Requiring a buyer to purchase a second product or service in order to get the first product. Tying arrangements may violate the federal antitrust laws. Synonyms: tying agreement, tie-in sale.

typing A laboratory method of determining the antigenic characteristics (type) of a blood or tissue sample, that is, of determining whether or not the blood or tissue taken is likely to cause a reaction if introduced into another person with whom the type can be compared.

U

UACDS See *Uniform Ambulatory Care Data Set* under *data set*.

UB-04 The uniform billing form created by the National Uniform Billing Committee to replace the *UB-92*, beginning in 2007. The UB-04 data set accommodates the National Provider Identifier (NPI) and incorporates a number of other important changes and improvements. Synonym: CMS-1450 form.

UB-82 Uniform Billing Code of 1982. See *National Uniform Billing Committee*.

UB-92 Uniform Billing Code of 1992. Also known as CMS-1450 (previously as HCFA-1450), the UB-92 is the form used by hospitals to bill for Medicare, Medicaid, and TRICARE. It was created by the National Uniform Billing Committee (NUBC), and contains the items from the *Uniform Hospital Discharge Data Set (UHDDS)* (see under *data set*) along with additional information. This was replaced in 2007 with *UB-04*.

UBI Unrelated Business Income. See *unrelated business income tax*.

UBIT See *unrelated business income tax*.

UCC See *Uniform Commercial Code*.

UCDS See *Uniform Clinical Data Set* under *data set*.

UCR Usual, customary, and reasonable (charge). See *customary, prevailing, and reasonable charge (or fee)*.

UDI See *unique device identifier*.

UDSMR See *Uniform Data System for Medical Rehabilitation*.

UGME See *undergraduate medical education* under *medical education*, under *education*.

UHDDS See *Uniform Hospital Discharge Data Set* under *data set*.

UHP See *unconventional healing practices*.

UIHP See *Urban Indian Health Program*.

UIN See *unique identifier number*.

ULR Universal leukoreduction. See *leukoreduction*.

ultrasonography See *sonography*.

ultrasound Sound with a pitch above human hearing (above 20,000 cycles per second). Ultrasound is used in an imaging technique called sonography and in some forms of therapy, such as phacoemulsification.

ultrasound practitioner (UP) A health professional who performs and interprets ultrasound procedures in primary or specialty care settings. See also *Advanced Practice Sonographer* under *diagnostic medical sonographer*.

ultrasound scan See *sonography*.

ultra vires "Outside the powers." A legal term referring to activities of a corporation that it is not authorized to do either by its charter or the laws of the state in which it is incorporated.

UM See *utilization management*.

umbrella coverage See under *insurance coverage*.

UMC See *Utilization Management Certified* under *utilization manager*.

UMDNS See *Universal Medical Device Nomenclature System*.

UMLS See *Unified Medical Language System*.

UMLS Metathesaurus A large, multipurpose, multilingual vocabulary database, part of the *Unified Medical Language System (UMLS)*, that contains information about biomedical and health-related concepts, their various names, and the relationships among them. It is built from the electronic versions of many different thesauri, classifications, code sets, and lists of controlled terms used in patient care, health services billing, public health statistics, indexing and cataloging biomedical literature, and basic, clinical, and health services research. These are called "source vocabularies." In the Metathesaurus, all the source vocabularies are available in a single, fully specified database format. Source vocabularies in 2007 included SNOMED CT, Logical Observation Identifiers Names and Codes (LOINC), RxNorm, MeSH, ICD-10, and over 100 other sources.

unanticipated outcome See under *outcome*.

unbundling Selling individual components of a service or product separately rather than as a package. Sometimes unbundling is done for the convenience of the customer, but often it is done in order to sell the same components for a greater total price than if they were packaged together (bundled). For example, a complete automobile can be purchased for far less than its parts. In health care, the care of a fracture, for example, may be priced to include the diagnosis, treatment, and aftercare as a single package (bundled); alternatively, diagnosis, setting of the fracture, applying the cast, removing the cast, and other services may be priced individually (unbundled). See also *bundling*.

uncompensated care Care for which no payment is expected or no charge is made.

unconventional healing practices (UHP) A classification introduced by Ted Kaptchuk and David Eisenberg in 2001 that contains two major groups: *complementary and alternative medicine (CAM)* and *parochial and unconventional medicine (PUM)*. Kaptchuk, T., & Eisenberg, D. "Varieties of Healing. 2: A Taxonomy of Unconventional Healing Practices." *Annals of Internal Medicine*, 2001;135(3):196–204.

undercoding See under *coding (billing)*.

undergraduate A student in an academic institution who has not achieved a given degree. The term most often refers to an individual before the bachelor's degree, but in medicine, the degree in question is the Doctor of Medicine (MD) or Doctor of Osteopathic Medicine (DO) degree.

undersea medicine The area of medicine concerned with the health of divers and with the effects of the undersea environment on health and safety. Sometimes called diving medicine. See also *hyperbaric medicine*.

underwriting Assuming a risk. In finance, it means assuming the risk of buying a new issue of securities directly from a corporation or government entity, and then reselling them to the public. In insurance, it means assuming the risk of loss in exchange for an amount of money (the premium).

medical underwriting A practice by healthcare insurers to reduce their risk by deciding who *needs* coverage and then denying it to them. The insurer uses the health status of groups and individuals to determine the rates, and whether to provide healthcare coverage and under what conditions.

negotiated underwriting A private sale of bonds by their issuer as contrasted with advertisement for public bids. Most hospital bond underwritings are negotiated because of special marketing considerations.

UNESCO See *United Nations Educational, Scientific and Cultural Organization*.

UNEX Unexplained Deaths Project. An interdisciplinary group at the Centers for Disease Control and Prevention (CDC) that examines cases where state and local health authorities, medical examiners, and sometimes private physicians have been unable to determine a cause of death. UNEX started in 1995 as a group of scientists trying to identify outbreaks of new infectious diseases before they reached epidemic proportions. It is now part of the National Center for Zoonotic, Vector-Borne and Enteric Diseases (NCZVED) and is composed of virologists, bacteriologists, epidemiologists, veterinarians, and clinicians.

unexpected adverse drug reaction Not synonymous with, but defined and discussed under, *adverse drug event*.

Unified Medical Language System (UMLS) A system maintained by the National Library of Medicine (NLM) containing a metathesaurus that links clinical terminology, semantics, and formats of the major clinical coding and reference systems. The UMLS links medical terms (e.g., ICD-9, CPT, SNOMED, DSM-IV) to the NLM's medical index subject headings (MeSH codes) and to each other. By mapping these differing biomedical terminologies to each other, it is hoped that patient records can be more effectively linked to decision support tools like clinical practice guidelines and MEDLINE. **www.nlm.nih.gov/research/umls**

Uniform Ambulatory Care Data Set (UACDS) See under *data set.*

uniform benefit package See *standard benefit package* under *benefit package.*

Uniform Billing Code See *National Uniform Billing Committee.*

Uniform Clinical Data Set (UCDS) See under *data set.*

Uniform Commercial Code (UCC) A compilation of laws governing commercial transactions including sales of goods, banking transactions, and secured transactions for personal property. The code has been adopted, with minor modifications, by all fifty states (Louisiana did not adopt the UCC in its entirety), the District of Columbia, Guam, Puerto Rico, and the U.S. Virgin Islands. The UCC has greatly facilitated interstate commerce.

Uniform Data System for Medical Rehabilitation (UDSMR) A system for documenting the severity of patient disability and outcomes of medical rehabilitation. It includes the world's largest database of medical rehabilitation outcomes. UDSMR is a division of UB Foundation Activities, Inc., a nonprofit organization affiliated with the University at Buffalo, The State University of New York. **www.udsmr.org**

Uniform Determination of Death Act (UDDA) This model act, followed by all fifty states and the District of Columbia, states that "an individual who has sustained either (1) irreversible cessation of circulatory and respiratory functions, or (2) irreversible cessation of all functions of the entire brain, including the brain stem, is dead. A determination of death must be made in accordance with accepted medical standards."

In cases where the dying patient is an organ donor, the technical determination of death is critical in terms of time because otherwise viable organs may no longer be suitable for transplanting after a certain amount of time has passed. See *anencephaly* for an example of this issue.

Uniform Hospital Discharge Data Set (UHDDS) See under *data set.*

uniform physician identifier number (UPIN) See *UPIN.*

uniform reporting Reporting of patient care information, financial information, or both under uniform definitions (and sometimes formats) in order to permit comparisons among hospitals or physicians.

unique device identifier (UDI) A unique *identifier* for *medical devices*, similar to the *National Drug Code (NDC)* used for drugs. See also *Universal Medical Device Nomenclature System.*

unique identifier number (UIN) Generally, a number assigned to patients, persons, or providers to uniquely identify them and their health information. Similar to a Social Security Number (SSN), such a number would be national in scope, be regulated in its use, and remain specific to a certain individual for his or her lifetime. Synonyms: unique health identifier (UHI), unique personal identifier (UPI) (but that gets confused with unique provider/physician identification number; see *UPIN*). See also *identifier.*

unique physician identifier number (UPIN) See *UPIN.*

unit See *patient care unit.*

unit clerk A person who performs clerical duties in a patient care unit. Synonyms: ward clerk, unit secretary.

United Nations Educational, Scientific and Cultural Organization (UNESCO) An international organization founded by the United Nations (UN) in 1945 to promote collaboration among nations through education, science, culture, and communication in order to further universal respect for justice, the rule of law, and human rights and fundamental freedoms. In 1997, UNESCO developed the "Universal Declaration on the Human Genome and Human Rights," which was endorsed by the UN. Headquartered in Paris, France, UNESCO has field offices and units in various parts of the world. **www.unesco.org**

United Network for Organ Sharing (UNOS) A national organ transplant network that facilitates organ sharing among transplant centers, organ procurement organizations, and histocompatibility laboratories across the United States. Its "Organ Center" matches donors to recipients and coordinates the organ-sharing process 24 hours a day, 365 days a year. Its technology group maintains the databases that contain all clinical transplant data for every transplant event that occurs in the United States, and its research department performs data analyses, fills data requests, produces data reports, and authors authoritative publications. UNOS also provides professional and patient services. It was established in 1982 as the Kidney Center. **www.unos.org**

United States Department See under "Department" for the specific federal department desired (e.g., *Department of Agriculture*, *Department of Energy*, etc.).

United States Health Information Knowledgebase (USHIK) A *metadata registry* of health information data element definitions, values, and information models that enable browsing, comparison, synchronization, and harmonization within a uniform query and interface environment. USHIK contains the data elements and information models of standards development organizations (SDOs) and other healthcare organizations so that public and private organizations can harmonize their information formats with healthcare standards. It also contains information for government initiatives such as HIPAA and the Consolidated Health Informatics (CHI) initiative. **www.ushik.org**

United States Medical Licensing Examination (USMLE) A single, uniform examination for medical licensure developed by the National Board of Medical Examiners (NBME) and the Federation of State Medical Boards (FSMB), implemented in 1994 and computerized in 1999. It replaced the Federation Licensing Examination (FLEX) and the certifying examinations of the NBME, Parts I, II, and III. **www.usmle.org**

United States Pharmacopeia (USP) The official public standards-setting authority for all prescription and over-the-counter medicines, dietary supplements, and other healthcare products manufactured and sold in the United States. USP sets standards for the quality of these products and works with healthcare providers to help them reach the standards. USP's standards are also recognized and used in more than 130 other countries.

Founded in 1820, the USP is an independent, nonprofit organization with about 450 members who represent U.S. colleges and state associations of medicine and pharmacy; governments of the United States and other countries; national and international health professional, scientific, and trade organizations; the pharmaceutical industry; and consumer organizations.

The USP annually revises and publishes the *United State Pharmacopeia—National Formulary (USP-NF)*. See also *MEDMARX*. **www.usp.org**

United States Pharmacopeia—National Formulary (USP-NF) The official compendia for drugs marketed in the United States. The USP-NF contains standards for medicines, dosage forms, drug substances, excipients (inert substances added to drugs), medical devices, and dietary supplements. It includes directions for drug preparation, and requirements as to their potency and purity. USP-NF standards are also recognized in more than 130 other countries. Originally published in 1820, it was made a legal standard in 1907. Published in print, CD, and online by the *United States Pharmacopeia (USP)*. **www.usp.org/USPNF**

unit manager The person in charge of a patient care unit. Synonym: ward manager.

unit record A single *medical record* in which are kept the records of all hospitalizations of the individual. This is the preferred method of filing medical records.

unit record system The system for filing *medical records* in which a separate file is kept for each individual patient, and the medical records of all hospitalizations of that individual are placed in the one file.

unit secretary See *unit clerk*.

universal coverage/universal insurance coverage See *coverage*.

universal design Designing living spaces and appliances in a way that makes them easier and safer to use, regardless of the inhabitants' physical size or capabilities. Many specialized designs have been encouraged by the Americans with Disabilities Act (ADA) in an effort to level the playing field for those with handicaps, but "universal design" says these designs are good for everyone.

Universal Medical Device Nomenclature System (UMDNS) A standard international nomenclature and computer coding system for *medical devices*. UMDNS has been officially adopted by many nations, including the entire European Union (EU). The purpose of UMDNS is to make it easier to exchange information about medical devices. The nomenclature is used in applications ranging from hospital inventory control to governmental regulation of medical devices. The U.S. National Library of Medicine (NLM) incorporates UMDNS into its Unified Medical Language System (UMLS). See also *unique device identifier*.

universal physician identifier number (UPIN) See *UPIN*.

universal precautions (UP) See under *precautions*.

Universal Product Code (UPC) The ubiquitous identifier found on almost all retail packaging, typically encoded in bar code format. This code should not be confused with the *Universal Product Number (UPN)* used in the healthcare industry. The UPC is maintained in the United States by the Uniform Code Council (UCC), and by the EAN internationally. See also *identifier*.

Universal Product Number (UPN) A unique, variable-length, alphanumeric identifier assigned to each medical product, allowing healthcare product manufacturers, vendors, and consumers to improve "supply chain management." This identifier compares to the *National Drug Code (NDC)* used to identify medications. To support the UPN, the health industry has asked that the Health Industry Business Communications Council (HIBCC) develop and administer the **UPN Repository**, a master list of medical/surgical products containing basic data elements such as UPN, manufacturer's name, part number and description, and unit of measure. The repository, freely available on the Internet (**www.upnrepository.org**), also allows the healthcare industry to cross-reference manufacturer part numbers to UPNs.

Even though the repository of UPN numbers in 2007 contained nearly 250,000 items, usage of UPNs was not universal, and there were reports of multiple items sharing the same UPN. Support for the use of the UPN is growing, however, and even now the Department of Defense (DoD) requires all manufacturers doing business with it to identify and bar code their products with the UPN. See also *identifier* and *unique device identifier*.

Universal Protocol Short for Universal Protocol for Preventing Wrong Site, Wrong Procedure, Wrong Person Surgery. The protocol calls for (1) a preoperative verification process, (2) marking the operative site, and (3) taking a "time-out" immediately before the procedure to verify the correct patient, procedure, site, and, as applicable, implants. Issued by the Joint Commission on Accreditation of Healthcare Organizations (JCAHO) and endorsed by more than forty professional medical associations and organizations. Not to be confused with *universal precautions* (see under *precautions*), which have to do with infection control.

Universal Service Administrative Company (USAC) An independent, nonprofit corporation designated as the administrator of the federal Universal Service Fund by the Federal Communications Commission (FCC). **www.usac.org**

Universal Service Fund (USF) A fund to promote nationwide access to quality telecommunications services at just, reasonable, and affordable prices. Universal Service was mandated by the Telecommunications Act of 1996, and the USF was created in 1997 by the Federal Communications Commission (FCC). All telecommunications carriers that provide service internationally and between states must pay contributions into the USF. They have the option of passing those costs on to their customers directly (for example, a "Universal Service" line item charge on telephone bills).

The USF has four programs:

High Cost: Ensures that consumers in rural areas have access to and pay rates for telecommunications services that are reasonably comparable to those in urban areas.

Low Income ("Lifeline" and "Link Up" programs): Provides discounts that make basic, local telephone service affordable for more than 7 million low-income consumers.

Rural Health Care: Provides reduced rates to rural healthcare providers for telecommunications and Internet services so they pay no more than their urban counterparts for the same or similar services.

Schools and Libraries ("E-Rate Support"): Provides affordable services to connect schools and libraries to the Internet.

The USF is administered by the Universal Service Administrative Company (USAC).

universe The term used to designate the kind of thing being considered. In health care, diagnoses (the terms applied to describe disorders of patients) form one universe. Other universes are the ages of patients, sexes, external forces such as those that cause injuries, surgical procedures—the list is virtually endless.

UNOS See *United Network for Organ Sharing*.

unrelated business income tax (UBIT) Tax paid by a nonprofit corporation on the profits of activities that are not "substantially related" to the nonprofit purpose of the corporation (the "unrelated business income," or UBI). A nonprofit corporation is normally exempt from taxation, but may engage in profit-making activities and pay taxes on those, while preserving its tax-exempt status, by complying with specific federal tax law requirements regarding unrelated business income.

UP See *universal precautions* (under *precautions*) and *ultrasound practitioner*.

UPC See *Universal Product Code*.

upcoding See under *coding (billing)*.

UPIN Unique Physician Identification Number. An identifier assigned by CMS to an individual physician, allowing nationwide, accurate access to information about healthcare providers. The UPIN was assigned only to physicians who handled Medicare patients, and it did not include nonphysicians. UPIN was replaced by the *National Provider Identifier (NPI)* in 2007. UPIN has also been used for various combinations of words—Uniform/Unique/Universal Physician/Provider/Patient Identification Number—but not necessarily with any defined meanings. See *identifier*.

UPN See *Universal Product Number*.

upskilling Adding an additional skill to one's professional repertoire, often in a field different from one's primary area. For example, a dietitian may train and become qualified to draw blood. Synonym: multiskilling.

UR See *utilization review*.

URAC A nonprofit organization formed in 1990 to set standards for the managed care industry (originally called the Utilization Review Accreditation Commission). It has accreditation programs for many types of healthcare organizations, including managed care organizations, health plans, and preferred provider organizations (PPOs). URAC also accredits vendors who sell to URAC-accredited organizations.

In 2001, URAC launched its Health Web Site Accreditation program, and by 2005 had accredited fifty web sites and 300 portals including WebMD, Healthwise, National Institutes of Health, National Library of Medicine, KidsHealth, and Consumer Health Interactive. The program evaluates web sites for their privacy and security policies, health content editorial processes, disclosure of financial relationships, linking policies, consumer complaints, and promoting emerging best practices.

URAC is also known as the American Accreditation HealthCare Commission, Inc. **www.urac.org**

Urban Indian Health Program (UIHP) A program of the Indian Health Service (IHS) to fund and support the delivery of health services to American Indians and Alaska Natives

(AI/AN) who reside in urban areas, away from reservations. In 2007 there were thirty-four urban health programs funded under Title V of the Indian Health Care Improvement Act (IHCIA). These programs provide comprehensive ambulatory care services, including pre-natal and postpartum care, women's health, immunizations for children and adults, pediatric care, chronic disease clinics (for example, diabetes), acute medical care, infectious disease treatment and control (tuberculosis, sexually transmitted diseases), and referral to special-ized providers when needed. Other services include dental services; community services; alcohol and drug abuse prevention, education, and treatment; AIDS and sexually transmitted disease education and prevention services; mental health services; nutrition education and counseling services; pharmacy services; health education; optometry services; social services; and home health care. Fifteen of the programs are designated as Federally Qualified Health Centers (FQHCs) and provide services to both Indians and non-Indians.

urbanized area According to the U.S. Department of Commerce, Census Bureau, an urban-ized area is defined as "A densely settled territory that contains 50,000 or more people." A "non-urbanized area" is an area that is outside of an urbanized area. A Rural Health Clinic (RHC) must be located in a non-urbanized area.

UR committee See *utilization review committee.*

UR coordinator See *utilization review coordinator.*

urgent A term that, in regard to a patient's condition, refers to a degree of illness that is less severe than an emergency, but that requires care within a reasonably short time (more quickly than elective care).

urgent care center A sort of competitor of an emergency department, but for less "emergent" problems. For example, a painful ear infection or sprained ankle requires quick attention, but it is not necessarily an emergency, requiring immediate attention in order to prevent death or severe disability. An urgent care center offers walk-in service, usually during extended hours. Sometimes it is stated that a facility, to be called an "urgent care center," must have certain laboratory and x-ray services on-site, but must not hold itself out as ready for emergencies such as those brought by ambulance or to provide continuity of care. An urgent care center may be free standing or a part of another facility.

urologic Having to do with the genitourinary tract in males and females, and the reproduc-tive system in males.

urologic associate A health professional who assists in serving the needs of urologic patients.

Certified Urologic Associate (CUA) A licensed practical/vocational nurse or other quali-fied, experienced health professional who has met the requirements of the Certification Board for Urologic Nurses and Associates (CBUNA). **www.suna.org**

urologic nursing The area of nursing focusing on the needs of urologic patients.

Certified Urologic Clinical Nurse Specialist (CUCNS) A clinical nurse specialist in uro-logic nursing who has passed an advanced examination of the Certification Board for Uro-logic Nurses and Associates (CBUNA). **www.suna.org**

Certified Urologic Nurse Practitioner (CUNP) A nurse practitioner in urologic nursing who has passed an advanced examination of the Certification Board for Urologic Nurses and Associates (CBUNA). **www.suna.org**

Certified Urologic Registered Nurse (CURN) A registered nurse who has passed a uro-logic nursing examination of the Certification Board for Urologic Nurses and Associates (CBUNA). **www.suna.org**

urologic physician's assistant A *physician assistant* (PA) who specializes in treating uro-logic patients.

Certified Urologic Physician's Assistant (CUPA) A licensed physician assistant who has passed an examination of the Certification Board for Urologic Nurses and Associates (CBUNA).

urology The study of diseases and disorders of the genitourinary tract in males and females, and the reproductive system in males.

USAC See *Universal Service Administrative Company*.

USDA See *Department of Agriculture*.

USDA National Nutrient Database for Standard Reference (SR) A database, developed by the Nutrient Data Laboratory (NDL) of the U.S. Department of Agriculture (USDA), that serves as the foundation of most food and nutrition databases in the United States, used in food policy, research, and nutrition monitoring. The SR is available free online with a searchable interface or may be downloaded at **www.ars.usda.gov/nutrientdata**. The database is being continually updated, and includes brand name foods. As of Release 19, issued in 2006, SR contained 7,293 food items. References to this database in the literature are frequently of the form "USDA SR19," here referring to release number 19. USDA food composition data are in the public domain, so there is no copyright, but the source of the data should be cited when used. The database was formerly published (until 2000) as the USDA's *Agriculture Handbook No. 8 (AH-8)*.

USDA SR See *USDA National Nutrient Database for Standard Reference*.

use effectiveness See *method effectiveness*.

use failure See *method effectiveness*.

USF See *Universal Service Fund*.

USFMG See *U.S. foreign medical graduate* under *foreign medical graduate*.

USHIK See *United States Health Information Knowledgebase*.

USMLE See *United States Medical Licensing Examination*.

USP See *United States Pharmacopeia—National Formulary*.

USPHS United States Public Health Service. See *Public Health Service*.

USP-NF See *United States Pharmacopeia—National Formulary*.

U.S. TAG A group formed by *ASTM* to develop the U.S. position on health information standards for submission to *ISO/TC 215*. Interested organizations may join upon payment of a fee. **www.astm.org**

usual, customary, and reasonable (UCR) See *customary, prevailing, reasonable charge (or fee)*.

utilization control Any effort to control or account for the provision of healthcare services, typically undertaken by the provider or the payer of the services. "Utilization control" is also mentioned in the context of Medicare and Medicaid, specifically Section 1902(a)(30) of the Social Security Act (42 U.S.C. § 1396(a)(30) (2004)), which has established procedures for reviewing the utilization of, and payment for, Medical Assistance services. See also *utilization management*.

utilization management (UM) A management initiative that seeks to ensure the efficiency and appropriateness of any healthcare service that may be provided to (utilized by) a healthcare consumer (patient). UM seeks to eliminate both over- and underutilization of medically necessary care. Before the era of managed care, utilization of healthcare resources tended to be done retrospectively, and was known as utilization review (UR). Increasingly the trend is towards utilization control, which is essentially prospective in nature. One major effort that is a component of utilization management is the use of *clinical practice guidelines* (see under *guidelines*).

utilization manager A health professional specializing in utilization management.

> **Certified Professional Utilization Management (CPUM)** A person who has completed a course of instruction in utilization management offered by InterQual, a division of McKesson. **www.interqual.com**

> **Utilization Management Certified (UMC)** A credential for health professionals (physicians, nurses, executives, respiratory therapists, social workers, pharmacists, etc.) who qualify in utilization management, offered by the American Institute of Outcomes Care Management (AIOCM). **www.aiocm.com**

utilization review (UR) The examination and evaluation of the efficiency and appropriateness of any healthcare service that has already been provided (utilized). Often the term applies to a concurrent process, one carried out during hospitalization, for determination of the individual patient's need for continued stay. Increasingly, in the era of managed care, this process is moving towards utilization control and utilization management.

Certified Professional Utilization Review (CPUR) A person who has completed a course of instruction in utilization review offered by InterQual, a division of McKesson. **www.interqual.com**

utilization review committee (UR committee) A committee, made up primarily of medical staff members, designated to carry out the utilization review function, that is, reviewing the appropriateness of hospitalizations and of the services used, and the lengths of stay of patients subject to such review.

utilization review coordinator (UR coordinator) A hospital employee, typically a medical record professional or a nurse, who coordinates the hospital's utilization review activities, gathers data from medical records and elsewhere for the use of the utilization review committee and others, and otherwise assists in utilization review. The UR coordinator may also have duties involving liaison with other community agencies regarding transfer of patients to other facilities or services, including home care.

V

VA See *Department of Veterans Affairs.*

vaccine A preparation that, when introduced into a human or other animal, stimulates the development of *active immunity* (see under *immunity*) against specific infections. Most vaccines are either (1) killed bacteria or viruses of strains that, when alive, are able to cause the disease in question, or (2) live bacteria or viruses of attenuated (weakened) strains of the disease-causing organism (closely related bacteria or viruses that are not able to cause the disease but are able to stimulate the production of the specific immunity required). Vaccines do not produce passive immunity; passive immunity is the result of introduction into the body of prefabricated immune serum that protects against the disease in question.

Vaccines for Children (VFC) A federal program that provides free vaccines to doctors who serve eligible children—those without health insurance or whose insurance does not cover vaccinations. It is administered by the Centers for Disease Control and Prevention (CDC) through the National Immunization Program (NIP).

VAD See *ventricular assist device.*

vaginal births after cesarean section (VBAC) A commonly computed hospital statistic.

valet See *resident valet.*

valley of death For pharmaceutical manufacturers, the time between early research on a new drug and the eventual payoff from sales of that drug (which can only happen after approval by the Food and Drug Administration (FDA)). It can take years and hundreds of millions of dollars to bridge this gap, which can slow down, stop, or even prevent research and development of needed drugs and vaccines. See also *Biomedical Advanced Research and Development Authority* and *orphan drug.*

value-added Reflecting the position that something done to a given product or service has increased its value. Value-added taxes indicate that a product is worth more, and thus can be subject to a higher tax, after something has been done to it, such as merely keeping it in stock for the convenience of the customer. An annotated bibliography could be termed a "value-added" bibliography, because the discussion added to the citation makes it more valuable. See also *value-added reseller.*

value-added reseller (VAR) A vendor of products and services who does more than simply buy products at wholesale from a manufacturer and resell them at retail to a consumer. In the healthcare industry, for example, a hospital might wish to buy a computer system. Instead of going to a computer store and buying brand X computer hardware, with brand Y software, the hospital might contact an information systems VAR specializing in health care. This VAR would not only sell the hospital brand X and Y hardware and software, but also the VAR's own brand Y software that added the special functionality required by this hospital. The VAR would also typically install, train, and support the entire installation, as well as provide ongoing support after the sale on a contractual basis.

value-added tax (VAT) A tax imposed on goods and services at each stage of production. The end result is similar to a sales tax, but usually produces much more revenue because the tax is not so "visible" and therefore is less painful. It has been discussed as one method of financing health care under healthcare reform.

value-based purchasing (VBP) Obtaining the highest quality health care at the most reasonable price. The concept links the payment for care with the quality of care, including patient outcomes and health status, and rewards cost-effective practices. For example, the employer or other purchaser of healthcare services contracts with the provider to pay for care that meets specific standards of quality, such as performance measures. See also *pay-for-performance.*

value-driven health care A healthcare system in which price and quality are made visible so that purchasers of care (consumers, employers, insurers, Medicare) can make choices based on value—presumably choosing the highest quality care at the lowest price. See **transparency initiative** and **transparent**.

value inventory A statement elicited from an individual as to that person's values with regard to living and functioning, for example, the person's tolerance for discomfort and pain, desire for personal mobility, willingness to be kept on life support systems, and similar matters. Value inventory questionnaires have been developed as adjuncts to advance directives to make those documents more likely to conform with the individual's own preferences.

values history See under **advance directive**.

VAR See **value-added reseller**.

vascular Having to do with blood vessels. See **cardiovascular**.

vascular neurology The medical discipline pertaining to neurological disorders involving the central nervous system (CNS) due to ischemia or hemorrhage—for example, strokes.

VAT See **value-added tax**.

VBAC See **vaginal births after cesarean section**.

VBP See **value-based purchasing**.

vector (epidemiology) An organism, such as an insect, bird, dog, or rodent, that is capable of carrying and transmitting a disease. For example, the vector for West Nile virus is the mosquito.

vector (genetics) An agent that carries a substance from one host to another. For example, a modified noninfectious virus used to deliver genetic material into the body for gene therapy.

vegetative state (VS) The American Academy of Neurology defines vegetative state as "a clinical condition of complete unawareness of the self and the environment accompanied by sleep-wake cycles with either complete or partial preservation of hypothalamic and brainstem autonomic functions."

permanent vegetative state A vegetative state that is irreversible. This assessment cannot be absolute, but only made with a "high degree of clinical certainty, i.e., when the chance of regaining consciousness is exceedingly rare" (American Academy of Neurology).

persistent vegetative state (PVS) A patient who has been in a vegetative state for at least a month. The acronym PVS is also sometimes used in reference to permanent vegetative state.

vendor managed inventory (VMI) See **Strategic National Stockpile**.

venereal disease See **sexually transmitted disease**.

venereology The study of **sexually transmitted disease**.

ventricular assist device (VAD) A mechanical device used to perform the pumping tasks of the heart during surgery or in an emergency while waiting for a heart transplant. This device does not replace the entire heart as does an artificial heart.

vertical transmission Transmission of a disease from one generation to another. Transmission of HIV infection (AIDS) from a mother to her offspring is vertical transmission. Horizontal transmission is from one individual to another in the *same* generation.

Veteran's Administration (VA) See **Department of Veterans Affairs**.

Veterinary Medical Assistance Team (VMAT) See under **National Disaster Medical System**.

VFC See **Vaccines for Children**.

VHA Inc. A nationwide alliance of nonprofit healthcare organizations. VHA was founded in 1977 dedicated to "the success of not-for-profit, community-based health care." Originally named Voluntary Hospitals of America, Inc., it had over 2,400 members in 2007, including approximately 1,400 hospitals. **www.vha.com**

viable (can live) Capable of living, as a baby born above a certain birth weight.

viable (can succeed) Capable of being carried out or of succeeding, for example, "viable plans."

viatical benefits Life insurance proceeds obtained while one is still alive by selling the policy for cash to a third party. The sale is called a "viatical settlement." See also *accelerated death benefit*.

vice president, medical affairs (VPMA) See *director of medical affairs*.

VIM See *Volunteers in Medicine Clinic*.

virology The study of viruses and the diseases caused by them.

Virtual Hospital A project by the Electric Differential Multimedia Laboratory in the Department of Radiology at the University of Iowa Medical School that created a link between academia and the practicing primary care physician. The Virtual Hospital combined a wide-area computer network (WAN) with a medical multimedia database to provide an online link between academia and primary care physicians. After thirteen years of service, on January 1, 2006, Virtual Hospital/Virtual Children's Hospital ceased operations after serving over 80 million users, due to a lack of funding. However, much of the content remains available online. **www.vh.org**

virtual merger A loosely defined concept in which healthcare companies, such as hospitals, agree to cooperate in some areas in which they had previously competed with one another. For example, two hospitals just a few miles apart might agree that one will offer obstetrics and the other will focus on neurosurgery, and neither will duplicate the services of the other. Unlike an actual merger, the individual companies retain their legal identities and responsibilities. They may also continue to compete in areas not covered by the "virtual merger" agreement.

This practice, although seemingly well suited to avoiding wasteful duplication of expensive resources, may easily run afoul of antitrust laws. This is because it involves two separate legal entities agreeing not to compete. The U.S. Federal Trade Commission (FTC) and the Department of Justice (DOJ) issued a joint document in 2000 called *Antitrust Guidelines for Collaboration Among Competitors*, in which they set out distinctions between true mergers and what they refer to as "collaborations."

virtual organization An arrangement among actual organizations (or some of their parts) and individuals that carries out functions as though they were provided by a single organization, although the arrangement is not a separate organization. Some emerging healthcare networks or their programs are virtual organizations. For example, some communities handle teenage pregnancy problems with physicians, the local hospital, the local health department, social welfare agencies, churches, and schools each providing some services, working together *seamlessly* as though the "teenage pregnancy program" were provided by a single organization.

The term may also be applied to an organization that does not have a central geographic location, but rather a number of individuals or departments that are connected via telecommunications.

virulence The ability of an organism to cause disease.

virus A microscopic living organism that cannot reproduce itself; reproduction is accomplished by invading a cell of another organism and using part of that cell's reproductive machinery.

Visible Human Project Includes "Visible Human Male" and "Visible Human Female." See *cybercadaver*.

vision rehabilitation therapist A health professional practicing vision rehabilitation therapy.

> **Certified Vision Rehabilitation Therapist (CVRT)** A vision rehabilitation therapist who has passed a certification examination of the Academy for Certification of Vision Rehabilitation and Education Professionals (ACVREP). **www.acvrep.org**

vision rehabilitation therapy (VRT) Education of people who are blind or visually impaired to assist them to lead safe, productive, and independent lives. Subjects taught include communication systems (Braille, assistive technology, etc.), personal management (grooming, clothing organization, social skills), home management (organization, labeling, budgeting, record keeping, repairs), activities of daily living (cooking, cleaning, shopping), leisure and recreation, psychosocial aspects of vision loss, medical management, and basic orientation and mobility skills. Formerly called rehabilitation teaching (RT).

visit In ordinary use a "visit" means, for example, the appearance of a patient in the emergency department or the appearance of a physician at the bedside. In health care, however, very specific definitions of "visit" are employed in calculation of statistics and in payment. Nevertheless, the use of the term "visit" is not uniform: The "visit" of a patient to an outpatient department in which a physician sees the patient, and then the patient goes to the laboratory and x-ray departments, may be considered one visit or three. Such definitions are often unique to the hospital, the departments involved, and the payment system; one must inquire as to exactly what is meant locally.

office visit All services provided a patient in the course of a single appearance for care at a physician's office.

outpatient visit All services provided an outpatient in the course of a single appearance for care.

visiting nurse association (VNA) A private nonprofit organization with the purpose of providing skilled nursing care and other healthcare services, primarily in the home, on an hourly basis. Most VNAs are classified as *home health agencies*.

VistA Veterans Health Information Systems and Technology Architecture. An integrated, enterprise-wide electronic health record system developed by the Department of Veterans Affairs (VA) for use in its veterans hospitals, outpatient clinics, and nursing homes. VistA's core is the **Computerized Patient Record System (CPRS)**, which provides a single interface for providers to review and update a patient's medical record and to place orders, including medications, special procedures, x-rays, nursing orders, diets, and laboratory tests. CPRS organizes and presents all relevant data on a patient in a way that directly supports clinical decision making. The "cover sheet" displays timely patient information including active problems, allergies, current medications, recent laboratory results, vital signs, hospitalization, and outpatient clinic history. CPRS capabilities include:

- A real-time order checking system that alerts clinicians during the ordering session that a possible problem (for example drug incompatibility) could exist if the order is processed.
- A notification system that immediately alerts clinicians about clinically significant events.
- A "patient posting" system that alerts clinicians to issues related specifically to the patient, including crisis notes, warnings, adverse reactions, and advance directives.
- A reminder system that allows caregivers to track and improve preventive health care for patients and ensure that timely clinical interventions are initiated.
- A remote data view functionality that allows clinicians to view a patient's medical history from other VA facilities.

Another component of the VistA system is **VistA Imaging**, which integrates medical images, including x-rays, pathology slides, video views, scanned documents, cardiology exam results, wound photos, dental images, endoscopies, and so forth, into the patient record.

VistA was originally developed in the early 1980s as the Decentralized Hospital Computer Program (DHCP). It is public domain software and freely available through the U.S. Freedom of Information Act (FOIA). A demo of the CPRS can be found at **www1.va.gov/CPRSdemo**. See also *Bar Code Medication Administration*, *HealtheVet*, and *VistA-Office Electronic Health Record*.

Hui OpenVistA A nonproprietary, open-source version of *VistA* originally developed by the Pacific Telehealth & Technology Hui, a joint venture of the Department of Veterans Affairs

(VA) and the Department of Defense (DoD), in collaboration with VistA developers and programmers in the open source community. ("Hui" is the Hawaiian word for partnership.) Development is now under the oversight of the Open Source Vista Governance Council. **openvista.pacifichui.org**

WorldVistA A nonprofit organization incorporated in 2002 dedicated to developing VistA beyond its uses in the Department of Veterans Affairs (VA)—for example, by developing packages for pediatrics, obstetrics, and other hospital services not present in veterans' hospitals—and making it available worldwide. WorldVistA is also the official vendor support organization (VSO) for the *VistA-Office Electronic Health Record*. **www.worldvista.org**

VistA Imaging See *VistA*.

VistA-Office Electronic Health Record (VOE) An adaptation of *VistA* software designed for use in small- to medium-sized physician practices, developed by CMS and the Department of Veterans Affairs (VA). VOE includes existing VistA functions such as order entry, documentation, and results reporting, and has been enhanced in the areas of physician-office patient registration, interfacing with existing billing systems, and reporting of quality measures. VOE was developed as an alternative to commercial products, although it is not entirely free. VOE operates on a Windows platform with Cache as the underlying database program. Licenses for certain code sets, such as Current Procedural Terminology (CPT), are also required. The software is not open source, but it is in the public domain. Synonyms: VistaOffice, VistA Office, VistA-Office EHR.

visually impaired Being unable to see better than 20/60 (perfect is 20/20) without glasses or contacts. Poor night vision, limited peripheral vision, double vision, and loss of vision in one eye are also forms of visual impairment. See also *blind* and *low vision*.

vital signs A medical term that has been traditionally used for four objective physical signs that are routinely monitored to give a quick picture of a patient's condition—temperature, blood pressure, pulse rate, and respiratory rate. Several states have passed legislation that also require the monitoring of the patient's subjective pain (for example, having the patient rate his or her pain on a scale from one to ten), in effect redefining "vital signs" to also include this item of information. In fact, pain is becoming known as the "fifth vital sign." Synonym: life signs.

vital statistics Statistics dealing with births, deaths, marriages, divorces, and fetal deaths, compiled from official registers. In the United States, legal authority for the registration of these vital events resides individually with the fifty states, two cities (Washington, DC, and New York City), and five territories (Puerto Rico, the Virgin Islands, Guam, American Samoa, and the Commonwealth of the Northern Mariana Islands). See also *National Vital Statistics System*.

vivisection The act of cutting into, dissecting, or otherwise injuring live animals for purposes of physiological or pathological research. Some use the term more broadly to include all painful or injurious experimentation on animals, such as for testing the safety of cosmetics. Hence the term antivivisectionism, which means against animal testing. See also *animal rights movement*.

VMAT See *Veterinary Medical Assistance Team* under *National Disaster Medical System*.

VMI Vendor managed inventory; see *Strategic National Stockpile*.

VNA See *visiting nurse association*.

vocabulary A set of words used (or available for use) by an individual or group, or within a particular type of work or field of knowledge. For people using the English language, every word found in the most comprehensive English dictionary constitutes one vocabulary. Teenagers have their own (constantly changing) vocabulary, as do dockworkers, singers, and computer users.

In the healthcare context, vocabulary typically means **controlled vocabulary**, a limited or restricted set of "preferred" words to be used within a specific context to represent specific ideas. This is an effort to control the expression of ideas in such a way that a specific idea is always expressed using exactly the same words.

The motivation to use controlled vocabularies is particularly strong when computers are used to process healthcare information, as in the trend towards using an electronic medical record (EMR). This is because computer systems still have relatively limited intelligence when it comes to processing "everyday" language (see *natural language*).

However, there are major problems in trying to use controlled vocabularies for the EMR. One is that some ideas that are *not identical* are likely to be expressed with the same words from the vocabulary, whose purpose is often to "group" (classify) similar ideas. The resulting misinformation, or loss of information, may not appear to be critical at the time; however, it may become so later when additional information becomes known about the idea, and it is then too late to go back and retrieve the actual, original words.

A second problem is that health care, like much of the rest of the world, is constantly changing, often in unforeseen ways. Natural language is very fluid (not always a good thing, as we say in the Preface to this book!), and as new ideas surface, the language adapts itself to being able to express these new ideas. With a controlled vocabulary, one is dependent on the controller of the vocabulary to make the necessary changes before the new ideas can be expressed.

Distinguish *nomenclature*, and see the diagram at *natural language*.

vocational rehabilitation counselor (VRC) See under *rehabilitation counselor*.

VOE See *VistA-Office Electronic Health Record*.

volume adjustment See *behavior offset*.

Voluntary Hospitals of America Former name of *VHA Inc*.

voluntary hospital system The national aggregate of private nonprofit hospitals and for-profit hospitals in the United States. As in the case of the term "*American Hospital System*," the voluntary hospital system is not a formal system, but a de facto one.

Voluntary Protection Program (VPP) A cooperative relationship between an employer and the Occupational Safety and Health Administration (OSHA). The VPP is designed to recognize and promote employee safety and health management. Under the VPP, if the employer implements a program that meets certain criteria, OSHA publicly recognizes the program and removes the employer's site from routine scheduled inspections.

OSHA will still investigate major accidents, formal employee complaints, and chemical spills at the employer's site. Reportedly, VPP sites experience about 50% fewer lost workdays attributable to injuries than comparable sites not participating in this program.

volunteer A person who performs services without pay. In the hospital, governing body members are often volunteers, as are persons who provide patient assistance services, as well as amenities and revenue-producing services such as the library and gift shop.

in-service volunteer A volunteer who performs services in the hospital that augment, but do not replace, those of paid personnel and professional staff.

Volunteer Protection Act of 1997 (VPA) A federal law granting immunity from lawsuits to volunteers, including board members, who contribute their time to nonprofit and governmental organizations. Volunteers are protected if they are acting within the scope of their duties and their simple negligence results in harm to someone. Even if they are grossly negligent, the VPA limits punitive damages to cases of willful or criminal misconduct, reckless misconduct, or conscious, flagrant indifference to the rights or safety of the person harmed. The law does not protect violent crimes, sexual offenses, or civil rights violations, nor harm resulting from operation of a motor vehicle, vessel, or aircraft. 42 U.S.C. § 14501 et seq. (2004).

volunteer services Services provided by volunteers.

volunteer services department A hospital department that coordinates volunteer services to the hospital.

Volunteers in Medicine (VIM) Clinic A free, nonprofit, outpatient clinic staffed by retired healthcare professionals. The first VIM clinic was established in Hilton Head Island, South Carolina, in 1992, when one out of three people living on the island had no access to health care. At the same time, a number of retired physicians, nurses, and dentists were expressing an interest in volunteering their time to help those without access to care. The Hilton Head VIM Clinic (**www.vimclinic.org**) began with fifty-five physicians, sixty-four nurses, and fifteen dentists, all of whom were retired. Initial obstacles included licensure and insurance. To overcome these, the VIM Clinic engineered a bill through the South Carolina General Assembly creating a "Special Volunteer License" for the practice of medicine for retired physicians who work in such clinics, with certain stipulations, including the restriction of their practice to volunteer services. The clinic obtained malpractice insurance through the Joint Underwriters Association of South Carolina. By 2007, over 200 retired medical professionals and 220 lay volunteers were providing free medical, dental, and mental health services to a population of about 13,000. VIM promotes a "Culture of Caring," as expressed by its mission statement:

> May we have eyes to see those who are rendered invisible and excluded,
> Open arms and hearts to reach out and include them,
> Healing hands to touch their lives with love,
> And in the process heal ourselves.

Due to interest in VIM, the **Volunteers in Medicine Institute (VIMI)** was formed to assist others to replicate the VIM Clinic model (**www.vimi.org**). The mission of VIMI is to promote and guide the development of a national network of free clinics emphasizing the use of retired medical and lay volunteers to care for the "working uninsured" within a "culture of caring" so that everyone in a community has access to health care. Its motto is, "A National Solution to America's Uninsured, One Community at a Time." By 2007 there were forty-six operating VIM clinics in the United States. Many more are in the planning stages. Because of this, Hilton Head is no longer the only town in the United States that can claim that every person who lives or works there has easy access to high quality health care.

VIM was originally the brainchild of Dr. Jack McConnell, who began the project after retiring to Hilton Head Island. A highly talented and energetic man, Dr. McConnell is widely recognized for other significant contributions to health care. He directed the development of the TB Tine Test used in the detection of tuberculosis, the development of Tylenol tablets, and a research program leading to the first commercially available MRI instrument in the United States. He also helped to write the enabling legislation to map the human genome. In his honor, the American Medical Association Foundation established the Jack B. McConnell, MD, Award for Excellence in Volunteerism.

vortal A vertical *portal*. The term was coined for portals that are geared toward a specific niche audience with focused content; for example, a portal for funeral directors or kite flyers. Some have compared the portal to the large television network, and the vortal to the small, specialized cable channel. For example, Health Technology Assessment International (HTAi) has a vortal at **www.htai.org/vortal**.

voucher A certificate that may be exchanged for a contract for care for a given period of time under a prepayment plan.

VPA See *Volunteer Protection Act of 1997*.

VPMA Vice president, medical affairs; see *director of medical affairs*.

VPP See *Voluntary Protection Program*.

VRC See *vocational rehabilitation counselor* under *rehabilitation counselor*.

VS See *vegetative state*.

vulnerable adult A grown-up who requires special protection. The definition of vulnerable adult varies. In Florida, a "vulnerable adult" is defined as "a person 18 years of age or older whose ability to perform the normal activities of daily living or to provide for his or her own care or protection is impaired due to a mental, emotional, long-term physical, or developmental disability or dysfunctioning, or brain damage, or the infirmities of aging" (Fla. Stat. § 415.102(26) (2006)). The Florida statute requires any person, including professionals engaged in the care of vulnerable adults, to report abuse, neglect, or exploitation to the central abuse hotline (Fla. Stat. § 415.1034(1)(a) (2006)). Laws in other states vary regarding the reporting of maltreatment of vulnerable adults.

W

wage index See under *index (numerical)*.

waiver A special permission, which frees a person or organization from something that would otherwise be required or prohibited. In health care, a common usage is exemption of a state from participating in the Medicare program under the prospective payment system (PPS) when the state has presented an alternate method of payment that the federal government has accepted. Similarly, Oregon has been granted a waiver of compliance with regulations as written so that it may use the Oregon Health Plan.

ward (person) A person for whom a guardian or conservator has been appointed by a court, to care for and make decisions concerning the ward's person, property, or both. The ward is legally incompetent to act on his or her own behalf, usually because of immaturity (age) or lack of mental capacity.

ward (room) See under *room*. See also *patient care unit*.

ward clerk See *unit clerk*.

ward manager See *unit manager*.

Warren Grant Magnuson Clinical Center See *Clinical Center* under *National Institutes of Health*.

WC See *workers' compensation* under *compensation*.

WCMSA Workers Compensation Medicare Set-Aside. See *Medicare Set-Aside*.

weapons of mass destruction (WMD) Means of killing extraordinarily large numbers of people, or killing indiscriminately (attacking civilian as well as military targets). The phrase is used to refer to four major categories of weapons: chemical, biological, radiological, and nuclear (CBRN).

WEDI See *Workgroup for Electronic Data Interchange*.

weighting A statistical method for combining numerical data from more than one source into a single value. Each value from a given source is usually multiplied by a factor (its "weight") that has been judged by the person producing the statistic to represent the importance of that factor in relation to the importance of the other factors going into the single final value. A simple example of the importance of weighting is found when it is necessary to "average averages" (it is usually stated that "you must *not* average averages").

For example, if a group of people was made up of 100 women with an average height of 5 feet and 200 men with an average height of 6 feet, it would be incorrect to simply add the two averages and divide by 2 (because there are two values going into the total): $(5 + 6) / 2 = 5.5$ feet (5'6"). The correct method is one of weighting: $(5 \times 100) + (6 \times 200) = 1,200$. Then 1,200 is divided by 300 (total persons). The weighted average is 5.66 feet (5'8").

welcome to Medicare examination The initial physical examination of a new Medicare beneficiary, instituted by the *Medicare Modernization Act*.

well-baby care Healthcare services to normal babies in order to detect any problems early and to give preventive advice. This is the counterpart of prenatal care for pregnant women.

wellness program See *health promotion*.

well-year The equivalent of one completely well-year of life, a measure designed to assess the benefits of health programs. The well-year value is derived from measures of (1) life expectancy and (2) health-related quality of life (HRQOL) during years before death. If an individual, for example, was judged to be functioning at a 60% level (as rated on the investigator's scale) for one year, he or she would be considered to have had 0.60 well-years of life.

wet location An area of a building so designated because it often has standing water or because the floor is regularly drenched to a greater degree than with ordinary floor cleaning.

WHCRA See *Women's Health and Cancer Rights Act*.

WHI Women's Health Initiative. See *National Heart, Lung, and Blood Institute* under *National Institutes of Health*.

whistleblower A person, usually an employee (or other insider), who reports wrongdoing by his or her employer (for example, dumping toxic waste). See *qui tam claimant*.

WHO See *World Health Organization*.

wholistic health See *holistic health*.

WHOQOL See under *quality of life scale*.

WIC See *Women, Infants, and Children*.

Wiley Act See *Federal Food and Drugs Act of 1906*.

will to live See *living will* under *advance directive*.

withhold The portion of a payment due a physician in a managed care plan that is held back by the plan in order to provide a contingency fund to be used in case (1) the usage under the plan exceeds the predictions under which the premiums were established, and the plan is unable to pay the full amount (the withheld money is needed for more claims or other unexpected costs), and/or (2) the plan has a system for releasing the withhold variably to different physicians under a formula that takes into account the relative productivity and performance of each physician. The withheld amount is typically about 20% of the claims, and is sometimes called the physician contingency reserve (PCR).

W.K. Kellogg Foundation A philanthropic organization dedicated to helping people help themselves through the practical application of knowledge and resources to improve their quality of life and that of future generations. It was founded by W.K. Kellogg, the cereal industry pioneer, in 1930, and has focused on building the capacity of individuals, communities, and institutions to solve their own problems. It has a strong interest in health and health care. **www.wkkf.org**

WMD See *weapons of mass destruction*.

WMS See *workload management system*.

WOC See *wound, ostomy and continence nursing*.

Women, Infants, and Children (WIC) A federally funded program within the Department of Health and Human Services (HHS) that provides specific food vouchers and nutrition education to "at risk" pregnant women and children five years old and under.

Women's Health and Cancer Rights Act (WHCRA) A federal law requiring health plans that provide coverage for mastectomies to also cover reconstructive surgery and related benefits. Prior to this law, a plan might pay for the mastectomy but not cover breast reconstruction. The act was part of an omnibus appropriations bill signed into law on October 21, 1998.

women's health care nursing The area of nursing focusing on the particular health needs of women.

Women's Health Care Nurse Practitioner (RNC) A nurse practitioner specializing in women's healthcare nursing, who has passed an examination of the National Certification Corporation (NCC) and received the credential Registered Nurse Certified (RNC). **www.nccnet.org**

Women's Health Initiative (WHI) See *National Heart, Lung, and Blood Institute* under *National Institutes of Health*.

woodwork effect From "coming out of the woodwork"; used in health care to mean the appearance of previously unidentified problems (unmet needs) when programs for them are announced. For example, when Medicare was initiated in the mid 1960s, an unexpected number of cataract and hernia operations were performed; people who had previously lived with these problems had them corrected when funds became available. The term is currently being used particularly as long-term care programs are being considered, and it is impossible to predict the load of patients who would appear and who (themselves or their families) would demand home or institutional care.

workers' compensation (WC) See under *compensation*.

Workgroup for Electronic Data Interchange (WEDI) An organization formed to foster widespread support for the adoption of electronic commerce within the healthcare industry. WEDI seeks to provide a forum for the definition of standards, the resolution of implementation issues, and the development and delivery of education and training programs. See also *Strategic National Implementation Process*. **www.wedi.org**

work hours See discussion under *chronobiology*, *chronohygiene*, and *patient safety*.

workload management system (WMS) A method for analyzing an institution or department's workload and calculating the staffing requirements. See *GRASP*.

workmen's compensation An obsolete term for *workers' compensation* (see under *compensation*).

World Health Organization (WHO) The division of the United Nations (UN) that is concerned with health. Headquartered in Geneva, Switzerland, WHO came into being in April 1948, when the United Nations ratified WHO's Constitution. Its objective is the attainment by all peoples of the highest possible level of health. It is governed by the World Health Assembly, which meets annually. Priorities endorsed at the 2006 assembly included urging immediate, voluntary compliance with the new *International Health Regulations (IHR)* related to avian and pandemic influenza; speeding up response to HIV/AIDS; promotion of breastfeeding; prevention and control of sexually transmitted diseases; intellectual property rights to promote research and development on new and essential medicines, vaccines, and diagnostics, particularly those most needed in the developing world; coordination on trade and health policies; training of health workers; and eradication of polio. WHO is also known by its French name, *l'Organisation mondiale de la Santé*. **www.who.ch**

WorldVistA See under *VistA*.

wound, ostomy, and continence nursing (WOC) The nursing specialty focused on the needs of patients who have had colostomies and other stoma, draining wounds, pressure and vascular ulcers, and problems with incontinence. Formerly called enterostomal therapy nursing (ETN). The Wound, Ostomy, and Continence Nursing Certification Board (WOCNCB) (**www.wocncb.org**) offers the following credentials for registered nurses who pass their examinations; an "Advanced Practice" (AP) credential is also available in each area:

Certified Continence Care Nurse (CCCN) A nurse specializing in the care of patients with urinary or fecal incontinence.

Certified Ostomy Care Nurse (COCN) A nurse specializing in the care of patients in the preoperative and postoperative phases of surgery for ileostomy, colostomy, urinary diversion, or fistula.

Certified Wound and Ostomy Nurse (CWON) A new, combined credential for nurses who have obtained both the Certified Wound Care Nurse (CWCN) and Certified Ostomy Care Nurse (COCN) credentials.

Certified Wound Care Nurse (CWCN) A nurse specializing in the care of patients with pressure ulcers, draining incisions, and wounds caused by traumatic injuries, venous and arterial disease, and diabetes.

Certified Wound, Ostomy, and Continence Nurse (CWOCN) A nurse who has completed the requirements for all of the other three WOC nursing specialty certificates; called a "tri-specialty" certificate. Formerly certified enterostomal therapy nurse (CETN).

wound specialist A health professional specializing in the treatment of wounds.

Certified Wound Specialist (CWS) A multidisciplinary credential offered by the American Academy of Wound Management (AAWM) to health professionals who qualify and pass an examination. **www.aawm.org**

wraparound coverage See under *insurance coverage*.

wrongful birth A type of lawsuit concerning a baby who would not have been born but for the existence of professional negligence. A wrongful birth action is brought by the parents on their own behalf, as opposed to a *wrongful life* action, which is brought by or on behalf of the child. Wrongful birth cases, which involve the birth of both healthy and unhealthy children, may allege contraceptive failure or unsuccessful sterilization, the failure to diagnose pregnancy, unsuccessful abortion, the failure to warn the parents of genetic risks, or the failure to timely diagnose (or inform the parents about) a birth defect or disease of the fetus. Not all states permit wrongful birth suits.

wrongful death A death for which there is legal liability; for example, one caused by professional negligence. Deaths are treated differently than injuries in the legal system. For example, a different statute of limitations may apply to a wrongful death action than to a negligence action, even though negligence may have been the cause of the wrongful death. Also, some states limit the amount of recovery to a specific dollar amount (for example, $50,000) in a wrongful death action.

wrongful discharge Termination of employment of an individual "employed at will" (see *employment at will*) when the discharge is against public policy, violates an implied contract, or is not carried out in "good faith and fair dealing." For example, firing an employee who reasonably refuses to do something dangerous may be against public policy. Also, certain laws protect "at will" employees from wrongful discharge; it may violate anti-discrimination laws or whistleblower statutes, which prohibit firing someone for reporting safety or other violations to the authorities.

wrongful life A type of lawsuit concerning a baby who would not have been born but for the existence of professional negligence. A wrongful life action is brought by (or on behalf of) the baby, where the child is suffering from a birth defect or genetic or other disease, as opposed to a *wrongful birth* action, which is brought by the parents and where the child may be healthy. Wrongful life cases may involve the failure to warn the parents of genetic risks, failure of contraception or sterilization, unsuccessful abortion, or the failure to timely diagnose (or inform the parents about) a birth defect or disease of the fetus. Not all states permit wrongful life suits.

X

xenograft An organ or tissue implanted (grafted) from one species to another. The Baby Fae case, in which the heart of a baboon was transplanted into a human baby, was a case in which a xenograft was used. Synonym: heterograft.

xenozoonosis See *zoonosis*.

X-linked disease A genetic disease caused by a mutation on the X chromosome. In the case of X-linked disease in a male, it is the mother who passes the mutated X chromosome to the affected son (a male has both an X and a Y chromosome, and the father contributes only the Y chromosome). Even a recessive X-linked disease will be expressed, because there is no compliment on the Y chromosome. An example is hemophilia. See also *Y-linked disease*.

x-ray (picture) An image on a sensitized surface of the pattern of transmission of x-rays through a person or object.

x-ray (process) The process of exposing a person or object to x-rays for the purpose of making an image on a sensitized surface of the transmission of the rays through the object.

x-ray (radiation) Electromagnetic radiation in a certain portion of the electromagnetic spectrum, used for diagnostic and treatment purposes. Synonym: Roentgen ray.

X12N The common name used to refer to *ANSI ASC X12N*.

Y

years of potential life lost (YPLL) See *potential years of life lost*.

Y-linked disease A genetic disease caused by a mutation on the Y chromosome. Only males, who have both an X and a Y chromosome, can have this disorder, and only fathers can pass it along to their sons. Females have only two X chromosomes, no Y, and so cannot carry the disease. Y-linked diseases are very rare. See also *X-linked disease*.

YPLL Years of potential life lost. See *potential years of life lost*.

Z

ZBB See *zero-based budget*.

ZBS See *zero-based standards*.

ZEBRA See *Zero Balance Reimbursement Account*.

Zero Balance Reimbursement Account (ZEBRA) A type of healthcare benefit plan provided by employers who are self-insured and pay for the care as it is given. The ceiling under such a plan is typically "unlimited." The Internal Revenue Service (IRS) has ruled that funds spent for a beneficiary (here an employee) under such a plan are taxable to the beneficiary, and that the employer is liable for withholding income tax on benefits, except for those benefits that are nontaxable under federal statutes. Distinguished from *cafeteria plans* because a ZEBRA does not qualify under Section 125 of the IRS Code.

zero-based Starting from scratch.

zero-based budget (ZBB) A budget wherein all expenditures are justified for each new budget period, rather than being based on past experience.

zero-based standards (ZBS) Standards rebuilt from the ground up, rather than relying on whatever was in place before.

zeumatography See *magnetic resonance imaging*.

zoonosis A disease or infection transmissible from an animal to a human under natural conditions. The plural of this term is "zoonoses," and it is "zoonotic" when used as an adjective. When a zoonosis results from a *xenograft*, the resulting disease is known as a "xeno-zoonosis." Avian influenza, HIV/AIDS, Ebola hemorrhagic fever, and West Nile fever are all zoonotic, caused by pathogens that have moved from animal populations to humans.

zymogen A chemical from which an enzyme is produced in the body (a precursor of the enzyme).

U.S. Health Care Time Line

1630–40   Massachusetts and Virginia enact laws regulating excessive fees for medical care.

1730   The colonies require sailors to pay taxes for hospital care.

1736   The first physician fee schedule is set up in Virginia to prevent excessive fees.

1747   John Wesley, the founder of the religion Methodism, publishes the first widely distributed book on patient empowerment, entitled *Primitive Physic*.

1752   America's first general hospital, created for the purpose of caring for the sick, is created in Philadelphia.

1765   Philadelphia strikes again—the precursor to the University of Pennsylvania opens the first medical school in America.

1772   The New Jersey Supreme Court becomes the first state medical board, even before New Jersey or any other colony is even a "state."

1790   There is one physician for every 950 people in the United States.

1798   The nation's first prepaid health plan comes into existence when Congress establishes the U.S. Marine Hospital Service. This program, later to become the Public Health Service, provides health care to sailors in exchange for taxes being paid.

1809   Massachusetts makes vaccinations against smallpox mandatory.

1847   The American Medical Association (AMA) and the first insurance company (Boston) to issue health insurance are established.

1849   The State of New York passes the first law specifically intended to regulate insurance and appoints the first full-time insurance commissioner ten years later (1859).

1850   There is one physician for every 600 people in the United States.

1855   Massachusetts creates the first state insurance department.

1863   Accident insurance for railway accidents is available from the Travelers Insurance Company (Hartford), followed by other forms of accident coverage. This was the first issuance of insurance similar to today's policies.

1870   The average length of stay (ALOS) at Boston City Hospital is twenty-seven days. There are fewer than 200 hospitals in the entire United States, and they are generally considered to be institutions in which patients die.

1877   The nation's very first telephone exchange hooks up a Hartford drug store with city doctors.

1879   Dr. William Mayo's farmhouse is connected to the downtown drug store with Rochester's (Minnesota) first telephone line.

1888   *Dent v. West Virginia*, a landmark U.S. Supreme Court case, applies physician licensure requirements equally on all applicants.

1896   Massachusetts General Hospital begins to report average length of stay (ALOS) in days instead of weeks.

1898   The U.S. Supreme Court affirms a state's authority to deny a physician a license based on the applicant's character.

1904   The *Journal of the American Medical Association* (JAMA) writes that the average annual salary for physicians is $750. This compares to $1,000 for federal employees, $759 for ministers, and $540 for non-farm workers. Health insurance is endorsed by the Socialists, the first American political party to do so.

1906   The Pure Food and Drug Act ushers in governmental oversight of what Americans eat and use as medicine, giving birth to what is now known as the Food and Drug Administration (FDA).

1910   There are now over 4,000 hospitals in the United States, compared to less than 200 forty years prior in 1870. The *Flexner Report*, commissioned by the Carnegie Foundation and produced with help from the AMA, proposes that medical education follow the "university-hospital" model used by Johns Hopkins University. This report is considered pivotal in the development of medicine in the United States. The report suggests the then-used "guild-apprenticeship" model be abolished.

1911   Montgomery Ward & Co. sets up an employee disability fund now generally considered to be the first group health insurance policy in the United States.

1912   Teddy Roosevelt is the first presidential candidate to endorse health insurance. Most states enact the National Association of Insurance Commissioners (NAIC) model law regarding health insurance.

1916   An AMA committee recommends compulsory health insurance. The National Association of Manufacturers and other business organizations oppose it.

1918   Military draft physicals from World War I suggest Americans need more medical care. Studies find that about half, or more, of draftees have medical problems. Mental health surfaces as an issue, and the states receive the first federal grants related to public health issues.

1919   Hospitals that want accreditation from the American College of Surgeons (ACS) are required to have their physicians form a medical staff and regulate their own activities with bylaws.

1920   The AMA opposes government health insurance. There are now over 6,000 hospitals in the United States, and one physician for every 730 people.

1921   The Maternity and Infancy Act (Sheppard-Towner Act) becomes the prototype for federal grants to the states by subsidizing maternity and children's health programs. The program dies eight years later due to opposition in Congress and from the AMA.

1929   Two physicians (Ross and Loos) contract with a Los Angeles utility company to provide both hospital and medical care to their 2,000 employees and dependents, creating in essence the country's first health maintenance organization (HMO).

1930   The Hygienic Laboratory becomes the (first) National Institute(s) of Health (NIH). The laboratory's roots go back to the bacteriological laboratory established in 1887 in the Marine Hospital on Staten Island. Health care begins to be seen as a necessity of life, and communities now supplement their welfare payments to cover medical costs.

1933   Money for emergency medical and dental care for the needy is made available to the states by the passage of the Federal Emergency Relief Act.

1935   The first government health insurance bill (the Epstein Bill) is introduced, and the Social Security Act (Public Law 74-271) becomes law.

1937   The National Cancer Institute becomes the first of the disease-specific institutes that make up the National Institutes of Health (NIH). The next, the National Heart Institute, comes eleven years later in 1948.

1940   The wage freezes of World War II result in health insurance becoming an important part of the bargaining process for employee benefits. In an effort to attract scarce workers, employers offer more and more fringe benefits, including healthcare benefits.

1945   President Harry S. Truman becomes the first U.S. president to propose national health insurance. Approximately one-tenth of healthcare costs are paid by employers.

1946   President Truman signs the Hospital Survey and Construction Act, better known as the Hill-Burton Act.

1953   The cabinet-level Department of Health, Education, and Welfare replaces the Federal Security Agency.

1954   Twenty-five percent of all health insurance bought in the United States is a direct result of labor union negotiations. Hill-Burton is expanded to include nursing homes and other facilities.

1955   The Commission on Professional and Hospital Activities (CPHA) is established, ushering in the use of computers to help build the knowledge base in health care.

1960   Congress passes the Kerr-Mills bill as Title XVI of the Social Security Act. By providing federal matching funds to the medically needy elderly, a major funding commitment is made.

1964   The food stamp program begins.

1965 Medicare and Medicaid are established (effective July 1, 1966), and "Caution: Cigarette Smoking May Be Hazardous to Your Health" now challenges advertising agencies in finding ways to hide warning messages.

1967 Thanks to the Age Discrimination in Employment Act (ADEA), "older" employees (ages forty to sixty-five) must receive the same benefits as younger ones.

1969 Environmental Impact Statements are now a prerequisite for some federal actions.

1972 Amendments to the Social Security Act create the professional standards review organizations (PSROs).

1973 A Patient's Bill of Rights is adopted by the American Hospital Association (AHA).

1975 Federal law now mandates a certificate of need (CON) for expanding any healthcare facility.

1976 Concern over fraud and abuse in Medicare and Medicaid results in the creation of the Office of Inspector General (OIG), and the Health Care Financing Administration (HCFA) is created to take over Medicare and Medicaid. It is no longer federal policy to increase the number of physicians.

1978 Amendments to the 1967 ADEA bump up the mandatory retirement age from sixty-five to seventy, and the Civil Rights Act of 1964 is amended to forbid discriminating against pregnant employees.

1980 Major changes to Medicare and Medicaid are made by the Omnibus Budget Reconciliation Act (OBRA) of 1980 (Public Law 96-499), and more in OBRA 1981 (Public Law 97-35).

1981 The IBM PC is introduced at a press conference in New York on August 12.

1982 The Tax Equity and Fiscal Responsibility Act (TEFRA) replaces PSROs with PROs (peer review organizations), puts a cap on hospital cost reimbursement under Medicare, and makes many other changes.

1985 Average length of stay (ALOS) is 6.5 days (7.6 days for Medicare enrollees).

1987 The healthcare industry is the country's third largest private employer.

1993 Forty-nine million Americans now receive their health care from 544 health maintenance organizations (HMOs).

1995 The Internet starts showing up on the healthcare radar screen.

1996 The Health Insurance Portability and Accountability Act of 1996 (HIPAA) is enacted into federal law. Although its primary purpose is to provide continuity of healthcare coverage, its privacy provisions are the major news generators.

1997 The Balanced Budget Act of 1997 (BBA 1997) creates many significant changes to federal and state health programs. It includes the creation of a $48 billion children's health insurance program and reforms aimed at extending the life of the Medicare Trust Fund. Some say the BBA's changes are the most significant in health reform in over thirty years.

1999   *To Err is Human: Building a Safer Health System*, published by the Institute of Medicine, reports that medical errors result in the deaths of between 44,000 and 98,000 people each year in U.S. hospitals.

2002   The Hospital Quality Alliance (HQA) is established to develop performance measures to look at hospital quality; soon after, the Hospital Compare web site is launched to display results of hospitals' performances to the world. PROs become QIOs (quality improvement organizations).

2003   The Medicare Modernization Act (MMA) gives Medicare beneficiaries a drug benefit for the first time.

2004   The U.S. Office of the National Coordinator for Health Information Technology (ONC) lays out a ten-year strategy to achieve the Nationwide Health Information Network (NHIN) and other national health information technology (HIT) goals. AQA is formed to develop performance measures for physicians; by 2007, more than eighty measures have been established.

2005   The Patient Safety and Quality Improvement Act creates a voluntary, confidential reporting system for medical errors.

2006   The Pandemic and All-Hazards Preparedness Act is enacted to bolster national preparedness for public health emergencies such as pandemics, terrorism, and mass disasters.

2007   The number of Americans without health insurance is at an all time high of more than 47 million people.

About the Authors

Debora A. Slee, JD, is an attorney, writer, and teacher with experience in healthcare law, quality management, and information systems. She received her bachelor's degree from the University of Michigan and juris doctor from William Mitchell College of Law in St. Paul, Minnesota. She is contributing author to *The Law of Hospital and Health Care Administration, Second Edition*, by Arthur F. Southwick.

Vergil N. Slee, MD, MPH, is Chairman of the Board of the Health Commons Institute and Emeritus Fellow of Estes Park Institute (EPI). He pioneered the Professional Activity Study (PAS) and founded the Commission on Professional and Hospital Activities (CPHA). Dr. Slee was president of the Council on Clinical Classifications, which, with the U.S. National Center for Health Statistics, created the *Clinical Modification of the International Classification of Diseases, Ninth Revision* (ICD-9-CM). He served for over twenty-five years as a member of the faculty of EPI. Dr. Slee is a Fellow of the American College of Physicians, a Fellow of the American Public Health Association, and an Honorary Fellow of the American College of Healthcare Executives. In 1998, the University of North Carolina at Chapel Hill established the Vergil N. Slee Distinguished Professorship in Healthcare Quality Management in the School of Public Health, Department of Health Policy and Administration.

H. Joachim ("HJ") Schmidt, JD, is an attorney-turned-computer jockey. He has a bachelor's degree from Yale University and a juris doctor from William Mitchell College of Law. He has been involved in numerous information management projects, including those concerning health maintenance organizations, air quality, traffic safety, performance management, and healthcare claims processing.

The three authors also collaborated on *The Endangered Medical Record: Ensuring Its Integrity in the Age of Informatics*.